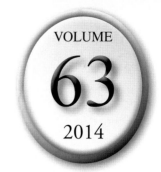

VOLUME

63

2014

INSTRUCTIONAL COURSE LECTURES

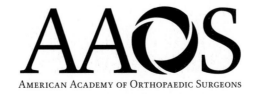

AMERICAN ACADEMY OF ORTHOPAEDIC SURGEONS

VOLUME

63

2014

INSTRUCTIONAL COURSE LECTURES

Edited by

Robert A. Hart, MD
Professor and Director
Spine Fellowship Program
Department of Orthopaedics and
  Rehabilitation
Oregon Health and Science University
Portland, Oregon

Craig J. Della Valle, MD
Associate Professor of Orthopaedic Surgery
Director, Adult Reconstructive Fellowship
Rush University Medical Center
Chicago, Illinois

Published 2014 by the
American Academy of
Orthopaedic Surgeons
6300 North River Road
Rosemont, IL 60018

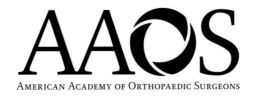

AMERICAN ACADEMY OF ORTHOPAEDIC SURGEONS

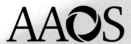

AAOS
AMERICAN ACADEMY OF ORTHOPAEDIC SURGEONS

Instructional Course Lectures Volume 63

The material presented in *Instructional Course Lectures, Volume 63* has been made available by the American Academy of Orthopaedic Surgeons for educational purposes only. This material is not intended to present the only, or necessarily best, methods or procedures for the medical situations discussed, but rather is intended to represent an approach, view, statement, or opinion of the author(s) or producer(s), which may be helpful to others who face similar situations.

Some drugs or medical devices demonstrated in Academy courses or described in Academy print or electronic publications have not been cleared by the Food and Drug Administration (FDA) or have been cleared for specific uses only. The FDA has stated that it is the responsibility of the physician to determine the FDA clearance status of each drug or device he or she wishes to use in clinical practice.

Furthermore, any statements about commercial products are solely the opinion(s) of the author(s) and do not represent an Academy endorsement or evaluation of these products. These statements may not be used in advertising or for any commercial purpose.

All rights reserved. No part of this publication may be reproduced, stored in a retrieval system, or transmitted, in any form, or by any means, electronic, mechanical, photocopying, recording, or otherwise, without prior written permission from the publisher.

Published 2014 by the
American Academy of Orthopaedic Surgeons
6300 North River Road
Rosemont, IL 60018

Copyright 2014 by the American Academy of Orthopaedic Surgeons

ISSN 0065-6895

ISBN 978-1-62552-129-3

Printed in the USA

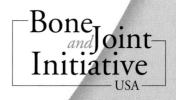

Contributors

Joshua M. Abzug, MD
Assistant Professor, Department of Orthopedics, University of Maryland School of Medicine, Baltimore, Maryland

Christoph E. Albers
Orthopaedic Resident, Department of Orthopaedic Surgery, University of Bern, Bern, Switzerland

Louis F. Amorosa, MD
Spine Fellow, Department of Orthopaedic Surgery, Rothman Institute, Thomas Jefferson University Hospital, Philadelphia, Pennsylvania

Paul A. Anderson, MD
Professor, Department of Orthopedic Surgery and Rehabilitation, University of Wisconsin, Madison, Wisconsin

Elizabeth A. Arendt, MD
Professor and Vice Chair, Department of Orthopaedic Surgery, University of Minnesota, Minneapolis, Minnesota

William V. Arnold, MD, PhD
Rothman Institute, Thomas Jefferson University Hospital, Philadelphia, Pennsylvania

Matthew S. Austin, MD
Associate Professor, Rothman Institute, Thomas Jefferson University Hospital, Philadelphia, Pennsylvania

B. Sonny Bal, MD, JD, MBA
Associate Professor, Department of Orthopaedic Surgery, Missouri Orthopaedic Institute, Columbia, Missouri

Joseph S. Barr Jr, MD
Department of Orthopaedic Surgery, Massachusetts General Hospital, Boston, Massachusetts

Asheesh Bedi, MD
Assistant Professor, Department of Orthopaedic Surgery, University of Michigan, Ann Arbor, Michigan

Joseph Benevenia, MD
Professor and Chair, Department of Orthopaedic Surgery, University of Medicine and Dentistry of New Jersey, New Jersey Medical School, Newark, New Jersey

Prosper Benhaim, MD
Associate Professor and Chief of Hand Surgery, Department of Orthopaedic Surgery and Division of Plastic Surgery, University of California Los Angeles Medical Center, Los Angeles, California

Patrick F. Bergin, MD
Assistant Professor, Department of Orthopaedic Surgery and Rehabilitation, University of Mississippi Medical Center, Jackson, Mississippi

Sigurd H. Berven, MD
Professor in Residence, Department of Orthopaedic Surgery, University of California, San Francisco, California

Stuart Blankenship, MD
Resident, Department of Orthopaedic Surgery, Southern Illinois University School of Medicine, Springfield, Illinois

Philip E. Blazar, MD
Associate Professor, Department of Orthopaedic Surgery, Brigham and Women's Hospital, Boston, Massachusetts

Michael R. Bloomfield, MD
Fellow, Adult Reconstruction, Rothman Institute, Thomas Jefferson University Hospital, Philadelphia, Pennsylvania

Pascal Boileau, MD
Chair, Department of Orthopaedic Surgery and Sports Traumatology, L'Archet 2 Hospital, University of Nice-Shophia Antipolis, Nice, France

Joseph A. Bosco III, MD
Vice Chair, Department of Orthopaedic Surgery, New York University Hospital for Joint Diseases, New York, New York

Michael J. Bosse, MD
Chief, Orthopaedic Trauma, Department of Orthopaedic Surgery, Carolinas Medical Center, Charlotte, North Carolina

Jonathan P. Braman, MD
Assistant Professor, Department of Orthopaedics, University of Minnesota, Minneapolis, Minnesota

Donita I. Bylski-Austrow, PhD
Research Associate Professor, Department of Orthopaedics, Cincinnati Children's Hospital Medical Center, Cincinnati, Ohio

Patrick J. Cahill, MD
Attending Orthopaedic Surgeon, Department of Orthopaedic Surgery, Shriners Hospitals for Children, Philadelphia, Pennsylvania

James Chang, MD
Professor and Chief, Department of Plastic Surgery, Stanford University Medical Center, Palo Alto, California

Nicholas M.P. Clarke, ChM, DM, FRCS, FRCS Ed
Professor and Consultant Orthopaedic Surgeon, Department of Child Health, University Hospital Southampton, Southampton, United Kingdom

Jacqueline Corona, MD
Orthopaedic Resident, Division of Orthopaedics and Rehabilitation, Department of Surgery, Southern Illinois University School of Medicine, Springfield, Illinois

R. Richard Coughlin, MD, MSc
Clinical Professor, Department of Orthopaedic Surgery, University of California, San Francisco, California

Edward V. Craig, MD, MPH
Attending Surgeon, Department of Orthopedics, Hospital for Special Surgery, New York, New York

Fred D. Cushner, MD
Surgeon, Department of Orthopaedics, North Shore-Long Island Jewish Health System, New York, New York

Brian Dahl, MD
Resident, Department of Orthopaedic Surgery, Southern Illinois University School of Medicine, Springfield, Illinois

Diane L. Dahm, MD
Associate Professor, Department of Orthopedic Surgery, Mayo Clinic, Rochester, Minnesota

David Dejour, MD
Surgeon, Knee Department, Lyon-Ortho-Clinic, Lyon, France

Elizabeth M. D'Elia, JD, RN
Associate General Counsel, Office of General Counsel, Memorial Sloan-Kettering Cancer Center, New York, New York

Craig J. Della Valle, MD
Associate Professor of Orthopaedic Surgery, Director, Adult Reconstructive Fellowship, Rush University Medical Center, Chicago, Illinois

Joshua S. Dines, MD
Surgeon, Department of Orthopedic Surgery, Hospital for Special Surgery, New York, New York

Jeffery S. Dlott, MD
Medical Director, Coagulation, Department of Laboratory Medicine, Quest Diagnostics Nichols Institute, Chantilly, Virginia

Paul J. Duwelius, MD
Adjunct Associate Professor, Oregon Health Services University, Orthopedic and Fracture Specialist, Portland, Oregon

Christopher J. Dy, MD, MSPH
Resident and Postdoctoral Research Fellow, Department of Orthopedic Surgery, Hospital for Special Surgery, New York, New York

Mark Eilers, MD
Resident, Department of Orthopaedic Surgery, Southern Illinois University School of Medicine, Springfield, Illinois

Iain S. Elliott, BS
Morgan and Madison McClellan Research Fellow, Institute for Global Orthopaedics and Traumatology, University of California, San Francisco, California

Jill A. Erickson, PA-C
Physician Assistant, Department of Orthopaedics, University of Utah, Salt Lake City, Utah

Lauren H. Fischer, MD
Resident, Department of Plastic Surgery, Stanford University Medical Center, Palo Alto, California

Donald C. Fithian, MD
Department of Orthopedics, Kaiser Permanente, El Cajon, California

Leesa M. Galatz, MD
Associate Professor, Department of Orthopaedic Surgery, Washington University, St. Louis, Missouri

Gary M. Gartsman, MD
Professor, Department of Orthopaedics, University of Texas Health Science Center, Houston, Texas

Jaime A. Gomez, MD
Orthopaedic Resident, Department of Orthopaedic Surgery, Columbia University Medical Center, New York, New York

Robert Goodkin, MD
Department of Neurological Surgery, University of Washington School of Medicine, Seattle, Washington

Vipool K. Goradia, MD
Orthopaedic Surgeon, Go Orthopedics, Chester, Virginia

Richard A. Gosselin, MD, MPH, MSC, FRCS
Lecturer, School of Public Health, University of California, Berkeley, California

Pamela K. Greenhouse, MBA
Executive Director, Patient and Family Care Centered Innovation Center, University of Pittsburgh Medical Center, Pittsburgh, Pennsylvania

Ranjan Gupta, MD
Professor and Chair, Department of Orthopaedic Surgery, University of California, Irvine, Orange, California

Pascal C. Haefeli, MD
Research Fellow, Department of Orthopaedic Surgery, University of Bern, Bern, Switzerland

Adam Hall, MD
Resident, Department of Orthopaedic Surgery, Southern Illinois University School of Medicine, Springfield, Illinois

Douglas P. Hanel, MD
Professor, Department of Orthopaedics and Sports Medicine, University of Washington, Seattle, Washington

Rachel Hansen, BS
Medical Student, Department of Orthopaedic Surgery, Southern Illinois University School of Medicine, Springfield, Illinois

Robert A. Hart, MD
Professor and Director, Spine Fellowship Program, Department of Orthopaedics and Rehabilitation, Oregon Health and Science University, Portland, Oregon

Nathanael Heckmann, MD
Resident Physician, Department of Orthopaedic Surgery, University of California, Irvine, Orange, California

Cynthia K. Hinds, CLU, ChFC, MSFS
President, Hinds Financial Group, Denver, Colorado

Wellington K. Hsu, MD
Assistant Professor, Department of Orthopaedic Surgery, Northwestern University, Chicago, Illinois

Lawrence C. Hurst, MD
Professor and Chair, Department of Orthopaedics and Hand Surgery, University of Stony Brook, Stony Brook, New York

Lorraine Hutzler, BA
Quality Project Manager, Department of Orthopaedic Surgery, New York University Hospital for Joint Diseases, New York University Langone Medical Center, New York, New York

Kenneth D. Illingworth, MD
Resident, Department of Orthopaedic Surgery, Southern Illinois University School of Medicine, Springfield, Illinois

Viral Jain, MD
Assistant Professor, Department of Orthopaedics, Cincinnati Children's Hospital Medical Center, Cincinnati, Ohio

Louis G. Jenis, MD
Associate Chair, Department of Orthopaedic Surgery, Newton Wellesley Hospital, Newton, Massachusetts

Norman A. Johanson, MD
Chairman, Department of Orthopaedic Surgery, Drexel University College of Medicine, Philadelphia, Pennsylvania

GaToya Jones, BS
Medical Student, Department of Orthopaedic Surgery, Southern Illinois University School of Medicine, Springfield, Illinois

Jesse B. Jupiter, MD
Hansjorg Wyss/AO Professor, Harvard Medical School, Massachusetts General Hospital, Boston, Massachusetts

Gregory Katz, MD
Medical Resident, Internal Medicine, New York University, New York, New York

Graham J.W. King, MD, MSc, FRCSC
Chief of Orthopaedic Surgery, Hand and Upper Limb Centre, St. Joseph's Health Care Centre, London, Ontario, Canada

Scott H. Kozin, MD
Chief of Staff, Department of Orthopaedic Surgery, Shriners Hospitals for Children, Philadelphia, Pennsylvania

Paul Kraemer, MD
Spine Surgeon, Assistant Professor, Department of Orthopaedics, Indiana Spine Group, Indiana University, Indianapolis, Indiana

John E. Kuhn, MD, MS
Chief of Shoulder Surgery, Vanderbilt Sports Medicine, Vanderbilt University Medical Center, Nashville, Tennessee

Michael Lapner, MD, BSc, FRCSC
Clinical Fellow, Hand and Upper Limb Centre, St. Joseph's Health Care Centre, London, Ontario, Canada

Amanda Le, BA
Medical Student, Division of Orthopaedics and Rehabilitation, Department of Surgery, Southern Illinois University School of Medicine, Springfield, Illinois

Paul E. Levin, MD
Vice-Chairman, Department of Orthopaedic Surgery, Montefiore Medical Center, The University Hospital for the Albert Einstein College of Medicine, Bronx, New York

Gregory Lopez, MD
Resident, University of California, Irvine, Orange, California

James H. Lubowitz, MD
Director, New Mexico Knee Surgery, Taos Orthopaedic Institute Research Foundation, Taos, New Mexico

Marios Lykissas, MD
Clinical Fellow in Spine Surgery, Department of Orthopedic Surgery, Hospital for Special Surgery, New York, New York

Steven J. MacDonald, MD, FRCSC
Professor, Division of Orthopaedic Surgery, Western University, London Health Sciences Centre-University Hospital, London, Ontario, Canada

Ellen J. MacKenzie, PhD
Fred and Julie Soper Professor and Chair, Department of Health Policy and Management, Johns Hopkins Bloomberg School of Public Health, Baltimore, Maryland

Melvin C. Makhni, MD, MBA
Orthopaedic Resident, Department of Orthopaedic Surgery, Columbia University Medical Center, New York, New York

William J. Maloney, MD
Orthopaedic Surgeon, Department of Orthopaedic Surgery, Stanford Medicine Outpatient Center, Redwood City, California

John J. Mangelson, MD
Orthopaedic Surgery Resident, Department of Orthopaedic Surgery, University of Cincinnati, Cincinnati, Ohio

Blaine T. Manning, BS
Researcher I, Division of Orthopaedics and Rehabilitation, Department of Surgery, Southern Illinois University School of Medicine, Springfield, Illinois

Brook I. Martin, PhD, MPH
Health Services Researcher, Dartmouth Institute of Health Policy and Clinical Practice, Geisel School of Medicine at Dartmouth, Lebanon, New Hampshire

Augustus D. Mazzocca, MD, MS
Associate Professor, Department of Orthopaedic Surgery, University of Connecticut Health Center, Farmington, Connecticut

Joseph C. McCarthy, MD
Vice Chairman Orthopaedic Surgery, Department of Orthopaedics, Massachusetts General Hospital, Newton-Wellesley Hospital, Boston Massachusetts

Michael J. McCaslin, BA, CPA
Principal, Health Care Team, Somerset Certified Public Accountants, Indianapolis, Indiana

Walter B. McClelland Jr, MD
Peachtree Orthopaedic Clinic, Atlanta, Georgia

Michael D. McKee, MD, FRCS(C)
Professor of Surgery, Division of Orthopaedics, Department of Surgery, St. Michael's Hospital and the University of Toronto, Toronto, Ontario, Canada

Christian McNeely, BS
Medical Student, Department of Orthopaedic Surgery, Southern Illinois University School of Medicine, Springfield, Illinois

John W. McNeil II, BA
Research Assistant, Department of Orthopaedics, Naval Medical Center, San Diego, California

Carissa Meyer, MD
Resident, Department of Orthopaedics, University of Maryland Medical Center, Baltimore, Maryland

William M. Mihalko, MD, PhD
Professor and J.R. Hyde Chair, Department of Orthopaedics and Biomedical Engineering, Campbell Clinic, University of Tennessee, Memphis, Tennessee

Sohail K. Mirza, MD, MPH
Professor and Chair, Department of Orthopaedic Surgery, Geisel School of Medicine at Dartmouth, Hanover, New Hampshire

Michael A. Mont, MD
Director, Center for Joint Preservation and Replacement, Sinai Hospital of Baltimore, Baltimore, Maryland

Brent J. Morris, MD
Orthopaedic Resident, Department of Orthopaedic Surgery, Vanderbilt University, Nashville, Tennessee

Carol D. Morris, MD, MS
Associate Professor, Department of Orthopaedic Surgery, Weill Cornell School of Medicine, Memorial Sloan-Kettering Cancer Center, New York, New York

Scott J. Mubarak, MD
Department of Orthopedics, Pediatric Orthopedic and Scoliosis Center, Rady Children's Hospital, University of California, San Diego, California.

Patrick Mulkey, MD
Adult Reconstruction Fellow, Department of Orthopaedics, University of Utah, Salt Lake City, Utah

G. Andrew Murphy, MD
Assistant Professor, Department of Orthopaedic Surgery, University of Tennessee, Campbell Clinic, Memphis, Tennessee

George A.C. Murrell, MD, PhD
Director, Orthopaedic Research Institute, St. George Hospital, Sydney, New South Wales, Australia

Peter O. Newton, MD
Director of Scoliosis and Orthopedic Research, Rady Children's Hospital, University of California, San Diego, California

Michael Nogler, MD, MA, MAS, MSc
Full Professor, Chairman, Department of Experimental Orthopaedics, Medical University of Innsbruck, Innsbruck, Austria

Sarah Nossov, MD
Resident, Department of Orthopaedic Surgery, University of Michigan, Ann Arbor, Michigan

Joseph R. O'Brien, MD, MPH
Assistant Professor, Department of Orthopaedic Surgery, George Washington University Medical Faculty Associates, Washington, DC

Crispin Ong, MD
Resident Physician, Department of Orthopaedic Surgery, New York University Hospital for Joint Diseases, New York, New York

A. Lee Osterman, MD
Professor of Hand and Orthopedic Surgery, Thomas Jefferson University, The Philadelphia Hand Center, Philadelphia, Pennsylvania

Wayne G. Paprosky, MD
Orthopaedic Surgeon, Midwest Orthopaedics, Winfield, Illinois

Christopher L. Peters, MD
Professor and Orthopaedic Surgeon, Department of Orthopaedics, University of Utah, Salt Lake City, Utah

Robert Pivec, MD
Research Fellow, Center for Joint Preservation
and Replacement, Sinai Hospital of Baltimore,
Baltimore, Maryland

David Pope, MD
Resident, Department of Orthopaedic Surgery,
Southern Illinois University School of Medicine,
Springfield, Illinois

Anish G. Potty, MD
Adult Reconstruction Fellow, Division of
Orthopaedics and Rehabilitation, Department of
Surgery, Southern Illinois University School of
Medicine, Springfield, Illinois

Cyrus M. Press, MD
Shoulder and Elbow Surgery Fellow, Foundation of
Orthopaedic Athletic and Reconstructive Research,
Texas Orthopedic Hospital, Houston, Texas

CDR Matthew T. Provencher, MD, MC, USN
Director of Orthopaedic Shoulder, Knee and Sports
Surgery, Department of Orthopaedic Surgery, Naval
Medical Center, San Diego, California

Robert H. Quinn, MD
Professor and Chair, Department of Orthopaedic
Surgery, University of Texas Health Science Center,
San Antonio, Texas

R. Lor Randall, MD
Professor, Department of Orthopaedics, University
of Utah, Salt Lake City, Utah

Kevin A. Raskin, MD
Attending Surgeon, Department of Orthopaedic
Surgery, Massachusetts General Hospital, Boston,
Massachusetts

Joshua A. Ratner, MD
Hand and Upper Extremity Center of Georgia,
Atlanta, Georgia

Michael D. Ries, MD
Orthopaedic Surgeon, Department of Orthopaedic
Surgery, University of California, San Francisco,
California

Marco Rizzo, MD
Associate Professor, Department of Orthopedic
Surgery, Mayo Clinic, Rochester, Minnesota

Brooke S. Robinson, MPH
Research Coordinator, Department of Orthopaedic
Surgery, Southern Illinois University School of
Medicine, Springfield, Illinois

Scott A. Rodeo, MD
Professor, Department of Orthopedic Surgery,
Hospital for Special Surgery, New York, New York

Reza Roghani, MD
Fellow, Department of Orthopaedic Surgery, New
York University Hospital for Joint Diseases, New
York, New York

David S. Ruch, MD
Professor and Director of Hand and Upper
Extremity Surgery, Department of Orthopaedics,
Duke University Medical Center, Durham, North
Carolina

Allison V. Ruel, BA
Research Coordinator, Office of Dr. Geoffrey
Westrich, Hospital for Special Surgery, New York,
New York

Adam P. Rumian, MD, FRCS (Tr&Orth)
Consultant Orthopaedic Surgeon, Department
of Trauma and Orthopaedics, East and North
Hertfordshire National Health Service Trust,
Stevenage, United Kingdom

Ranjan Sachdev, MD, MBA, CHC
Founder, Sachdev Orthopaedics LLC, Easton,
Pennsylvania

**Khaled J. Saleh, BSc, MD, MSc, FRCS(C),
MHCM**
Professor and Chair, Division of Orthopaedic
Surgery, Southern Illinois University School of
Medicine, Springfield, Illinois

Rick C. Sasso, MD
Professor, Chief of Spine Surgery, Department of
Clinical Orthopaedic Surgery, Indiana University
School of Medicine, Indiana Spine Group,
Indianapolis, Indiana

Andrew H. Schmidt, MD
Faculty, Department of Orthopaedic Surgery,
Hennepin County Medical Center, Minneapolis,
Minnesota

Louis A. Shapiro
President and Chief Executive Officer, Hospital for Special Surgery, New York, New York

Mark E. Shirtliff, PhD
Associate Professor, Department of Microbial Pathogenesis, Dental School, Department of Microbiology and Immunology, School of Medicine, University of Maryland, Baltimore, Maryland

Klaus A. Siebenrock, MD
Professor of Orthopaedic Surgery, Department of Orthopaedic Surgery, University of Bern, Bern, Switzerland

Edwin E. Spencer Jr, MD
Attending Surgeon, Department of Shoulder and Elbow Service, Knoxville Orthopaedic Clinic, Knoxville, Tennessee

John W. Sperling, MD, MBA
Consultant, Department of Orthopedic Surgery, Mayo Clinic, Rochester, Minnesota

David Spiegel, MD
Department of Orthopaedic Surgery, Children's Hospital of Philadelphia, Philadelphia, Pennsylvania

Spencer M. Stein, BA
Medical Student, Department of Orthopaedics, New York University Hospital for Joint Diseases, New York, New York

Bryon F. Stephens, MD
Orthopaedic Surgery Resident, Department of Orthopaedic Surgery, Campbell Clinic, University of Tennessee, Memphis, Tennessee

Simon D. Steppacher, MD
Orthopaedic Resident, Department of Orthopaedic Surgery, University of Bern, Bern, Switzerland

Peter J. Stern, MD
Professor and Chairman, University of Cincinnati School of Medicine, Cincinnati, Ohio

Paul Stoodley, PhD
Associate Professor, Microbial Tribology, National Centre for Advanced Tribology, Engineering and the Environment, University of Southampton, Southampton, Hampshire, United Kingdom

Benjamin M. Stronach, MS, MD
Assistant Professor, Department of Orthopaedic Surgery, University of Mississippi Medical Center, Jackson, Mississippi

Peter F. Sturm, MD
Professor, Pediatric Orthopaedic Surgery, Director Crawford Spine Center, Department of Orthopaedic Surgery, Cincinnati Children's Hospital Medical Center, Cincinnati, Ohio

Moritz Tannast, MD
Attending Orthopaedic Surgeon, Department of Orthopaedic Surgery, University of Bern, Bern, Switzerland

Thomas (Quin) Throckmorton, MD
Associate Professor, Campbell Clinic, University of Tennessee, Memphis, Tennessee

John M. Tokish, MD
Director Orthopaedic Surgical Residency, Department of Surgery, Section of Orthopaedics, Tripler Army Medical Center, Honolulu, Hawaii

Paul Tornetta III, MD
Orthopaedic Surgeon, Department of Orthopaedics, Boston Medical Center, Boston, Massachusetts

Peter G. Trafton, MD
Professor, Department of Orthopaedic Surgery, Alpert Medical School of Brown University, Providence, Rhode Island

Per Trobisch, MD
Attending Spine Surgeon, Orthopädische Klinik, Otto-von-Guericke Universität, Magdeburg, Germany

Anthony S. Unger, MD
Clinical Professor, Department of Orthopaedic Surgery, George Washington University, Washington, DC

Alexander R. Vaccaro, MD, PhD
Professor, Department of Orthopaedics and Neurosurgery, Rothman Institute, Thomas Jefferson University Hospital, Philadelphia, Pennsylvania

Thomas Parker Vail, MD
Professor and Chairman, Department of Orthopaedic Surgery, University of California, San Francisco, California

Edward M. Vasarhelyi, MD, MSc, FRCSC
Assistant Professor, Division of Orthopaedic Surgery, Western University, London Health Sciences Centre, University Hospital, London, Ontario, Canada

Nikhil N. Verma, MD
Assistant Professor, Department of Orthopaedic Surgery, Rush University Medical Center, Chicago, Illinois

Michael G. Vitale, MD, MPH
Chief, Pediatric Spine and Scoliosis Service, Associate Chief of Pediatrics, Department of Pediatric Orthopaedics, Morgan Stanley Children's Hospital, New York Presbyterian Hospital, New York, New York

Nathan Wachter, BS
Medical Student, Department of Orthopaedic Surgery, Southern Illinois University School of Medicine, Springfield, Illinois

Eric J. Wall, MD
Director, Sports Medicine, Department of Orthopaedics, Cincinnati Children's Hospital Medical Center, Cincinnati, Ohio

Kenneth D. Weeks III, MD
Resident, Department of Orthopedic Surgery, Hospital for Special Surgery, New York, New York

Stuart L. Weinstein, MD
Ignacio V. Ponseti Chair and Professor of Orthopaedic Surgery, University of Iowa Hospitals and Clinics, Iowa City, Iowa

Dennis R. Wenger, MD
Director, Orthopedic Training Program, Department of Orthopedics, Rady Children's Hospital, San Diego, California

Geoffrey H. Westrich, MD
Orthopedic Surgeon, Department of Total Joint Replacement, Hospital for Special Surgery, New York, New York

Peter G. Whang, MD, FACS
Associate Professor, Department of Orthopaedics and Rehabilitation, Yale University School of Medicine, New Haven, Connecticut

Brent B. Wiesel, MD
Chief Shoulder Service and Assistant Professor of Orthopaedic Surgery, Department of Orthopaedic Surgery, Georgetown University School of Medicine, Washington, DC

Gerald R. Williams Jr, MD
Professor, Director of the Shoulder and Elbow Center, Department of Orthopaedic Surgery, Rothman Institute, Thomas Jefferson University Hospital, Philadelphia, Pennsylvania

Scott W. Wolfe, MD
Professor of Orthopedic Surgery and Attending Physician, Division of Hand and Upper Extremity Surgery, Hospital for Special Surgery, New York, New York

Matthew S. Zimmerman, MD
Hand Fellow, The Philadelphia Hand Center, Jefferson Medical College, Thomas Jefferson University Hospital, Philadelphia, Pennsylvania

Dan A. Zlotolow, MD
Associate Professor, Department of Orthopaedic Surgery, Temple University, Shriners Hospitals for Children, Philadelphia, Pennsylvania

Joseph D. Zuckerman, MD
Professor and Chair, Department of Orthopaedic Surgery, New York University Hospital for Joint Diseases, New York, New York

Preface

This 63rd volume of the Instructional Course Lectures series arrives at a time of transition for the practice of medicine and for orthopaedic surgery in particular. Beyond the technical know-how, knowledge base, and communication skills required of orthopaedic surgeons, we are increasingly required to interpret and respond to an array of quality metrics from hospitals and payers. Several chapters in this book not only acknowledge this transition but hopefully also lay the groundwork for understanding how to participate and shape this process, specifically as it relates to orthopaedics. I am 100% confident that no group is better qualified or positioned than practicing orthopaedic surgeons to drive positive change in the practice of our medical specialty.

It has been my great pleasure and privilege to serve on the American Academy of Orthopaedic Surgeons (AAOS) Central Instructional Course Committee over the past several years. I gratefully acknowledge Dr. John Tongue for this opportunity. It was consistently stimulating and fun to work with the overlapping members during my time on the committee, including Mary I. O'Connor, Mark W. Pagnano, Craig J. Della Valle, Thomas (Quin) Throckmorton, Dempsey S. Springfield, Kenneth A. Egol, and Paul Tornetta III. Steven Frick was an outstanding partner in working out the content and schedule of the 2013 AAOS Annual Meeting.

I also want to acknowledge the incredible support given to the committee by Kathie Niesen, April Holmes, and Scottie Rangel. They are incredibly practiced at executing the daunting efforts needed each year to organize and produce an amazing educational program of instructional courses and symposia. From the publications side, Kathleen Anderson, Senior Editor, has kept me on task and, even more remarkably, more or less on schedule with this project. Katie Hovany, Digital Media Specialist, made the selection of video supplements a breeze. I also want to acknowledge Craig J. Della Valle who ably shouldered a substantial workload as the Assistant Editor of *Instructional Lectures, Volume 63*. Of course, my thanks also go to the more than 160 authors who share their knowledge and expertise in the 47 chapters that comprise this book.

Finally, I want to thank my wife, Susan Orloff, and our children, Annie and Jackson, for their consistent support and tolerance of the time away from them. They are simultaneously my harshest critics, my best friends, and my greatest joys.

Robert A. Hart, MD
Portland, Oregon

Table of Contents

Section 3: Hand and Wrist

Section 4: Adult Reconstruction: Hip and Knee

Section 5: Spine

Section 6: Pediatrics

Section 7: Sports Medicine

Section 8: Orthopaedic Medicine

Section 9: The Practice of Orthopaedics

Symposium

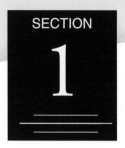

Trauma

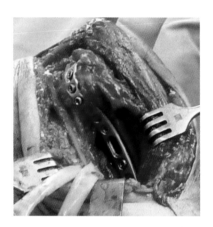

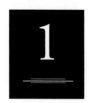

Radial Head Fractures

Michael Lapner, MD, BSc, FRCSC
Graham J.W. King, MD, MSc, FRCSC

Abstract

The radial head is the most commonly fractured bone of the elbow, with most fractures occurring in women older than 50 years. The radial head is an important stabilizer for valgus, axial, and posterolateral rotational forces. Loss of articular segments of the radial head negatively affects elbow kinematics and stability. Most fractures are treated nonsurgically. Indications for nonsurgical treatment include nondisplaced and isolated displaced fractures without a block to motion. Fragment excision is indicated when a mechanical block from a small, displaced fragment impedes elbow motion. If technically possible, open reduction and internal fixation is preferred for larger fragments, whereas radial head arthroplasty is reserved for comminuted fractures if reconstruction of the fragments is not possible. Radial head excision can be considered for isolated, displaced, and comminuted fractures in patients with low functional demands; in the presence of infection; or after other treatment modalities have failed. Complications include stiffness, heterotopic ossification, infection, and instability. The indications for surgical versus nonsurgical management of radial head fractures remain controversial.

Instr Course Lect 2014;63:3-13.

Epidemiology

Radial head fractures constitute 3% of all fractures, making them the most common fracture of the elbow in adults.[1,2] A retrospective epidemiologic study from the Netherlands noted that the incidence of radial head fractures was 2.8 per 10,000 inhabitants per year.[3] The male-to-female ratio was 2:3. The mean age was 43 years.

Anatomy and Biomechanics

The elbow has three separate articulations: the ulnohumeral, radiocapitellar, and proximal radioulnar articulations. The medial collateral ligament (MCL) resists valgus, whereas the lateral collateral ligament (LCL) resists varus and posterolateral instability.[4,5] The radial head is an important stabilizer for valgus, axial, and posterolateral rotational forces.

An increasing size of the radial head fracture fragment alters radiocapitellar stability and kinematics because of the loss of concavity-compression, which may cause painful clicking. Stability is restored with open reduction and internal fixation (ORIF) or radial head replacement.[6-8]

Radial head excision alters elbow stability, even with intact ligaments, and radial head arthroplasty restores normal kinematics.[9,10] With an MCL injury, radial head excision further exacerbates valgus instability, whereas radial head arthroplasty restores stability similar to the native radial head.[9,11,12] Bipolar radial head implants are less stable than monopolar implants in cadaver studies, suggesting that monopolar implants may be preferred in treating complex elbow instability.[13,14]

Anthropometric studies have shown that the radial head has a variably elliptic shape.[11,15] The radial head is variably offset from the radial neck, which is important because most current radial head arthroplasty and plate designs do not replicate anatomic characteristics.[16]

Dr. King or an immediate family member has received royalties from Wright Medical Technology and Tenet Medical, serves as a paid consultant to or is an employee of Wright Medical Technology and Tornier, and serves as a board member, owner, officer, or committee member of the American Shoulder and Elbow Surgeons. Neither Dr. Lapner nor any immediate family member has received anything of value from or has stock or stock options held in a commercial company or institution related directly or indirectly to the subject of this chapter.

The radial head articulates with the lesser sigmoid notch of the proximal part of the ulna and has articular and nonarticular surfaces. The nonarticular zone can be identified by a 110° arc from 65° anterolaterally to 45° posterolaterally with the forearm in neutral rotation.[17-19]

Classification System

The optimal classification and characterization for radial head fractures are debatable.[20] Mason[1] classified radial head fractures as nondisplaced, displaced, and displaced and comminuted. This classification system was modified by Broberg and Morrey[21] to include parameters of displacement and size. However, these classifications have poor interobserver reliability and do not direct treatment.[22-24]

This chapter's authors prefer to consider radial head fractures as partial articular (wedge) or complete articular, nondisplaced or displaced, with or without comminution. The treatments described in this chapter reflect this classification.

History and Physical Examination

Patient age, occupation, date of the injury, and treatment history are obtained. The location of pain and mechanism of injury may assist in determining associated injuries along with a history of dislocation or instability. Neurologic symptoms are elicited. The medical, surgical, anesthetic, and social history, as well as medication and allergy history, are reviewed.

A thorough physical examination begins with inspection of the upper extremity and elbow for alignment, soft-tissue injury, and osseous injuries. Laterally, the epicondyle, capitellum, and radial head and neck are palpated. Medially, the epicondyle, sublime tubercle, and proximal part of the ulna are palpated. The wrist and distal radioulnar joint are assessed to rule out con-

comitant distal injuries. Elbow motion is assessed and, if restricted, is reevaluated after evacuation of the hematoma and intra-articular injection of local anesthetic.[24,25] A mechanical block to forearm rotation is an indication for surgical treatment.

Associated Injuries

Minimally displaced or nondisplaced fractures do not usually have associated injuries.[25] Displaced, unstable, or comminuted radial head fractures have a high prevalence of an associated fracture or ligamentous injury.[26,27] More complex radial head fractures are commonly seen with posterior dislocation, LCL and/or MCL disruption, capitellar fracture, terrible triad injury, posterior transolecranon fracture-dislocation (posterior Monteggia), and interosseous membrane disruption (Essex-Lopresti injury).[26] Higher-energy injuries are associated with more comminuted radial head fractures and concomitant distal radial, scaphoid, and proximal humeral fractures.[14,28,29]

Imaging

AP, lateral, and oblique elbow radiographs are made. Improved characterization of the radial head is possible with CT; however, CT does not improve classification.[20] CT aids in detecting concomitant fractures of the coronoid and capitellum. If a block to motion is present, but there is no obvious mechanical cause visible on radiographs, CT may help to identify the pathology. If the CT does not confirm a cause, an interposed cartilage fragment should be suspected.[30]

Management

The management of radial head fractures includes nonsurgical and surgical treatment (**Figure 1**). Surgical options include fragment excision, radial head excision, radial head arthroplasty, and ORIF. There is controversy regarding

the indications for surgery among elbow surgeons.

Nonsurgical Treatment
Indications

Nonsurgical treatment of radial head fractures may be used for nondisplaced and isolated displaced fractures, which do not block motion[21,31] (**Figure 2**). The amount of displacement and fracture fragment size that allow a good outcome with nonsurgical treatment is controversial. Some physicians have recommended that fractures involving less than 25% of the radial head and depressed less than 2 mm be treated nonsurgically, whereas fractures that are larger and more displaced be treated surgically, even without a block to motion.[1,21,25,31-41] Other physicians have reported that even large displaced fractures, which do not interfere with rotation, can be successfully managed nonsurgically with early motion.[32]

Treatment

Early motion is essential to prevent stiffness. A period of immobilization, typically 5 to 7 days, is useful if the patient has pain. The patient is managed with a collar and cuff with instructions to begin active flexion, extension, pronation, and supination. The collar and cuff is discarded when the pain resolves. Patients are evaluated for fracture position at 2 weeks and to document if motion is improving. By 6 weeks, the patient should have recovered full or nearly full elbow motion. If stiffness persists, a referral to a therapist is indicated for passive stretching and static progressive splinting.

Outcomes

The long-term outcome for nonsurgical treatment has been favorable. In one study, 40 of 49 patients had no subjective complaints at 19 years; however, 6 patients had radial head excision for suboptimal outcomes.[32] In an-

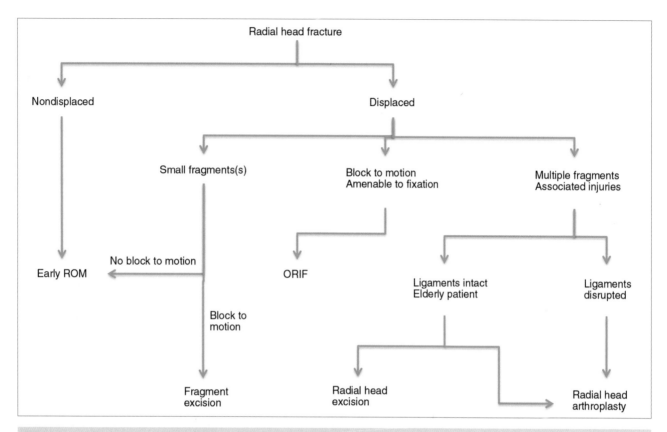

Figure 1   Summary flowchart of the management of radial head fractures. ROM = range of motion.

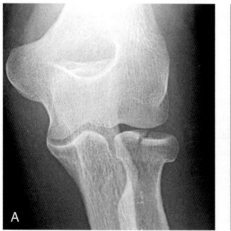
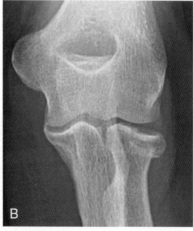

Figure 2   Radiographs of the elbow of an 18-year-old woman with a partial articular fracture without a block to motion. **A,** AP radiograph made at the time of presentation. **B,** AP radiograph made 1 year after nonsurgical treatment. The patient had full range of motion and excellent function.

other study, 32 patients were evaluated at 21 years after nonsurgical treatment of displaced radial head fractures.[31] Twenty-nine patients had good or ex-cellent results, and none had under-gone surgery. Asymptomatic radio-graphic degeneration in the injured elbow was seen in 27 patients, whereas only 1 patient had degenerative chang-es in the uninjured elbow. Radial head excision or arthroplasty are effective options if nonsurgical treatment fails.[42,43]

A retrospective study comparing nonsurgical treatment with surgical fixation of displaced and comminuted radial head fractures noted similar functional outcomes between groups.[44]

Painful malunion with clicking, fracture displacement, nonunion, and arthritis can occur with nonsurgical management. Late treatment options include fragment excision, radial head osteotomy, radial head excision, and radial head arthroplasty.[45]

Surgical Options
Surgical Approach
A posterior or lateral skin incision may be used, depending on surgeon prefer-

ence and the presence of concomitant injuries. With a posterior incision, there are fewer crossing cutaneous nerves and better cosmesis, but there is an increased risk of seroma and flap necrosis.[46] The patient is positioned supine with the arm over the chest with an arm bolster or on an arm table. A common extensor tendon-splitting approach is used if the LCL is intact. This protects the lateral ulnar collateral ligament, which lies posterior to the capsular incision and provides improved anterior exposure. The extensor carpi ulnaris-anconeus interval is further posterior and is preferred if the LCL is ruptured.[45] The main risk during lateral surgical exposures of the elbow is to the posterior interosseous nerve.[47] Maneuvers to decrease injury to the posterior interosseous nerve include pronating the forearm and avoiding anterior and medial retractors.

LCL injuries are repaired after the surgical treatment of the radial head and any associated fractures. The isometric point of the LCL origin and flexion-extension axis is selected by determining the center of a circle continuing from the capitellum anteroinferiorly. The LCL and common extensor origin are repaired with heavy, nonabsorbable braided sutures. The elbow is tested for stability in all forearm positions, and the wound is closed in layers. Repair of associated injuries to the coronoid, proximal part of the ulna, or MCL are performed as indicated.

Fragment Excision
Indications: Fragment excision is indicated when there is a mechanical block from a small, displaced fragment that impedes elbow motion. If technically possible, ORIF is preferred for larger fragments. Excision of fragments that are larger than 25% of the radial head should be avoided because of the risk

of painful clicking or symptomatic instability.[6,48]

Technique: Fragment excision is performed surgically or arthroscopically. With the patient under anesthesia, the elbow is examined for stability. Posterolateral capitellar fractures from impaction of the dislocated radial head may be excised if they involve less than 25% of capitellar surface area. A secure lateral ligament repair is essential to avoid posterolateral rotatory instability.[49,50]

Outcomes: There is limited literature available. In one case series of two patients, both did well.[40] However, other series have reported less promising results, with good or excellent outcomes in 17 of 33 patients, although these included patients with excision of fragments involving more than 33% of the radial head.[33,51] To the knowledge of this chapter's authors, results of arthroscopic fragment excision have not been reported.

Complications of fragment excision include clicking and instability, for which treatment options include radial head excision, radial head arthroplasty, and/or ligament reconstruction.

Radial Head Excision
Indications: Radial head excision has been used to treat isolated, displaced, and comminuted fractures.[52] Radial head excision should be performed only on stable elbows; however, given that most comminuted radial head fractures are associated with concomitant fractures and ligamentous injuries, this is not a common clinical scenario. Excision may be considered in patients with low functional demands, in those with infection, or after other treatment modalities have failed. The results of delayed radial head excision are comparable with those after acute excision.[42]

Technique: After the radial head is exposed, typically through a common

extensor-splitting incision (this can also be done arthroscopically), the radial head fragments and bone are excised to the head-neck junction. Forearm rotation is carefully evaluated to check for impingement of the proximal radial stump with the ulna. Forearm and elbow stability are examined (with fluoroscopy, if necessary) to confirm that a radial head implant is not required.

Outcomes: Multiple studies have supported radial head excision as an effective option to manage isolated comminuted fractures.[37] In a review of 26 patients younger than 40 years, with a minimum follow-up of 15 years after treatment with primary radial head excision, good to excellent results were reported for 24 patients, and none had subsequent surgery.[53] In nonrandomized studies in which ORIF was compared with excision of the radial head for comminuted displaced fractures, better functional outcomes and a lower prevalence of arthritis were found after ORIF.[41,54,55] There is a high prevalence of asymptomatic arthritis after radial head excision, but good longterm clinical results.[21,37,52,53,56,57] Less optimal outcomes, including subjective limitation in the activities of daily living and at work, have been reported.[58,59]

Limited results of early and late arthroscopic excision indicate it is a safe procedure with outcomes similar to the open resection, with possibly faster healing times.[60]

Valgus and axial instability is the most common complication of radial head excision. Excision alters elbow kinematics, even with intact ligaments, and is contraindicated in the setting of ligament injuries.[11] If resection is limited to 2 cm or less, the results are more favorable.[61] Proximal radioulnar impingement syndrome may occur if excessive resection is performed.[52,59,61] An anconeus interposition arthroplasty or radial head arthroplasty may be used to treat radioulnar impingement.[62]

Radial Head Arthroplasty

Indications: Radial head arthroplasty is indicated for the management of comminuted displaced radial head fractures if stable internal fixation is not achievable at surgery (**Figure 3**). Radial head excision is also indicated in cases of instability following radial head excision, malunion, and nonunion.

Technique: The surgical technique depends on the prosthesis used. Monopolar and bipolar designs, modular prostheses, and different implant materials are available.[14,63-66]

The articular fragments should be kept to ensure all fragments are removed and to determine the optimal radial head diameter and length. Fragments are reassembled on the back table. A radial head implant diameter that is too large may lead to pain and arthrosis. Because the native radial head is typically elliptic, the minor (smaller) diameter of the radial head is selected as the appropriate implant size if an axisymmetric implant is used.[67]

The height of the excised radial head is used to estimate the size of the implant. Instability, pain, and arthrosis may result from over or underlengthening the radial head prosthesis.[9,11,67-70] To confirm the correct implant length, the implant should articulate at the level of the proximal radioulnar joint, typically 1 to 2 mm distal to the tip of the coronoid.[71] Length cannot be accurately judged by assessing congruity of the lateral aspect of the lateral ulnohumeral facet radiographically because of normal anatomic variability.[68,72] The medial ulnohumeral facet is normally parallel, but it may not show radiographic signs of lateral widening until substantial overlengthening is present[70] (**Figure 4**). Contralateral

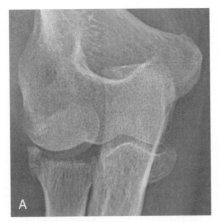
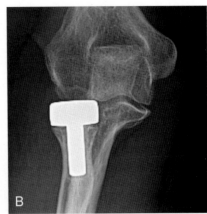

Figure 3   Radiographs of the elbow of a 60-year-old woman who sustained a comminuted, displaced, multifragmented radial head fracture. **A,** AP radiograph made at the time of presentation. **B,** AP radiograph made after treatment with modular radial head arthroplasty and LCL repair. Note the correct sizing of the implant with symmetric medial ulnohumeral joint space.

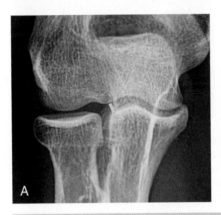
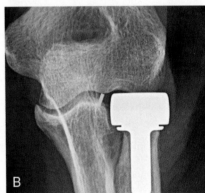

Figure 4   Overlengthening of the radial head is best diagnosed with the use of comparative radiographs of the contralateral (**A**) and involved (**B**) elbows. Overlengthening of the radial head is shown by an increase in the lateral ulnohumeral joint space (yellow lines).

elbow radiographs can be used to reliably diagnose overlengthening from the radial head implant.[68]

Elbow and forearm motion and stability are tested using fluoroscopy after insertion of the trial implant. The distal radioulnar joint is tested for instability and ulnar variance. The definitive implant is inserted according to the manufacturer's recommended technique.

Outcomes: The outcomes of radial head arthroplasty in the medium term are favorable, with limited longer-term data available.[14,63,69,73-79] Results appear to be better if surgery is per-

formed early (less than 10 days from injury) and less favorable with concomitant unrepaired ligamentous instability.[69,73] Grewal et al[63] reported on 26 patients with unreconstructible radial head fractures that were treated with radial head arthroplasty with use of a modular, monopolar prosthesis with a loose press-fit stem. Patient satisfaction was high, with a mean Mayo Elbow Performance Index score of 83 at the time of the 2-year follow-up. Asymptomatic mild arthritis was seen in five patients at the time of the 2-year follow-up. In an evaluation of a

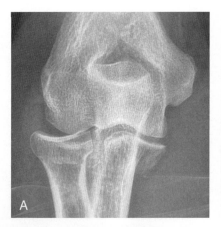
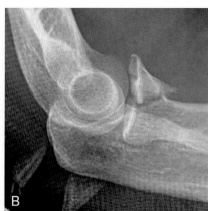
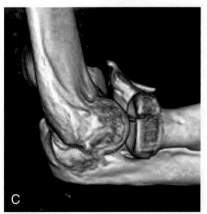
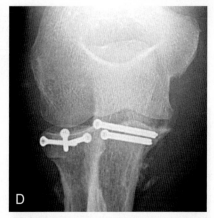
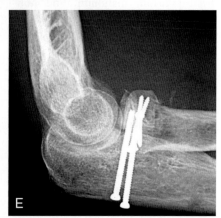

Figure 5 Imaging studies from a 63-year-old man who sustained a displaced, partial articular radial head fracture with associated coronoid fracture and elbow instability. AP (**A**) and lateral (**B**) radiographs made at the time of presentation. **C,** CT scan showing a comminuted displaced coronoid fracture and a partial articular radial head fracture resulting in elbow instability. AP (**D**) and lateral (**E**) radiographs made 2 months after ORIF of the radial head and coronoid as well as a transosseous LCL repair. The patient had a good functional outcome.

bipolar prosthesis with a loose stem in 29 patients with a mean follow-up of 34 months, Zunkiewicz et al[14] reported a mean Mayo Elbow Performance Index score of 92, with only two patients needing further surgery: one for gross instability and one for overlengthening from the radial head implant. Studies evaluating pyrocarbon implants have reported good short-term results; however, dissociation at the head-neck junction has been observed.[64,65]

Complications of radial head arthroplasty include radiocapitellar arthritis, stem loosening, failed and/or fractured components, instability, dislocation, and infection.[69] Radiolucencies surrounding a smooth stem are common,

with up to 94% in one study; however, they do not appear to correlate with forearm pain or elbow function.[80] Implant wear and osteolysis have been reported in fixed bipolar implants. In one study of 51 patients with a mean follow-up interval of 8.4 years, 37 patients had progressive radiographic osteolysis, which suggests some caution is required when these implants are used.[81] However, there were no revisions for prosthetic loosening. Capitellar erosion caused by metal radial heads does not appear to be correlated with clinical symptoms, but overlengthening should be avoided.[63,69,82]

In a study of 47 elbows with a failed radial head prosthesis, the most common cause of revision was painful

aseptic loosening, which occurred in 31 elbows.[79] Instability was the cause of revision in nine elbows (19%). In a study reviewing the outcomes of metallic press-fit implants in 37 patients with a mean follow-up of 50 months, one third of the patients had early symptomatic loosening, necessitating implant removal in 9 of them.[83]

Open Reduction and Internal Fixation
Indications: Indications for ORIF include displaced, noncomminuted fractures with a block to rotation[26,39] (**Figure 5**). ORIF is also performed as part of the management of more complex, unstable fracture-dislocations, in which restoration of articular congru-

ity is important to render the elbow stable. An articular fracture involving more than 30% of the radial head and with more than mm of displacement has been suggested as an indication for ORIF, but this is controversial.

Technique: The goals of treatment are to obtain a stable anatomic reduction with preservation of the soft-tissue attachments to the fragments, where possible, and to allow for early mobilization of the elbow. Most partial articular radial head fractures are located in the anterolateral quadrant, as seen in 22 of 24 displaced radial head fractures in one series.[84] Consequently, when the LCL is intact, a common extensor tendon-splitting approach is recommended for better visualization of the fragment(s), rather than the use of a more posterior extensor carpi ulnaris-anconeus interval.

Care should be taken to protect the periosteum on the fragments to preserve the vascular supply and avoid having fragments fall out of the elbow during surgery.[85] Reduction is facilitated by the use of a dental pick or small Kirschner wires. Impacted partial articular fractures should be restored with the intact head used as a scaffold. If bone graft is required, the olecranon or lateral humeral epicondylar region is available. Small headless or countersunk headed screws (1.5-to-2.5 mm) should be used.

Complete articular radial head fractures are more challenging to reduce and secure than partial articular fractures. None of the available plating systems are perfect because of the highly variable anatomy of the radial neck; even precontoured plates may need to be contoured to conform to patient anatomy.[85] Plates are placed on the nonarticulating safe zone of the radial head with as little soft-tissue stripping as possible.[18,86]

An alternative to using a plate for noncomminuted neck fractures is to use the bouquet technique with obliquely oriented countersunk cannulated screws.[87] Clinical results have suggested that there is less stiffness and a decreased need for implant removal with screw fixation relative to plates.[88]

Outcomes: The results of ORIF are favorable for noncomminuted displaced fractures.[34,35] In a study of 20 radial head fractures (displaced [Mason type 2] or displaced and comminuted fractures [Mason type 3]) treated with ORIF and followed for a mean of 7 years, all patients had good or excellent outcomes.[34] The same study also noted that in the setting of radial head fracture-dislocations (Mason type 4), good results were achieved in only four of six patients. Further surgery was required in two patients. These outcomes are supported in other reviews.[40,50] Ring[26] concluded that ORIF may be less optimal with greater than three fragments.

Stiffness may result from adhesions, migration of internal fixation, nonunion, degenerative arthritis, and osteonecrosis.[19,26] Adhesions may initially be treated nonsurgically. Nonunion, osteonecrosis, and arthritis may require a radial head arthroplasty, radial head excision, or total elbow arthroplasty.

General Complications of Radial Head Fractures

Elbow and/or forearm stiffness is a common complication.[26] Capsular tightness and/or adhesions are the usual cause. Physical examination reveals whether motion end points are soft or firm. If soft end points are noted, passive stretching and static progressive or turnbuckle splinting should be initiated after secure fracture healing.[89] A firm or solid-feeling end point suggests mature contracture, impinging implants, or heterotopic ossification; therapy is less likely to be successful. If therapy fails, open or arthroscopic

contracture releases are usually successful. Risk factors for heterotopic ossification include floating elbow fractures, repeated surgery, delay to surgery, and prolonged immobilization. The overall incidence of heterotopic ossification was 7% of all elbow fractures in one series.[90] Indomethacin or radiation can be used to prevent heterotopic ossification; however, its effectiveness has not been validated for the elbow. Caution is warranted if radiation is used because it is detrimental to fracture-healing.[91]

Infection should be considered when the patient presents postoperatively with elbow pain, stiffness, or radiographic lucencies around implants. A history, physical examination, and review of imaging accompanied by erythrocyte sedimentation rate and C-reactive protein level will aid in making the diagnosis along with joint aspiration. Patients with an acute postoperative infection are treated with irrigation, débridement, and antibiotics. Patients with chronic infections are treated with removal of internal fixation, débridement, antibiotic-loaded cement spacers, and staged revision or resection arthroplasty.[92]

The ulnar and posterior interosseous nerves are most commonly injured.[27,55,93] Most nerve injuries are transient. Treatment of ongoing ulnar nerve symptoms includes ulnar nerve decompression and/or transposition and has been reported to yield favorable results.[31,56]

A static or dynamic external fixator can be used for elbows that are persistently unstable despite the repair of concomitant fractures and the collateral ligaments. If an articulated external fixator is used, it is important to correctly identify the axis of motion through the capitellum and trochlea; otherwise, the fixator may promote persistent articular maltracking. Static external fixation may be preferable when acute traumatic instability is being treated because it is more forgiving, particularly in the hands of surgeons less experienced with articulated devices.

Postoperative Management

The postoperative management is based on the injury pattern, particularly the status of any associated fractures and collateral ligament injuries. The elbow is immobilized and elevated for the first week to allow swelling to resolve.[94] Self-directed or therapist-supervised activity starts after 7 to 10 days.

If the LCL was repaired and the MCL is intact, active flexion-extension exercises should be performed with the forearm in pronation. With the elbow at 90° of flexion, pronation and supination may be performed.[95] It should be emphasized to the patient that shoulder abduction and varus stress should be avoided. With combined MCL and LCL injuries, active flexion-extension exercises are performed with the forearm in neutral. If the MCL is injured but the LCL is intact or stably repaired, active flexion-extension is performed in supination. Full extension should be avoided if ligament injuries are present. Initially, extension should be limited to the position in which the elbow was stable during the examination under anesthesia. A gradual increase in extension is permitted each week; full extension is allowed by 4 weeks. After 6 weeks, passive range-of-motion exercises are initiated. At the 6-week follow-up visit, if range of motion has failed to progress, static progressive extension splinting or turnbuckle orthoses are added. Strengthening begins at 8 to 12 weeks, depending on the status of fracture healing.

Summary

Radial head fractures are common. Most fractures can be treated nonsurgically. The surgical indications remain controversial in patients without a mechanical block to motion. Treatment options include nonsurgical treatment, fragment excision, radial head excision, radial head arthroplasty, and ORIF.

References

1. Mason ML: Some observations on fractures of the head of the radius with a review of one hundred cases. *Br J Surg* 1954;42(172): 123-132.

2. Duckworth AD, Clement ND, Jenkins PJ, Aitken SA, Court-Brown CM, McQueen MM: The epidemiology of radial head and neck fractures. *J Hand Surg Am* 2012;37(1):112-119.

3. Kaas L, van Riet RP, Vroemen JP, Eygendaal D: The epidemiology of radial head fractures. *J Shoulder Elbow Surg* 2010;19(4):520-523.

4. Galik K, Baratz ME, Butler AL, Dougherty J, Cohen MS, Miller MC: The effect of the annular ligament on kinematics of the radial head. *J Hand Surg Am* 2007;32(8):1218-1224.

5. Morrey BF, An KN: Articular and ligamentous contributions to the stability of the elbow joint. *Am J Sports Med* 1983;11(5):315-319.

6. Beingessner DM, Dunning CE, Gordon KD, Johnson JA, King GJ: The effect of radial head fracture size on elbow kinematics and stability. *J Orthop Res* 2005;23(1): 210-217.

7. Johnson JA, Beingessner DM, Gordon KD, Dunning CE, Stacpoole RA, King GJ: Kinematics and stability of the fractured and implant-reconstructed radial head. *J Shoulder Elbow Surg* 2005; 14(1):195S-201S.

8. Shukla DR, Fitzsimmons JS, An KN, O'Driscoll SW: Effect of radial head malunion on radiocapitellar stability. *J Shoulder Elbow Surg* 2012;21(6):789-794.

9. Beingessner DM, Dunning CE, Gordon KD, Johnson JA, King GJ: The effect of radial head excision and arthroplasty on elbow kinematics and stability. *J Bone Joint Surg Am* 2004;86(8):1730-1739.

10. Jensen SL, Olsen BS, Søjbjerg JO: Elbow joint kinematics after excision of the radial head. *J Shoulder Elbow Surg* 1999;8(3):238-241.

11. King GJ, Patterson SD: Metallic radial head arthroplasty. *Tech Hand Up Extrem Surg* 2001;5(4): 196-203.

12. Pomianowski S, Morrey BF, Neale PG, Park MJ, O'Driscoll SW, An KN: Contribution of monoblock and bipolar radial head prostheses to valgus stability of the elbow. *J Bone Joint Surg Am* 2001; 83(12):1829-1834.

13. Moon JG, Berglund LJ, Zachary D, An KN, O'Driscoll SW: Radiocapitellar joint stability with bipolar versus monopolar radial head prostheses. *J Shoulder Elbow Surg* 2009;18(5):779-784.

14. Zunkiewicz MR, Clemente JS, Miller MC, Baratz ME, Wysocki RW, Cohen MS: Radial head replacement with a bipolar system: A minimum 2-year follow-up. *J Shoulder Elbow Surg* 2012;21(1): 98-104.

15. van Riet RP, Van Glabbeek F, Neale PG, Bortier H, An KN, O'Driscoll SW: The noncircular shape of the radial head. *J Hand Surg Am* 2003;28(6):972-978.

16. Burkhart KJ, Nowak TE, Kim YJ, Rommens PM, Müller LP: Anatomic fit of six different radial head plates: Comparison of precontoured low-profile radial head plates. *J Hand Surg Am* 2011; 36(4):617-624.

17. Caputo AE, Mazzocca AD, Santoro VM: The nonarticulating portion of the radial head: Anatomic and clinical correlations for internal fixation. *J Hand Surg Am* 1998;23(6):1082-1090.

18. Giannicola G, Manauzzi E, Sacchetti FM, et al: Anatomical variations of the proximal radius and their effects on osteosynthesis. *J Hand Surg Am* 2012;37(5): 1015-1023.

19. Smith GR, Hotchkiss RN: Radial head and neck fractures: Anatomic guidelines for proper placement of internal fixation. *J Shoulder Elbow Surg* 1996;5(2 pt 1): 113-117.

20. Guitton TG, Ring D; Science of Variation Group: Interobserver reliability of radial head fracture classification: Two-dimensional compared with three-dimensional CT. *J Bone Joint Surg Am* 2011; 93(21):2015-2021.

21. Broberg MA, Morrey BF: Results of treatment of fracture-dislocations of the elbow. *Clin Orthop Relat Res* 1987;216:109-119.

22. Matsunaga FT, Tamaoki MJ, Cordeiro EF, et al: Are classifications of proximal radius fractures reproducible? *BMC Musculoskelet Disord* 2009;10:120.

23. Morgan SJ, Groshen SL, Itamura JM, Shankwiler J, Brien WW, Kuschner SH: Reliability evaluation of classifying radial head fractures by the system of Mason. *Bull Hosp Jt Dis* 1997;56(2):95-98.

24. Sheps DM, Kiefer KR, Boorman RS, et al: The Hotchkiss modification of the Mason classification and the AO classification systems. *Can J Surg* 2009;52(4):277-282.

25. Davidson PA, Moseley JB Jr, Tullos HS: Radial head fracture: A potentially complex injury. *Clin Orthop Relat Res* 1993;297:224-230.

26. Ring D: Displaced, unstable fractures of the radial head: Fixation vs. replacement. What is the evidence? *Injury* 2008;39(12):1329-1337.

27. van Riet RP, Morrey BF: Documentation of associated injuries occurring with radial head fracture. *Clin Orthop Relat Res* 2008; 466(1):130-134.

28. Rineer CA, Guitton TG, Ring D: Radial head fractures: Loss of cortical contact is associated with concomitant fracture or dislocation. *J Shoulder Elbow Surg* 2010; 19(1):21-25.

29. Kaas L, Turkenburg JL, van Riet RP, Vroemen JP, Eygendaal D: Magnetic resonance imaging findings in 46 elbows with a radial head fracture. *Acta Orthop* 2010; 81(3):373-376.

30. Caputo AE, Burton KJ, Cohen MS, King GJ: Articular cartilage injuries of the capitellum interposed in radial head fractures: A report of ten cases. *J Shoulder Elbow Surg* 2006;15(6):716-720.

31. Herbertsson P, Josefsson PO, Hasserius R, Karlsson C, Besjakov J, Karlsson MK: Displaced Mason type I fractures of the radial head and neck in adults: A fifteen- to thirty-three-year follow-up study. *J Shoulder Elbow Surg* 2005;14(1): 73-77.

32. Akesson T, Herbertsson P, Josefsson PO, Hasserius R, Besjakov J, Karlsson MK: Primary nonoperative treatment of moderately displaced two-part fractures of the radial head. *J Bone Joint Surg Am* 2006;88(9):1909-1914.

33. Carstam N: Operative treatment of fractures of the head and neck of the radius. *Acta Orthop Scand* 1950;19(4):502-526.

34. Esser RD, Davis S, Taavao T: Fractures of the radial head treated by internal fixation: Late results in 26 cases. *J Orthop Trauma* 1995;9(4):318-323.

35. Iacobellis C, Visentin A, Aldegheri R: Open reduction and internal fixation of radial head fractures. *Musculoskelet Surg* 2012; 96(suppl 1):S81-S86.

36. Johnston GW: A follow-up of one hundred cases of fracture of the head of the radius with a review of the literature. *Ulster Med J* 1962; 31:51-56.

37. Karlsson MK, Herbertsson P, Nordqvist A, Hasserius R, Besjakov J, Josefsson PO: Long-term outcome of displaced radial neck fractures in adulthood: 16-21 year follow-up of 5 patients treated with radial head excision. *Acta Orthop* 2009;80(3):368-370.

38. Radin EL, Riseborough EJ: Fractures of the radial head: A review of eighty-eight cases and analysis of the indications for excision of the radial head and non-operative treatment. *J Bone Joint Surg Am* 1966;48(6):1055-1064.

39. Ring D, Quintero J, Jupiter JB: Open reduction and internal fixation of fractures of the radial head. *J Bone Joint Surg Am* 2002; 84(10):1811-1815.

40. Wexner SD, Goodwin C, Parkes JC, Webber BR, Patterson AH: Treatment of fractures of the radial head by partial excision. *Orthop Rev* 1985;14:83-86.

41. Zarattini G, Galli S, Marchese M, Mascio LD, Pazzaglia UE: The surgical treatment of isolated mason type 2 fractures of the radial head in adults: Comparison between radial head resection and open reduction and internal fixation. *J Orthop Trauma* 2012; 26(4):229-235.

42. Broberg MA, Morrey BF: Results of delayed excision of the radial head after fracture. *J Bone Joint Surg Am* 1986;68(5):669-674.

43. Shore BJ, Mozzon JB, MacDermid JC, Faber KJ, King GJ: Chronic posttraumatic elbow disorders treated with metallic radial head arthroplasty. *J Bone Joint Surg Am* 2008;90(2):271-280.

44. Duckworth AD, Clement ND, Jenkins PJ, Will EM, Court-Brown CM, McQueen MM: Socioeconomic deprivation predicts outcome following radial head and neck fractures. *Injury* 2012; 43(7):1102-1106.

45. Husband JB, Hastings H II: The lateral approach for operative release of post-traumatic contracture of the elbow. *J Bone Joint Surg Am* 1990;72(9):1353-1358.

46. Dowdy PA, Bain GI, King GJ, Patterson SD: The midline posterior elbow incision: An anatomical appraisal. *J Bone Joint Surg Br* 1995;77(5):696-699.

47. Witt JD, Kamineni S: The posterior interosseous nerve and the posterolateral approach to the proximal radius. *J Bone Joint Surg Br* 1998;80(2):240-242.

48. King GJ, Evans DC, Kellam JF: Open reduction and internal fixation of radial head fractures. *J Orthop Trauma* 1991;5(1):21-28.

49. Osborne G, Cotterill P: Recurrent dislocation of the elbow. *J Bone Joint Surg Br* 1966;48(2):340-346.

50. Jeon IH, Micic ID, Yamamoto N, Morrey BF: Osborne-Cotterill lesion: An osseous defect of the capitellum associated with instability of the elbow. *AJR Am J Roentgenol* 2008;191(3):727-729.

51. Parasa RB, Maffulli N: Surgical management of radial head fractures. *J R Coll Surg Edinb* 2001;46(2):76-85.

52. Iftimie PP, Calmet Garcia J, de Loyola Garcia Forcada I, Gonzalez Pedrouzo JE, Giné Gomà J: Resection arthroplasty for radial head fractures: Long-term follow-up. *J Shoulder Elbow Surg* 2011;20(1):45-50.

53. Antuña SA, Sánchez-Márquez JM, Barco R: Long-term results of radial head resection following isolated radial head fractures in patients younger than forty years old. *J Bone Joint Surg Am* 2010;92(3):558-566.

54. Ikeda M, Sugiyama K, Kang C, Takagaki T, Oka Y: Comminuted fractures of the radial head: Comparison of resection and internal fixation. *J Bone Joint Surg Am* 2005;87(1):76-84.

55. Lindenhovius AL, Felsch Q, Doornberg JN, Ring D, Kloen P: Open reduction and internal fixation compared with excision for unstable displaced fractures of the radial head. *J Hand Surg Am* 2007;32(5):630-636.

56. Herbertsson P, Hasserius R, Josefsson PO, et al: A 14- to 46-year follow-up study. *J Bone Joint Surg Br* 2009;91(11):1499-1504.

57. Janssen RP, Vegter J: Resection of the radial head after Mason type-III fractures of the elbow: Follow-up at 16 to 30 years. *J Bone Joint Surg Br* 1998;80(2):231-233.

58. Fuchs S, Chylarecki C: Do functional deficits result from radial head resection? *J Shoulder Elbow Surg* 1999;8(3):247-251.

59. Mikíc ZD, Vukadinović SM: Late results in fractures of the radial head treated by excision. *Clin Orthop Relat Res* 1983;181:220-228.

60. Wijeratna M, Bailey KA, Pace A, Tytherleigh-Strong G, Van Rensburg L, Kent M: Arthroscopic radial head excision in managing elbow trauma. *Int Orthop* 2012;36(12):2507-2512.

61. Schiffern A, Bettwieser SP, Porucznik CA, Crim JR, Tashjian RZ: Proximal radial drift following radial head resection. *J Shoulder Elbow Surg* 2011;20(3):426-433.

62. Morrey BF, Schneeberger AG: Anconeus arthroplasty: a new technique for reconstruction of the radiocapitellar and/or proximal radioulnar joint. *J Bone Joint Surg Am* 2002;84(11):1960-1969.

63. Grewal R, MacDermid JC, Faber KJ, Drosdowech DS, King GJ: Comminuted radial head fractures treated with a modular metallic radial head arthroplasty: Study of outcomes. *J Bone Joint Surg Am* 2006;88(10):2192-2200.

64. Lamas C, Castellanos J, Proubasta I, Dominguez E: Comminuted radial head fractures treated with pyrocarbon prosthetic replacement. *Hand (N Y)* 2011;6(1):27-33.

65. Sarris IK, Kyrkos MJ, Galanis NN, Papavasiliou KA, Sayegh FE, Kapetanos GA: Radial head replacement with the MoPyC pyrocarbon prosthesis. *J Shoulder Elbow Surg* 2012;21(9):1222-1228.

66. Smets S, Govaers K, Jansen N, Van Riet R, Schaap M, Van Glabbeek F: The floating radial head prosthesis for comminuted radial head fractures: A multicentric study. *Acta Orthop Belg* 2000;66(4):353-358.

67. Van Glabbeek F, Van Riet RP, Baumfeld JA, et al: Detrimental effects of overstuffing or understuffing with a radial head replacement in the medial collateral-ligament deficient elbow. *J Bone Joint Surg Am* 2004;86(12):2629-2635.

68. Athwal GS, Rouleau DM, MacDermid JC, King GJ: Contralateral elbow radiographs can reliably diagnose radial head implant overlengthening. *J Bone Joint Surg Am* 2011;93(14):1339-1346.

69. Doornberg JN, Parisien R, van Duijn PJ, Ring D: Radial head arthroplasty with a modular metal spacer to treat acute traumatic elbow instability. *J Bone Joint Surg Am* 2007;89(5):1075-1080.

70. Frank SG, Grewal R, Johnson J, Faber KJ, King GJ, Athwal GS: Determination of correct implant size in radial head arthroplasty to avoid overlengthening. *J Bone Joint Surg Am* 2009;91(7):1738-1746.

71. Doornberg JN, Linzel DS, Zurakowski D, Ring D: Reference points for radial head prosthesis size. *J Hand Surg Am* 2006;31(1):53-57.

72. Rowland AS, Athwal GS, MacDermid JC, King GJ: Lateral ulnohumeral joint space widening is not diagnostic of radial head arthroplasty overstuffing. *J Hand Surg Am* 2007;32(5):637-641.

73. Ashwood N, Bain GI, Unni R: Management of Mason type-III radial head fractures with a titanium prosthesis, ligament repair, and early mobilization. *J Bone Joint Surg Am* 2004;86(2): 274-280.

74. Chapman CB, Su BW, Sinicropi SM, Bruno R, Strauch RJ, Rosenwasser MP: Vitallium radial head prosthesis for acute and chronic elbow fractures and fracture-dislocations involving the radial head. *J Shoulder Elbow Surg* 2006; 15(4):463-473.

75. Dotzis A, Cochu G, Mabit C, Charissoux JL, Arnaud JP: Comminuted fractures of the radial head treated by the Judet floating radial head prosthesis. *J Bone Joint Surg Br* 2006;88(6):760-764.

76. El Sallakh S: Radial head replacement for radial head fractures. *J Orthop Trauma* 2013;27(6): e137-e140.

77. Harrington IJ, Sekyi-Otu A, Barrington TW, Evans DC, Tuli V: The functional outcome with metallic radial head implants in the treatment of unstable elbow fractures: A long-term review. *J Trauma* 2001;50(1):46-52.

78. Moro JK, Werier J, MacDermid JC, Patterson SD, King GJ: Arthroplasty with a metal radial head for unreconstructible fractures of the radial head. *J Bone Joint Surg Am* 2001;83(8):1201-1211.

79. van Riet RP, Sanchez-Sotelo J, Morrey BF: Failure of metal radial head replacement. *J Bone Joint Surg Br* 2010;92(5):661-667.

80. Fehringer EV, Burns EM, Knierim A, Sun J, Apker KA, Berg RE: Radiolucencies surrounding a smooth-stemmed radial head component may not correlate with forearm pain or poor elbow function. *J Shoulder Elbow Surg* 2009;18(2):275-278.

81. Popovic N, Lemaire R, Georis P, Gillet P: Midterm results with a bipolar radial head prosthesis: Radiographic evidence of loosening at the bone-cement interface. *J Bone Joint Surg Am* 2007; 89(11):2469-2476.

82. Van Riet RP, Van Glabbeek F, Verborgt O, Gielen J: Capitellar erosion caused by a metal radial head prosthesis: A case report. *J Bone Joint Surg Am* 2004;86(5): 1061-1064.

83. Flinkkilä T, Kaisto T, Sirniö K, Hyvönen P, Leppilahti J: Short- to mid-term results of metallic press-fit radial head arthroplasty in unstable injuries of the elbow. *J Bone Joint Surg Br* 2012;94(6): 805-810.

84. van Leeuwen DH, Guitton TG, Lambers K, Ring D: Quantitative measurement of radial head fracture location. *J Shoulder Elbow Surg* 2012;21(8):1013-1017.

85. Koslowsky TC, Schliwa S, Koebke J: Presentation of the microscopic vascular architecture of the radial head using a sequential plastination technique. *Clin Anat* 2011; 24(6):721-732.

86. Kuhn S, Burkhart KJ, Schneider J, et al: Implications on fracture implant design. *J Shoulder Elbow Surg* 2012;21(9):1247-1254.

87. Neumann M, Nyffeler R, Beck M: Comminuted fractures of the radial head and neck: Is fixation to the shaft necessary? *J Bone Joint Surg Br* 2011;93(2):223-228.

88. Smith AM, Morrey BF, Steinmann SP: Low profile fixation of radial head and neck fractures: Surgical technique and clinical experience. *J Orthop Trauma* 2007;21(10):718-724.

89. Szekeres M, Chinchalkar SJ, King GJ: Optimizing elbow rehabilitation after instability. *Hand Clin* 2008;24(1):27-38.

90. Bauer AS, Lawson BK, Bliss RL, Dyer GS. Risk factors for posttraumatic heterotopic ossification of the elbow: Case-control study. *J Hand Surg Am* 2012;37(7): 1422-1429.

91. Hamid N, Ashraf N, Bosse MJ, et al: Radiation therapy for heterotopic ossification prophylaxis acutely after elbow trauma: A prospective randomized study. *J Bone Joint Surg Am* 2010;92(11):2032-2038.

92. Lindenhovius AL, Felsch Q, Ring D, Kloen P: The long-term outcome of open reduction and internal fixation of stable displaced isolated partial articular fractures of the radial head. *J Trauma* 2009;67(1):143-146.

93. Geel CW, Palmer AK, Ruedi T, Leutenegger AF: Internal fixation of proximal radial head fractures. *J Orthop Trauma* 1990;4(3):270-274.

94. Liow RY, Cregan A, Nanda R, Montgomery RJ: Early mobilisation for minimally displaced radial head fractures is desirable: A prospective randomised study of two protocols. *Injury* 2002;33(9):801-806.

95. Dunning CE, Zarzour ZD, Patterson SD, Johnson JA, King GJ: Muscle forces and pronation stabilize the lateral ligament deficient elbow. *Clin Orthop Relat Res* 2001;388:118-124.

Video Reference

King GJW: Video. Excerpt. *Radial Head Arthroplasty.* Arlington, TN, Wright Medical, 2013.

2

Elbow Arthroplasty for Distal Humeral Fractures

Michael Lapner, MD, BSc, FRCSC
Graham J.W. King, MD, MSc, FRCSC

Abstract

The treatment of comminuted, distal humeral fractures in elderly patients with osteoporotic bone is challenging. Total elbow arthroplasty or hemiarthroplasty are reliable treatment options with favorable outcomes for fractures that are not amenable to open reduction and internal fixation. Total elbow arthroplasty is a reliable option for a comminuted distal humeral fracture in an elderly patient with osteoporosis and low functional demands. Longer-term studies have shown good to excellent results and a low risk of complications. Specific indications for hemiarthroplasty are evolving, but include comminuted coronal shear or low transverse fractures in patients who have higher functional demands than those that can be met by total elbow arthroplasty. Further studies with longer-term follow-ups are needed to compare the benefits of hemiarthroplasty with total elbow arthroplasty.

Instr Course Lect 2014;63:15-26.

Historically, complex distal humeral fractures were treated nonsurgically with either cast immobilization or early motion in a sling; this was termed the bag of bones treatment.[1,2] Other treatment options have included arthrodesis or interposition arthroplasty.[3,4] Multiple studies have shown that open reduction and internal fixation (ORIF) achieves better outcomes than nonsurgical treatment.[5-12] The treatment of comminuted, distal humeral fractures in patients older than 65 years with osteoporosis continues to

be challenging. Surgical treatment with ORIF in elderly patients has a high risk of complications, including poor functional outcomes, persistent pain, infection, stiffness, nonunion, ulnar neuropathy, internal fixation failure, and heterotopic ossification.[13-15] Jupiter and Morrey[16] reported a 20% rate of unsatisfactory outcomes in 846 distal humeral fractures in adults treated with ORIF. Because of poorer outcomes in elderly patients with osteoporosis, there has been increasing interest in hemiarthroplasty and total elbow

arthroplasty as more reliable alternatives to ORIF and nonsurgical treatment.

Hemiarthroplasty of the distal humerus has evolved from early custom acrylic devices to anatomically designed, commercially available, metallic implant systems. In 1947, Mellen and Phalen[17] reported on hemiarthroplasty of the distal humerus for difficult or unreconstructable distal humeral fractures. In 1952, Venable[18] reported good short-term pain relief with humeral hemiarthroplasty. Recently, there has been renewed interest in hemiarthroplasty for distal humeral fractures because of the high complication rates reported in ORIF and possible complications of total elbow arthroplasty in younger patients.[7,19,20]

Total elbow arthroplasty has achieved increasingly favorable results over the past 40 years because of better available implants and surgical techniques and appropriate patient selection.[9,15,21-32] Morrey et al[33] and, later, Figgie et al[28] were early pioneers of elbow arthroplasty for distal humeral fractures. In 1997, Cobb and Morrey[25] reported good or excellent outcomes in all 20 elderly patients (21 elbows) with distal humeral fractures treated with total elbow arthroplasty. Two patients had minor complications (one ulnar

Dr. King or an immediate family member has received royalties from Wright Medical Technology, Tornier, and Tenet Medical; serves as a paid consultant to Wright Medical Technology and Tornier; and serves as a board member, owner, officer, or committee member of the American Shoulder and Elbow Surgeons. Neither Dr. Lapner nor any immediate family member has received anything of value from or owns stock in a commercial company or institution related directly or indirectly to the subject of this chapter.

neurapraxia and one complex regional pain syndrome).

Epidemiology

Distal humeral fractures account for 0.5% to 2% of all fractures and have a higher incidence in females (71%).[34,35] The incidence is bimodal, with these fractures occurring most frequently in young patients during the second decade of life and in elderly patients (typically women). In a Finnish study of elderly women, the age-adjusted incidence of distal humeral fractures increased 395% from 1970 to 2000 and increased 838% in women older than 80 years.[36] These results likely reflect a more active aging population and longer life expectancy. These changing demographics suggest that fragility fractures of the distal humerus will continue to increase in the future.

Classification

The Orthopaedic Trauma Association system is the most widely used for classifying distal humeral fractures. Fractures are divided into three main categories: type A, extra-articular; type B, partial articular; and type C, complete articular.[37] Further subclassifications are based on the fracture's complexity and comminution. Other classification systems are available but are rarely used.[9,38]

Patient Evaluation

History

A detailed patient history should be obtained regarding the mechanism and timing of the injury and any associated injuries. In an elderly patient, the most common injury mechanism is a fall from a standing height.[34,36] Fractures from higher-energy mechanisms are more common in younger patients and may indicate injuries to other systems. The patient's past medical history is needed for surgical opti-

mization; medical or anesthesia consultations should be done as required. Patients should be informed of the options for surgical or nonsurgical care, with an explanation of the benefits and the risks of each treatment. A social history regarding ambulatory aids, mental status, the ability to comply with rehabilitation, living arrangements, and functional level will assist in the decision process.

Physical Examination

A screening orthopaedic physical examination should be performed to rule out other injuries, with a low threshold for radiographic studies as required. The elbow should be examined to document the soft-tissue status, open wounds, and neurologic function. Transient ulnar neurapraxia has been associated with distal humeral fractures in up to 26% of patients.[5]

Imaging

Standard elbow radiographs are recommended for distal humeral fractures. Because the morphology of these fractures in elderly patients is often complicated by articular comminution, traditional traction radiographs have been largely replaced by CT to better delineate the fracture pattern and assist the surgeon in recommending nonsurgical treatment, ORIF, hemiarthroplasty, or total elbow arthroplasty. The use of plain radiographs and two-dimensional CT versus three-dimensional CT has been evaluated.[39] Three-dimensional reconstructions improve the reliability but not the accuracy of fracture morphology and classification.

Indications for Elbow Arthroplasty

Total elbow arthroplasty for the treatment of distal humeral fractures is indicated in elderly, low-demand patients and those with osteoporosis,

preexisting inflammatory arthritis, osteoarthritis, or a reduced life expectancy.[22,40] It is also indicated for comminuted and nonrepairable articular surfaces, pathologic fractures, and fracture nonunions (**Figure 1**). Specific indications for hemiarthroplasty in distal humeral fractures are evolving but currently include comminuted coronal shear or low transverse fractures in patients with higher functional demands than can be accommodated by total elbow arthroplasty[41] (**Figure 2**). An algorithm of arthroplasty options is shown in **Figure 3**.

Contraindications for arthroplasty generally include local or distant infection, a neuropathic joint, and a poor soft-tissue envelope. Arthroplasty is also contraindicated in patients who cannot comply with the restrictions of an elbow arthroplasty. Arthroplasty should not be considered in young, active patients in whom good outcomes can be obtained with ORIF.[5,9,35] Contraindications specific to hemiarthroplasty include unreconstructable columns, preexisting arthritis, and concomitant coronoid fractures.[41]

Surgical Technique

The patient is placed in a supine or lateral decubitus position. The arm is draped free, allowing full mobility of the elbow for intraoperative assessment. A sterile tourniquet is applied and inflated, and a posterior skin incision is placed just medial to the olecranon. Full-thickness, fasciocutaneous flaps are developed medially and laterally as required. The ulnar nerve is identified and transposed.

Many deep surgical approaches are available to treat distal humeral fractures. A triceps-on or paratricipital approach is preferred for total elbow arthroplasty because the displaced condyles allow for good exposure for inserting the implants and this approach avoids triceps weakness. Excis-

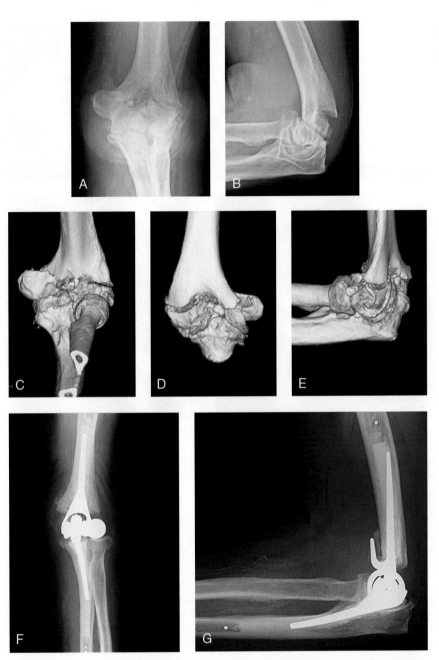

Figure 1   AP (**A**) and lateral (**B**) radiographs of the elbow of a 75-year-old man with vasculopathy, a comminuted distal humeral fracture, and preexisting osteoarthritis. **C** through **E,** Three-dimensional CT reconstructions show extensive arthritis. AP (**F**) and lateral (**G**) radiographs 2 months postoperatively show condylar excision and a linked total elbow arthroplasty. The patient regained functional range of motion.

are intact; however, it is not recommended if conversion to total elbow arthroplasty is a possibility because of fixation problems and the risk of nonunion after insertion of an ulnar component.[43,44] Alternatively, the triceps can be detached from the olecranon by splitting it centrally and elevating the triceps medially to laterally (Bryan-Morrey approach) or from laterally to medially (extended Kocher approach).[33] With the aforementioned options, the triceps is released from the attachment to the olecranon by dividing the Sharpey fibers and later reattached with bone tunnels through the olecranon.

Hemiarthroplasty is more technically challenging because the integrity of the collateral ligaments must be restored at the conclusion of the procedure. In T-condylar fractures, the fractured condyles can be retracted medially or laterally, thus preserving soft-tissue and ligament attachments for later column reconstruction and allowing access to the humeral canal. In coronal shear fractures, the joint may be hinged open on the medial collateral ligament after releasing the lateral collateral ligament from the lateral epicondyle. If necessary, the medial collateral ligament can be sharply released from the origin off the medial epicondyle facilitating exposure during the paratricipital approach.

After accessing the joint, the articular segments are removed. The distal humeral articular segments, radial head, and olecranon/coronoid are used to template the implant size. The humeral canal is opened, reamed, and broached. If performing a total elbow arthroplasty, the ulna is prepared using the appropriate instrumentation. The radial head should only be excised if it is fractured or arthritic; otherwise it is retained. Radial head replacement is not required because a linked total elbow arthroplasty is typically used for

ing the fractured condyles during total elbow arthroplasty further improves the exposure of the proximal ulna for placing the total elbow prosthesis and does not result in weakness.[42] A paratricipital approach can be used for

a hemiarthroplasty if the condyles are fractured; however, the condyles must be retained and fixed in humeral hemiarthroplasty to restore elbow stability. An olecranon osteotomy can be used for a hemiarthroplasty if the condyles

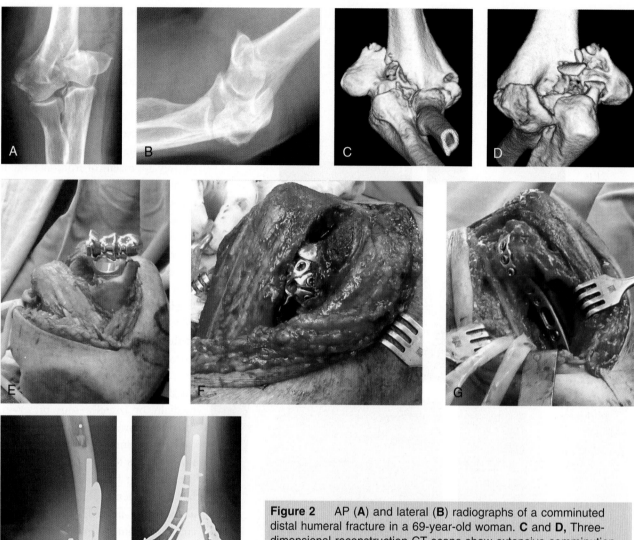

Figure 2 AP (**A**) and lateral (**B**) radiographs of a comminuted distal humeral fracture in a 69-year-old woman. **C** and **D,** Three-dimensional reconstruction CT scans show extensive comminution of the articulation. **E,** Intraoperative photograph showing anatomic distal humeral hemiarthroplasty through a paratricipital approach. **F,** The lateral column is repaired with plate and sutures for ligament fixation. **G,** The medial column is fixed, and the ulnar nerve is transpositioned. Lateral (**H**) and AP (**I**) radiographs taken 2 months postoperatively. The patient had a good functional outcome.

distal humeral fractures. If performing a distal humeral hemiarthroplasty, the radial head should be retained or should be replaced to maintain elbow stability and load distribution across the elbow. A trial prosthesis is inserted and tested for stability, length, and alignment. If the length of the implant is difficult to determine because of extensive comminution, a trial prosthesis can be inserted and the soft-tissue tension tested with the elbow extended.

Placement of the yoke of the humeral component and the anterior flange at the level of the top of the olecranon fossa is a useful landmark for humeral length. The humeral component should be internally rotated 14° relative to the flat spot on the distal humerus to correctly align the flexion-extension axis.[45] Cement restrictors are placed in the medullary canals, and antibiotic cement is inserted using a retrograde technique with a cement

gun. The components are inserted and held firmly until the cement has set.

The implants are coupled if a linked, total elbow arthroplasty is performed. The columns and/or collateral ligaments are repaired in distal humeral hemiarthroplasty. This may be accomplished using a variety of techniques, including plates, sutures, or tension-band wiring.[41] Unicortical screws may be sufficient for plate fixation, or screws can be placed anterior

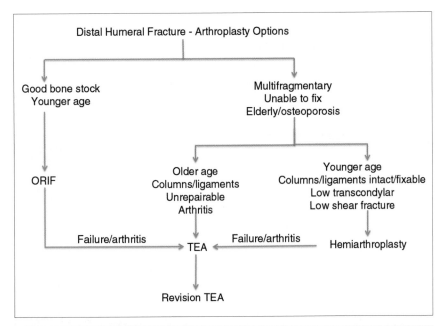

Figure 3   Arthroplasty options for distal humeral fractures. TEA = total elbow arthroplasty.

or posterior to the stem into the cement mantle.

If the triceps was detached during the surgical approach, it is repaired to the olecranon using transosseous drill tunnels. The wound is closed in layers after secure hemostasis. A drain may be used at the surgeon's discretion and removed at 24 to 48 hours postoperatively.

Postoperative Management

After total elbow arthroplasty, the elbow is splinted in full extension using an anterior plaster slab to avoid posterior wound pressure. After hemiarthroplasty, the elbow is immobilized at 70° to maintain stability and protect internal fixation. Edema is controlled with elevation and ice for the first 48 hours. The initial splint is removed after 10 days when skin healing is secure. An extension splint is made by the therapist to be worn at night, and a collar and cuff is used between exercises. Shoulder, wrist, and hand range-of-motion exercises should be started early. If a triceps-on approach was used, active flexion and extension are

performed. If a triceps-detaching approach was used, active flexion is allowed, but full flexion is avoided and active extension is not permitted until the extension mechanism has healed (typically at 6 weeks). If hemiarthroplasty was performed, abduction of the shoulder and full terminal extension is avoided for 6 weeks to protect the collateral ligament repairs and/or condylar reconstruction.

Results

A literature review of elbow arthroplasty for distal humeral fractures is summarized in **Table 1**.[22,25,29-31,40,46,47] Functional outcomes of acute distal humeral fractures treated with total elbow arthroplasty were good to excellent based on mean Mayo Elbow Performance Scores ranging from 82 to 94. The outcomes appear to be consistent regardless of the timing of the surgery.[47] Distal humeral fractures in patients with rheumatoid arthritis have been treated successfully with total elbow arthroplasty, with good to excellent results in most patients.[25,40,46,48,49]

The treatment of symptomatic distal humeral fracture nonunions with total elbow arthroplasty have also yielded good outcomes.[27] Figgie et al[28] reported good or excellent results in most patients treated with total elbow arthroplasty for nonunion about the elbow. Morrey et al[33] reported an 86% success rate for total elbow arthroplasty in the treatment of distal humeral nonunions in patients with posttraumatic arthritis.

Column fixation combined with total elbow arthroplasty was evaluated in 32 patients treated with an unlinked Souter elbow arthroplasty (Stryker-Howmedica-Osteonics).[48] The authors reported a 37.5% nonunion rate. Subsequent studies have shown that column fixation may not be necessary, and column excision is an acceptable treatment with a linked total elbow prosthesis.[42] In the context of distal humeral hemiarthroplasty, ORIF for column fixation appears to have a high rate of union; however, further studies are needed to verify this finding.[41]

Two studies compared ORIF and total elbow arthroplasty[15,26] (**Table 2**). In a 2009 randomized trial, McKee et al[15] reported that total elbow arthroplasty achieved substantially better functional outcomes in elderly patients and had faster surgical times and a lower incidence of complications compared with ORIF. The Mayo Elbow Performance Score was 86 in the total elbow arthroplasty group compared with 73 in the ORIF group at 2-year follow-up. There was a 12% revision rate in the total elbow arthroplasty group, including revisions for infection, stiffness, and ulnar neuropathy. The revision rate in the ORIF group was 27%. Five patients were moved from the ORIF group to the total elbow arthroplasty group at the time of surgery because of inability to reconstruct the fracture. In the total elbow arthroplasty group, two patients with

Table 1

Results of Elbow Arthroplasty for Distal Humeral Fractures

Study (Year)	Mean Age (Years)	Implant	No. of Patients	Indications
Ali et al[22] (2010)	72	Coonrad-Morrey (Zimmer)	26	Acute fracture, noninflammatory arthritis
Burkhart et al[46] (2010)	72	Latitude Total Elbow (Tornier)	15	Acute fracture, nonunion, posttraumatic osteoarthritis, rheumatoid arthritis
Prasad and Dent[47] (2008)	75	Coonrad-Morrey	32	Acute fracture versus delayed (failed nonarthroplasty treatment)
Lee et al[31] (2006)	73	Coonrad-Morrey	7	Acute/subacute distal humeral fractures
Kamineni and Morrey[40] (2004)	67	Coonrad-Morrey	43	Acute fracture, failed ORIF, inflammatory arthritis, osteopenia
Garcia et al[30] (2002)	73	Coonrad-Morrey	19	Acute fracture: 2 type A3 2 type B2 11 type C3 1 unclassified
Gambirasio et al[29] (2001)	85	Coonrad-Morrey	10	Acute fracture, osteopenia, comminuted fracture
Cobb and Morrey[25] (1997)	72	Coonrad-Morrey	21	Acute inflammatory and noninflammatory arthritis

UNP = ulnar neuropathy, CRPS = complex regional pain syndrome, HO = heterotopic ossification, ASL = aseptic loosening, ROM = range of motion, MEPS = Mayo Elbow Performance Score.

Table 2

Results of Total Elbow Arthroplasty Versus ORIF for Distal Humeral Fractures

Study (Year)	Mean Age (Years)	Implant	Number of Patients	Indications
Egol et al[26] (2011)	79	Coonrad-Morrey and Solar (Stryker)	TEA 9 ORIF 11	Age older than 60 years
McKee et al[15] (2009)	77	Coonrad-Morrey	42 ORIF 15 TEA 25 Excluded 2	Age older than 65 years Displaced, comminuted, intra-articular fractures of distal humerus (OTA type 13C) Closed or Gustilo grade 1 open fractures treated within 12 hours

TEA = total elbow arthroplasty, ORIF = open reduction and internal fixation, OTA = Orthopaedic Trauma Association, ROM F/E = range-of-motion flexion-extension arc, DASH = Disabilities of the Arm, Shoulder and Hand score (mean).

Table 1 (continued)
Results of Elbow Arthroplasty for Distal Humeral Fractures

Follow-up (Years)	MEPS	ROM Measurements (Mean)	Notes
5	92 (mean)	Flexion arc 28°– 125° Pronation = 74° Supination = 78°	2 HO 2 transient neurapraxias
1.1	89 (mean)	Flexion arc = 15°– 119° Pronation = 78° Supination = 79°	6 hemiarthroplasties 2 linked 6 unlinked
5.5	82% good or excellent scores	Flexion arc = 26°– 119° Pronation = 70° Supination = 80°	92% subjective satisfaction 1 CRPS 2 ASLs 2 radiographic lucent lines 2 UNPs 2 infections 1 HO 93% survivorship at 88 months No difference in groups
2	94 (mean)	Arc of flexion = 89°	1 superficial infection
7	93 (mean)	Flexion arc = 24°– 131°	2 component fractures 3 revisions for loosening 2 wound dehiscence s1 hardware removal 3 drainage of hematomas
3	93 (mean)	Flexion arc = 24°– 125° Supination = 90° Pronation = 70°	15 of 16 patients satisfied with outcome
1	94 (mean)	Arc of flexion = 125° Loss of extension = 24°	High satisfaction rate in elderly patients 1 infection
3.3	82	Flexion arc = 25°– 130°	1 fractured ulnar component (fall) 3 UNPs 1 CRPS

UNP = ulnar neuropathy, CRPS = complex regional pain syndrome, HO = heterotopic ossification, ASL = aseptic loosening, ROM = range of motion, MEPS = Mayo Elbow Performance Score.

Table 2 (continued)
Results of Total Elbow Arthroplasty Versus ORIF for Distal Humeral Fractures

Follow-up (Weeks)	MEPS (TEA vs ORIF)	ROM F/E Arc (Mean)	Notes
64	79 vs 85	TEA 92° ORIF 98°	1 TEA revised 2 ORIF stiffness releases TEA – DASH = 30 ORIF–DASH = 32
6 12 26 52 104	73 vs 62 86 vs 65[a] 86 vs 68[a] 88 vs 72[a] 86 vs 73[a]	TEA 107° ORIF 95°	5 ORIFs converted to TEA due to extensive comminution, inability to obtain fixation Operating room time 32 minutes; faster in TEA TEA decreased revision rate (3/25 vs 4/15)

[a]significant, TEA = total elbow arthroplasty, ORIF = open reduction and internal fixation, OTA = Orthopaedic Trauma Association, ROM F/E = range-of-motion flexion-extension arc, DASH = Disabilities of the Arm, Shoulder and Hand score (mean).

Table 3
Results of Hemiarthroplasty for Distal Humeral Fractures

Study (Year)	Mean Age (Years)	Implant	Number of Patients	Indications
Adolfsson and Nestorson[51] (2012)	79	Kudo (Biomet) with radial head resection	8	Osteopenia, intra-articular fracture, collaterals intact or repairable, no arthritis, 5 with failed ORIFs
Burkhart et al[52] (2011)	75	Latitude	10	Osteopenia, elderly patients, 2 with failed ORIFs
Adolfsson and Hammer[50] (2006)	80	Kudo with radial head resection	4	OTA 1.3 C2/C3 fractures
Parsons et al[41] (2005)	61	Sorbie–Questor (Wright Medical Technology)	8	4 acute and 4 nonacute fractures

MEPS = Mayo Elbow Performance Score, ROM = range of motion, UH = ulnohumeral, UNP = ulnar neuropathy, HO = heterotopic ossification, ASES = American Shoulder and Elbow Surgeons score.

elbow stiffness were treated with capsular release and excision of heterotopic ossification, one infection was treated with staged revision, and one patient with ulnar neuropathy was treated with ulnar neurolysis.

There are a limited number of studies in the literature reporting the outcomes of hemiarthroplasty[41,50-52] (Table 3). Although the short-term results of hemiarthroplasty are favorable, longer-term follow-up studies are needed. Burkhart et al[52] reported that the treatment of complex intra-articular fractures of the distal humerus with an anatomic distal humeral hemiarthroplasty implant had good to excellent results in 90% of patients at 1-year follow-up. No revision surgeries were needed, but progressive symptomatic osteoarthritis developed in one patient. Attempts to achieve good outcomes with nonanatomic hemiarthroplasty implants have not been as successful and have shown ulnohumeral wear.[51,53]

Complications

Soft-tissue complications include delayed wound healing, flap necrosis, triceps failure, and ulnar neuropathy. Delayed wound healing may be caused by seroma or hematoma formation in the early postoperative period. This complication may be prevented by meticulous hemostasis and the use of a postoperative drain. Using a soft, bulky dressing to prevent undue pressure or stress on the posterior tissue is also helpful. Limiting medial and lateral dissection and keeping the arm relatively extended until the wound has closed may prevent flap necrosis. Flap necrosis is best treated with local or free flaps because delayed wound healing may result in secondary infection of the prosthesis.[54] Ulnar neuropathy is typically transient; however, persistent ulnar neuropathy can be treated with ulnar nerve neurolysis and revision transposition.[21,49,55,56] The prevention of extensor mechanism failure may include a triceps-preserving approach.[57,58] Extensor mechanism failure can be treated nonsurgically in a well-functioning patient or with primary repair or reconstruction in symptomatic patients.[59] Excessive humeral shortening caused by placing the implant more than 2 cm proximal to the olecranon fossa may interfere with triceps function.[60]

Soft-tissue contractures requiring surgery are uncommon. Heterotopic ossification has been reported after total elbow arthroplasty and hemiarthroplasty for distal humeral fractures.[47,52] The administration of 25 mg indomethacin three times a day may prevent heterotopic ossification; however, because it has not been proven effective and has a higher complication rate in elderly patients, it is not typically used.[5] In hemiarthroplasty with column fixation, union may be impaired by radiotherapy.[61]

Infection remains a difficult complication to treat.[62] In acute infections, irrigation and débridement may be sufficient to eradicate the infection if accompanied by appropriate antibiotic therapy. In delayed infections, staged revision is recommended. Before reimplantation, a 3-month prosthesis-free interval is suggested along with return of normal inflammatory markers.

Complications specific to the use of linked total elbow prostheses for distal humeral fractures include implant loosening, periprosthetic fracture, polyethylene wear, and component fracture.[47,63,64] A detailed evaluation

Table 3 (continued)

Results of Hemiarthroplasty for Distal Humeral Fractures

Mean Follow-up (Years)	MEPS	ROM Measurements (Mean)	Notes
4.5	8 excellent or good	Flexion arc = 31°– 126°	1 stiffness 3 of 5 patients had radiographic signs of UH wear but were asymptomatic
1	9 excellent or good, 1 fair	Flexion arc = 18°– 125° Pronation = 80° Supination = 80°	1 triceps weakness 1 UNP 1 superficial infection 2 HO 1 UH arthritis
0.9	3 excellent, 1 good	Flexion arc = 20°– 125° Pronation = 80° Supination = 78°	Ligaments preserved Column fractures stabilized
short-term		Flexion arc = 22°– 126°	ASES 80.6 1 UNP 3 removals of fixation (wires) 1 progressive arthritis

MEPS = Mayo Elbow Performance Score, ROM = range of motion, UH = ulnohumeral, UNP = ulnar neuropathy, HO = heterotopic ossification, ASES = American Shoulder and Elbow Surgeons score.

of the elbow and radiographic imaging are helpful in diagnosing the etiology of the complication. Revision arthroplasty may be performed in symptomatic patients after infection is ruled out; however, this is often a technically challenging procedure, and functional results are not as good as those achieved with primary surgery.[64]

Complications specific to distal humeral hemiarthroplasty include ulnar arthritis, bony erosion, instability, humeral stem loosening, and prominence or failure of internal fixation.[41,51,52] Internal fixation prominence for column ORIF may necessitate removal. Failed column fixation is treated by revision ORIF or conversion to a linked total elbow arthroplasty. Instability is treated by reconstruction or repair of the collateral ligaments or revision to a linked total elbow arthroplasty. Radiographic ulnohumeral arthritis and ulnar erosion have been reported but are not correlated with clinical symptoms.[51] In a study by Adolfsson and Nestorson,[51] 3 of 11 patients with distal humeral fractures treated with primary hemiarthroplasty had ulnohumeral arthritis. Another study reported ulnohumeral arthritis in 1 in 11 patients treated with distal humeral hemiarthroplasty.[41] In symptomatic patients with ulnohumeral arthritis, conversion to a total elbow arthroplasty should be considered; a convertible implant is helpful in this situation.

Summary

The treatment of distal humeral fractures is often challenging, particularly in osteoporotic and highly comminuted articular surfaces. ORIF is the gold standard in younger patients and should be the first-line treatment in elderly patients. Total elbow arthroplasty or hemiarthroplasty are dependable treatment options with good to excellent outcomes for humeral fractures not amenable to ORIF.

References

1. Brown RF, Morgan RG: Intercondylar T-shaped fractures of the humerus: Results in ten cases treated by early mobilisation. *J Bone Joint Surg Br* 1971;53(3):425-428.

2. Zagorski JB, Jennings JJ, Burkhalter WE, Uribe JW: Comminuted intraarticular fractures of the distal humeral condyles: Surgical vs. nonsurgical treatment. *Clin Orthop Relat Res* 1986;202:197-204.

3. Hughes RE, Schneeberger AG, An KN, Morrey BF, O'Driscoll SW: Reduction of triceps muscle force after shortening of the distal humerus: A computational model. *J Shoulder Elbow Surg* 1997;6(5):444-448.

4. McAuliffe JA, Burkhalter WE, Ouellette EA, Carneiro RS: Compression plate arthrodesis of the elbow. *J Bone Joint Surg Br* 1992;74(2):300-304.

5. Gofton WT, Macdermid JC, Patterson SD, Faber KJ, King GJ: Functional outcome of AO type C distal humeral fractures. *J Hand Surg Am* 2003;28(2):294-308.

6. Huang TL, Chiu FY, Chuang TY, Chen TH: The results of open reduction and internal fixation in elderly patients with severe fractures of the distal humerus: A critical analysis of the results. *J Trauma* 2005;58(1):62-69.

7. Korner J, Lill H, Müller LP, et al: Results after open reduction and internal fixation. *Osteoporos Int* 2005;16(suppl 2):S73-S79.

8. McKee MD, Wilson TL, Winston L, Schemitsch EH, Richards RR: Functional outcome following surgical treatment of intra-articular distal humeral fractures through a posterior approach. *J Bone Joint Surg Am* 2000; 82(12):1701-1707.

9. Mehlhoff TL, Bennett JB: Distal humeral fractures: Fixation versus arthroplasty. *J Shoulder Elbow Surg* 2011;20(2):S97-S106.

10. Riseborough EJ, Radin EL: Intercondylar T fractures of the humerus in the adult: A comparison of operative and non-operative treatment in twenty-nine cases. *J Bone Joint Surg Am* 1969;51(1): 130-141.

11. Sanchez-Sotelo J, Torchia ME, O'Driscoll SW: Complex distal humeral fractures: Internal fixation with a principle-based parallel-plate technique. Surgical technique. *J Bone Joint Surg Am* 2008;90(suppl 2 pt 1):31-46.

12. Srinivasan K, Agarwal M, Matthews SJ, Giannoudis PV: Fractures of the distal humerus in the elderly: Is internal fixation the treatment of choice? *Clin Orthop Relat Res* 2005;434:222-230.

13. Jupiter JB, Neff U, Holzach P, Allgöwer M: Intercondylar fractures of the humerus: An operative approach. *J Bone Joint Surg Am* 1985;67(2):226-239.

14. Kundel K, Braun W, Wieberneit J, Rüter A: Intraarticular distal humerus fractures: Factors affecting functional outcome. *Clin Orthop Relat Res* 1996;332:200-208.

15. McKee MD, Veillette CJ, Hall JA, et al: A multicenter, prospective, randomized, controlled trial of open reduction internal fixation versus total elbow arthroplasty for displaced intra-articular distal humeral fractures in elderly patients. *J Shoulder Elbow Surg* 2009;18(1):3-12.

16. Jupiter J, Morrey BF: *The Elbow and Its Disorders*, ed 3. Philadelphia, PA, WB Saunders, 2000, pp 293-330.

17. Mellen RH, Phalen GS: Arthroplasty of the elbow by replacement of the distal portion of the humerus with an acrylic prosthesis. *J Bone Joint Surg Am* 1947; 29(2):348-353.

18. Venable CS: An elbow and an elbow prosthesis: Case of complete loss of the lower third of the humerus. *Am J Surg* 1952;83(3): 271-275.

19. Hausman M, Panozzo A: Treatment of distal humerus fractures in the elderly. *Clin Orthop Relat Res* 2004;425(425):55-63.

20. John H, Rosso R, Neff U, Bodoky A, Regazzoni P, Harder F: Operative treatment of distal humeral fractures in the elderly. *J Bone Joint Surg Br* 1994;76(5):793-796.

21. Aldridge JM III, Lightdale NR, Mallon WJ, Coonrad RW: Total elbow arthroplasty with the Coonrad/Coonrad-Morrey prosthesis: A 10- to 31-year survival analysis. *J Bone Joint Surg Br* 2006;88(4):509-514.

22. Ali AS, Shahane S, Stanley D: Total elbow arthroplasty for distal humeral fractures: Indications, surgical approach, technical tips, and outcome. *J Shoulder Elbow Surg* 2010;19(2):53-58.

23. Armstrong AD, Yamaguchi K: Total elbow arthroplasty and distal humerus elbow fractures. *Hand Clin* 2004;20(4):475-483.

24. Chalidis B, Dimitriou C, Papadopoulos P, Petsatodis G, Giannoudis PV: Total elbow arthroplasty for the treatment of insufficient distal humeral fractures: A retrospective clinical study and review of the literature. *Injury* 2009;40(6):582-590.

25. Cobb TK, Morrey BF: Total elbow arthroplasty as primary treatment for distal humeral fractures in elderly patients. *J Bone Joint Surg Am* 1997;79(6):826-832.

26. Egol KA, Tsai P, Vazques O, Tejwani NC: Comparison of functional outcomes of total elbow arthroplasty vs plate fixation for distal humerus fractures in osteoporotic elbows. *Am J Orthop (Belle Mead NJ)* 2011;40(2): 67-71.

27. Espiga X, Antuña SA, Ferreres A: Linked total elbow arthroplasty as treatment of distal humerus nonunions in patients older than 70 years. *Acta Orthop Belg* 2011; 77(3):304-310.

28. Figgie MP, Inglis AE, Mow CS, Figgie HE III: Salvage of nonunion of supracondylar fracture of the humerus by total elbow arthroplasty. *J Bone Joint Surg Am* 1989;71(7):1058-1065.

29. Gambirasio R, Riand N, Stern R, Hoffmeyer P: Total elbow replacement for complex fractures of the distal humerus: An option for the elderly patient. *J Bone Joint Surg Br* 2001;83(7):974-978.

30. Garcia JA, Mykula R, Stanley D: Complex fractures of the distal humerus in the elderly: The role of total elbow replacement as primary treatment. *J Bone Joint Surg Br* 2002;84(6):812-816.

31. Lee KT, Lai CH, Singh S: Results of total elbow arthroplasty in the treatment of distal humerus fractures in elderly Asian patients. *J Trauma* 2006;61(4):889-892.

32. Ray PS, Kakarlapudi K, Rajsekhar C, Bhamra MS: Total elbow arthroplasty as primary treatment for distal humeral fractures in elderly patients. *Injury* 2000; 31(9):687-692.

33. Morrey BF, Adams RA, Bryan RS: Total replacement for posttraumatic arthritis of the elbow. *J Bone Joint Surg Br* 1991;73(4): 607-612.

34. Court-Brown CM, Caesar B: Epidemiology of adult fractures: A review. *Injury* 2006;37(8): 691-697.

35. Robinson CM: Fractures of the distal humerus, in Bucholz RW, Heckman JD, Court-Brown C, eds: *Rockwood and Green's Fractures in Adults*, ed 6. Philadelphia, PA, Lippincott, Williams, & Wilkins, 2006, pp 1052-1116.

36. Palvanen M, Niemi S, Parkkari J, Kannus P: Osteoporotic fractures of the distal humerus in elderly women. *Ann Intern Med* 2003; 139(3):W-W61.

37. Orthopaedic Trauma Association Committee for Coding and Classification: Fracture and dislocation compendium. *J Orthop Trauma* 1996;10(suppl 1):v-ix, 1-154.

38. Jupiter JB, Mehne DK: Fractures of the distal humerus. *Orthopedics* 1992;15(7):825-833.

39. Doornberg J, Lindenhovius A, Kloen P, van Dijk CN, Zurakowski D, Ring D: Two and three-dimensional computed tomography for the classification and management of distal humeral fractures: Evaluation of reliability and diagnostic accuracy. *J Bone Joint Surg Am* 2006;88(8): 1795-1801.

40. Kamineni S, Morrey BF: Distal humeral fractures treated with noncustom total elbow replacement. *J Bone Joint Surg Am* 2004; 86(5):940-947.

41. Parsons M, O'Brien RJ, Hughes JS: Elbow hemiarthroplasty for acute and salvage reconstruction of intra-articular distal humerus fractures. *Tech Shoulder Elbow Surg* 2005;6(2):87-97.

42. McKee MD, Pugh DM, Richards RR, Pedersen E, Jones C, Schemitsch EH: Effect of humeral condylar resection on strength and functional outcome after semiconstrained total elbow arthroplasty. *J Bone Joint Surg Am* 2003;85(5): 802-807.

43. Bailey CS, MacDermid J, Patterson SD, King GJ: Outcome of plate fixation of olecranon fractures. *J Orthop Trauma* 2001; 15(8):542-548.

44. Hewins EA, Gofton WT, Dubberly J, MacDermid JC, Faber KJ, King GJ: Plate fixation of olecranon osteotomies. *J Orthop Trauma* 2007;21(1):58-62.

45. Sabo MT, Athwal GS, King GJ: Landmarks for rotational alignment of the humeral component during elbow arthroplasty. *J Bone Joint Surg Am* 2012;94(19):1794-1800.

46. Burkhart KJ, Müller LP, Schwarz C, Mattyasovszky SG, Rommens PM: [Treatment of the complex intraarticular fracture of the distal humerus with the latitude elbow prosthesis]. *Oper Orthop Traumatol* 2010;22(3):279-298.

47. Prasad N, Dent C: Outcome of total elbow replacement for distal humeral fractures in the elderly: A comparison of primary surgery and surgery after failed internal fixation or conservative treatment. *J Bone Joint Surg Br* 2008;90(3): 343-348.

48. Ikävalko M, Lehto MU: Fractured rheumatoid elbow: Treatment with Souter elbow arthroplasty. A clinical and radiologic midterm follow-up study. *J Shoulder Elbow Surg* 2001;10(3):256-259.

49. Morrey BF, Adams RA: Semiconstrained arthroplasty for the treatment of rheumatoid arthritis of the elbow. *J Bone Joint Surg Am* 1992;74(4):479-490.

50. Adolfsson L, Hammer R: Elbow hemiarthroplasty for acute reconstruction of intraarticular distal humerus fractures: A preliminary report involving 4 patients. *Acta Orthop* 2006;77(5):785-787.

51. Adolfsson L, Nestorson J: The Kudo humeral component as primary hemiarthroplasty in distal humeral fractures. *J Shoulder Elbow Surg* 2012;21(4):451-455.

52. Burkhart KJ, Nijs S, Mattyasovszky SG, et al: Distal humerus hemiarthroplasty of the elbow for comminuted distal humeral fractures in the elderly patient. *J Trauma* 2011;71(3):635-642.

53. Swoboda B, Scott RD: Humeral hemiarthroplasty of the elbow joint in young patients with rheumatoid arthritis: A report on 7 arthroplasties. *J Arthroplasty* 1999; 14(5):553-559.

54. Choudry UH, Moran SL, Li S, Khan S: Soft-tissue coverage of the elbow: An outcome analysis and reconstructive algorithm. *Plast Reconstr Surg* 2007;119(6): 1852-1857.

55. Hildebrand KA, Patterson SD, Regan WD, MacDermid JC, King GJ: Functional outcome of semiconstrained total elbow arthroplasty. *J Bone Joint Surg Am* 2000; 82(10):1379-1386.

56. Kasten MD, Skinner HB: Total elbow arthroplasty: An 18-year experience. *Clin Orthop Relat Res* 1993;290:177-188.

57. Pierce TD, Herndon JH: The triceps preserving approach to total elbow arthroplasty. *Clin Orthop Relat Res* 1998;354:144-152.

58. Prokopis PM, Weiland AJ: The triceps-preserving approach for semiconstrained total elbow arthroplasty. *J Shoulder Elbow Surg* 2008;17(3):454-458.

59. Celli A, Arash A, Adams RA, Morrey BF: Triceps insufficiency following total elbow arthroplasty. *J Bone Joint Surg Am* 2005;87(9): 1957-1964.

60. Ramsey ML, Adams RA, Morrey BF: Instability of the elbow treated with semiconstrained total elbow arthroplasty. *J Bone Joint Surg Am* 1999;81(1):38-47.

61. Hamid N, Ashraf N, Bosse MJ, et al: Radiation therapy for heterotopic ossification prophylaxis acutely after elbow trauma: A prospective randomized study. *J Bone Joint Surg Am* 2010;92(11):2032-2038.

62. Spormann C, Achermann Y, Simmen BR, et al: Treatment strategies for periprosthetic infections after primary elbow arthroplasty. *J Shoulder Elbow Surg* 2012;21(8): 992-1000.

63. Goldberg SH, Urban RM, Jacobs JJ, King GJ, O'Driscoll SW, Cohen MS: Modes of wear after semiconstrained total elbow arthroplasty. *J Bone Joint Surg Am* 2008;90(3):609-619.

64. Kim JM, Mudgal CS, Konopka JF, Jupiter JB: Complications of total elbow arthroplasty. *J Am Acad Orthop Surg* 2011;19(6): 328-339.

3

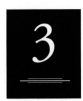

Distal Radius Fractures: Strategic Alternatives to Volar Plate Fixation

Christopher J. Dy, MD MSPH
Scott W. Wolfe, MD
Jesse B. Jupiter, MD
Philip E. Blazar, MD
David S. Ruch, MD
Douglas P. Hanel, MD

Abstract

Volar locking plates have provided surgeons with enhanced capability to reliably repair both simple and complex fractures and avoid the hardware-related complications associated with dorsal plating. However, there have been an increasing number of published reports on the frequency and types of complications and failures associated with volar locked plating of distal radius fractures. An informed, critical assessment of distal radius fracture characteristics will allow surgeons to select an individualized treatment strategy that maximizes the likelihood of a successful outcome. Knowledge of the anatomy, patterns, and characteristics of the diverse types of distal radius fractures and the complications and failures associated with volar locked plating will be helpful to orthopaedic surgeons who treat patients with these injuries.

Instr Course Lect 2014;63:27-37.

Fractures of the distal radius are common, and the incidence of these injuries continues to increase.[1] A broad range of individuals are affected, from young patients with high-energy injuries to elderly patients with osteoporotic fragility fractures. Treatment strategies have evolved along with an understanding of these injuries, with recent epidemiologic studies indicating the growing use of internal fixation.[2,3] Volar locking plates have provided surgeons with enhanced capability to reliably repair both simple and complex fractures while avoiding the hardware-related complications associated with dorsal plating.[4] However, there is a growing body of literature reporting the frequency and types of complications and failures associated with distal radius fracture fixation with volar locking plates.[5] An assessment of fracture characteristics will allow the surgeon to select an individualized treatment strategy that maximizes the chances of success.

Dr. Dy or an immediate family member serves as a board member, owner, officer, or committee member of the Accreditation Council for Graduate Medical Education. Dr. Wolfe or an immediate family member has received royalties from Extremity Medical; is a member of a speakers' bureau or has made paid presentations on behalf of TriMed; serves as a paid consultant to or is an employee of Extremity Medical; has received research or institutional support from Integra AxoGen; and serves as a board member, owner, officer, or committee member of the New York Society for Surgery of the Hand. Dr. Jupiter or an immediate family member serves as a paid consultant to or is an employee of OHK; serves as an unpaid consultant to Synthes TriMed; has received research or institutional support from the AO Foundation; has stock or stock options held in OHK; and is a member of a speakers' bureau or has made paid presentations on behalf of the AAHS Board Curriculum Committee. Dr. Blazar or an immediate family member serves as a paid consultant to or is an employee of Auxillium Pharmaceuticals and has received research or institutional support from Auxillium Pharmaceuticals. Dr. Ruch or an immediate family member has received research or institutional support from Synthes and serves as a board member, owner, officer, or committee member of the American Society for Surgery of the Hand. Dr. Hanel or an immediate family member serves as a paid consultant to or is an employee of Aptis Medical.

Table 1

Complications of Volar Plate Fixation

Study (Year)	Number of Patients	Reported Complications
Extensor tendon-related		
Arora et al[20] (2007)	141	2 EPL ruptures 4 extensor tenosynovitis
Rampoldi and Marsico[22] (2007)	90	3 extensor tendon irritations or ruptures
Soong et al[23] (2011)	321	1 extensor tendon irritation
Flexor tendon-related		
Arora et al[20] (2007)	141	2 FPL ruptures 9 flexor tendon irritations
Rampoldi and Marsico[22] (2007)	90	2 flexor tendon irritations
Soong et al[23] (2011)	321	13 flexor tendon irritations
Loss of volar tilt		
Rozental and Blazar[21] (2006)	41	2 cases
Loss of lunate facet fixation		
Rozental and Blazar[21] (2006)	41	2 cases
Rampoldi and Marsico[22] (2007)	90	1 case
Harness et al[37] (2004)	NA (case report series)	7 cases

EPL = extensor pollicis longus, FPL = flexor pollicis longus, NA = not available.

Anatomic and Biomechanical Considerations

Current approaches to the management of distal radius fractures are based on the principle that restoration of normal anatomy will facilitate an expeditious return to function.[6,7] Careful consideration of the anatomy and biomechanics of the injury will help the surgeon choose a treatment strategy to restore the normal stability and load-bearing characteristics of the wrist.

The three-column theory of the distal radius and ulna is particularly helpful in understanding the biomechanical rationale for treating distal radius fractures.[8,9] The lateral (radial) column, composed of the radial styloid and the scaphoid fossa, provides radiocarpal stability through the styloid's osseous buttress and the origin of the palmar radiocarpal ligaments. Restoring the intermediate column, composed of the lunate fossa and sigmoid notch, reestablishes the primary load-bearing surface of the radiocarpal joint.[9] Reducing the articular surface of the sigmoid notch provides congruity to the distal radioulnar joint (DRUJ) and tensions its soft-tissue attachments.[10,11] Restoring the volar lunate facet provides radiocarpal stability via a bony buttress (the teardrop or critical corner) and the ligamentous support of the short radiolunate ligament.[12] Restoring the integrity of the medial (or ulnar) column, composed of the distal ulna and triangular fibrocartilage complex (TFCC), allows it to serve as a fulcrum for rotating the radius and share in load transmission from the carpus.[9]

The optimal management of a distal radius fracture will ensure restoration of each column. The radial and intermediate columns are anatomically reduced and rigidly fixed, and the medial column is stabilized as necessary through bony fixation, TFCC repair, and/or immobilization.[8] During preoperative planning, careful attention should be paid to fractures that are particularly prone to radiocarpal instability (such as articular shearing fractures),[13] loss of fixation (such as lunate facet fractures), and fractures that may require direct articular visualization and reconstruction (such as extensively impacted articular fractures). Each of these fracture characteristics should alert the surgeon that adequate fracture fixation may not be possible using only volar plating; however, the fracture can be successfully managed if these characteristics are recognized preoperatively or intraoperatively.[14,15]

Complications Associated With Volar Locking Plates

Since their introduction, volar locking plates have been reliably used to treat displaced distal radius fractures.[16,17] The fixed-angle construct minimizes the load transmitted to the often-comminuted metaphysis while decreasing the risks of screw loosening and loss of reduction.[18] Successful reports of fixation with volar plating were contemporaneous with the increasing frequency of hardware-related complications from dorsal plating, leading to the rapid adoption of volar plating to fix dorsally angulated fractures.[4,19]

Although volar plates are increasingly used to manage many injury patterns, complications are associated with these implants. These complications can be divided into two main categories: tendon-related and loss of fixation (**Table 1**). Other complications, including complex regional pain syndrome and neurologic injury, occur less frequently and are less directly related to the hardware.[5,20,21]

Tendon-Related Complications
Extensor Tendons
Although avoidance of extensor tendon irritation was seen as a key advan-

tage of volar locking plate fixation for dorsally displaced fractures, damage to the extensor tendons still occurs from drill tips, prominent screws, and displaced bony fragments (**Figure 1**). Arora et al[20] reported 2 ruptures of the extensor pollicis longus and 4 patients with extensor tenosynovitis in a series of 141 consecutive patients with dorsally displaced distal radius fractures treated with a volar locking plate. In a study of 90 patients with distal radius fractures treated with volar plate fixation, Rampoldi and Marisco[22] reported 3 extensor tendon irritations or ruptures.[22] In the largest series of patients followed for complications after volar plating, Soong et al[23] reported that 1 of 321 patients had plate-related extensor tendon irritation.

Despite its relative rarity, this chapter's authors attempt to prevent intraoperative extensor tendon damage and postoperative extensor tendon irritation by drilling only the volar cortex and inserting unicortical locked screws that are slightly shorter than the measured amount, particularly in the setting of dorsal comminution. Alternatively, if the fracture necessitates bicortical fixation, full-length smooth pegs are preferred. This practice is substantiated by a biomechanical study by Wall et al[24] that reported no difference in axial or sagittal stiffness force among full-length bicortical screws, unicortical screws (full length, 75% length, and 50% length), and unicortical pegs in an osteoporotic distal radius model.

Flexor Tendons

The placement of hardware within the volar concavity of the distal radius minimizes the risk of flexor tendon irritation. This innate advantage is present only if the plate is positioned proximal to the transverse ridge at the distal extent of the pronator fossa (the so-called watershed line).[25] Placing the plate distal to the ridge allows greater capability in securing distal subchondral fragments but leaves the plate and screw heads in close proximity to the flexor tendons and at increased risk for

postoperative flexor tendon rupture[26] (**Figure 2, A**). Distal plate placement does not allow the hardware to be fully covered by the pronator quadratus (**Figure 2, B**). Arora et al[20] reported 2 flexor pollicis longus ruptures and 9 cases of flexor tendon tenosynovitis in their study of 141 patients with unstable distal radius fractures treated with a fixed-angle plate. Two cases of

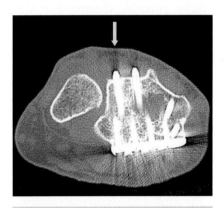

Figure 1 CT scan showing the risk of injury to extensor tendons (arrow) from prominent locking screws. (Courtesy of Philip E. Blazar, MD, Boston, MA.)

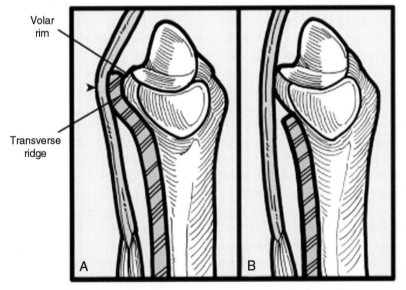

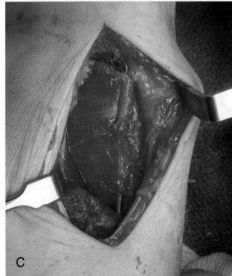

Figure 2 Distal placement of a volar locking plate puts the hardware in close proximity to the flexor tendons. **A,** In this illustration, the position of the volar plate is too distal, placing the flexor tendons at increased risk for irritation from the hardware. **B,** Illustration showing the appropriate position of the volar plate within the concavity of the distal radius. (Reproduced with permission from Wolfe SW: Distal radius fractures, in Wolfe SW, Hotchkiss RN, Pederson WC, Kozin SH, eds: *Green's Operative Hand Surgery*, ed 6. Philadelphia, PA, Elsevier, 2010, pp 561-638.) **C,** Distal placement of a volar locking plate does not allow the hardware to be fully covered by closure of the pronator quadratus. (Courtesy of Philip E. Blazar, MD, Boston, MA.)

flexor tendon irritation in 90 patients were reported by Rampoldi and Marsico,[22] and 13 cases of plate-related flexor tendon irritation were reported in 321 patients by Soong et al.[23] Given that delayed flexor tendon rupture has been reported up to 5 years after volar plating,[27] there should be a low threshold of consideration for hardware removal if there is concern about flexor tendon irritation. Ultrasound or MRI can be useful in identifying synovitis or attritional changes in at-risk flexor tendons. Retained drilling guides from screw insertion and loosening of improperly engaged locking screws have been reported as mechanisms for flexor tendon irritation after volar plating.[20,28]

Loss of Fixation After Volar Plating
Loss of Volar Tilt

The restoration of radiocarpal alignment in the sagittal plane substantially influences functional outcomes and grip strength after distal radius fracture treatment.[29] After achieving intraoperative reduction of anatomic sagittal tilt, the volar fixed-angle construct can be used to secure reduction without applying an implant to the dorsal surface. However, long-term clinical success has been correlated with maintenance of sagittal collinearity of the radius and the carpus.[29] The biomechanical stability of the construct is contingent on the distance of the distal screws from subchondral bone, with the highest resistance to metaphyseal settling seen with screws inserted as close to subchondral bone as possible.[30] Because fractures with extensive dorsal comminution are believed to be at greatest risk for loss of volar tilt, multiple fluoroscopic views should be used to maximize subchondral screw purchase distal to the zone of comminution.[21,31]

Loss of Fixation in the Lunate Facet

The importance of the volar lunate facet as the cornerstone of stability for the radiocarpal joint and the DRUJ was reported by Melone.[10] The effects of this fragment on radiocarpal instability have been emphasized, and awareness of its importance for DRUJ stability is increasing.[32-35] The volar aspect of the lunate facet contains a radiographic prominence (teardrop) that provides stability against volar subluxation by serving as a bony buttress at the origin of the short radiolunate ligament.[12,36] Loss of fixation of the volar lunate facet has been widely recognized as a mechanism of failure after volar plating.[21,22,37] Because the teardrop is less than 5 mm wide and has a relatively steep volar slope, it is difficult for the ulnar limb of volar locking plates to provide adequate stabilization.[37,38] This chapter's authors believe that at least two points of fixation are needed within this critical corner of the intermediate column. The newest volar locking plates feature two distal rows of multiaxial locking screws, providing the potential to achieve additional screw purchase within the volar lunate facet.[39] However, it is unlikely that the additional proximal row of screws provides sufficient distal capture for this small fragment, and distal placement of the entire plate comes at the expense of potential flexor tendon irritation. Given this risk, alternate methods of fixation are often preferred to secure the volar lunate facet fragment. Plating of the intermediate column can be accomplished through a volar-ulnar incision using a buttress pin, a mini plate-and-screw construct, or a tension banding technique.[14,34,40,41] These fixation techniques can be used as part of a multicolumn internal fixation approach or an approach augmented by external fixation.[8,34]

What Cannot Be Fixed With a Volar Plate?
Dorsal Ulnar Fragment

The displaced dorsal ulnar fragment is particularly challenging to control with a volar implant. Although not all dorsal ulnar fragments require stabilization, it is important to recognize that this fragment comprises a portion of both the radiolunate and radioulnar articular surfaces, and displacement of larger fragments can lead to instability of either joint. The inability to secure the dorsal ulnar fragment, depending on its size, can prevent the maintenance of adequate sagittal radiocarpal alignment and predispose the fracture to dorsal collapse. Although dorsal comminution and articular impaction can be addressed using an extended flexor carpi radialis approach,[42] this technique relies on indirect articular reduction and gaining adequate indirect purchase of the dorsal fragments with volarly to dorsally placed screws. A dorsal approach provides the surgeon with the advantage of visualizing and directly reducing the articular surface, often through a limited and targeted approach. The application of a dorsally based implant also provides a buttress against dorsal fragment displacement, which decreases the risk of secondary collapse.

As previously mentioned, the frequency of hardware-related irritation of the extensor tendons was a major limitation of conventional dorsally applied implants. This prompted the development of low-profile dorsal plates; however, these plates had inherently less material strength. In recognizing the need to strategically apply these smaller plates, Rikli and Regazzoni[8] introduced the concept of multicolumn fixation. They achieved stable fixation and promising clinical results using 2.0-mm plates positioned on the lateral and intermediate columns at 50° to 70° from each other.[8,43] Biomechanical studies supported the multi-column strategy, with superior stiffness compared with both augmented external fixation and conventional dorsal plates.[44,45] Because of persistent implant irritation, a system of even lower-profile pin-plates and wireforms was developed.[40,43,46] This fragment-specific implant system allows the surgeon greater versatility in selecting implants for challenging fracture patterns, such as those that include a dorsal ulnar fragment. Using a pin-plate to secure the dorsal ulnar corner allows buttressing of the deformity while minimizing the risk of soft-tissue irritation. Multicolumn fixation with fragment-specific implants has been used with good to excellent results and no reported extensor tendon ruptures.[40,47,48]

The specific utility of multicolumn fixation for stabilizing the dorsal ulnar fragment is substantiated by biomechanical testing. During loads expected in the rehabilitation phase, the dorsal ulnar pin-plate provided a buttress effect against dorsal closure of the osteotomy that was not provided by the volar locking plate.[49] A biomechanical evaluation by Taylor et al[50] demonstrated that a multicolumn approach using a dorsal ulnar pin-plate provided greater stiffness for the ulnar-sided fracture fragment than a volar locking plate. When viewed in conjunction, these studies indicate that multicolumn plating provides an advantage over volar locking plates in securing the intermediate column and opposing dorsal fracture collapse.

Volar Ulnar Fragment

As previously mentioned, the volar ulnar fragment is regarded as the cornerstone of the radiocarpal joint and the DRUJ because it plays critical roles in maintaining sagittal alignment, transmitting the load from the carpus, and providing sigmoid notch congru-

ity.[9,10,37] The challenges of securing the volar ulnar fragment with a volar locking plate mainly arise from the small size and sloping morphology of the fragment.[38] Given the contour of currently available volar locking plates, it is difficult to achieve multiple points of fixation within the volar ulnar fragment. Moving the plate more distally puts the flexor tendons at increased risk for irritation, whereas using a multiaxial guide to obtain more distal and ulnar screw trajectories increases the risk of screw placement within the radiocarpal joint or the DRUJ. The shortcomings of using volar locking plate fixation in this situation have been recognized along with the need for smaller implants that can be placed more distally.[21,37] It has been reported that Kirschner wires, tension-band wiring, and miniplates provide adequate fixation of the volar ulnar corner.[34,41] The volar buttress pin has been reported to provide rapid and secure fixation of small critical corner fragments.[14,15,40] Provisional fixation of the fragment is performed with a Kirschner wire, and sagittal radiocarpal alignment and stability are carefully assessed. The buttress pin has two prongs that provide fixed-angle support within the subchondral bone (**Figure 3**). The proximal aspect of the volar buttress pin implant is secured to the intact diaphysis with 2.0-mm screws and washers. Although the implant can be applied through the standard volar approach, a limited approach between the flexor tendons and the ulnar neurovascular bundle is helpful when performing multicolumn fixation with multiple incisions.[14,15] Care must be taken to avoid traction on the median nerve and the palmar cutaneous branch if applying an ulnar-sided implant through a standard Henry approach.

Marginal Articular Shear Fractures

Marginal shearing fractures (Fernandez type II) are difficult to treat with volar locking plates for many of the same reasons described for dorsal and volar ulnar fragments[13] (**Figure 4**). Dorsal shearing fractures (reverse Barton fractures) are associated with radiocarpal subluxation or dislocation. These fractures are relatively uncommon; are usually caused by high-energy mechanisms; and often have a spectrum of associated volar injuries, including carpal ligament tears, articular impaction, and volar marginal shearing.[51] Because of the direction of the associated radiocarpal instability, these injuries are often best approached from the dorsal side. Articular impaction can be directly assessed from this approach, and bone grafting is often helpful to provide subchondral support. The fracture is then buttressed with a dorsally based implant to minimize the risk of recurrent instability.[51] Low-profile implants of various sizes, ranging from 2.0-mm to 3.5-mm dorsal plates to fragment-specific pin-plates or wireforms can be used (**Figure 4**). The surgeon chooses the implant based on the fracture characteristics and the soft-tissue coverage capability. Volar shearing fractures (and the treatment of volar injuries associated with dorsal marginal shearing fractures) require an analogous approach. Larger fragments can be stabilized with volar locking plates; however, marginal shear fragments typically require the use of low-profile, distally positioned implants to buttress the articular surface.

Unstable Radial Styloid

The radial styloid plays a critical role in radiocarpal stability, providing both an osseous buttress and the ligamentous origin of the stout palmar radiocarpal ligaments.[9] Reduction of the ra-

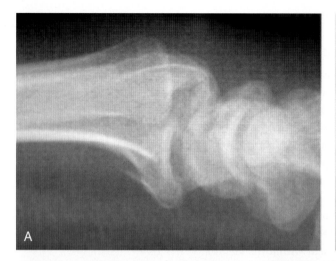

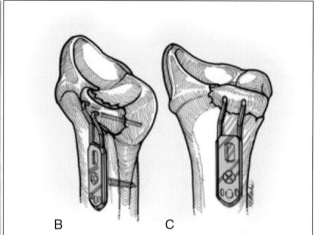

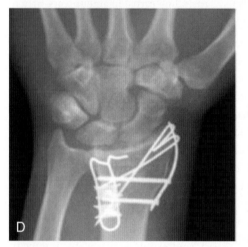

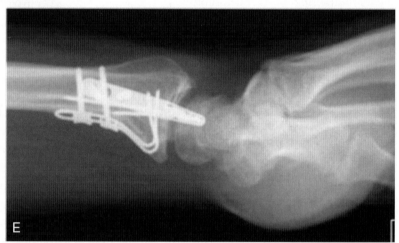

Figure 3 A volar buttress pin can be used to secure the volar ulnar corner of the distal radius. **A,** Radiograph showing volar subluxation of the carpus. Oblique view (**B**) and frontal view (**C**) of a volar buttress pin applied to secure the volar-ulnar corner. AP (**D**) and lateral (**E**) intraoperative radiographs of multicolumn fixation, including a volar buttress pin. (Reproduced with permission from Wolfe SW: Distal radius fractures, in Wolfe SW, Hotchkiss RN, Pederson WC, Kozin SH, eds: *Green's Operative Hand Surgery*, ed 6. Philadelphia, PA, Elsevier, 2010, pp 561-638.)

dial styloid is essential to ensure appropriate restoration of radial inclination and the length and congruity of the radioscaphoid articulation. Two or more points of fixation can usually be obtained for large radial styloid fragments within the radial-sided distal screws of the volar locking plate. However, if anatomic reduction and solid fixation of the radial styloid cannot be confidently obtained because of comminution, small fragment size, or instability from shearing, the application of a 2.0-mm plate should be considered along the radial column.[8,40] The plate provides addi-

tional coronal plane compression to close articular gaps and aids in supporting a comminuted articular surface (**Figure 5**). This plate can be used in combination with a volar locking plate or intermediate column-specific, low-profile implants.[40,52,53] Mechanical studies support the addition of a radial column plate to enhance the stability of a volar locking plate for comminuted articular fractures.[54]

Central Impaction

The dorsal approach provides a distinct advantage if there is substantial

central impaction of the articular surface. Because of the volar radiocarpal ligaments, the volar approach requires indirect visualization and reduction techniques. Alternatively, an extended Henry approach allows visualization but entails considerable periosteal stripping.[42] Using a targeted dorsal approach, the articular surface is directly reduced and reconstructed. Bone graft may be used to fill subchondral and metaphyseal voids to aid in supporting small impacted articular fragments. If the subchondral bone has sufficient integrity, a dorsal plate is applied for

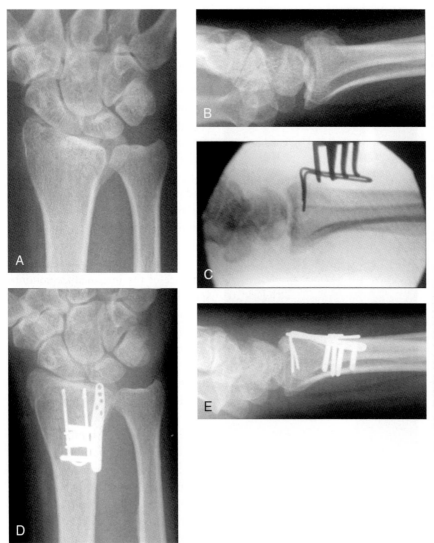

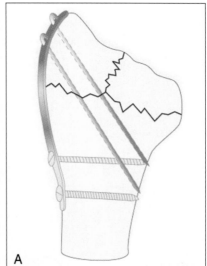

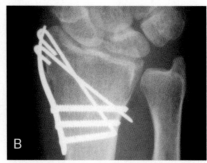

Figure 4 Preoperative (**A**) and lateral (**B**) radiographs of a dorsal marginal shear fracture. **C,** Intraoperative lateral fluoroscopic view. The fracture was reduced and secured with dorsal wireform implants. AP (**D**) and lateral (**E**) radiographs taken 1 month postoperatively.

Figure 5 Illustration (**A**) and radiograph (**B**) of a radial styloid plate used to stabilize an unstable radial styloid fracture and to close an articular gap. (Panel 5A reproduced with permission from Wolfe SW: Distal radius fractures, in Wolfe SW, Hotchkiss RN, Pederson WC, Kozin SH, eds: *Green's Operative Hand Surgery*, ed 6. Philadelphia, PA, Elsevier, 2010, pp 561-638. Panel 5B copyright Scott Wolfe, MD, New York, NY.)

fracture fixation. If bone stock is severely compromised from a high-energy injury, a spanning dorsal plate can be used in a bridging fashion to neutralize the compressive forces on the articular surface[55,56] (**Figure 6**). The plate, which essentially serves as an internally placed external fixator, is placed along the dorsal wrist and beneath the extensor retinaculum. Fixation screws are placed far from the zone of injury, in the radial diaphysis and the metacarpal, to increase the rigidity of the construct.[57] Different plates and hardware positions have been reported, with the original description of a 3.5-mm plate applied under the fourth dorsal compartment.[58] Hanel et al[59] described the use of a 2.4- to 2.7-mm combiplate applied under the second dorsal compartment. Three screws each are placed on the distal and proximal sides using a combination of locking and cortical screws.[60] In addition to its use for centrally impacted articular injuries, this technique is useful in the polytrauma setting (limited surgical time, bilateral fractures, and fractures with severe comminution or osteoporosis).[56,59,61] Consolidation of the fracture typically occurs at a mean of 110 days; the distraction plate can be removed shortly thereafter.[56] The clinical results are comparable to other fixation techniques. The complication profile is safe, with the need for staged plate removal being the major limitation.[62]

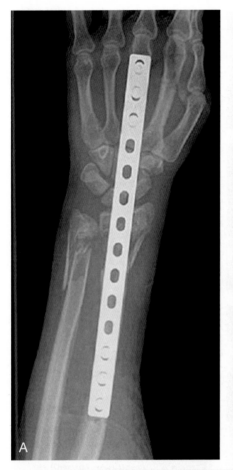 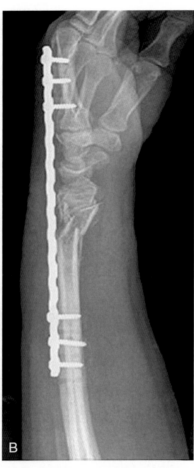

Figure 6 AP (**A**) and lateral (**B**) radiographic views of a spanning plate used to bridge a comminuted articular surface. Fixation points are placed far from the zone of injury. (Reproduced with permission from Ruch DS, Ginn TA, Yang CC, Smith BP, Rushing J, Hanel DP: Use of a distraction plate for distal radial fractures with metaphyseal and diaphyseal comminution. *J Bone Joint Surg Am* 2005;87(5):945-954.)

DRUJ Instability

Volar plating alone cannot treat DRUJ instability. Stabilization of the intermediate column may help improve DRUJ stability in two ways: by (1) restoring articular congruency of the sigmoid notch to provide a seat for the distal ulna and (2) tensioning the TFCC and the surrounding soft-tissue stabilizers of the DRUJ. In each instance, stability of the ulnar column should be assessed immediately after the lateral and intermediate columns have been stabilized. Injury patterns with TFCC avulsions or basilar styloid fractures or fractures with proximal extension are at highest risk

for DRUJ instability.[35] If the DRUJ is unstable, forearm rotation should be examined to find a position of stability for postoperative immobilization. Ten to 14 days of above-elbow immobilization is generally sufficient to achieve adequate stability to begin active forearm rotation exercises. If a stable position cannot be identified, TFCC repair and/or open reduction and internal fixation of the basilar styloid or ulnar head fracture should be performed using Kirschner wires or styloid-specific plates. In the setting of persistent instability, dual 0.062-inch Kirschner wire fixation can be used to temporar-

ily fix the radius and the ulna in supination.

Summary

Although most distal radius fractures can be treated reliably with volar locking plates, each fracture should be carefully assessed to ensure that alternative strategies are not needed. When using volar locking plates, the risk of tendon-related complications can be minimized by drilling in a unicortical fashion, inserting less than full-length distal locking screws, and avoiding distal positioning of the plate. The importance of the intermediate column, specifically the volar and dorsal ulnar fragments of the distal radius, cannot be overemphasized. Inadequate fixation of these fragments can have adverse implications on radiocarpal alignment, radioulnar stability, and functional outcome. Marginal shearing fractures are difficult to secure with volar locking plates. Multicolumn fixation techniques can be used to fix volar and dorsal ulnar fragments and buttress marginal shearing fractures. Dorsal approaches can be useful in reconstructing impacted articular fractures, with dorsal plating or distraction plating used for definitive fixation. The ulnar column needs to be assessed after osteosynthesis of the distal radius is complete, with stabilization if necessary via styloid plating, TFCC repair, or supine immobilization. Adherence to these principles will maximize the opportunity for the restoration of normal anatomy and function after a distal radius fracture.

References

1. Nellans KW, Kowalski E, Chung KC: The epidemiology of distal radius fractures. *Hand Clin* 2012; 28(2):113-125.

2. Koval KJ, Harrast JJ, Anglen JO, Weinstein JN: Fractures of the

distal part of the radius: The evolution of practice over time. Where's the evidence? *J Bone Joint Surg Am* 2008;90(9):1855-1861.

3. Chung KC, Shauver MJ, Birkmeyer JD: Trends in the United States in the treatment of distal radial fractures in the elderly. *J Bone Joint Surg Am* 2009;91(8): 1868-1873.

4. Orbay JL, Fernandez DL: Volar fixation for dorsally displaced fractures of the distal radius: A preliminary report. *J Hand Surg Am* 2002;27(2):205-215.

5. Berglund LM, Messer TM: Complications of volar plate fixation for managing distal radius fractures. *J Am Acad Orthop Surg* 2009;17(6):369-377.

6. Gartland JJ Jr, Werley CW: Evaluation of healed Colles' fractures. *J Bone Joint Surg Am* 1951;33(4): 895-907.

7. McQueen M, Caspers J: Colles fracture: Does the anatomical result affect the final function? *J Bone Joint Surg Br* 1988;70(4): 649-651.

8. Rikli DA, Regazzoni P: Fractures of the distal end of the radius treated by internal fixation and early function: A preliminary report of 20 cases. *J Bone Joint Surg Br* 1996;78(4):588-592.

9. Rikli DA, Honigmann P, Babst R, Cristalli A, Morlock MM, Mittlmeier T: Intra-articular pressure measurement in the radioulnocarpal joint using a novel sensor: In vitro and in vivo results. *J Hand Surg Am* 2007;32(1):67-75.

10. Melone CP Jr: Articular fractures of the distal radius. *Orthop Clin North Am* 1984;15(2):217-236.

11. Moritomo H: The distal interosseous membrane: Current concepts in wrist anatomy and biomechanics. *J Hand Surg Am* 2012;37(7):1501-1507.

12. Medoff RJ: Essential radiographic evaluation for distal radius fractures. *Hand Clin* 2005;21(3): 279-288.

13. Fernández DL: Fractures of the distal radius: Operative treatment. *Instr Course Lect* 1993;42:73-88.

14. Wolfe SW: *Green's Operative Hand Surgery*, ed 6. Philadelphia, PA, Elsevier, 2010.

15. Lam JW, Wolfe SW: Distal radius fractures: What cannot be fixed with a volar plate? The role of fragment-specific fixation in modern fracture treatment. *Oper Tech Sports Med* 2010;18(3):181-188.

16. Gesensway D, Putnam MD, Mente PL, Lewis JL: Design and biomechanics of a plate for the distal radius. *J Hand Surg Am* 1995;20(6):1021-1027.

17. Orbay JL: The treatment of unstable distal radius fractures with volar fixation. *Hand Surg* 2000; 5(2):103-112.

18. Orbay JL, Touhami A: Current concepts in volar fixed-angle fixation of unstable distal radius fractures. *Clin Orthop Relat Res* 2006; 445:58-67.

19. Drobetz H, Kutscha-Lissberg E: Osteosynthesis of distal radial fractures with a volar locking screw plate system. *Int Orthop* 2003;27(1):1-6.

20. Arora R, Lutz M, Hennerbichler A, Krappinger D, Espen D, Gabl M: Complications following internal fixation of unstable distal radius fracture with a palmar locking-plate. *J Orthop Trauma* 2007;21(5):316-322.

21. Rozental TD, Blazar PE: Functional outcome and complications after volar plating for dorsally displaced, unstable fractures of the distal radius. *J Hand Surg Am* 2006;31(3):359-365.

22. Rampoldi M, Marsico S: Complications of volar plating of distal radius fractures. *Acta Orthop Belg* 2007;73(6):714-719.

23. Soong M, van Leerdam R, Guitton TG, Got C, Katarincic J, Ring D: Fracture of the distal radius: Risk factors for complications after locked volar plate fixation. *J Hand Surg Am* 2011; 36(1):3-9.

24. Wall LB, Brodt MD, Silva MJ, Boyer MI, Calfee RP: The effects of screw length on stability of simulated osteoporotic distal radius fractures fixed with volar locking plates. *J Hand Surg Am* 2012;37(3):446-453.

25. Orbay J: Volar plate fixation of distal radius fractures. *Hand Clin* 2005;21(3):347-354.

26. Soong M, Earp BE, Bishop G, Leung A, Blazar P: Volar locking plate implant prominence and flexor tendon rupture. *J Bone Joint Surg Am* 2011;93(4):328-335.

27. Koo SC, Ho ST: Delayed rupture of flexor pollicis longus tendon after volar plating of the distal radius. *Hand Surg* 2006;11(1-2): 67-70.

28. Bhattacharyya T, Wadgaonkar AD: Inadvertent retention of angled drill guides after volar locking plate fixation of distal radial fractures: A report of three cases. *J Bone Joint Surg Am* 2008;90(2): 401-403.

29. McQueen MM, Hajducka C, Court-Brown CM: Redisplaced unstable fractures of the distal radius: A prospective randomised comparison of four methods of treatment. *J Bone Joint Surg Br* 1996;78(3):404-409.

30. Drobetz H, Bryant AL, Pokorny T, Spitaler R, Leixnering M, Jupiter JB: Volar fixed-angle plating of distal radius extension fractures: Influence of plate position on secondary loss of reduction. A biomechanic study in a cadaveric model. *J Hand Surg Am* 2006; 31(4):615-622.

31. Soong M, Got C, Katarincic J, Akelman E: Fluoroscopic evaluation of intra-articular screw placement during locked volar plating of the distal radius: A cadaveric study. *J Hand Surg Am* 2008; 33(10):1720-1723.

32. Apergis E, Darmanis S, Theodoratos G, Maris J: Beware of the ulno-palmar distal radial fragment. *J Hand Surg Br* 2002;27(2):139-145.

33. Smith RS, Crick JC, Alonso J, Horowitz M: Open reduction and internal fixation of volar lip fractures of the distal radius. *J Orthop Trauma* 1988;2(3):181-187.

34. Ruch DS, Yang C, Smith BP: Results of palmar plating of the lunate facet combined with external fixation for the treatment of high-energy compression fractures of the distal radius. *J Orthop Trauma* 2004;18(1):28-33.

35. Cole DW, Elsaidi GA, Kuzma KR, Kuzma GR, Smith BP, Ruch DS: Distal radioulnar joint instability in distal radius fractures: The role of sigmoid notch and triangular fibrocartilage complex revisited. *Injury* 2006;37(3):252-258.

36. Berger RA, Landsmeer JM: The palmar radiocarpal ligaments: A study of adult and fetal human wrist joints. *J Hand Surg Am* 1990;15(6):847-854.

37. Harness NG, Jupiter JB, Orbay JL, Raskin KB, Fernandez DL: Loss of fixation of the volar lunate facet fragment in fractures of the distal part of the radius. *J Bone Joint Surg Am* 2004;86(9):1900-1908.

38. Andermahr J, Lozano-Calderon S, Trafton T, Crisco JJ, Ring D: The volar extension of the lunate facet of the distal radius: A quantitative anatomic study. *J Hand Surg Am* 2006;31(6):892-895.

39. Buzzell JE, Weikert DR, Watson JT, Lee DH: Precontoured fixed-angle volar distal radius plates: A comparison of anatomic fit. *J Hand Surg Am* 2008;33(7):1144-1152.

40. Konrath GA, Bahler S: Open reduction and internal fixation of unstable distal radius fractures: Results using the trimed fixation system. *J Orthop Trauma* 2002;16(8):578-585.

41. Chin KR, Jupiter JB: Wire-loop fixation of volar displaced osteochondral fractures of the distal radius. *J Hand Surg Am* 1999;24(3):525-533.

42. Orbay JL, Badia A, Indriago IR, et al: A new perspective for the distal radius fracture. *Tech Hand Up Extrem Surg* 2001;5(4):204-211.

43. Jakob M, Rikli DA, Regazzoni P: Fractures of the distal radius treated by internal fixation and early function: A prospective study of 73 consecutive patients. *J Bone Joint Surg Br* 2000;82(3):340-344.

44. Dodds SD, Cornelissen S, Jossan S, Wolfe SW: A biomechanical comparison of fragment-specific fixation and augmented external fixation for intra-articular distal radius fractures. *J Hand Surg Am* 2002;27(6):953-964.

45. Peine R, Rikli DA, Hoffmann R, Duda G, Regazzoni P: Comparison of three different plating techniques for the dorsum of the distal radius: A biomechanical study. *J Hand Surg Am* 2000;25(1):29-33.

46. Leslie BM, Medoff RJ: Fracture specific fixation of distal radius fractures. *Tech Orthop* 2000;15(4):336-352.

47. Benson LS, Minihane KP, Stern LD, Eller E, Seshadri R: The outcome of intra-articular distal radius fractures treated with fragment-specific fixation. *J Hand Surg Am* 2006;31(8):1333-1339.

48. Gerostathopoulos N, Kalliakmanis A, Fandridis E, Georgoulis S: Trimed fixation system for displaced fractures of the distal radius. *J Trauma* 2007;62(4):913-918.

49. Cooper EO, Segalman KA, Parks BG, Sharma KM, Nguyen A: Biomechanical stability of a volar locking-screw plate versus fragment-specific fixation in a distal radius fracture model. *Am J Orthop (Belle Mead NJ)* 2007;36(4):E46-E49.

50. Taylor KF, Parks BG, Segalman KA: Biomechanical stability of a fixed-angle volar plate versus fragment-specific fixation system: Cyclic testing in a C2-type distal radius cadaver fracture model. *J Hand Surg Am* 2006;31(3):373-381.

51. Lozano-Calderón SA, Doornberg J, Ring D: Fractures of the dorsal articular margin of the distal part of the radius with dorsal radiocarpal subluxation. *J Bone Joint Surg Am* 2006;88(7):1486-1493.

52. Tang P, Ding A, Uzumcugil A: Radial column and volar plating (RCVP) for distal radius fractures with a radial styloid component or severe comminution. *Tech Hand Up Extrem Surg* 2010;14(3):143-149.

53. Bae DS, Koris MJ: Fragment-specific internal fixation of distal radius fractures. *Hand Clin* 2005;21(3):355-362.

54. Grindel SI, Wang M, Gerlach M, McGrady LM, Brown S: Biomechanical comparison of fixed-angle volar plate versus fixed-angle volar plate plus fragment-specific fixation in a cadaveric distal radius fracture model. *J Hand Surg Am* 2007;32(2):194-199.

55. Ginn TA, Ruch DS, Yang CC, Hanel DP: Use of a distraction plate for distal radial fractures with metaphyseal and diaphyseal comminution: Surgical technique. *J Bone Joint Surg Am* 2006;88(suppl pt 1):29-36.

56. Ruch DS, Ginn TA, Yang CC, Smith BP, Rushing J, Hanel DP: Use of a distraction plate for distal radial fractures with metaphyseal and diaphyseal comminution. *J Bone Joint Surg Am* 2005;87(5):945-954.

57. Behrens F, Johnson W: Unilateral external fixation: Methods to in-

crease and reduce frame stiffness. *Clin Orthop Relat Res* 1989;241: 48-56.

58. Burke EF, Singer RM: Treatment of comminuted distal radius with the use of an internal distraction plate. *Tech Hand Up Extrem Surg* 1998;2(4):248-252.

59. Hanel DP, Lu TS, Weil WM: Bridge plating of distal radius fractures: The Harborview method. *Clin Orthop Relat Res* 2006;445:91-99.

60. Wolf JC, Weil WM, Hanel DP, Trumble TE: A biomechanic comparison of an internal radiocarpal-spanning 2.4-mm locking plate and external fixation in a model of distal radius fractures. *J Hand Surg Am* 2006;31(10):1578-1586.

61. Richard MJ, Katolik LI, Hanel DP, Wartinbee DA, Ruch DS: Distraction plating for the treatment of highly comminuted distal radius fractures in elderly patients.

J Hand Surg Am 2012;37(5): 948-956.

62. Hanel DP, Ruhlman SD, Katolik LI, Allan CH: Complications associated with distraction plate fixation of wrist fractures. *Hand Clin* 2010;26(2):237-243.

Improving Outcomes: Understanding the Psychosocial Aspects of the Orthopaedic Trauma Patient

Paul E. Levin, MD
Ellen J. MacKenzie, PhD
Michael J. Bosse, MD
Pamela K. Greenhouse, MBA

Abstract

The care of orthopaedic trauma patients with multiple injuries has dramatically improved in the past 25 years. The understanding of the physiology of trauma has evolved, new surgical approaches have been developed, and technologic advances have created better implants. New methods of treating fractures include fluoroscopic and computer-assisted imaging. Surgical interventions have changed from extensive and prolonged dissections to more limited and effective percutaneous and minimally invasive techniques. The lives of patients are being saved, and radiographic outcomes are improving; however, medical and surgical advances that achieve better radiographic and anatomic outcomes do not always improve functional outcomes. Understanding and optimizing the management of the psychosocial factors that affect trauma patients can improve outcomes.

Instr Course Lect 2014;63:39-48.

Understanding and identifying the psychological and social factors that affect a patient's recovery from traumatic injuries has been shown to improve outcomes.[1-3] Many centers have recognized that psychosocial problems are important clinical features that can adversely affect a successful recovery. Strategies and programs are being developed to identify psychosocial problems early and successfully address these issues. Patients with multiple traumatic injuries and those with severe isolated musculoskeletal injuries are subjected to immediate social and psychological stresses that affect recovery. The Lower Extremity Assessment Project (LEAP) identified psychological and social characteristics and comorbidities as more predictive of outcome after a severe open tibial fracture than either amputation or limb salvage.[1-3]

One possible explanation for this dichotomy of physical recovery versus functional outcomes is the failure to recognize the differences between treating a disease and treating an illness.[4,5] A disease is a specific, usually identifiable pathology that the physician can treat in caring for his or her patient. In orthopaedic trauma, the pathology may be a specific fracture, a soft-tissue injury, or multiple injuries. Illness is the gamut of psychosocial concerns and pathologies that are commonly seen in trauma patients. The symptoms of an illness include fear of the loss of social support, poor self-efficacy, concerns about finances and the ability to return to work or recreational activities, pain, narcotic dependence, acute anxiety, phobias, catastrophizing, posttraumatic stress, and depression.[6,7] Illnesses can affect both the patient and his or her family and may lead to secondary disease, which can compromise a patient's

Dr. Levin or an immediate family member serves as a board member, owner, officer, or committee member of the American Academy of Orthopaedic Surgeons Committee on Ethics, the American Academy of Orthopaedic Surgeons Trauma Program Subcommittee, and the American Academy of Orthopaedic Surgeons Resolution Committee. Dr. MacKenzie or an immediate family member serves as a board member, owner, officer, or committee member of the National Trauma Institute. Neither of the following authors nor any immediate family member has received anything of value from or has stock or stock options held in a commercial company or institution related directly or indirectly to the subject of this chapter: Dr. Bosse and Ms. Greenhouse.

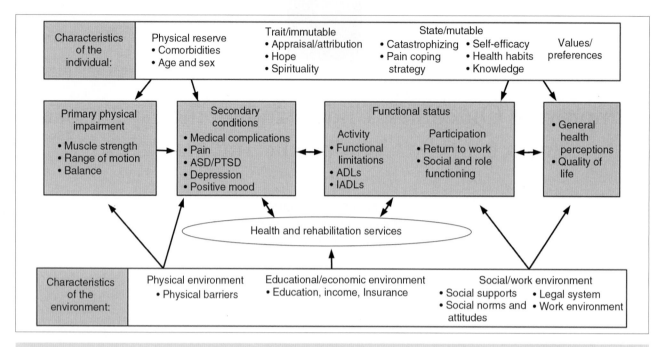

Figure 1 Physical and psychosocial factors affecting a patient's outcome after a traumatic injury. ASD = acute stress disorder, PTSD = posttraumatic stress disorder, ADLs = activities of daily living, IADLs = instrumental activities of daily living.

ultimate recovery. When illnesses are not identified and addressed or are ignored because of the belief that they will resolve with functional recovery, patients may experience irreversible psychosocial decline. Peabody,[8] an early 20th century Harvard medical professor, stated it best: "The treatment of the disease must be completely impersonal; the treatment of the patient must be completely personal."

Lessons Learned From LEAP and Other Orthopaedic Outcome Studies

A growing body of literature on patient outcomes indicates that many factors influence functional outcomes and quality of life in addition to the initial treatment of the injury and the extent of residual impairment.[1,9-18] Although the relationships among these factors are multivariate and complex, principal relationships and a framework for opportunities for intervention can be identified (**Figure 1**). This framework acknowledges that

secondary conditions, including medical complications, pain, posttraumatic stress disorder, and depression, can affect functional status and participation in life roles, which influence general health perceptions and the overall quality of life.

Characteristics of the individual and the environment influence the prevalence of these secondary conditions and their effect on function and quality of life. Some of these characteristics, such as age, sex, comorbidities, personal traits, economic resources, and social support networks are difficult or impossible to change. Other characteristics, such as self-efficacy and coping abilities, are mutable. Focusing on these latter characteristics provides opportunities to improve long-term outcomes after a traumatic injury.

Results from the LEAP study underscore these lessons.[1-3,7,19,20] In a prospective longitudinal observational outcomes study, 569 patients with severe lower extremity injuries who were treated with amputation or reconstruc-

tion were assessed using the Sickness Impact Profile and the Brief Symptom Inventory health measures to help determine if functional outcomes are improved by amputation or limb salvage.[1] The Sickness Impact Profile consists of 136 statements about limitations in 12 domains and asks about multiple aspects of both physical and psychosocial functioning. The Brief Symptom Inventory is used to assess the psychological symptoms of psychiatric and medical patients as well as individuals from the general population.[1] At 2 and 7 years after injury, both groups had similar outcomes as measured by the Sickness Impact Profile. Forty-two percent of the patients reported moderate to severe disabilities.[1,2] Only 51% of those working before being injured had returned to work at the time of the 2-year follow-up.

In addition to difficulties with physical activities, the patients had high rates of psychosocial disability. Forty-eight percent of the patients had positive results on a screening for a likely psychological disorder at 3 months after injury, and 42% had positive findings at 24 months after injury. Two years after the injury, almost 20% of the patients reported severe phobic anxiety and/or depression.[19] The LEAP study also reported that outcomes were more affected by the patient's economic, social, and personal resources than by the initial treatment of the injury, specifically amputation versus reconstruction and the level of amputation. Patients with a baseline report of low self-efficacy; a weak social support system; and high levels of depression, anxiety, and pain were significantly more likely to have poor long-term outcomes.

Self-efficacy refers to confidence in the ability to perform specific tasks or activities. Individuals with low self-efficacy are more likely to disengage from the coping process because failure is expected. The negative effect of posttraumatic stress and anxiety on a patient's ability to recover was also identified. Unfortunately, only a few of the LEAP patients who screened positive for a likely psychological disorder reported receiving mental health services after their injuries.[19]

Several conclusions can be drawn from the LEAP study. Orthopaedic surgeons are adept at treating musculoskeletal pathology and its associated complications but are often unable or untrained in identifying and addressing other factors that may improve a patient's functional outcome. Major improvements in functional outcomes may be achieved by placing a greater emphasis on nonclinical psychosocial interventions along with the early and aggressive engagement of vocational rehabilitation. Targeted therapy can improve self-efficacy deficiencies and psychosocial disability. Because orthopaedic surgeons play a central role in coordinating care for patients who sus-

tain severe lower extremity injuries, it is imperative that they consider screening these patients for psychosocial problems.

The Role of the Orthopaedic Surgeon

The LEAP study highlighted many factors involved in recovering from physical trauma, which is often associated with psychological trauma. Some individuals are much better equipped than others to overcome these events. Social support from friends and family can make a substantial difference in facilitating a full recovery. Guiding patients through recovery may simply mean that orthopaedic surgeons should be more readily available to counsel patients when concerns arise. It clearly means that family and friends should be actively recruited to aid in the recovery process.

Although severe, unrelenting psychological and social problems requiring professional care may develop in some patients, other patients will not require special assistance. It is likely that a combination of an empathetic and understanding relationship with the treating orthopaedic surgeon along with an institutional commitment in supporting patients and their families can improve outcomes. Family and patient-centered care, including meeting the psychosocial needs of the patient and his or her family, have been shown to be highly successful in improving satisfaction and outcomes. Although clinical studies have not specifically demonstrated the benefit of psychosocial support in patients with orthopaedic trauma, it is clear that the lack of support has a deleterious effect on outcomes.[2,18,19] Researchers in this field strongly believe that the early institution of social and psychological support and early interventions (if necessary) will help prevent the downward spiral of anxiety, depression, and pain

management frequently encountered in the multiply-injured trauma patient.[18] The orthopaedic surgeon can become a source of support by helping recruit and maintain the involvement of a patient's social support network and by enlisting support from other professionals to create an environment that recognizes and addresses the importance of psychosocial factors in optimizing patient care.

Humanize the Patient

Orthopaedic surgeons are adept at solving medical problems but may forget the unique individual characteristics of the injured patient. It is helpful to remember that the patient in the trauma bay with a femoral fracture, a pelvic fracture, and pneumothorax has a unique personality, occupation, vocation, family, friends, and idiosyncrasies. When the individual characteristics of a patient are ignored, the disease, not the illness created by the disease, is being treated.[5] Showing empathy to the patient and the family provides the crucial support necessary to maximize a patient's likelihood of recovery. Professional, detached concern should be replaced with emotional attunement.[21] Routinely requesting a psychiatry consultation for a patient is not a substitute for providing assistance and guidance to the patient and his or her family. Many concerns and fears that arise during recovery are better addressed and explained by an experienced orthopaedic traumatologist than a psychotherapist.

Communication

The life of the patient and his or her family immediately and permanently changes when a traumatic injury occurs. The patient and/or family may be frightened, possibly worried about life-threatening injuries, and emotionally overwhelmed. Information is vital. When possible, the orthopaedic surgeon should sit next to the patient and provide comfort and empathy (possibly resting a hand on the patient's shoulder or holding a hand). Time should also be spent with family members to review the patient's injuries and explain treatment plans. Information should be honest and as reassuring as possible. Definitive predictions should be avoided, unless the outcome is certain.

The American Academy of Orthopaedic Surgeons in conjunction with the Institute for Health Care Communication recommends that four principles be incorporated into an ambulatory patient visit: engagement, empathy, education, and enlistment (NM Nanchoff, PhD, et al, Germantown, WI, unpublished data presented at the Institute for Health Care Communications workshop, September 2012).[22] Although the traumatic injury scenario is different, these four steps can be helpful in initial encounters with the patient and his or her family.

A patient often has difficulty remembering information that is given when he or she is experiencing pain, fear, and extreme stress; however, the general impression of kindness and empathy may be recalled. Developing a good relationship and understanding with the patient and his or her family as soon as possible may be instrumental in working as a team and helping the patient recover. Ideally, either the orthopaedic surgeon or a trauma coordinator should meet with the patient and his or her family daily to review the diagnoses and treatment plans. These sessions should allow time for questions and expressions of concern. Keeping the patient fully informed and involved in the decision-making process can help prevent unnecessary anxiety and psychological stress and can prevent medical errors. It is much better to ask specific questions than to simply ask "do you have any ques-

tions?" Conversation with the patient about family, work, pets, or hobbies can improve the doctor-patient relationship, and shared decision making can forge a partnership that can improve adherence to the treatment recommendation and maximize positive outcomes.[23-25]

Residents and fellows should be present during meetings with patients and families to develop appropriate skills; however, the staff orthopaedic surgeon should take the lead in guiding his or her patient through the recovery process.[26-28]

Managing Pain

Dependence on narcotic pain medications and physical therapy services are commonplace after multiple traumatic injuries.[29] These issues should be discussed early in the recovery period, with strategies to taper the use of pain medications and therapy services. Patients should be encouraged to begin a self-directed exercise program to decrease the need for physical therapy. The appropriate use of pain medications to assist rehabilitation should be discussed, along with the need to decrease narcotic use during recovery. The hard work required by the patient to recover should be stressed so the patient and his or her family can maintain their commitment, focus on the recovery process, and not become discouraged.

Recruiting the Family

A growing body of evidence in the care of hospitalized children and adults in both general ward and intensive care settings has shown improved patient satisfaction and adherence to the treatment regimen when there is active family involvement by the care team.[30-34] In the trauma setting, it is often the most junior member of the team who is available to communicate with the family during the critical re-

covery period.[35] The presence of family members during a patient's hospitalization, including the time spent in the intensive care unit, improves clinical outcomes; however, the presence of family members also can create conflict with the medical staff.[18,36-43]

Most patients have personal relationships and social support structures. The surgeon should ask the patient's permission to inform the family about the patient's condition. If the patient is unconscious, a reasonable assumption can be made that information can be shared with people who have appropriately identified themselves as friends or family. If no family or friends are initially available, the surgeon should ask the patient for the names of people to be notified about the injury. Every effort should be made to contact family members.

Family members and friends of the patient may be unfamiliar with and intimidated by the hospital environment. Many hospitals foster these feelings by establishing visiting hours and asking family members to leave the patient's room during examinations and other activities. Family members and friends should be allowed and encouraged to visit for as long as possible, including overnight. The family should also be invited to stay for patient rounds.[30,34,42] The inclusion of the family can help ensure that all concerned parties understand the medical issues and the treatment plan. Family members may require instructions on how to participate in a patient's care. Initially, this may be providing company and holding a hand, but later they may provide assistance in rehabilitation exercises and during meals.

Patient- and Family-Centered Care Methodology

In 2006, DiGioia developed methodology for patient- and family-centered care (PFCC) to create a system that viewed care from the perspectives of the patient and the family.[37,44-46] It was found that these methods optimized the patient and family experience of care and led to excellent patient satisfaction, better clinical outcomes and efficiency, and decreased cost.[37,44-48] Because of the promising results with PFCC at the Magee Women's Hospital at the University of Pittsburgh Medical Center, DiGioia refined the methodology based on the work of experts in the fields of design science, business, organizational behavior, leadership, and marketing.[49-54] The methodology has since been exported to other healthcare settings nationally and internationally. PFCC methodology and practice have been adopted in nearly 60 different clinical areas of University of Pittsburgh Medical Center, in areas as varied as two men's cancer care services, outpatient mental health services, surgical services, and adult level I trauma services.[46] The success of the PFCC method of practice has been recognized by the Picker Institute, the Joint Commission, and the Institute for Healthcare Improvement.[47,55-57]

PFCC Concept and Method

Although many healthcare organizations have successfully implemented improvements in care delivery, sustaining these initiatives and disseminating them across organizations has proven problematic. Barriers include hierarchic and functional silos, staff desensitization, staffing shortages, and budget pressures.

The PFCC methodology and practice was designed as a new operating system for providing health care. With tools from the PFCC toolkit (such as shadowing and care experience flow mapping), caregivers (defined broadly as both clinical staff, such as doctors, nurses, therapists and technicians, and nonclinical staff, such as parking atten-

Table 1	
The Three Central Elements of PFCC Methodology and Practice	
Element	**Results/Implementation**
View the care experience through the eyes of the patient and family.	The PFCC toolkit provides simple tools that allow caregivers to real-time view care as patients and families experience it. This leads to understanding, emotional connections, and urgency to drive change.
Engage patients and families as full partners with the physician in designing a patient's care.	The care provided is exactly what patients and families want and need, no more and no less. Patients and families relate their current experience and help guide caregivers toward the ideal experience.
Provide simple approaches to overcome challenges in a complex system.	The PFCC methodology is simple to learn, is simple to implement, and uses resources that already exist rather than requiring new resources.

PFCC = patient- and family-centered care.

dants, appointment schedulers, housekeepers, and billing representatives) can identify the current care experience as defined by patients and families, imagine an ideal experience as defined by patients and families, and then form cross-functional and cross-hierarchic working groups to close the gap between the two concepts.[37,46]

PFCC working groups are permanent groups that are charged with continually identifying new gaps between current care and ideal care. When gaps are identified, PFCC project teams work toward developing solutions to close the gaps. This system creates sustainability because gaps between current and ideal experiences continually evolve and require resolution. PFCC methodology and practice will spread through organizations as caregivers at all levels of the organization become involved in PFCC working groups and project teams. The three central elements of PFCC methodology and practice are shown in **Table 1**.

PFCC in the Trauma Setting

PFCC methods and practice can lower costs and achieve substantial benefits in the trauma setting as evidenced by results achieved at the University of Pittsburgh Medical Center This adult level I trauma center achieved a 50% reduction in the time from a patient's admission for treatment to cervical spine clearance and collar removal. This was accomplished as the result of cross-functional communication between radiology and orthopaedic physicians based on recommendations of PFCC working groups and the implementation of changes by the project teams.[46]

The University of Pittsburgh Medical Center also has implemented other policies and initiatives to support PFCC. A computer laptop with Health Insurance Portability and Accountability Act–approved webcam functionality visually connects adult trauma patients with their children injured in the same traumatic event who are being treated at Children's Hospital of Pittsburgh (several miles away). The adult patient is also connected with the child's healthcare team.

Dissatisfaction with the lack of communication between trauma teams led to the development of three primary trauma teams, each of which follows its assigned patients from admission to discharge. This approach led to improved continuity of care; communication between patients, families, and caregivers; patient satisfaction; discharge efficiency; and resident work hour compliance. A screening and psychiatric referral process also was implemented for all discharged trauma patients who return for follow-up care in the trauma clinic.[58]

A living history project was started to emphasize that every patient is a patient first, not a diagnosis or a room number. The project uses storytelling and interview techniques, which establish a stronger connection between caregivers, patients, and families.

Annually, one in three people older than 65 years will fall. Forty-two percent of patients admitted to the hospital have an injury caused by a fall.[59] The readmission rate in the first 3 months after hip fracture surgery is reported to be 19%, including 54.8% for medical comorbidities, 31% for infection, 23.8% for failure of rehabilitation, and 19% for orthopaedic complications.[60] Based on these findings, a geriatric fall prevention program was started to provide education on fall prevention at home and during hospitalization. Home health and physical therapy consultations were also implemented. Other PFCC trauma care projects include real-time patient and family advisory councils, information on transitioning from the intensive care unit, discussions on living at home after a traumatic event, improved hospital and rehabilitation discharge instructions, and a resident orientation program on providing trauma care.

Promoting Peer Support and Self-Management

Establishing a peer visitation program within a trauma center can help patients cope with the aftermath of a sudden injury. Peer visitation offers the opportunity for patients to talk with trained volunteers who have lived through the trauma recovery experience, including the rescue scene, hospitalization, and rehabilitation. These volunteers can connect with trauma patients on a deeply personal level. When a new trauma patient expresses anxieties regarding the long recovery ahead or the frustrations of dealing with the medical system, the peer visitor can offer sympathy and tips for coping with the upcoming challenges. Peer visitation programs also provide survivors with an opportunity to give back and help others. However, appropriate training for peer visitors is critical. The Amputee Coalition of America[61] and the American Trauma Society[62] provide resources for implementing peer visitation programs.

Because most of the recovery process takes place outside the doctor's office, patients need tools to build self-efficacy, make good decisions, and follow through on behaviors that will promote good outcomes. A substantial body of research has shown that self-management interventions based on cognitive-behavioral theory are particularly effective in achieving these goals and improving overall function and quality of life.[63-67] Cognitive-behavioral theory helps patients (1) appreciate the relationship between their thoughts, feelings, and behaviors and (2) identifies self-defeating patterns of thought and replaces them with adaptive thoughts and behaviors to achieve better outcomes. Self-management programs address the core value of patient-centered care and have gained widespread application in chronic conditions in which pain and physical disability are common. Self-management programs empower patients to become active participants in their care and recovery. In this way, patients along with care providers are held accountable for good outcomes.

The NextSteps Program is a self-management program designed specifically for trauma patients. One barrier to fully implementing this program in trauma centers has been the cost of training and supporting individuals to run the required classes. Many trauma centers also find it difficult to recruit enough trauma survivors (ideally 9 to 12) at any given time who can commit to the 6-week program. A new online version of the NextSteps program overcomes these barriers and provides a cost-effective strategy for connecting trauma survivors from around the country and teaching them the essential skills of self-management.[68]

Participants are enrolled into the online NextSteps program in groups of 9 to 12 survivors. Before starting the program, participants are introduced over the telephone to the class facilitator who provides an overview of the program. Over the next 6 weeks, participants are asked to work through weekly online lessons (two lessons per week). Each lesson is facilitated by interactive didactics, self-monitoring with feedback, videos (of survivors and content experts), exercises to reinforce key messages, and relaxation exercises. At the end of each week, participants are encouraged to take part in a facilitated online discussion or chat group. Each week's discussion has a theme based on the lesson content from that week. NextSteps provides the opportunity for participants to keep a private journal, where they can write down thoughts and feelings they experience as they work through the program. There are also community forums where participants can connect with NextSteps classmates and people in other classes. The lessons cover the essential elements of self-management described here.

Week 1: Taking Stock

Lessons 1 and 2 include a review of how the injury has affected the survivor's life in how things are done and what can be done. The concept of self-management is introduced to show how survivors are an important component in directing their own treatment. Week 1 also includes education about the types of communication (aggressive, passive, and assertive) and introduces regular relaxation and visual imagery exercises that accompany each lesson.

Week 2: Moving Forward

Week 2 of the program includes lessons 3 and 4, which focus on identifying problems, changing perspectives, and viewing problems as challenges or goals that can be attained. These goals are saved and monitored throughout the program and can be modified, revised, or changed. Participants are shown how to track and measure progress toward their goals.

Week 3: Managing Emotions I

Week 3 of the program includes lessons 5 and 6, which focus on the emotional consequences of physical trauma. Didactic education covers the differences between normal adjustment and major depression (including diagnostic methods to screen the severity of symptoms). Strategies to help improve mood are included.

Week 4: Managing Emotions II

Lessons 7 and 8, presented in week 4 of the program, focus on educating the participant about the body's natural stress response and its relationship to anxiety. Diagnostic screening for posttraumatic stress disorder is included, with relevant treatment recommendations. Relaxation training using progressive muscle relaxation, guided imagery, deep breathing, and brief relaxation are included.

Week 5: Family and Friends

Lessons 9 and 10, presented in week 5, include reviews of the different ways

that individual trauma affects significant others, family members, and relationships. The concepts of helpful and unhelpful assistance are discussed, and participants are provided with guides in asking for help, showing appreciation, and declining help when necessary. Survivors also review ways that they might be contributing to the stress of others and how to help alleviate caregiver stress.

Week 6: Moving Forward

In lessons 11 and 12, presented in week 6, participants reflect on their future goals and the steps they need to take to prepare for and manage setbacks.

Summary

Orthopaedic trauma is a life-altering experience for patients as well as their family and friends. Improved survival rates have resulted from the dramatic advances made in understanding the physiology of trauma, such as the successful repair of fractures that previously could not be treated surgically. Unfortunately, our understanding of the critical importance of the psychosocial aspect of traumatic injuries has lagged behind advances in the medical and surgical care of trauma patients. A failure of psychosocial recovery can prevent full functional recovery even when musculoskeletal injuries have successfully healed. To achieve optimal patient outcomes, many trauma centers and orthopaedic surgeons are analyzing the evidence and developing strategies to address psychosocial factors that can derail a successful functional recovery.

References

1. Bosse MJ, MacKenzie EJ, Kellam JF, et al: An analysis of outcomes of reconstruction or amputation after leg-threatening injuries. *N Engl J Med* 2002;347(24): 1924-1931.

2. MacKenzie EJ, Bosse MJ, Pollak AN, et al: Long-term persistence of disability following severe lower-limb trauma. Results of a seven-year follow-up. *J Bone Joint Surg Am* 2005;87(8):1801-1809.

3. MacKenzie EJ, Bosse MJ, Kellam JF, et al: Early predictors of long-term work disability after major limb trauma. *J Trauma* 2006; 61(3):688-694.

4. Cousins N: Anatomy of an illness (as perceived by the patient). *N Engl J Med* 1976;295(26): 1458-1463.

5. Helman CG: Disease versus illness in general practice. *J R Coll Gen Pract* 1981;31(230):548-552.

6. Crichlow RJ, Andres PL, Morrison SM, Haley SM, Vrahas MS: Depression in orthopaedic trauma patients: Prevalence and severity. *J Bone Joint Surg Am* 2006;88(9): 1927-1933.

7. McCarthy ML, MacKenzie EJ, Edwin D, Bosse MJ, Castillo RC, Starr A; LEAP study group: Psychological distress associated with severe lower-limb injury. *J Bone Joint Surg Am* 2003;85(9):1689-1697.

8. Peabody FW: The care of the patient. *JAMA* 1927;88:877-882.

9. Mock C, MacKenzie E, Jurkovich G, et al: Determinants of disability after lower extremity fracture. *J Trauma* 2000;49(6): 1002-1011.

10. MacKenzie EJ, Morris JA Jr, Jurkovich GJ, et al: The role of economic, social, and job-related factors. *Am J Public Health* 1998; 88(11):1630-1637.

11. Holbrook TL, Hoyt DB, Stein MB, Sieber WJ: Perceived threat to life predicts posttraumatic stress disorder after major trauma: Risk factors and functional outcome. *J Trauma* 2001;51(2):287-292, discussion 292-293.

12. Michaels AJ, Michaels CE, Moon CH, Zimmerman MA, Peterson C, Rodriguez JL: Psychosocial

factors limit outcomes after trauma. *J Trauma* 1998;44(4): 644-648.

13. Michaels AJ, Michaels CE, Moon CH, et al: Impact on general health outcome and early risk assessment. *J Trauma* 1999;47(3): 460-466, discussion 466-467.

14. Landsman IS, Baum CG, Arnkoff DB, et al: The psychosocial consequences of traumatic injury. *J Behav Med* 1990;13(6):561-581.

15. Franche RL, Krause N: Readiness for return to work following injury or illness: Conceptualizing the interpersonal impact of health care, workplace, and insurance factors. *J Occup Rehabil* 2002; 12(4):233-256.

16. Ponzer S, Bergman B, Brismar B, Johansson LM: A study of patient-related characteristics and outcome after moderate injury. *Injury* 1996;27(8):549-555.

17. Kempen GI, Scaf-Klomp W, Ranchor AV, Sanderman R, Ormel J: Social predictors of recovery in late middle-aged and older persons after injury to the extremities: A prospective study. *J Gerontol B Psychol Sci Soc Sci* 2001; 56(4):S229-S236.

18. MacKenzie EJ, Bosse MJ: Factors influencing outcome following limb-threatening lower limb trauma: Lessons learned from the Lower Extremity Assessment Project (LEAP). *J Am Acad Orthop Surg* 2006;14(10 Spec No.):S205-S210.

19. McCarthy ML, MacKenzie EJ, Edwin D, Bosse MJ, Castillo RC, Starr A; LEAP study group: Psychological distress associated with severe lower-limb injury. *J Bone Joint Surg Am* 2003;85(9):1689-1697.

20. Castillo RC, MacKenzie EJ, Wegener ST, Bosse MJ; LEAP Study Group: Prevalence of chronic pain seven years following limb threatening lower extremity trauma. *Pain* 2006;124(3):321-329.

21. In Focus: Patient encounters of a difficult kind. FOJP website. 2009. http://www.fojp.com/ sites/default/files/ inFocus%20Spring09.pdf. Accessed October 2, 2013.

22. Tongue JR, Epps HR, Forese LL: Communication skills for patient-centered care: Research-based, easily learned techniques for medical interviews that benefit orthopaedic surgeons and their patients. *J Bone Joint Surg Am* 2005;87: 652-658.

23. Silver RC: Clarifying the presence of posttraumatic stress symptoms following orthopaedic trauma. *J Bone Joint Surg Am* 2005;87(3): 673-675.

24. Adams RJ, Smith BJ, Ruffin RE: Impact of the physician's participatory style in asthma outcomes and patient satisfaction. *Ann Allergy Asthma Immunol* 2001;86(3): 263-271.

25. DiMatteo MR, Giordani PJ, Lepper HS, Croghan TW: Patient adherence and medical treatment outcomes: A meta-analysis. *Med Care* 2002;40(9):794-811.

26. Kenny NP, Mann KV, MacLeod H: Role modeling in physicians' professional formation: Reconsidering an essential but untapped educational strategy. *Acad Med* 2003;78(12):1203-1210.

27. Pinney SJ, Mehta S, Pratt DD, et al: Applying the principles of adult education to teaching orthopaedic residents. *J Bone Joint Surg Am* 2007;89(6):1385-1392.

28. Pratt DD, Arseneau R, Collins JB: Reconsidering "good teaching" across the continuum of medical education. *J Contin Educ Health Prof* 2001;21(2):70-81.

29. Castillo RC, MacKenzie EJ, Webb LX, Bosse MJ, Avery J; LEAP Study Group: Use and perceived need of physical therapy following severe lower-extremity trauma. *Arch Phys Med Rehabil* 2005; 86(9):1722-1728.

30. Rosen P, Stenger E, Bochkoris M, Hannon M, Kwoh K: Family-centered multidisciplinary rounds enhance the team approach in pediatrics. *Pediatrics* 2009;124(4): e603-e608.

31. Carr DD: Building collaborative partnerships in critical care: The RN case manager/social work dyad in critical care. *Prof Case Manag* 2009;14(3):121-132.

32. Drageset J, Eide GE, Nygaard HA, Bondevik M, Nortvedt MW, Natvig GK: The impact of social support and sense of coherence on health-related quality of life among nursing home residents: A questionnaire survey in Bergen, Norway. *Int J Nurs Stud* 2009; 46(1):65-75.

33. Joosten EA, DeFuentes-Merillas L, de Weert GH, Sensky T, van der Staak CP: de long CA: Systematic review of the effects of shared decision-making on patient satisfaction, treatment adherence and health status. *Psychother Psychosom* 2008;77(4):219-226.

34. Frazee S: Goal of the day: Initiating goal of the day to improve patient- and family-centered care. *Dimens Crit Care Nurs* 2011; 30(6):326-330.

35. Mangram AJ, McCauley T, Villarreal D: Families' perception of the value of timed daily "family rounds" in a trauma ICU. *Am Surg* 2005;71(10):886-891.

36. Carlson B, Riegel B, Thomason T: Visitation: policy versus practice. *Dimens Crit Care Nurs* 1998; 17(1):40-47.

37. DiGioia AM III, Greenhouse PK: Patient and family shadowing: Creating urgency for change. *J Nurs Adm* 2011;41(1):23-28.

38. Fedor MC, Leyssene-Ouvrard C: "Integration of families in hospital": Expectations and reticence of patients, relatives and nursing staff? A study in progress at the Clermont-Ferrand academic medical center. *Rech Soins Infirm* 2007;89(89):58-75.

39. Geary PA, Tringali R, George E: Social support in critically ill adults: A replication. *Crit Care Nurs Q* 1997;20(2):34-41.

40. Giuliano KK, Giuliano AJ, Bloniasz E, Quirk PA, Wood J: A quality-improvement approach to meeting the needs of critically ill patients and their families. *Dimens Crit Care Nurs* 2000;19(1):30-34.

41. Hammond F: Involving families in care within the intensive care environment: A descriptive survey. *Intensive Crit Care Nurs* 1995; 11(5):256-264.

42. Rotman-Pikielny P, Rabin B, Amoyal S, Mushkat Y, Zissin R, Levy Y: Participation of family members in ward rounds: Attitude of medical staff, patients and relatives. *Patient Educ Couns* 2007; 65(2):166-170.

43. Söderström IM, Saveman BI, Benzein E: Interactions between family members and staff in intensive care units: An observation and interview study. *Int J Nurs Stud* 2006;43(6):707-716.

44. DiGioia AM III, Greenhouse PK: Care experience-based methodologies: Performance improvement roadmap to value-driven health care. *Clin Orthop Relat Res* 2012; 470(4):1038-1045.

45. DiGioia AM III, Greenhouse PK, Levison TJ: Patient and family-centered collaborative care: An orthopaedic model. *Clin Orthop Relat Res* 2007;463(463):13-19.

46. DiGioia AM III, Lorenz H, Greenhouse PK, Bertoty DA, Rocks SD: A patient-centered model to improve metrics without cost increase: Viewing all care through the eyes of patients and families. *J Nurs Adm* 2010;40(12): 540-546.

47. The patient and family centered care methodology and practice, in Bisognano M, Kenney C: *Pursuing the Triple Aim: Seven Innovators Show the Way to Better Care, Better Health, and Lower Costs.*

San Francisco, CA, John Wiley & Sons, 2012, pp 199-230.

48. Meyer H: At UPMC, improving care processes to serve patients better and cut costs. *Health Aff (Millwood)* 2011;30(3):400-403.

49. Brown T: *Change by Design: How Design Thinking Transforms Organizations and Inspires Innovation.* New York, NY, Harper Collins, 2009.

50. Denning S: *The Leader's Guide to Storytelling.* San Francisco, CA, Jossey-Bass, 2005.

51. Simon H: *The Sciences of the Artificial.* Cambridge, MA, MIT Press, 1996.

52. Christensen C: *The Innovator's Dilemma: The Revolutionary Book That Will Change the Way You Do Business.* New York, NY, Harper Collins, 2003.

53. Kotter JP: *A Sense of Urgency.* Boston, MA, Harvard Business School Press, 2008.

54. Pine BJ, Gilmore JH: *The Experience Economy.* Boston, MA, Harvard Business School Press, 1999.

55. Shaller D, Darby C: *High Performing Patient-and-Family-Centered Academic Medical Centers: Cross-Site Summary of Six Case Studies.* Picker Institute Report, July 2009. http://www.upstate.edu/gch/about/special/picker_report_7_09.pdf. Accessed July 25, 2013.

56. The Joint Commission: *Putting the Care in Health Care: Improving the Patient Experience. Putting Compassionate Care Into Practice: Case Studies.* Oak Brook, IL, Joint Commission Resources, 2009.

57. Martin LA, Neumann CW, Mountford J, Bisognano M, Nolan TW: *Increasing Efficiency and Enhancing Value in Health Care: Ways to Achieve Savings in Operating Costs Per Year.* Cambridge,

MA, Institute for Healthcare Improvement, 2009.

58. Alarcon LH, Germain A, Clontz AS, et al: Predictors of acute post-traumatic stress disorder symptoms following civilian trauma: Highest incidence and severity of symptoms after assault. *J Trauma Acute Care Surg* 2012;72(3):629-635, discussion 635-637.

59. Falls in older adults: An overview. Centers for Disease Control and Prevention. 2013. http://www.cdc.gov/Homeand Recreational Safety/Falls/index.html. Accessed October 2, 2013.

60. Hahnel J, Burdekin H, Anand S: Re-admissions following hip fracture surgery. *Ann R Coll Surg Engl* 2009;91(7):591-595.

61. Amputee Coalition website. http://www.amputee-coalition.org/support-groups-peer-support/certified-peer-visitor-program/. Accessed August 26, 2013.

62. America Trauma Society: Trauma Survivors Network. http://www.traumasurvivorsnetwork.org/pages/for-trauma-centers. Accessed August 26, 2013.

63. Lorig KR, Holman H: Self-management education: History, definition, outcomes, and mechanisms. *Ann Behav Med* 2003; 26(1):1-7.

64. Lorig K, Holman H: Arthritis self-management studies: A twelve-year review. *Health Educ Q* 1993;20(1):17-28.

65. Lorig KR, Sobel DS, Stewart AL, et al: Evidence suggesting that a chronic disease self-management program can improve health status while reducing hospitalization: A randomized trial. *Med Care* 1999; 37(1):5-14.

66. Norris SL, Engelgau MM, Narayan KM: Effectiveness of self-management training in type 2 diabetes: A systematic review of randomized controlled

trials. *Diabetes Care* 2001;24(3): 561-587.

67. Wegener ST, Mackenzie EJ, Ephraim P, Ehde D, Williams R: Self-management improves outcomes in persons with limb loss. *Arch Phys Med Rehabil* 2009; 90(3):373-380.

68. NextSteps website. http://www.nextstepsonline.org/. Accessed August 26, 2013.

Geriatric Trauma: The Role of Immediate Arthroplasty

Andrew H. Schmidt, MD

Jonathan P. Braman, MD

Paul J. Duwelius, MD

Michael D. McKee, MD, FRCS(C)

Abstract

Periarticular fractures in elderly patients are challenging to manage because the fractures are typically comminuted and the bone is osteopenic, which often result in the failure of internal fixation. Patients who sustain these fractures demand immediate mobilization or they often do not recover their preinjury level of function. In geriatric patients, immediate arthroplasty provides an alternative to internal fixation for many periarticular fractures of the shoulder, elbow, and hip.

Instr Course Lect 2014;63:49-59.

Periarticular fractures in elderly patients are difficult to stabilize, and nonsurgical treatment is not well tolerated. Surgery is usually indicated, but standard techniques of internal fixation often fail in patients in this age group because of osteopenic bone and fracture comminution. These factors often prevent sufficient fixation to allow early weight bearing, which is of critical importance in the geriatric patient.

In contrast, immediate arthroplasty of periarticular fractures in an elderly patient allows immediate mobilization of the patient. This chapter reviews the role of immediate arthroplasty in four common fractures that occur in elderly patients: the proximal and distal end of the humerus, the acetabulum, and the proximal part of the femur.

Shoulder Arthroplasty for Proximal Humeral Fractures

Proximal humeral fractures are the third most common fracture in elderly patients after wrist and hip fractures. They have a substantial effect on quality of life even when they are minimally displaced and do not require surgery.[1] Factors consistently associated with poor outcomes after either nonsurgical management or open reduction and internal fixation (ORIF) are advanced patient age, fracture comminution, varus angulation of the humeral head, and osteoporosis.[2-7] Appropriate indications for shoulder arthroplasty in patients with a complex proximal humeral fracture are a dysvascular humeral head, a patient who cannot tolerate the limitations that accompany nonsurgical treatment, and a comminuted and/or varus displaced fracture pattern, especially when associated with poor bone quality that precludes ORIF.

Shoulder function after hemiarthroplasty depends on achieving ana-

Dr. Schmidt or an immediate family member has received royalties from Smith & Nephew and CFI Medical Solutions; is a member of a speakers' bureau or has made paid presentations on behalf of Medtronic; serves as a paid consultant to Medtronic, DGIMED Ortho, AGA, and Smith & Nephew; serves as an unpaid consultant to Twin Star Medical and Conventus Orthopaedics; has stock or stock options held in Twin Star Medical, Anthem Orthopedics, Conventus Orthopaedics, the International Spine and Orthopedic Institute, and Exos; has received research or institutional support from Twin Star Medical; and serves as a board member, owner, officer, or committee member of the Orthopaedic Trauma Association. Dr. Braman or an immediate family member serves as a board member, owner, officer, or committee member of the American Academy of Orthopaedic Surgeons. Dr. Duwelius or an immediate family member has received royalties from Zimmer; is a member of a speakers' bureau or has made paid presentations on behalf of Accellero; serves as a paid consultant to Accellero; has received research or institutional support from Zimmer; and serves as a board member, owner, officer, or committee member of Freedom to Move Medical Missions. Dr. McKee or an immediate family member has received royalties from Stryker; is a member of a speakers' bureau or has made paid presentations on behalf of Synthes and Zimmer; serves as a paid consultant to Synthes and Zimmer; has received research or institutional support from Wright Medical Technology and Zimmer; and serves as a board member, owner, officer, or committee member of the American Shoulder and Elbow Surgeons, the Orthopaedic Trauma Association, and the Canadian Orthopaedic Association.

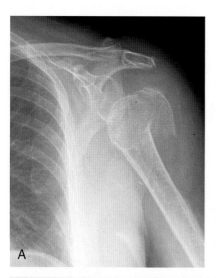
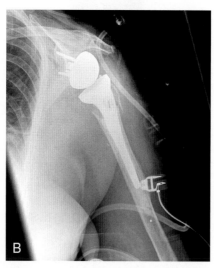

Figure 1 A 75-year-old woman sustained a four-part fracture of the proximal part of the humerus, including comminution of the humeral head and displacement of the tuberosities, in a fall from a standing height that involved her nondominant arm. **A,** Preoperative AP radiograph of the injured shoulder. **B,** Radiograph made after reverse total shoulder arthroplasty.

tomic reduction and secure, stable tuberosity fixation.[8] Reverse total shoulder arthroplasty is an attractive option for elderly patients with displaced proximal humeral fractures because restoration of rotator cuff function is not as critical. Expected patient activity level and longevity are the primary considerations for choosing between reverse total shoulder arthroplasty and shoulder hemiarthroplasty: reverse total shoulder arthroplasty is better for sedentary and elderly patients, whereas shoulder hemiarthroplasty is better for patients with higher activity levels[9,10] (**Figure 1**). Although short- and intermediate-term results of reverse total shoulder arthroplasty are reasonable, no long-term data that estimate the longevity of these devices in these patients are available, and salvage options are limited.

Hemiarthroplasty of the Shoulder

Surgery is performed using a long (15-cm) deltopectoral approach with the patient in the beach chair position. The coracoacromial ligament is preserved be-

cause this is an important secondary restraint preventing anterosuperior escape of the humeral head if the greater tuberosity does not heal. This chapter's authors tenodese the biceps tendon. Large sutures are placed at the bone-tendon interface of the greater and lesser tuberosities to provide control of the greater and lesser tuberosity fragments. External rotation of the arm improves reduction of the greater tuberosity. If there is a periosteal sleeve that remains in place, attempts are made to leave it to facilitate reduction and stability. However, in fractures that are more than a few days old, contracture of the periosteum can preclude reduction of the tuberosities, and release may be needed. A fracture-specific stem may improve the outcome and should allow conversion to a reverse total shoulder arthroplasty if necessary.[11-13] Suture fixation must provide interfragmentary compression fixation between tuberosity fragments, between the tuberosities and the humeral shaft, and around the neck of the implant.[14]

Proper positioning of the stem can be difficult because the normal osseous

landmarks of the proximal part of the humerus no longer exist. Achieving both the correct retroversion and height of the humeral head are critical for restoring shoulder biomechanics and function. Typically, the prosthetic humeral head should be placed in slightly less than anatomic retroversion (20°) to reduce tension on the greater tuberosity repair. Restoration of the height of the humeral head is also challenging. Krishnan et al[15] described the Gothic arch to help obtain the correct hemiarthroplasty height. Fortunately, the pectoralis major tendon is rarely torn in this injury, and both Murachovsky et al[16] and Greiner et al[17] described its use as a landmark for assessing humeral head height. According to Murachovsky et al,[16] the mean distance (and 95% confidence interval) between the top of the humeral head and the top of the pectoralis major tendon is 5.6 ± 0.5 cm, which will help in the accurate restoration of the humeral head position. Stems should be cemented to obtain rotational control.

Total Shoulder Arthroplasty

Many surgeons perform reverse total shoulder arthroplasty through the deltopectoral interval because of their comfort with this approach. ORIF can be performed using the same approach, facilitating conversion from one procedure to the other if intraoperative findings warrant. Other authors have preferred the superolateral approach for reverse total shoulder arthroplasty.[9] This approach releases the anterior deltoid muscle from the acromion and uses a split in the anterolateral raphe of the deltoid for access to the humeral shaft. The humerus is exposed and reamed, and the glenoid is addressed. Excellent en face glenoid access is imperative for reverse total shoulder arthroplasty. The height of the implant is determined by assessing tension in the deltoid and coracobrachialis muscles, which should be tight enough so that the implants do not dislocate but are not difficult to reduce. Tuberosity fixation is important in reverse total shoulder arthroplasty following fracture because it allows proper rotational control of the arm after healing. Consequently, secure suture repair of the tuberosities to the humeral shaft, humeral stem, and to each other is performed. Humeral stems should be cemented in reverse total shoulder arthroplasty to provide rotational stability of the construct.

Overview

Reverse total shoulder arthroplasty and shoulder hemiarthroplasty are both surgical options for comminuted fractures of the proximal part of the humerus in elderly patients with a dysvascular humeral head and/or severe fracture comminution. Younger patients should be treated with ORIF whenever possible. Patients who are more active or physiologically younger should undergo shoulder hemiarthroplasty with a convertible implant. Reverse total shoulder arthroplasty may be more predictable for restoring the ability to perform the activities of daily living for elderly or sedentary patients with this injury, especially those with an expected life span of less than 10 years.

Total Elbow Arthroplasty for Fractures of the Distal End of the Humerus

Improved surgical techniques, triceps-sparing approaches, and anatomic precontoured plates have improved outcomes following ORIF of intraarticular distal humeral fractures. However, complications remain frequent in elderly patients with severe fracture comminution and poor bone quality. Suboptimal plate fixation in osteopenic bone often leads to nonunion and more complications. Non-

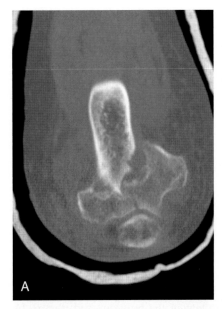 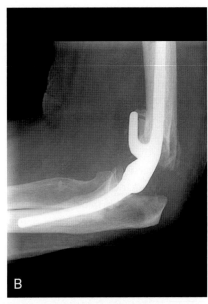

Figure 2   A 90-year-old man sustained an intra-articular distal humeral fracture. **A,** Preoperative axial CT showing the displaced distal humeral fragments. **B,** Lateral elbow radiograph made 3 months after total elbow reconstruction.

union or malunion of the distal end of the humerus causes substantial impairment in the functional ability and level of independence of a patient.[18]

Total elbow arthroplasty is an alternative to ORIF for comminuted, intra-articular distal humeral fractures in elderly patients (**Figure 2**). Total elbow arthroplasty is reserved for elderly patients only; it is not an option for younger, higher-demand individuals. Primary total elbow arthroplasty for elbow fracture was first reported, based on the knowledge of this chapter's authors, in 1997 by Cobb and Morrey,[19] who described 21 elbows in 20 patients (mean age, 72 years) with comminuted distal humeral fractures that were managed with a primary total elbow arthroplasty, resulting in a good or excellent outcome in 95% of the 20 elbows with complete data and only 1 reoperation in the entire cohort. Other retrospective reviews from single centers have confirmed similar, consistently reliable results.[20,21] In the first comparative study, Frankle et al[22]

performed a retrospective comparison of ORIF and total elbow arthroplasty for intra-articular distal humeral fractures in 24 women older than 65 years. At the time of the short-term follow-up, the patients who had total elbow arthroplasty had excellent or good results, with improved range of motion and less need for physical therapy than those who had ORIF, and 25% of patients treated with ORIF had a mechanical failure that required revision to total elbow arthroplasty. Recently, in a randomized prospective trial comparing ORIF and total elbow arthroplasty for comminuted intra-articular distal humeral fractures in elderly patients, McKee et al[23] reported that total elbow arthroplasty improved functional outcomes compared with ORIF on the basis of both objective elbow performance scores and patient-rated upper extremity disability and symptoms. They emphasized that the mean age of the patients in their study was close to 80 years, and that this procedure is not suitable for younger patients.

Indications and Contraindications

Although total elbow arthroplasty produces reliably good results in the appropriate patient, careful adherence to patient selection and surgical technique are critical.

Total elbow arthroplasty is indicated in low-demand patients older than 65 years; patients with preexisting, symptomatic arthritis of the elbow; those with articular comminution (typically three or more articular fragments); patients with a closed or a type 1 open fracture (if the arthroplasty is done within 8 to 12 hours of injury and satisfactory débridement is obtained);[24] patients with delayed presentation and articular fragmentation rendering reconstruction unfeasible; and those with associated severe ligamentous damage and/or elbow instability.

Total elbow arthroplasty is contraindicated in patients with active infection or insufficient soft-tissue coverage; those with advanced dementia or noncompliance issues (such as substance abuse); patients with extensor mechanism disruption (a relative contraindication); those with a type 2 or 3 open fracture; young, active, high-demand patients; and those with a simple fracture pattern (such as two articular fragments).

Technique

Total elbow arthroplasty for a fracture requires the correct implant, equipment, and an experienced operating-room staff and surgeon. The fracture is splinted until conditions are optimized for surgery; a wait of up to 14 days is rarely detrimental if required. A cemented, linked, or semiconstrained prosthesis is the treatment of choice for total elbow arthroplasty after a distal humeral fracture. Although some promising preliminary results are available for distal humeral hemiarthro-plasty (typically with an anatomic distal humeral replacement) that may extend the indications for this procedure to younger patients, such an approach should be considered experimental at present.[25]

The patient is placed in the lateral decubitus position with the affected arm free-draped over a bolster, with a tourniquet applied. A posterior approach is used; the ulnar nerve is identified and protected. The olecranon is not osteotomized; this compromises the insertion and stability of the ulnar component. When the fractured articular fragments or condyles are excised, this creates a so-called working space, allowing the humerus and ulna to be instrumented and the components inserted without detaching the triceps. Condylar resection does not appear to negatively affect forearm or wrist strength, and the condyles are not required for ligament attachment or stability when a linked prosthesis is used.[26] If greater exposure is required, the triceps can be split or peeled from the olecranon.[27,28] After insertion of the prosthesis, thorough irrigation and standard closure are performed: the ulnar nerve remains in a tension-free position medially. A major benefit of the linked total elbow arthroplasty in general and the so-called triceps-on approach in particular is the ability to allow immediate full range of active motion postoperatively. This enhances the elbow-specific outcome, rapidly restores independent function to the patient, and minimizes hospital and rehabilitation time.

Overview

Primary semiconstrained total elbow arthroplasty has a role in the treatment of comminuted intra-articular fractures of the distal end of the humerus in selected elderly patients. In this specific group, it results in improved patient outcomes compared with ORIF, enhances the return to independent function, and minimizes the hospital stay and rehabilitation time.

ORIF and Immediate Total Hip Replacement for the Management of Selected Displaced Acetabular Fractures

The recommended treatment for most displaced acetabular fractures is ORIF.[29,30] Acetabular fractures in elderly patients are an increasingly common injury pattern.[31-33] In elderly patients, these fractures are more likely the result of a low-energy fall than high-energy trauma,[33,34] yet they are often comminuted with major displacement and impaction of the articular surface.[31,32,35] Early mobilization of these fragile patients is of primary importance in restoring them to their preinjury level of function, as well as preventing complications from prolonged recumbency.[36] The difficulty of obtaining a satisfactory result with internal fixation and the common need for a delayed total hip replacement to treat failed internal fixation in these patients makes initial prosthetic replacement attractive.[37-42] One approach is to initially manage these patients nonsurgically, performing delayed total hip replacement after the fracture has healed in symptomatic patients.[35] However, delayed arthroplasty after acetabular fracture in elderly patients has inferior results compared with primary arthroplasty for degenerative disease.[40] Immediate total hip replacement with acetabular reconstruction allows early mobilization and lessens the risk of subjecting the patient to two major surgical procedures in a relatively short time period (**Figure 3**).

The challenge of immediate total hip replacement is to obtain stable acetabular component fixation and allow the patients early activity without

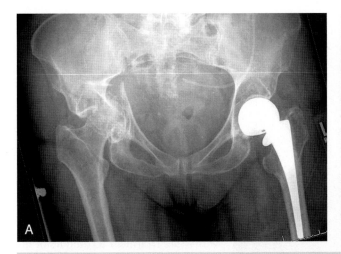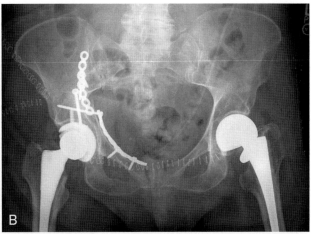

Figure 3   A 76-year-old woman with osteoporosis sustained a displaced acetabular fracture on the right side. **A,** Pre-operative AP pelvic radiograph showing the displaced acetabular fracture with the femoral head protruding into the fracture site. **B,** AP pelvic radiograph after internal fixation and immediate total hip replacement.

compromising fixation of the implants or hip stability. In fact, reports of this approach published several decades ago noted problems with fixation of the cemented acetabular component.[43] In the last decade, there has been renewed interest in treating selected acetabular fractures with early total hip replacement.[32,41,44-47] Beaulé et al[45] reported the cases of 10 patients managed with open reduction and acute total hip replacement utilizing a direct anterior surgical approach for anterior wall or column fractures in elderly patients. At an average follow-up of 3 years, none of the patients had nonunion, component loosening, or migration. One patient had an anterior dislocation that was treated successfully with closed reduction and immobilization. The average Merle d'Aubigné and Postel score was 16, indicating a good outcome. More recently, Boraiah et al[47] described 18 patients who were treated by a protocol very similar to that of this chapter's authors and were followed for at least 1 year; those authors also reported one early acetabular failure requiring revision surgery, whereas 81% of their patients had good or excellent results according to the Harris hip score.

ORIF of the acetabulum and immediate total hip replacement is a complex procedure that should be performed by surgeons adept at both surgical fixation of acetabular fractures and total hip replacement. Published results have indicated that functional outcomes are similar to those after primary total hip replacement for osteoarthritis.[34,45]

Technique

Patients undergo surgery as soon as possible after admission and thorough evaluation by the orthopaedic, trauma, and/or internal medicine services as indicated by their injuries and medical comorbidities (if any). Surgical procedures are usually done within 2 to 4 days. Patients with fracture-dislocations have their hip reduced immediately in the emergency department with deep intravenous sedation. If the hip is unstable after closed reduction, skeletal traction is placed, typically through the distal end of the femur. Subcutaneous heparin (5,000 units three times daily) and pneumatic compression stockings are routinely used for prophylaxis against venous thromboembolism.

This chapter's authors initially repair the acetabular fracture using standard techniques of internal fixation as appropriate for the fracture pattern. The goal of the internal fixation is to reduce and stabilize the anterior and/or posterior columns, not to restore the articular surface. In patients with major displacement of the anterior column, an ilioinguinal approach or Stoppa approach with the patient supine is used to reduce and plate the pelvic brim (**Figure 3**). Next, or for fractures primarily involving the posterior wall and/or column, a Kocher-Langenbeck approach is used with the patient in the lateral decubitus position. After exposure of the greater trochanter, the short external rotators are released and tagged with suture for later repair. A hip capsulotomy is performed, maintaining capsular flaps for later repair. The femoral head is dislocated, the femoral neck cut, and the femoral head removed in the standard fashion. A cobra retractor is placed over the anterior wall of the acetabulum, and any posterior wall fragments are identified. The acetabular labrum is excised. If there is a fracture of the posterior column, the posterior column is carefully exposed and reduced with clamps. If the posterior wall requires reconstruction, an acetabular

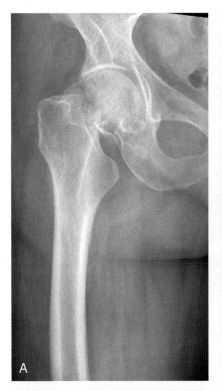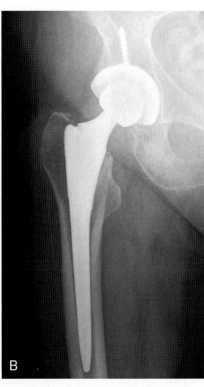

Figure 4 Preoperative (**A**) and postoperative (**B**) radiographs of a displaced femoral neck fracture in a 73-year-old woman who was treated with primary total hip arthroplasty.

trial that is similar in size to the resected femoral head is selected and placed in the acetabulum for use as a template for reconstruction. The posterior wall fragment(s) are repositioned against the acetabular trial component, and the posterior wall and column of the acetabulum are stabilized with a posterior buttress plate.

After the posterior wall and/or column are stabilized, any residual bone defects resulting from articular impaction or comminution are bone grafted using cancellous bone from the patient's femoral head. After repairing the acetabulum, a total hip arthroplasty is then performed through the same incision. The acetabulum is prepared with standard reaming with medialization of the cup to the floor of the cotyloid fossa. For uncemented cups, once bleeding subchondral bone is reached, a cup 1 mm larger than the outside diameter of the last reamer is

selected and implanted with an interference fit. The acetabular component is anchored with additional screw fixation into the ilium. Standard femoral canal preparation and femoral stem placement are used; uncemented, proximally porous-coated implants are used in most patients (**Figure 3**).

Postoperative Treatment

Patients receive prophylactic antibiotics for 24 hours and are started on warfarin or low-molecular-weight heparin postoperatively, which is continued for 4 weeks after discharge. Prophylaxis against heterotopic ossification using low-dose radiation (a single dose of 600 Gy) is recommended for male patients who have a posterior fracture-dislocation. Patients with displaced anterior or posterior column fractures are mobilized with crutches or a walker for 6 weeks. Patients with isolated posterior wall fractures are allowed full

weight bearing immediately. Patients are instructed to avoid hip flexion beyond 90° and to sleep with a pillow between their legs.

Displaced Femoral Neck Fractures: The Case for Total Hip Replacement

Total hip replacement for the treatment of displaced femoral neck fractures (**Figure 4**) in the elderly leads to improved outcomes, fewer complications, and decreased cost compared with other treatment techniques of internal fixation or hemiarthroplasty. The incidence of hip fractures in the United States in 1996 was approximately 250,000 cases, with projections that this would increase to 500,000 fractures per year by 2040.[48] Thus, the management of femoral neck fractures in a cost-effective manner is of societal importance, not to mention the consequences for the individual patient when complications of care occur.

This section reviews the role of arthroplasty in the management of fractures of the femoral neck: when to replace the hip, which device to use, and whether to cement or press fit the implant. Hemiarthroplasty has been the preferred management for femoral neck fractures that are not ideal for internal fixation because of advanced patient age and/or osteopenia. The advantages of hemiarthroplasty compared with total hip arthroplasty are the quick and relatively simple surgical technique and a documented low risk of dislocation.[49] The main disadvantages of hemiarthroplasty include the potential for rapid wear of acetabular articular cartilage (requiring conversion to total hip replacement) and pain related to the metallic femoral head against the host acetabulum (chondrolysis).

The justification for prosthetic replacement in the treatment of femoral neck fractures resides in the fact that arthroplasty provides optimal functional recovery. The literature overwhelmingly supports arthroplasty for the treatment of the displaced femoral neck fracture in elderly patients.[50-64] Complications and the need for multiple procedures are decreased when total hip replacement is used over other treatment options.

Schmidt et al[62] recently provided a comprehensive review of the literature regarding the optimal arthroplasty for displaced femoral neck fractures. Iorio et al[65] conducted a survey in 2006 that revealed that most surgeons preferred treating geriatric patients with displaced femoral neck fractures with bipolar arthroplasty. However, at the time of their survey, surgical practice was changing because of the recent introduction of highly cross-linked polyethylene and larger femoral heads to decrease dislocation rates. Newer stem designs also were proven to be successful in elderly patients with femoral neck fractures.[66] The Displaced Femoral (neck fracture) Arthroplasty Consortium for Treatment and Outcomes reported the results of their prospective, multicenter randomized clinical trial comparing hemiarthroplasty and total hip arthroplasty in 2008, finding that total hip replacement had superior results.[57]

Treatment choices for displaced femoral neck fractures might differ depending on which outcome criteria are considered. Possible criteria include complication rates, cost-effectiveness, and short- and long-term outcomes. Iorio et al[67] presented a cost-effectiveness analysis of four surgical treatments for a displaced femoral neck fracture. This series considered initial hospital costs, rehabilitation costs, and costs of reoperations and complications. Those authors determined that cemented total hip replacement was the most cost-effective treatment, and internal fixation was the most expensive option.[67]

The Scottish Trial of Arthroplasty or Reduction (STARS) for subcapital femoral neck fractures is a highly compelling study.[56] This multicenter randomized study showed that long-term function was best after total hip replacement. The STARS study reported an incidence of osteonecrosis of 20% and nonunion rates of 30% in the ORIF group, which was consistent with prior studies. The reoperation rate was much higher for the internal fixation group, which had a failure rate of 37%. Chondrolysis, which generally manifested as pain, occurred in 20% of the bipolar-monopolar treatment group, with a reoperation rate of 5%. A systematic review of fixation options indicated that cemented hip replacement is associated with less pain than uncemented hip replacement in patients with a hip fracture.[68] This finding was further substantiated in a recent study supporting cemented stems as being superior to bone ingrowth stems.[69] In the STARS study, the total hip replacement treatment group had the best functional outcome and the least pain, the lowest cost, and a reoperation rate of 9%. Healy and Iorio[70] also reported better results and lower cost with total hip replacement. Several randomized prospective series lend credence to the fact that arthroplasty leads to better results than internal fixation of displaced femoral neck fractures.[54-57,59,61,63]

Displaced femoral neck fractures pose certain problems for the treating surgeon. The randomized controlled trial by Blomfeldt et al,[71] which compared bipolar hemiarthroplasty with total hip replacement for displaced intracapsular fractures of the femoral neck in elderly patients, revealed superior results in the total hip replacement group in all outcomes parameters compared with the bipolar group, using the anterolateral approach in all cases to reduce the risk of dislocation typically

associated with posterior approaches. However, capsular repair and the use of a large femoral head may mitigate the dislocation risk when posterior approaches are done.[60,72] Berry et al[73] further described how the dislocation rate can be decreased with careful attention to detail, such as using larger femoral heads, highly cross-linked polyethylene, and capsular closure. The surgeon may use the surgical approach he or she is most comfortable with. Surgical techniques are more difficult in displaced femoral neck fractures compared with elective total hip replacement. Poor bone quality, intraoperative instability, and difficulties with abnormal anatomy resulting from the displaced fracture present unique problems. The surgeon can base his or her preoperative plan on the nonfractured side to best evaluate for stem size, head center, limb length, and offset. Technical pearls include the use of a larger femoral head, careful reaming, restoration of appropriate limb length and offset, repair of the hip capsule, and use of multiple acetabular screws with compromised bone quality. Controversy remains about whether to cement or press fit the femoral component.[52,69,71]

The treatment of these difficult fractures involves certain parameters that are outside the surgeon's control, such as the patient's age, mental status, bone quality, fracture pattern, time to diagnosis, and comorbidities. However, the surgeon does have control over many factors that are critical in the treatment of these fractures. These include the timing of surgery, the choice of the surgical approach, the restoration of the hip center, the use of larger femoral heads to decrease the prevalence of dislocation, the capsular closure, and the surgical experience. No single approach works best for all fracture types. However, for displaced femoral neck fractures, the surgeon should give strong consideration to the treatment of these difficult fractures with a total hip replacement to decrease cost, lower complications, and restore the best postoperative function.

References

1. Calvo E, Morcillo D, Foruria AM, Redondo-Santamaría E, Osorio-Picorne F, Caeiro JR; GEIOS-SECOT Outpatient Osteoporotic Fracture Study Group: Nondisplaced proximal humeral fractures: High incidence among outpatient-treated osteoporotic fractures and severe impact on upper extremity function and patient subjective health perception. *J Shoulder Elbow Surg* 2011; 20(5):795-801.

2. Brorson S, Rasmussen JV, Frich LH, Olsen BS, Hróbjartsson A: Benefits and harms of locking plate osteosynthesis in intraarticular (OTA Type C) fractures of the proximal humerus: A systematic review. *Injury* 2012;43(7):999-1005.

3. Hardeman F, Bollars P, Donnelly M, Bellemans J, Nijs S: Predictive factors for functional outcome and failure in angular stable osteosynthesis of the proximal humerus. *Injury* 2012;43(2): 153-158.

4. Krappinger D, Bizzotto N, Riedmann S, Kammerlander C, Hengg C, Kralinger FS: Predicting failure after surgical fixation of proximal humerus fractures. *Injury* 2011;42(11):1283-1288.

5. Ong C, Bechtel C, Walsh M, Zuckerman JD, Egol KA: Three- and four-part fractures have poorer function than one-part proximal humerus fractures. *Clin Orthop Relat Res* 2011;469(12): 3292-3299.

6. Osterhoff G, Hoch A, Wanner GA, Simmen HP, Werner CM: Calcar comminution as prognostic factor of clinical outcome after

7. Südkamp NP, Audigé L, Lambert S, Hertel R, Konrad G: Path analysis of factors for functional outcome at one year in 463 proximal humeral fractures. *J Shoulder Elbow Surg* 2011;20(8):1207-1216.

8. Liu JLi SH, Cai ZD, et al: Outcomes, and factors affecting outcomes, following shoulder hemiarthroplasty for proximal humeral fracture repair. *J Orthop Sci* 2011; 16(5):565-572.

9. Gallinet D, Clappaz P, Garbuio P, Tropet Y, Obert L: Three or four parts complex proximal humerus fractures: Hemiarthroplasty versus reverse prosthesis. A comparative study of 40 cases. *Orthop Traumatol Surg Res* 2009;95(1): 48-55.

10. Garrigues GE, Johnston PS, Pepe MD, Tucker BS, Ramsey ML, Austin LS: Hemiarthroplasty versus reverse total shoulder arthroplasty for acute proximal humerus fractures in elderly patients. *Orthopedics* 2012;35(5):e703-e708.

11. Dines DM, Warren RF: Modular shoulder hemiarthroplasty for acute fractures: Surgical considerations. *Clin Orthop Relat Res* 1994;307:18-26.

12. Kaback L, Aaron DL, Neviaser AS, et al: Abstract: Functional and radiographic outcomes using a tantalum porous implant in the treatment of three and four part proximal humerus fractures. *ASES 2011 Annual Meeting*. Rosemont, IL, American Shoulder and Elbow Surgeons, 2011, p 60.

13. Krishnan SG, Reineck JR, Bennion PD, Feher L, Burkhead WZ Jr: Shoulder arthroplasty for fracture: Does a fracture-specific stem make a difference? *Clin Orthop Relat Res* 2011;469(12):3317-3323.

14. Boileau P, Pennington SD, Alami G: Proximal humeral frac-

tures in younger patients: Fixation techniques and arthroplasty. *J Shoulder Elbow Surg* 2011; 20(2)S47-S60.

15. Krishnan SG, Bennion PW, Reineck JR, Burkhead WZ: Hemiarthroplasty for proximal humeral fracture: Restoration of the Gothic arch. *Orthop Clin North Am* 2008;39(4):441-450, vi.

16. Murachovsky J, Ikemoto RY, Nascimento LG, Fujiki EN, Milani C, Warner JJ: Pectoralis major tendon reference (PMT): A new method for accurate restoration of humeral length with hemiarthroplasty for fracture. *J Shoulder Elbow Surg* 2006;15(6):675-678.

17. Greiner SH, Kääb MJ, Kröning I, Scheibel M, Perka C: Reconstruction of humeral length and centering of the prosthetic head in hemiarthroplasty for proximal humeral fractures. *J Shoulder Elbow Surg* 2008;17(5):709-714.

18. McKee M, Jupiter J, Toh CL, Wilson L, Colton C, Karras KK: Reconstruction after malunion and nonunion of intra-articular fractures of the distal humerus: Methods and results in 13 adults. *J Bone Joint Surg Br* 1994;76(4): 614-621.

19. Cobb TK, Morrey BF: Total elbow arthroplasty as primary treatment for distal humeral fractures in elderly patients. *J Bone Joint Surg Am* 1997;79(6):826-832.

20. Garcia JA, Mykula R, Stanley D: Complex fractures of the distal humerus in the elderly: The role of total elbow replacement as primary treatment. *J Bone Joint Surg Br* 2002;84(6):812-816.

21. Lee KT, Lai CH, Singh S: Results of total elbow arthroplasty in the treatment of distal humerus fractures in elderly Asian patients. *J Trauma* 2006;61(4):889-892.

22. Frankle MA, Herscovici D Jr, Vasey MB, Sanders RW: A comparison of open reduction and internal fixation and primary total

elbow arthroplasty in the treatment of intraarticular distal humerus fractures in women older than age 65. *J Orthop Trauma* 2003;17(7):473-480.

23. McKee MD, Veillette CJ, Hall JA, et al: Internal fixation versus total elbow arthroplasty for displaced intra-articular distal humeral fractures in elderly patients. *J Shoulder Elbow Surg* 2009;18(1):3-12.

24. Gustilo RB, Anderson JT: Prevention of infection in the treatment of one thousand and twenty-five open fractures of long bones: Retrospective and prospective analyses. *J Bone Joint Surg Am* 1976; 58(4):453-458.

25. Adolfsson L, Nestorson J: The Kudo humeral component as primary hemiarthroplasty in distal humeral fractures. *J Shoulder Elbow Surg* 2012;21(4):451-455.

26. McKee MD, Pugh DM, Richards RR, Pedersen E, Jones C, Schemitsch EH: Effect of humeral condylar resection on strength and functional outcome after semiconstrained total elbow arthroplasty. *J Bone Joint Surg Am* 2003;85(5): 802-807.

27. Morrey BF, Sanchez-Sotelo J: Approaches for elbow arthroplasty: How to handle the triceps. *J Shoulder Elbow Surg* 2011;20(2): S90-S96.

28. Nauth A, McKee MD, Ristevski B, Hall J, Schemitsch EH: Distal humeral fractures in adults. *J Bone Joint Surg Am* 2011;93(7): 686-700.

29. Letournel E: Acetabulum fractures: Classification and management. *Clin Orthop Relat Res* 1980; 151:81-106.

30. Matta JM: Fractures of the acetabulum: Accuracy of reduction and clinical results in patients managed operatively within three weeks after the injury. *J Bone Joint Surg Am* 1996;78(11):1632-1645.

31. Anglen JO, Burd TA, Hendricks KJ, Harrison P: The gull sign: A

harbinger of failure for internal fixation of geriatric acetabular fractures. *J Orthop Trauma* 2003; 17(9):625-634.

32. Mears DC: Surgical treatment of acetabular fractures in elderly patients with osteoporotic bone. *J Am Acad Orthop Surg* 1999;7(2): 128-141.

33. Vanderschot P: Treatment options of pelvic and acetabular fractures in patients with osteoporotic bone. *Injury* 2007;38(4):497-508.

34. Mears DC, Velyvis JH: Acute total hip arthroplasty for selected displaced acetabular fractures: Two to twelve-year results. *J Bone Joint Surg Am* 2002;84(1):1-9.

35. Spencer RF: Acetabular fractures in older patients. *J Bone Joint Surg Br* 1989;71(5):774-776.

36. Helfet DL, Borrelli J Jr, Sanders R: Stabilization of acetabular fractures in elderly patients. *J Bone Joint Surg Am* 1992;74(5): 753-765.

37. Bellabarba C, Berger RA, Bentley CD, et al: Cementless acetabular reconstruction after acetabular fracture. *J Bone Joint Surg Am* 2001;83(6):868-876.

38. Boardman KP, Charnley J: Low-friction arthroplasty after fracture-dislocations of the hip. *J Bone Joint Surg Br* 1978;60(4):495-497.

39. Huo MH, Solberg BD, Zatorski LE, Keggi KJ: Total hip replacements done without cement after acetabular fractures: A 4- to 8-year follow-up study. *J Arthroplasty* 1999;14(7):827-831.

40. Romness DW, Lewallen DG: Total hip arthroplasty after fracture of the acetabulum: Long-term results. *J Bone Joint Surg Br* 1990;72(5):761-764.

41. Sermon A, Broos P, Vanderschot P: Total hip replacement for acetabular fractures: Results in 121 patients operated between 1983 and 2003. *Injury* 2008; 39(8):914-921.

42. Weber M, Berry DJ, Harmsen WS: Total hip arthroplasty after operative treatment of an acetabular fracture. *J Bone Joint Surg Am* 1998;80(9):1295-1305.

43. Coventry MB: The treatment of fracture-dislocation of the hip by total hip arthroplasty. *J Bone Joint Surg Am* 1974;56(6):1128-1134.

44. Mears DC, Shirahama M: Stabilization of an acetabular fracture with cables for acute total hip arthroplasty. *J Arthroplasty* 1998; 13(1):104-107.

45. Beaulé PE, Griffin DB, Matta JM: The Levine anterior approach for total hip replacement as the treatment for an acute acetabular fracture. *J Orthop Trauma* 2004; 18(9):623-629.

46. Tidermark J, Blomfeldt R, Ponzer S, Söderqvist A, Törnkvist H: Primary total hip arthroplasty with a Burch-Schneider antiprotrusion cage and autologous bone grafting for acetabular fractures in elderly patients. *J Orthop Trauma* 2003;17(3):193-197.

47. Boraiah S, Ragsdale M, Achor T, Zelicof S, Asprinio DE: Open reduction internal fixation and primary total hip arthroplasty of selected acetabular fractures. *J Orthop Trauma* 2009;23(4): 243-248.

48. Cummings SR, Rubin SM, Black D: The future of hip fractures in the United States: Numbers, costs, and potential effects of postmenopausal estrogen. *Clin Orthop Relat Res* 1990;252:163-166.

49. Carroll C, Stevenson M, Scope A, Evans P, Buckley S: Hemiarthroplasty and total hip arthroplasty for treating primary intracapsular fracture of the hip: A systematic review and cost-effectiveness analysis. *Health Technol Assess* 2011; 15(36):1-74.

50. Bhandari M, Matta J, Ferguson T, Matthys G: Predictors of clinical and radiological outcome in patients with fractures of the ac-

etabulum and concomitant posterior dislocation of the hip. *J Bone Joint Surg Br* 2006;88(12):1618-1624.

51. Cho MR, Lee HS, Lee SW, Choi CH, Kim SK, Ko SB: Results after total hip arthroplasty with a large head and bipolar arthroplasty in patients with displaced femoral neck fractures. *J Arthroplasty* 2011;26(6):893-896.

52. Dorr LD, Glousman R, Hoy AL, Vanis R, Chandler R: Treatment of femoral neck fractures with total hip replacement versus cemented and noncemented hemiarthroplasty. *J Arthroplasty* 1986;1(1):21-28.

53. Haidukewych GJ, Israel TA, Berry DJ: Long-term survivorship of cemented bipolar hemiarthroplasty for fracture of the femoral neck. *Clin Orthop Relat Res* 2002;403:118-126.

54. Hedbeck CJ, Enocson A, Lapidus G, et al: Comparison of bipolar hemiarthroplasty with total hip arthroplasty for displaced femoral neck fractures: A concise four-year follow-up of a randomized trial. *J Bone Joint Surg Am* 2011;93(5):445-450.

55. Johansson T, Jacobsson SA, Ivarsson I, Knutsson A, Wahlström O: Internal fixation versus total hip arthroplasty in the treatment of displaced femoral neck fractures: A prospective randomized study of 100 hips. *Acta Orthop Scand* 2000;71(6):597-602.

56. Keating JF, Grant A, Masson M, Scott NW, Forbes JF: Randomized comparison of reduction and fixation, bipolar hemiarthroplasty, and total hip arthroplasty: Treatment of displaced intracapsular hip fractures in healthy older patients. *J Bone Joint Surg Am* 2006;88(2):249-260.

57. Macaulay W, Nellans KW, Garvin KL, Iorio R, Healy WL, Rosenwasser MP; other members of the DFACTO Consortium: Prospective randomized clinical trial comparing hemiarthroplasty to total hip arthroplasty in the treatment of displaced femoral neck fractures: Winner of the Dorr Award. *J Arthroplasty* 2008;23(6):2-8.

58. Parker MJ, Khan RJ, Crawford J, Pryor GA: Hemiarthroplasty versus internal fixation for displaced intracapsular hip fractures in the elderly: A randomised trial of 455 patients. *J Bone Joint Surg Br* 2002;84(8):1150-1155.

59. Ravikumar KJ, Marsh G: Internal fixation versus hemiarthroplasty versus total hip arthroplasty for displaced subcapital fractures of femur: 13 year results of a prospective randomised study. *Injury* 2000;31(10):793-797.

60. Ricci WM, Langer JS, Leduc S, Streubel PN, Borrelli JJ: Total hip arthroplasty for acute displaced femoral neck fractures via the posterior approach: A protocol to minimise hip dislocation risk. *Hip Int* 2011;21(3):344-350.

61. Rogmark C, Carlsson A, Johnell O, Sernbo I: A prospective randomised trial of internal fixation versus arthroplasty for displaced fractures of the neck of the femur: Functional outcome for 450 patients at two years. *J Bone Joint Surg Br* 2002;84(2):183-188.

62. Schmidt AH, Leighton R, Parvizi J, Sems A, Berry DJ: Optimal arthroplasty for femoral neck fractures: Is total hip arthroplasty the answer? *J Orthop Trauma* 2009;23(6):428-433.

63. Tidermark J, Ponzer S, Svensson O, Söderqvist A, Törnkvist H: Internal fixation compared with total hip replacement for displaced femoral neck fractures in the elderly: A randomised, controlled trial. *J Bone Joint Surg Br* 2003;85(3):380-388.

64. Zi-Sheng A, You-Shui G, Zhi-Zhen J, Ting Y, Chang-Qing Z: Hemiarthroplasty vs primary total hip arthroplasty for displaced fractures of the femoral neck in the elderly: A meta-analysis. *J Arthroplasty* 2012;27(4):583-590.

65. Iorio R, Schwartz B, Macaulay W, Teeney SM, Healy WL, York S: Surgical treatment of displaced femoral neck fractures in the elderly: A survey of the American Association of Hip and Knee Surgeons. *J Arthroplasty* 2006;21(8):1124-1133.

66. Klein GR, Parvizi J, Vegari DN, Rothman RH, Purtill JJ: Total hip arthroplasty for acute femoral neck fractures using a cementless tapered femoral stem. *J Arthroplasty* 2006;21(8):1134-1140.

67. Iorio R, Healy WL, Lemos DW, Appleby D, Lucchesi CA, Saleh KJ: Displaced femoral neck fractures in the elderly: Outcomes and cost effectiveness. *Clin Orthop Relat Res* 2001;383:229-242.

68. Parker MJ, Gurusamy KS, Azegami S: Arthroplasties (with and without bone cement) for proximal femoral fractures in adults. *Cochrane Database Syst Rev* 2010;6:CD001706.

69. Taylor F, Wright M, Zhu M: Hemiarthroplasty of the hip with and without cement: A randomized clinical trial. *J Bone Joint Surg Am* 2012;94(7):577-583.

70. Healy WL, Iorio R: Total hip arthroplasty: Optimal treatment for displaced femoral neck fractures in elderly patients. *Clin Orthop Relat Res* 2004;429:43-48.

71. Blomfeldt R, Törnkvist H, Eriksson K, Söderqvist A, Ponzer S, Tidermark J: A randomised controlled trial comparing bipolar hemiarthroplasty with total hip replacement for displaced intracapsular fractures of the femoral neck in elderly patients. *J Bone Joint Surg Br* 2007;89(2):160-165.

72. Sierra RJ, Raposo JM, Trousdale RT, Cabanela ME: Dislocation of primary THA done through a posterolateral approach in the

elderly. *Clin Orthop Relat Res* 2005;441:262-267.

73. Berry DJ, von Knoch M, Schleck CD, Harmsen WS: Effect of femoral head diameter and operative approach on risk of dislocation after primary total hip arthroplasty. *J Bone Joint Surg Am* 2005; 87(11):2456-2463.

Video Reference

Matsen KD, Natarajn V, Carnahan C, Stas V, Duwelius PJ: Video. *Treatment of Displaced Femoral Neck With Total Hip Arthroplasty.* Portland, OR, 2013.

Shoulder

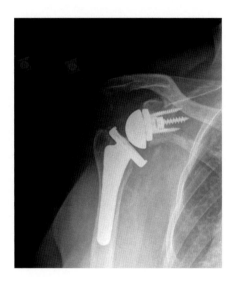

From Platelet-Rich Plasma to the Reverse Prosthesis: Controversies in Treating Rotator Cuff Pathology

Edward V. Craig, MD, MPH
Leesa M. Galatz, MD
John W. Sperling, MD, MBA

Abstract

Rotator cuff pathology and tearing remains a common cause of shoulder pain and disability. Although little controversy and disagreement exists regarding the treatment of small to moderate size tears in good quality tissue without retraction, there is difficulty in agreeing on the ideal treatment of the largest tears, particularly because those tears may be accompanied by widely variable levels of pain and function. Clinical decision making is made more difficult because of the variable presentations observed in patients with a documented full-thickness rotator cuff tear: some have good function and no pain, some have good function and pain, some have poor function and no pain, and some have both poor function and pain.

The role of biologics as an adjunct in treating most rotator cuff tears remains unclear, with ongoing exploration of the roles of stem cells, growth factors, and platelet-rich plasma. In patients with unreconstructable tears with marked weakness in external rotation but good elevation, a latissimus transfer may restore rotation. Patches may play a role in partial repairs while serving as both a lattice for healing and a biomechanical anchoring point for sutures. In patients with massive tears and arthritis and in many who have rotator cuff insufficiency, pseudoparalysis, or anterosuperior escape without arthritis, reverse shoulder arthroplasty has led to improvements in pain and strength and revolutionized the treatment of rotator cuff tears.

Instr Course Lect 2014;63:63-70.

The role of rotator cuff surgery is to repair the cuff to restore its primary function of maintaining a centered humeral head in the glenoid during elevation of the arm. In small or moderate tears with good tissue, healing rates appear to be high, with restoration of function and relief of pain predictable sequelae of surgical repair. Large and massive tears have proven to be a challenge for clinicians because the potential for healing and the predictability of the repair are often compromised by the older age of patients, the poor quality of tendon and muscle, medical comorbidities, and a poor biologic healing environment. Adding biologic augmentation to the treatment armamentarium to improve patient outcomes has generated intense interest.

In a massive rotator cuff tear, the loss of anterosuperior rotator cuff function may result in instability and humeral head escape from the coracoacromial arch, and superior and posterior rotator cuff loss may result in marked superior instability. In either clinical situation, the stable fulcrum, which is important for effective deltoid function, is lost. The loss of balance between the deltoid and rotator cuff

Dr. Craig or an immediate family member has received royalties from Biomet; is a member of a speakers' bureau or has made paid presentations on behalf of Biomet; serves as a paid consultant to or is an employee of Biomet; and serves as a board member, owner, officer, or committee member of the American Academy of Orthopaedic Surgeons and the American Shoulder and Elbow Surgeons. Dr. Galatz or an immediate family member serves as an unpaid consultant to Tornier and serves as a board member, owner, officer, or committee member of the American Shoulder and Elbow Surgeons, the American Orthopaedic Association, and the American Academy of Orthopaedic Surgeons. Dr. Sperling or an immediate family member has received royalties from Biomet and DJ Orthopaedics; serves as a paid consultant to or is an employee of Tornier; and has stock or stock options held in Emerge Medical and Tornier.

function results in dramatic diminution of the ability to position the arm in space. In some instances, this balance may be restored by standard rotator cuff reconstruction, biologic patch augmentation, or muscle transfer techniques. In clinical situations in which the rotator cuff is believed to be irreparable and function cannot be restored, prosthetic arthroplasty plays a role for patients disabled by pain and/or loss of function.

Because of the complexity in decision-making, the difficulty of predicting results in larger tears, and technologic advances applicable to rotator cuff pathology, treatment controversies have been the focus of recent clinical and basic science studies.

Biologic Augmentation

Massive rotator cuff tears pose an important clinical problem. Historically, rotator cuff repair had a high clinical success rate;[1-3] however, it is well known that failure of healing occurs at a surprisingly high rate, especially in patients with larger rotator cuff tears.[4] Several patient-related factors contribute to the complexity of larger tears. Tear size and chronicity affect the reparability and healing potential of rotator cuff tears. Larger tears have a higher failure rate, and healing is known to benefit from a stronger repair in the clinical setting. Like all musculoskeletal tissues, tendon and muscle are designed to bear load. When unloaded, degenerative changes occur in the tendon and muscle resulting in loss of compliance and a decrease in the biologic tendency for healing. Patient age is arguably the most important factor.[3,5,6] Patients older than 60 years have a lower rate of healing. Age is also a colinear factor that correlates with tear size and chronicity in many circumstances, but when extrapolated, has an effect. Medical comorbidities, such as diabetes, hypercholesterolemia,

and smoking, have been shown to decrease healing in animal models.[7-9] These findings have spurred an intense interest in rotator cuff healing and the potential of biologic augmentation.

Platelet-Rich Plasma

Platelet-rich plasma (PRP) is a treatment modality that has been used to enhance tendon-to-bone healing. PRP is an autologous blood sample with a concentration of platelets three to four times above the baseline value. Platelets, best known for their role in blood clotting, are nonnucleated bodies containing alpha granules. These granules contain growth factors, cytokines, and proteins, which have been associated with angiogenesis and cell recruitment and proliferation. Theoretically, PRP provides a vehicle for delivering beneficial factors to the healing site.

PRP is created from a sample of autologous blood. The blood is centrifuged and the red blood cells and, sometimes, the white blood cells are removed. PRP can be activated or nonactivated. Clotting leads to activation; therefore, bovine thrombin is applied to induce clotting in some systems. After activation, the alpha granules degranulate, releasing 70% of the stored factors in 10 minutes and approximately 100% in 1 hour. Because platelets live for 8 to 10 days, very small amounts of stored factors may be released later.

A similar product, platelet-rich fibrin matrix (PRFM), is created when calcium chloride is added to the second centrifugation step. This process stimulates autogenous thrombin, and a fibrin matrix is formed with the platelets inside. This matrix results in slower release of growth factor from the fibrin scaffold as it is absorbed, which, theoretically, makes this delivery mechanism more compelling. Because numerous commercial systems are available (each with small proprie-

tary variances), the surgeon should evaluate each system to learn about product characteristics before use.

Clinical results of PRP and PRFM augmentation have been somewhat disappointing. In a prospective randomized trial of 88 patients treated with PRP augmentation after rotator cuff repair, Castricini et al[10] reported no difference in Constant scores or MRI findings. A randomized controlled trial using PRFM showed no difference in rotator cuff tendon strength, healing, vascularity, or clinical outcome scores, and regression analysis suggested that PRFM actually decreased healing.[11] A level II cohort study by Bergeson et al[12] reported no improvement in clinical or structural outcomes with PRFM augmentation for rotator cuff tears.

Some promising results have been reported. In a nonrandomized study by Barber et al,[13] 20 of 40 patients undergoing rotator cuff repair were treated with PRFM augmentation. The patients treated with PRFM showed no difference in clinical outcome but had a higher healing rate in tears larger than 3 cm than the group that did not receive PRFM. Another randomized controlled trial using PRP in 53 patients treated with arthroscopic rotator cuff repair showed modest improvements in pain during the very early postoperative period; however, follow-up MRIs showed no difference in the healing rates of the tears.[14]

Overall, there is little evidence at this time to support the routine use of PRP or PRFM for rotator cuff repair. The fairest assessment is that its ability to enhance tendon healing and its cost effectiveness is unsubstantiated.

Mesenchymal Stem Cells

Mesenchymal stem cells are pluripotential cells with the ability to differentiate into multiple different musculoskeletal tissues. They can be obtained from bone marrow and adipose or tendon tissue. Native stem cells can be used by themselves, but their value is probably enhanced by the ability to transfect them to produce other components, including growth factors, transcription factors, and membrane proteins.

Several limitations exist in the use of stem cells. Specifically, huge numbers of stem cells are required because cell death occurs after implantation. The cells must adhere to a surface to survive and further differentiate. Many other processes, including angiogenesis and growth factor production, must be present to allow the cells to develop into mature tissues. Research of the role of mesenchymal stem cells in the field of rotator cuff repair is in its infancy, but a few studies have evaluated the use of stem cells at the tendon enthesis.

Gulotta et al[15] used stem cells in a rodent model of rotator cuff injury and repair. Bone marrow–derived cells alone had no effect, whereas cells transfected with membrane type I matrix metalloproteinase resulted in improved insertion-site characteristics and biomechanical properties of the healing tissue.[16] Using the same animal model, stem cells transfected with scleraxis[17] (a transcription factor associated with tendon development) resulted in some improvement. Thus far, only one study has been published on the use of stem cells in human rotator cuff tears. Autologous bone marrow–derived cells were applied in 14 patients.[18] Because there was no control group for comparison, better results were not proven; however, there were no adverse effects. Further research is necessary before the routine use of stem cells can be advocated in the clinical setting.

Patches

Healing problems after rotator cuff repair are well recognized. The literature reports that 10% to 90% of rotator cuffs are not intact after repair.[4] Studies have demonstrated that patients with retears have worse clinical outcomes than those with intact rotator cuffs.[5,19,20] The American Shoulder and Elbow Surgeons (ASES) score and the Constant score are lower in patients with retears, and range of motion and strength are also lower.[5,20]

One of the primary reasons that tears do not heal is certain biologic and mechanical changes occur after the tendon is torn. There is a change in the stiffness of the tendon with tearing as well as associated muscle atrophy and fatty infiltration.[21] Tears in rotator cuff tendons frequently occur through diseased tissues, which may have a poor blood supply. In addition, diseased rotator cuff tendons may exhibit degenerative changes with inferior material properties compared with normal tendons. Other factors associated with poor healing of the rotator cuff tendon include associated patient comorbidities, such as smoking, diabetes, obesity, and advanced age.[22] Most repair failures occur within the first several months.[23]

Because the high failure rate of rotator cuff surgery may be caused by poor quality tissue and a poor mechanical environment, patches have been designed to improve the mechanical strength and biologic environment of the repair to improve healing. The ideal patch material to augment rotator cuff repairs should be biocompatible and biologically active and should produce a low immune response to minimize associated inflammation, which has been shown to be a critical factor in the failure or success of patch materials.[24] The patch should have material properties that are similar to those of rotator cuff tendon. Appropriate construct properties and high suture retention to mechanically augment the repair are optimal characteristics. Ide-

ally, the patch would also play a biologic role in attracting host cells into the scaffold.

Biomechanical and Clinical Studies

The patch should play an important mechanical role in load sharing and decreasing gap formation and should increase the ultimate load to failure. In a biomechanical cadaver model, Shea et al[25] reported a 40% decrease in gap formation and found that load to failure was significantly higher in the patch group (429 ± 69 N) compared with the control group (335 ± 57 N) ($P < 0.05$). In a biomechanical study on rotator cuff augmentation, Barber et al[26] tested 10 matched pairs of human cadaver supraspinatus muscles and tendons. The authors found that the addition of a patch increased the initial strength of the repair. The mean failure strength for the control group was 273 ± 116 N compared with 325 ± 74 N in the augmented group ($P = 0.047$). Walton et al[24] published one of the first clinical studies on the use of a patch material for rotator cuff surgery. The investigators looked at the outcome of using porcine submucosa to reinforce rotator cuff repairs. An increased inflammatory response was noted, which led to the recognition of the potential immune response to graft materials.

In a 2008 study, Bond et al[27] reported on newer patch materials in 16 arthroscopic repairs for massive rotator cuff tears. The authors reported substantial improvement in University of California Los Angeles, Constant, and Simple Shoulder Test scores. Thirteen of 16 patients had MRI evidence of graft incorporation at a mean follow-up of 26.8 months (range, 12 to 38 months). In a study of the outcome of arthroscopic repair of large to massive rotator cuff tears, Barber et al[28] reported on 20 control patients

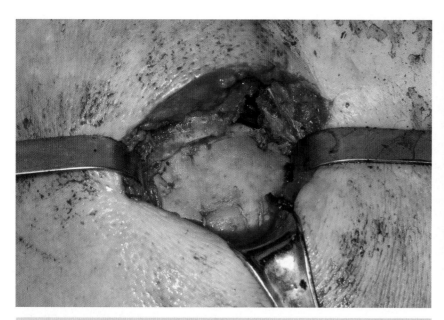

Figure 1 A synthetic patch may be added to a rotator cuff repair to provide anatomic and biomechanical advantages.

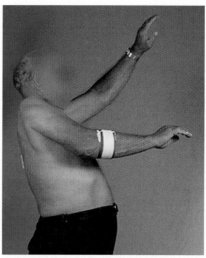

Figure 2 In a patient with pseudoparalysis, the deltoid acts unopposed and represents vertical muscle imbalance. (Reproduced with permission from Craig EV, Stein BE: *Atlas of Orthopedic Surgery: A Guide to Management and Practice.* Florence, KY, CRC Press, 2004, pp 46-74.)

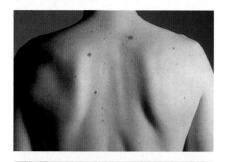

Figure 3 Supraspinatus and infraspinatus muscle atrophy of long-standing duration is an indication of rotator cuff irreparability.

and 22 patients treated with a patch. The investigators reported that 85% of the rotator cuff repairs with a patch were intact versus 40% of the repairs in the control patients at a mean follow-up of 24 months (range, 12 to 38 months).

Patch augmentation offers a potential solution to some of the mechanical and biologic problems of rotator cuff repair. Mechanically, patches can help decrease gap formation and increase the load to failure (**Figure 1**). From a biologic perspective, patches require a low immune response and the poten-tial for incorporation. Although recent clinical studies have reported encouraging results, additional studies are needed to further refine the indications for patch use in rotator cuff repair.

Reverse Shoulder Arthroplasty

Reverse arthroplasty plays an important role in treating an irreparable rotator cuff (one that can neither be repaired nor reconstructed). This implant may assist in restoring deltoid tension, moving the center of rotation within the glenohumeral joint, and providing a stable fulcrum to restore shoulder function.

Clinical signs that a rotator cuff cannot be repaired include pseudoparalysis with attempted active motion (**Figure 2**), marked supraspinatus and/or infraspinatus fossa atrophy (**Figure 3**), and anterosuperior humeral head escape. Radiographic signs include marked diminution of the acromiohumeral interval, static superior migration of the humeral head (**Figure 4**), anterosuperior subluxation, and an MRI showing a large (> 5 cm) tear of two or more tendons with a high degree (> 50%) of fatty infiltration of the rotator cuff muscle (Goutallier grade 3 or 4) (**Figure 5**).

Rotator cuff tear arthropathy is perhaps the clearest indication for reverse shoulder arthroplasty because other arthroplasty solutions have been shown to be suboptimal. Total shoulder replacement in the absence of a functioning rotator cuff is unpredictable in restoring a balanced centered shoulder, and glenoid longevity has been questioned because of the inability of the rotator cuff to center the humeral head (rocking horse glenoid). Hemiarthroplasty, with or without soft-tissue interposition, has mixed results and does little to recenter the humeral head; a few studies have reported improvement in active motion and functional scores.[29,30]

Several studies have shown that reverse shoulder arthroplasty can predictably restore function (including

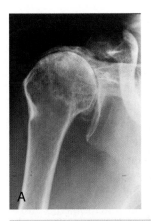

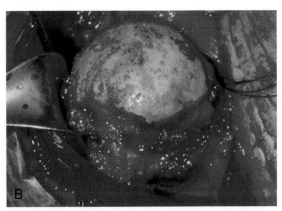

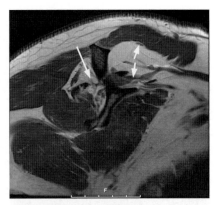

Figure 4 **A,** Radiograph showing superior migration and articulation with the acromion, which is typical in rotator cuff tear arthropathy. **B,** Intraoperative photograph of rotator cuff tear arthropathy, arthritic changes, and a massive tear.

Figure 5 MRI of a patient with a massive rotator cuff tear of long duration shows severe atrophy of the supraspinatus and infraspinatus muscles (short arrows) and evidence of fatty infiltration (long arrow).

overhead elevation), relieve pain, and increase external rotation, particularly if there is a functioning teres minor[31,32] (**Figures 6** and **7**). Some implant designs with a more lateral center of rotation appear to recruit the posterior deltoid to restore external rotation. Some studies have suggested that external rotation may be reestablished by adding a latissimus transfer to the reverse shoulder prosthesis.[33,34] Several recent clinical studies have shown that patients with rotator cuff tear arthropathy treated with reverse shoulder arthroplasty had substantial increases in active shoulder elevation and improvement in Constant or ASES scores.[31,35,36]

Success in treating rotator cuff tear arthropathy has encouraged the use of the reverse implant in patients with massive rotator cuff tears and poor function, even in the absence of arthritis. In the presence of a massive rotator cuff tear, some patients are able to compensate for the rotator cuff dysfunction and can maintain surprisingly good function. In the absence of arthritis, particularly if pseudoparalysis is not present, it is reasonable to attempt to restore muscle function through rehabilitation and recruitment of accessory muscles. In the presence of a mas-

sive rotator cuff tear, poor function, and pain without significant glenohumeral disease, options other than reverse shoulder arthroplasty can include partial or complete repair, arthroscopic débridement, and biceps tenotomy.

Pseudoparalysis, by definition, is equated with the loss of a fulcrum for effective deltoid function. The deltoid acts unopposed, leading to superior migration with loss of the lever arm. One goal of reverse shoulder arthroplasty is to restore the fulcrum to a stable, functional location.

Anterosuperior escape is a particularly disabling condition resulting from the loss of both the superior and the anterior rotator cuff, and it is often associated with prior surgery and compromise of the coracoacromial arch. Only a reverse prosthesis can provide the mechanical stability and fulcrum to treat this condition. A reverse prosthesis can reduce pain and improve function in patients with a massive tear and elevation less than 90°, particularly in the presence of anterosuperior humeral head escape. Several studies have shown an increase in active elevation from 50° to 80°, improvement in outcome scores (such as Constant, ASES, and Simple Shoulder Test scores) and a high degree of patient

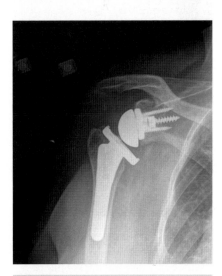

Figure 6 Radiograph of a reverse shoulder arthroplasty.

satisfaction.[32,35,37] The rate of short-to intermediate-term (2- to 10-year) implant survival has been reported to be 95%.[38] Patients with more than 90° of elevation may be less satisfied after reverse shoulder arthroplasty than those who begin with less active elevation.

Reverse shoulder arthroplasty has also played an important role in treating "massive rotator cuff tear equivalent," which can be defined as a standard arthroplasty that fails because of tuberosity nonunion or prosthetic in-

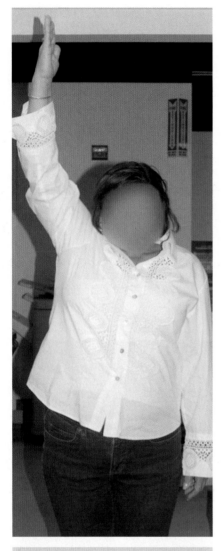

Figure 7 Photograph of a patient showing the postoperative clinical degree of active elevation after reverse shoulder arthroplasty for rotator cuff tear arthropathy.

stability. In the absence of a greater tuberosity attachment to the proximal humerus, with its associated loss of the supraspinatus, the infraspinatus, and the teres minor muscle attachment site, the patient has symptoms similar to those with a massive rotator cuff tear, superior instability, and pseudoparalysis. Reverse shoulder arthroplasty can potentially restore the fulcrum for deltoid function and provide the clinician with an acceptable option for treating tuberosity nonunion, exci-

sion, or dissolution, which can result in primary arthroplasty failure. Many patients have improvement in all shoulder scores with the reverse prosthesis.[38]

Although reverse shoulder arthroplasty has revolutionized the treatment of the rotator cuff–deficient shoulder, particularly in the presence of arthritis, complication rates have been high (10% to 47%), including dislocation (0% to 9%), infection (1% to 15%), loosening (1% to 25%), scapula notching (0% to 86%), and scapula fracture (3% to 5%).[39] Evaluating the extent and incidence of reported complications can be difficult because some studies report minor complications (such as hematoma) even if outcome is unaffected, whereas other studies do not report such complications.

Because major complications can have a substantial effect on clinical success, it is recommended that surgeons adhere to proper patient selection, have a thorough knowledge of the implantation technique, and closely examine the potential benefits versus risks for the individual patient.

Summary

Failure of rotator cuff repair occurs at a substantial rate, particularly in large tears and in elderly patients. Biologic augmentation, such as stem cells, growth factors, and PRP, have been explored as possible means of increasing healing potential, but research is still needed to identify the precise growth factors and concentrations needed to achieve consistent and predictable outcomes. In the presence of rotator cuff tears with poor native tissue, patch augmentation offers a potential solution from a biologic and mechanical perspective. Although recent clinical studies have been promising, further research is also needed to refine the indications for patch use.

In the presence of an unreconstructable rotator cuff, particularly when there is substantial external rotation deficiency (the hornblower sign), latissimus dorsi and teres major transfer may play an important role in overcoming functional deficits. In some cases, even after multiple surgeries, a patient with a rotator cuff–deficient shoulder may present with pain and severe functional deficits, such as pseudoparalysis and anterosuperior instability and escape. Prior to the introduction of the reverse prosthesis, there was often no good treatment option for these patients. The noted improvements in pain and function in patients with rotator cuff tear arthropathy have encouraged clinicians to extend the indications for the reverse prosthesis to patients with massive tears without arthritis.

References

1. Lafosse L, Brozska R, Toussaint B, Gobezie R: The outcome and structural integrity of arthroscopic rotator cuff repair with use of the double-row suture anchor technique. *J Bone Joint Surg Am* 2007; 89(7):1533-1541.

2. Charousset C, Bellaïche L, Kalra K, Petrover D: Arthroscopic repair of full-thickness rotator cuff tears: Is there tendon healing in patients aged 65 years or older? *Arthroscopy* 2010;26(3):302-309.

3. Boileau P, Brassart N, Watkinson DJ, Carles M, Hatzidakis AM, Krishnan SG: Arthroscopic repair of full-thickness tears of the supraspinatus: Does the tendon really heal? *J Bone Joint Surg Am* 2005;87(6):1229-1240.

4. Galatz LM, Ball CM, Teefey SA, Middleton WD, Yamaguchi K: The outcome and repair integrity of completely arthroscopically repaired large and massive rotator cuff tears. *J Bone Joint Surg Am* 2004;86(2):219-224.

5. Lichtenberg S, Liem D, Magosch P, Habermeyer P: Influence of tendon healing after arthroscopic rotator cuff repair on clinical outcome using single-row Mason-Allen suture technique: A prospective, MRI controlled study. *Knee Surg Sports Traumatol Arthrosc* 2006;14(11):1200-1206.

6. Tashjian RZ, Hollins AM, Kim H-M, et al: Factors affecting healing rates after arthroscopic double-row rotator cuff repair. *Am J Sports Med* 2010;38(12):2435-2442.

7. Abboud JA, Kim JS: The effect of hypercholesterolemia on rotator cuff disease. *Clin Orthop Relat Res* 2010;468(6):1493-1497.

8. Bedi A, Fox AJ, Harris PE, et al: Diabetes mellitus impairs tendon-bone healing after rotator cuff repair. *J Shoulder Elbow Surg* 2010;19(7):978-988.

9. Galatz LM, Silva MJ, Rothermich SY, Zaegel MA, Havlioglu N, Thomopoulos S: Nicotine delays tendon-to-bone healing in a rat shoulder model. *J Bone Joint Surg Am* 2006;88(9):2027-2034.

10. Castricini R, Longo UG, De Benedetto M, et al: Platelet-rich plasma augmentation for arthroscopic rotator cuff repair. A randomized controlled trial. *Am J Sports Med* 2011;39(2):258-265.

11. Rodeo SA, Delos D, Williams RJ, Adler RS, Pearle A, Warren RF: The effect of platelet-rich fibrin matrix on rotator cuff tendon healing: A prospective, randomized clinical study. *Am J Sports Med* 2012;40(6):1234-1241.

12. Bergeson AG, Tashjian RZ, Greis PE, Crim J, Stoddard GJ, Burks RT: Effects of platelet-rich fibrin matrix on repair integrity of at-risk rotator cuff tears. *Am J Sports Med* 2012;40(2):286-293.

13. Barber FA, Hrnack SA, Snyder SJ, Hapa O: Rotator cuff repair healing influenced by platelet-rich plasma construct augmentation. *Arthroscopy* 2011;27(8):1029-1035.

14. Randelli P, Arrigoni P, Ragone V, Aliprandi A, Cabitza P: Platelet rich plasma in arthroscopic rotator cuff repair: A prospective RCT study, 2-year follow-up. *J Shoulder Elbow Surg* 2011;20(4):518-528.

15. Gulotta LV, Kovacevic D, Ehteshami JR, Dagher E, Packer JD, Rodeo SA: Application of bone marrow-derived mesenchymal stem cells in a rotator cuff repair model. *Am J Sports Med* 2009;37(11):2126-2133.

16. Gulotta LV, Kovacevic D, Montgomery S, Ehteshami JR, Packer JD, Rodeo SA: Stem cells genetically modified with the developmental gene MT1-MMP improve regeneration of the supraspinatus tendon-to-bone insertion site. *Am J Sports Med* 2010; 38(7):1429-1437.

17. Gulotta LV, Kovacevic D, Packer JD, Deng X-H, Rodeo SA: Bone marrow-derived mesenchymal stem cells transduced with scleraxis improve rotator cuff healing in a rat model. *Am J Sports Med* 2011;39(6):1282-1289.

18. Ellera Gomes JL, da Silva RC, Silla LM, Abreu MR, Pellanda R: Conventional rotator cuff repair complemented by the aid of mononuclear autologous stem cells. *Knee Surg Sports Traumatol Arthrosc* 2012;20(2):373-377.

19. Zumstein MA, Jost B, Hempel J, Hodler J, Gerber C: The clinical and structural long-term results of open repair of massive tears of the rotator cuff. *J Bone Joint Surg Am* 2008;90(11):2423-2431.

20. Bishop J, Klepps S, Lo IK, Bird J, Gladstone JN, Flatow EL: Cuff integrity after arthroscopic versus open rotator cuff repair: A prospective study. *J Shoulder Elbow Surg* 2006;15(3):290-299.

21. Barry JJ, Lansdown DA, Cheung S, Feeley BT, Ma CB: The relationship between tear severity, fatty infiltration, and muscle atrophy in the supraspinatus. *J Shoulder Elbow Surg* 2013;22(1):18-25.

22. Tashjian RZ, Hollins AM, Kim HM, et al: Factors affecting healing rates after arthroscopic double-row rotator cuff repair. *Am J Sports Med* 2010;38(12): 2435-2442.

23. Miller BS, Downie BK, Kohen RB, et al: When do rotator cuff repairs fail? Serial ultrasound examination after arthroscopic repair of large and massive rotator cuff tears. *Am J Sports Med* 2011; 39(10):2064-2070.

24. Walton JR, Bowman NK, Khatib Y, Linklater J, Murrell GA: Restore orthobiologic implant: Not recommended for augmentation of rotator cuff repairs. *J Bone Joint Surg Am* 2007;89(4):786-791.

25. Shea KP, Obopilwe E, Sperling JW, Iannotti JP: A biomechanical analysis of gap formation and failure mechanics of a xenograft-reinforced rotator cuff repair in a cadaveric model. *J Shoulder Elbow Surg* 2012;21(8):1072-1079.

26. Barber FA, Herbert MA, Boothby MH: Ultimate tensile failure loads of a human dermal allograft rotator cuff augmentation. *Arthroscopy* 2008;24(1):20-24.

27. Bond JL, Dopirak RM, Higgins J, Burns J, Snyder SJ: Arthroscopic replacement of massive, irreparable rotator cuff tears using a GraftJacket allograft: Technique and preliminary results. *Arthroscopy* 2008;24(4):403-409, e1.

28. Barber FA, Burns JP, Deutsch A, Labbé MR, Litchfield RB: A prospective, randomized evaluation of acellular human dermal matrix augmentation for arthroscopic rotator cuff repair. *Arthroscopy* 2012;28(1):8-15.

29. Goldberg SS, Bell JE, Kim HJ, Bak F, Levine WN, Bigliani LU: Hemiarthroplasty for the rotator cuff-deficient shoulder. *J Bone

Joint Surg Am 2008;90(3): 554-559.

30. Sanchez-Sotelo J, Cofield RH, Rowland CM: Shoulder hemiarthroplasty for glenohumeral arthritis associated with severe rotator cuff deficiency. *J Bone Joint Surg Am* 2001;83(12):1814-1822.

31. Frankle M, Levy JC, Pupello D, et al: The reverse shoulder prosthesis for glenohumeral arthritis associated with severe rotator cuff deficiency: A minimum two-year follow-up study of sixty patients surgical technique. *J Bone Joint Surg Am* 2006;88(suppl 1 pt 2): 178-190.

32. Mulieri P, Dunning P, Klein S, Pupello D, Frankle M: Reverse shoulder arthroplasty for the treatment of irreparable rotator cuff tear without glenohumeral arthritis. *J Bone Joint Surg Am* 2010; 92(15):2544-2556.

33. Puskas GJ, Catanzaro S, Gerber C: Clinical outcome of reverse total shoulder arthroplasty combined with latissimus dorsi transfer for the treatment of chronic combined pseudoparesis of elevation and external rotation of the shoulder. [published online ahead of print June 18, 2013.] *J Shoulder Elbow Surg.* PMID: 23790326.

34. Boileau P, Chinard C, Roussanne Y, Neyton L, Trojani C: Modified latissimus dorsi and teres major transfer through a single deltopectoral approach for external rotation deficit of the shoulder: As an isolated procedure or with a reverse arthroplasty. *J Shoulder Elbow Surg* 2007;16(6):671-682.

35. Werner CM, Steinmann PA, Gilbart M, Gerber C: Treatment of painful pseudoparesis due to irreparable rotator cuff dysfunction with the Delta III reverse-ball-and-socket total shoulder prosthesis. *J Bone Joint Surg Am* 2005;87(7):1476-1486.

36. Boileau P, Watkinson D, Hatzidakis AM, Hovorka I: The Grammont reverse shoulder prosthesis: Results in cuff tear arthritis, fracture sequelae, and revision arthroplasty. *J Shoulder Elbow Surg* 2006;15(5):527-540.

37. Boileau P, Gonzalez JF, Chuinard C, Bicknell R, Walch G: Reverse total shoulder arthroplasty after failed rotator cuff surgery. *J Shoulder Elbow Surg* 2009;18(4): 600-606.

38. Feeley BT, Gallo RA, Craig EV: Cuff tear arthropathy: Current trends in diagnosis and surgical management. *J Shoulder Elbow Surg* 2009;18(3):484-494.

39. Cheung E, Willis M, Walker M, Clark R, Frankle MA: Complications in reverse total shoulder arthroplasty. *J Am Acad Orthop Surg* 2011;19(7):439-449.

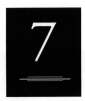

Massive Irreparable Rotator Cuff Tears: How to Rebalance the Cuff-Deficient Shoulder

Pascal Boileau, MD
Walter B. McClelland Jr, MD
Adam P. Rumian, MD, FRCS (Tr&Orth)

Abstract

In its natural state, the shoulder is unbalanced in both the vertical and horizontal planes because the deltoid is stronger than the rotator cuff muscles and the internal rotator muscles are stronger than the external rotator muscles. With aging, this muscle imbalance can become worse, leading to tendon wear, irreversible fatty infiltration of the rotator cuff muscles, and upward migration of the humeral head. Most shoulders with tendon wear are functional and asymptomatic. A traumatic event (such as a fall onto the upper limb) can lead to rotator cuff tearing and a shoulder that becomes symptomatic and nonfunctional. Symptomatic massive irreparable rotator cuff tears present in one of four recognizable patterns depending on the muscular imbalance that occurs and the symptoms that are present: painful loss of active elevation, with conserved muscle balance; isolated loss of active elevation, with loss of vertical muscle balance; isolated loss of external rotation, with loss of horizontal muscle balance; and combined loss of elevation and external rotation, with loss of vertical and horizontal muscle balance. Assessing the plane of shoulder muscle imbalance is a key feature in the decision-making process. Classifying and understanding these tears allows surgeons to select the correct treatment (conservative measures, arthroscopic techniques, reverse shoulder arthroplasty, or tendon transfers) to restore shoulder balance and function.

Instr Course Lect 2014;63:71-83.

The prevalence of massive irreparable rotator cuff tears reported in the literature has ranged from 10% to 40%; however, there is no consensus regarding the definition of a irreparable massive rotator cuff tear.[1-6] Both clinical and experimental studies have shown that isolated supraspinatus tears or paralysis does not disrupt glenohumeral kinematics.[6-11] Conversely, it has been shown that a substantial extension of a rotator cuff tear into the infraspinatus tendon disrupts the transverse force couple, and the stable fulcrum for glenohumeral abduction may be lost.[8,10,12] A rotator cuff tear is defined as massive if it involves the detachment of two or more entire tendons, typically beginning with the supraspinatus and infraspinatus. A rotator cuff tear is defined as irreparable when there is tendon retraction to the glenoid level or beyond (stage 3 or 4),[13] severe fatty infiltration of the cuff muscles (Goutallier stage 3 or 4),[14,15] or upward migration of the humeral head under the acromial arch (acromiohumeral distance < 7 mm) on an AP radiograph with the arm in neutral rotation.[16-20]

Most massive rotator cuff tears are chronic; occur in elderly, less active patients; and are often asymptomatic because they correspond to progressive tendon wear under the acromial arch.[3,4,6,20,21] Many symptomatic patients are best treated nonsurgically,[22-25] but the indications for surgical treatment are not clearly

Dr. Boileau or an immediate family member has received royalties from Tornier; serves as a paid consultant to or is an employee of Smith & Nephew; and serves as a board member, owner, officer, or committee member of the European Society for Surgery of the Shoulder and the Elbow. Neither of the following authors nor any immediate family member has received anything of value from or has stock or stock options held in a commercial company or institution related directly or indirectly to the subject of this chapter: Dr. McClelland and Dr. Rumian.

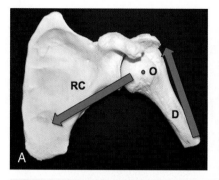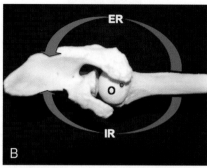

Figure 1   Illustration of the fragile shoulder muscle balance in the vertical (**A**) and horizontal (**B**) planes. With aging, the rotator cuff muscles become weaker, whereas the deltoid muscle remains strong. The external rotator muscles, already inferior in number, become weaker than the internal rotator muscles. O = center of rotation, RC = rotator cuff, D = deltoid, ER = external rotation, IR = internal rotation.

defined.[1,5,6,26-28] Many surgical treatment options have been suggested, including palliative management (including biceps tenotomy and cuff débridement), partial rotator cuff repair, muscle-tendon transfer, reverse shoulder arthroplasty, and combined procedures.

This chapter describes the current muscle balance–based classification for shoulders with massive irreparable rotator cuff tears and presents a treatment algorithm based on this classification.

Muscle Imbalance of the Shoulder

The shoulder is a complex joint affected by a variety of opposing muscular forces. The concept of glenohumeral force couples emphasizes the existence of vertical and horizontal or transverse force couples.[29] It is important to recognize that, in its natural state, the shoulder is unbalanced in both the vertical and horizontal planes (**Figure 1**). Vertically, the power of the deltoid exceeds that of the rotator cuff muscles. Horizontally, the number of internal rotator muscles exceeds the number of external rotator muscles.[30,31] As shoulder pathology ensues, the tenuous relationship that

keeps the shoulder pain free and functional can be disrupted. Consideration of the natural relationship of opposing forces around the shoulder will allow surgeons to appropriately evaluate pathologic disorders and devise treatments to restore shoulder function.

Vertical Muscle Imbalance

With aging, the rotator cuff muscles weaken, whereas the deltoid muscle remains strong. The head-elevating effect of the deltoid begins to overpower the head-depressing effect of the rotator cuff tendons. As this process continues, the rotator cuff tendons are compressed against the undersurface of the acromion, leading to anterosuperior impingement and, ultimately, rotator cuff wear. This pathology is often misrepresented as a rotator cuff tear by surgeons and radiologists, when the pathology is actually a slow progressive erosion of the tendon as opposed to an acute injury. Retraction of the torn rotator cuff tendons is followed by fatty infiltration of the muscles and proximal migration of the humeral head under the acromial arch. With time, this process transforms the shoulder joint into one that looks like a hip joint, and pain may be present. The shoulder is no longer a noncon-

strained joint and becomes a constrained joint (**Figure 2**). On radiographs, the acetabulization of the acromial arch (rounding of the acromion and ossification of the coracoacromial ligament) can be observed, as well as the femoralization of the humeral head (ossification and rounding of the greater tuberosity to articulate with the arch).

Horizontal Muscle Imbalance

In the normally functioning shoulder, four internal rotator muscles (subscapularis, pectoralis major, latissimus dorsi, and teres major) oppose only two external rotator muscles (infraspinatus and teres minor) (**Figure 3**). As the rotator cuff deteriorates with age, the relative effect on the external rotators exceeds that on the internal rotators. This imbalance is evident in the rotator cuff–deficient shoulder as a rotator cuff tear extends posteriorly. If the infraspinatus is torn, four muscles are working against one. The teres minor is the key muscle in maintaining external rotation of the shoulder, providing 40% of the strength in this plane.[32]

A recent MRI study found that 24% of patients with two-tendon rotator cuff tears (supraspinatus and infraspinatus) had associated atrophy of the teres minor.[33] The suggested injury mechanism was traction damage to the teres minor branch of the axillary nerve resulting from the proximal migration of the humeral head. Atrophy of the teres minor appears to be a turning point in the natural history of the disease because of the absence of external rotator muscles to counteract the action of the internal rotator muscles (four muscles working against zero muscles) leads to complete horizontal muscle imbalance. Until recently, the importance of active external rotation has been underestimated. Patients who have marked external rotation weak-

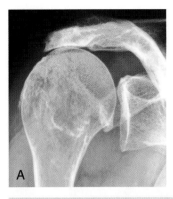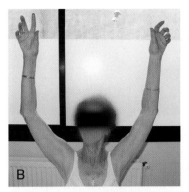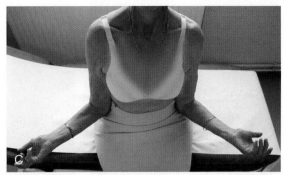

Figure 2   An example of a well-balanced "shoulder-hip joint." **A,** Radiograph showing a massive rotator cuff tear, with femoralization of the proximal humerus and acetabulization of the acromion (Hamada stage 3). Clinically, the shoulder remains well balanced in the vertical plane with normal active elevation (**B**) and in the horizontal plane with normal active external rotation (**C**). The shoulder is pain free because of a spontaneous rupture of the long head of the biceps.

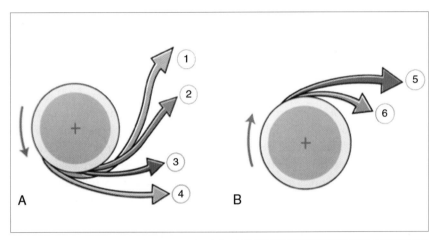

Figure 3   Illustrations of natural horizontal muscle imbalance. **A,** There are four internal rotator muscles: 1= latissimus dorsi, 2 = teres major, 3 = subscapularis, and 4 = pectoralis major. **B,** There are only two external rotator muscles: 5 = infraspinatus and 6 = teres minor.

Table 1

Classification of Patients With Symptomatic Irreparable Massive Rotator Cuff Tears

Patient Group	Symptoms/Shoulder Function
Group 1: Painful loss of active elevation	Pain and temporary vertical muscle imbalance
Group 2: Pseudoparalyzed shoulder or isolated loss of active elevation (See **Figure 4, A**.)	Definitive vertical muscle imbalance
Group 3: Isolated loss of external rotation (See **Figure 4, B**.)	Definitive horizontal muscle imbalance
Group 4: Combined loss of elevation and external rotation (See **Figure 4, C**)	Definitive vertical and horizontal muscle imbalance

ness caused by infraspinatus and teres minor tendon tears will lose the ability to control the positioning of their arms in space.[7,30,34]

Classification of the Rotator Cuff–Deficient Shoulder Based on Muscle Balance

With aging, the already fragile shoulder muscular imbalance can become worse, often because of a traumatic injury, such as a fall onto the upper limb. The clinical evaluation of shoulder muscle balance is easy to perform and allows differentiation of different groups of patients with massive irreparable rotator cuff tears.[7,30] From a biomechanical and surgical standpoint, patients with massive irreparable rotator cuff tears may be categorized into four groups: (1) those with painful loss of active elevation, (2) those with shoulder pseudoparalysis or isolated loss of active elevation, (3) those with an isolated loss of active external rotation, and (4) those with combined loss of active elevation and external rotation.[33] This classification system, which has been used since 2005 in the department of orthopaedic surgery at the L'Archet 2 Hospital (Nice, France), has helped this chapter's authors in the surgical decision-making process to achieve optimal shoulder reconstructions and

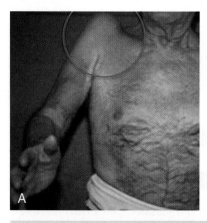
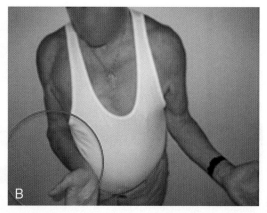
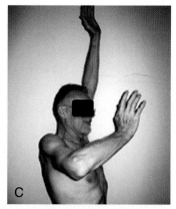

Figure 4 Clinical photographs of patients with shoulder muscle imbalance. **A,** A patient with isolated loss of active elevation resulting from muscle imbalance in the vertical plane. **B,** A patient with isolated loss of external rotation resulting from muscle imbalance in the horizontal plane. **C,** A patient with combined loss of elevation and external rotation resulting from muscle imbalance in both planes.

outcomes (**Table 1**, **Figure 4**). Patients who report painful loss of both active and passive elevation (those with a stiff and so-called frozen shoulder in the absence of degenerative changes) are excluded from initial surgical treatment because they must first be treated with nonsurgical modalities and rehabilitation therapy.

Clinical Presentation and Surgical Management

The clinical presentation of patients with massive irreparable rotator cuff tears depends on the presence or the absence of shoulder muscle balance in one or two planes. If the force couples are no longer balanced, there may be a loss of vertical, horizontal, or both types of muscle balance. In many instances, however, the loss of muscle balance is not definitive but temporary. The shoulder dysfunction can be related to pain, muscle sideration, and/or extension of the tear. A classification system based on muscle balance allows a surgical procedure to be tailored to the patient's symptoms and the type of shoulder muscle imbalance.

Painful Loss of Active Elevation

Patients with rotator cuff tear arthropathy may retain a surprising degree of

function and motion if they have an intact deltoid and acceptable fixed-fulcrum mechanics. However, some patients have pain and a functional deficit. Clinically, these patients demonstrate normal or near normal active external rotation with pain-limited active elevation. The vertical shoulder imbalance is perceived rather than real, and surgeons must realize that these shoulders will elevate if the source of pain is addressed. Usually, active elevation or abduction is more than 90°. Progressive recovery of shoulder elevation is commonly obtained with time, physical therapy, and a decrease in the initial level of pain.

On imaging studies, both the supraspinatus and the infraspinatus are atrophied and have fatty infiltration (Goutallier grade 3 or 4); the teres minor is normal or hypertrophic; and the subscapularis is normal or partially torn, thereby maintaining horizontal balance. Definitive loss of active elevation after a trauma is rare and often temporary. Even in patients with pseudoparalysis, a new shoulder muscle balance often can be achieved with time and rehabilitation.

The shoulder pain cannot be related to the so-called acromial impingement because the bone-to-bone

contact (between the humeral head and the acromion) has been present for many years, as proven by the decreased acromiohumeral space and the fatty infiltration of the rotator cuff muscles. The pain also cannot be related to the rotator cuff tear because the tear also has been present for years. The reasons for pain in massive irreparable rotator cuff tears are not yet fully understood, but the biceps tendon is often a source of pain.[21,35-37]

The surgeon should be sure that the pain and mechanical locking caused by the biceps tendon will not prevent full recovery. Two types of biceps pathology can cause pain and prevent restoration of a new muscle balance: a hypertrophic, entrapped hourglass biceps or an unstable (subluxated or dislocated) biceps.[21,35,36,38] Patients with either of these pathologies are best treated with an arthroscopic biceps tenotomy or tenodesis.[21,35,37] In a partial cuff repair, the goal is not to close the defect but rather restore a stable fulcrum to the glenohumeral joint.[29,39-41] Margin convergence sutures (without closing the superior defect) may improve the mechanical advantage of the rotator cuff and can restore the balance of coronal and transverse force couples.[29,39] For example, isolated repair of the in-

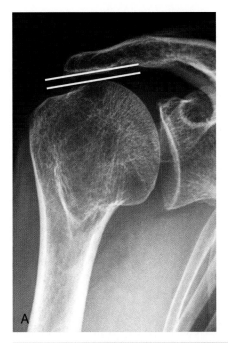
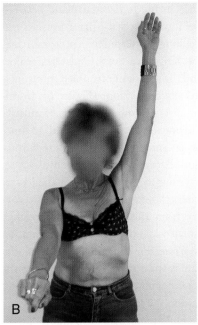
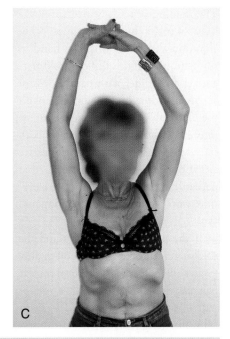

Figure 5   Definitive vertical muscle imbalance results in isolated loss of active elevation. **A,** Preoperative AP radiograph of a massive cuff tear with decreased (< 7 mm) acromiohumeral distance (two parallel lines). **B,** Postoperative clinical photograph of a patient with shoulder pseudoparalysis. Before arthroscopic surgery and acromioplasty to repair an irreparable rotator cuff tear, the patient had active shoulder elevation. **C,** Passive elevation is conserved, thus confirming that this is not a stiff shoulder but a shoulder with definitive loss of the vertical muscle balance.

fraspinatus tendon to bone can substantially improve external rotation strength and functional outcomes, even if the supraspinatus tendon cannot be repaired. The same is true when repairing a partially torn subscapularis tendon.

It is important for the surgeon to be aware of treatments that are contraindicated in patients with massive rotator cuff tears. Because the acromiohumeral distance is 7 mm or less, an acromioplasty is not recommended, and it is even contraindicated in the opinion of this chapter's authors because it can compromise the superior fulcrum and may lead to a loss of active elevation (such as a shoulder with pseudoparalysis). A complete rotator cuff repair is also contraindicated in a massive chronic rotator cuff tear with upward migration of the humerus and fatty infiltration of the rotator cuff muscles. Such a repair should not be used for the following four reasons: (1)

The acromiohumeral distance is decreased, and it is almost impossible to make a rotator cuff repair without performing an acromioplasty, which would compromise the superior fulcrum and may ultimately lead to a shoulder with pseudoparalysis.[8] (2) The tendons are retracted or almost absent. Their reinsertion into the greater tuberosity may ultimately lead to a stiff shoulder and/or increased osteoarthritis.[42,43] (3) The fatty infiltration of the rotator cuff muscles is irreversible, so the tendon repair will not improve muscle status and function.[6,15,17,44] (4) Because the humeral head has been upward migrated for months or years and the rotator cuff muscles lack adequate strength (fatty infiltrated), lowering of the humeral head cannot be achieved, which will ultimately lead to a failed repair.[19,27,35,45,46]

Although some surgeons defend the concept of "rotator cuff repair at all

cost,"[26] the clinical experiences of this chapter's authors have shown that performing surgery on the shoulder of a patient with normal or near normal elevation prior to surgery can result in a shoulder with pseudoparalysis after surgery because of an unrealistic attempt to close a rotator cuff defect[42] (**Figure 5**).

The Shoulder With Pseudoparalysis or Isolated Loss of Active Elevation

Patients with shoulder pseudoparalysis have muscular imbalance in the vertical plane between the intact deltoid muscle and the nonfunctional rotator cuff muscles. As the humeral head migrates superiorly, the glenohumeral center of rotation is altered, and the shoulder is destabilized. Clinical examination reveals that the patient is unable to elevate or abduct the arm to 90°; attempts to do so result in anterosuperior escape of the humeral head.

The landing test is positive (impossibility of maintaining the arm at 90° in elevation/abduction with the hand in supination).[35] If it is difficult to differentiate a shoulder with painful loss of active elevation from a shoulder with pseudoparalysis, the shoulder can be injected with Xylocaine (AstraZeneca). If the pain relief restores active elevation/abduction, this means that patient has painful loss of active elevation, not a shoulder with pseudoparalysis.

If the patient is seen early and the rotator cuff muscles are of good quality (as in sudden loss of the vertical muscle balance after severe trauma), a rotator cuff repair can be attempted (specifically, in young patients) to restore vertical muscle balance. However, most patients with massive cuff tears are seen late, after complete atrophy and fatty infiltration of the rotator cuff muscles. In those instances, a reverse shoulder arthroplasty resolves the problem of vertical muscle imbalance by providing a fixed center of rotation and increasing the deltoid tension and strength to compensate for the weak or torn rotator cuff muscles.[6,30,47-51] Because the results of the reverse shoulder arthroplasty are essentially superior to those reported with hemiarthroplasty, this chapter's authors no longer use the latter procedure.[52-56]

Muscle transfers, such as latissimus dorsi or pectoralis major transfers, have not proved reliable enough to stabilize the shoulder and restore active elevation in patients with shoulder pseudoparalysis.[6,57-59] Muscle transfers are rarely indicated and their use is limited to some salvage procedures in young patients with massive irreparable cuff tears.[55,59-64]

Isolated Loss of Active External Rotation

Patients with isolated loss of active external rotation have muscular imbalance in the horizontal plane between the intact internal rotator muscles (remaining subscapularis, pectoralis major, latissimus dorsi, and teres major) and the absent or atrophied infraspinatus and teres minor (**Figure 6**). In this condition, four functional muscles provide internal rotation, and no functional muscles provide external rotation. Because there are no muscles remaining to compensate for the loss of external rotation, spontaneous recovery from this deficit is not possible. Isolated loss of active external rotation is a rare but disabling condition that results from posterior extension of the rotator cuff tear to involve the teres minor.

Functionally, any attempt at shoulder elevation or abduction results in the forearm swinging inward toward the trunk, resulting in an inability for these patients to control the spatial positioning of their upper limb.[7] Simple activities of daily living, such as shaking hands, drinking, and brushing teeth or hair, become difficult or impossible.[7,65] Rehabilitation is not helpful because there are no external rotator cuff muscles to compensate for the absent infraspinatus and teres minor. The posterior deltoid is not strong enough to compensate for the horizontal muscle deficit. These patients have an external rotation lag sign and a hornblower sign (the need to abduct the arm with the elbow flexed to reach the head).[32,66] In the experience of this chapter's authors, patients with isolated loss of external rotation rarely show spontaneous recovery despite rehabilitation.[7]

A latissimus dorsi and teres major transfer, first described by L'Episcopo,[67] restores external rotation and solves the problem of horizontal muscle imbalance (**Figure 7**). The muscle-tendon transfer alone can rebalance the shoulder in the horizontal plane, resulting in two internal and two external rotators (two against two). The L'Episcopo transfer is performed through a single deltopectoral approach because it is simpler and does not compromise active elevation because the acromial arch remains intact.[7] Alternatively, a latissimus dorsi transfer can be performed.[58,59] Reverse shoulder arthroplasty is not indicated because active elevation is conserved. If pain is present, an associated tenotomy of the long head of the biceps is performed. The isolated L'Episcopo procedure is reserved to treat patients with isolated loss of external rotation who do not have osteoarthritis (Hamada stage 1 and 2).[7] In the rare instances in which the acromial arch is not intact (Hamada stage 3) or the glenohumeral joint is arthritic (Hamada stages 4 and 5), this chapter's authors perform an associated reverse shoulder arthroplasty despite the conserved elevation because possible rapid degradation of the shoulder joint has been observed in patients with advanced stages of the disease.[7]

Combined Loss of Active Elevation and External Rotation

In patients with combined loss of active elevation and external rotation, there is both vertical and horizontal muscle imbalance (**Figure 8**). A reverse shoulder arthroplasty can address the problem of vertical muscle imbalance, but in the presence of an absent or fatty-infiltrated infraspinatus and teres minor, prosthetic lateralization alone is not sufficient to provide active external rotation.[7] For this subgroup of patients, a L'Episcopo transfer should be combined with the reverse shoulder arthroplasty.[7,33,68] Alternatively, a latissimus dorsi transfer can be associated to the reverse shoulder arthroplasty, as proposed by Gerber et al.[69] The tendon transfer eliminates the tendency of the arm to swing inward toward the

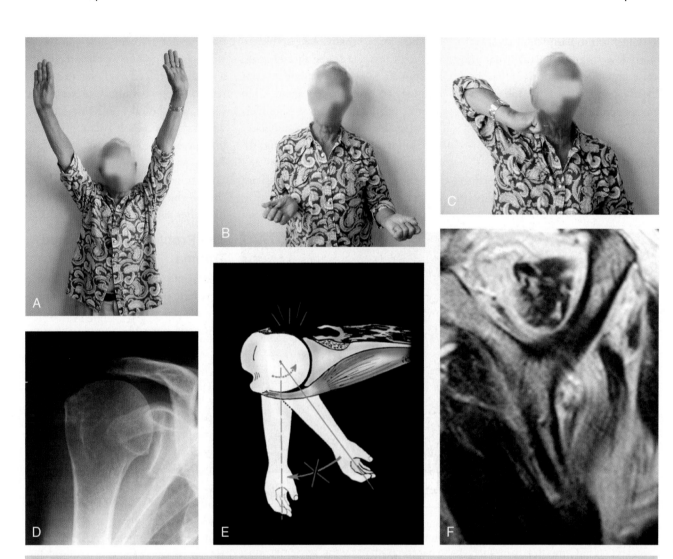

Figure 6 Definitive horizontal muscle imbalance results in isolated loss of active elevation. **A,** The patient has conserved and normal anterior active elevation. **B,** Active external rotation with the arm at the side has been definitively lost. **C,** External rotation is also lost in elevation, leading to an inability to control the positioning of the arm in space and requiring the patient to abduct his arm to reach his head (hornblower sign). **D,** AP radiograph shows upward migration of the humerus, which indicates at least a two-tendon tear (supraspinatus and infraspinatus). **E,** The absence or atrophy of external rotator cuff muscles (with conserved internal rotator muscles) explains the definitive loss of active external rotation. **F,** Sagittal MRI scan confirms the complete atrophy and fatty infiltration of the supraspinatus, infraspinatus, and teres minor muscles.

trunk during abduction or elevation, thereby improving spatial control of the limb and restoring the ability to perform the activities of daily living (**Figure 9**).

The combined procedure, performed in the same session through a deltopectoral approach, is indicated in a select subgroup of patients with a rotator cuff–deficient shoulder and an absent or atrophied infraspinatus and teres minor. It is important to realize

that patients who are able to maintain a minimum of neutral rotation with the arm at the side do not have combined loss of active elevation and external rotation. In addition, this disorder should not be confused with stiffness, which results in loss of active and passive external rotation.[7,33,68]

Most authors report external rotation as an amount of rotation measured in degrees with the arm by the side. However, the importance of ac-

tive external rotation is its function in acting as an antagonist to the force of gravity on the upper limb when the limb is positioned away from the trunk. If there is no active external rotation, gravity drives the arm inward and toward the trunk without control. This effect can be accentuated after reverse shoulder arthroplasty for rotator cuff tear arthropathy.[33,68] If the stiff arthritic rotator cuff–deficient shoulder is replaced by a low-friction reverse shoulder arthroplasty, this may reveal a hornblower sign and actually compromise shoulder function. It has been clearly demonstrated that the results of reverse shoulder arthroplasty are inferior if the teres minor is deficient.[7,50]

Algorithm for Treatment

The surgeon should consider three questions when treating a patient with a symptomatic massive irreparable rotator cuff tear. (1) Is the shoulder still functional? (Has the shoulder joint adapted to become a good "hip joint"?) In such a case, the "shoulder-hip" must be respected. Acromioplasty (risk of losing active elevation) and rotator cuff repair (risk of stiffness and worsening osteoarthritis) should not be performed. (2) If the shoulder is functional but painful, is the biceps still present? In such a case, the problem can be solved easily by an arthroscopic biceps tenotomy or tenodesis. (3) If the shoulder is nonfunctional, which type of muscle balance (vertical, horizontal, or both) has been lost? Based on the answers to these questions, the surgeon will be able to choose the best treatment option for his or her patient (**Figures 10** and **11**).

The Problem of Associated Trauma

The fragile shoulder muscle balance in an elderly patient with a massive rotator cuff tear is often lost after a minor traumatic event. As a result, the clinical picture may become more complex; both rotator cuff wear and tear are responsible for the symptoms and the impairment. For example, a pseudoparalytic shoulder is commonly seen immediately after a traumatic event. It may be challenging to determine if this is a real pseudoparalytic shoulder (isolated loss of active elevation) with definitive loss of the fragile muscle balance or a temporary loss of muscle balance related to pain, muscular sideration, or tear extension (painful loss of active elevation). The surgeon must

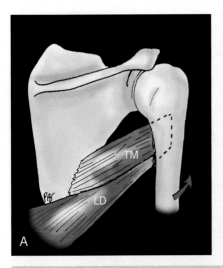
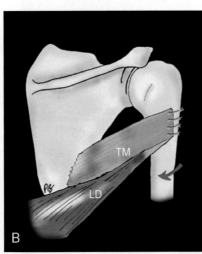

Figure 7   Illustration of the modified L'Episcopo transfer used to rebalance the shoulder in the horizontal plane. **A,** The latissimus dorsi (LD) and teres major (TM) muscles are harvested as a single musculotendinous unit. **B,** Transfer to the posterolateral humerus changes the vector to exert external rotation on the arm. Internal rotation is still accomplished by the pectoralis major and subscapularis muscles.

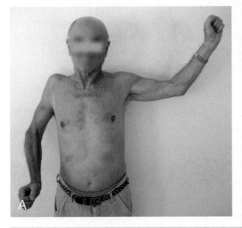
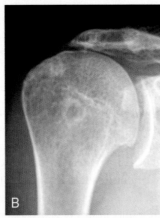
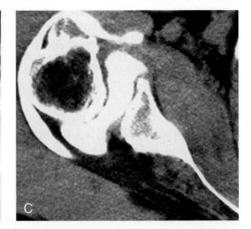

Figure 8   Definitive horizontal and vertical muscle imbalance results in a combined loss of active elevation and external rotation. **A,** Clinical photograph of a patient who is unable to elevate, abduct, and externally rotate his arm because of a definitive loss of vertical and horizontal muscle balance. **B,** Radiograph shows proximal humeral migration (Hamada and Fukuda stage 3 rotator cuff tear arthropathy). This "shoulder-hip joint" is not functional. **C,** Axial CT arthrogram shows complete atrophy and fatty infiltration (Goutallier stage 4) of the infraspinatus and teres minor muscles.

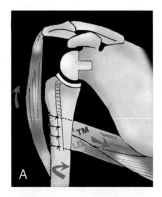
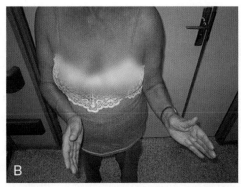
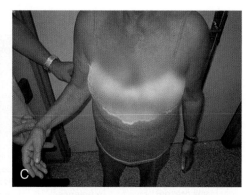

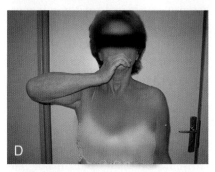
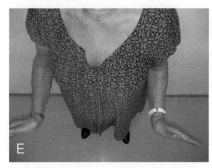

Figure 9   A combined procedure (reverse shoulder arthroplasty and L'Episcopo transfer) is used to rebalance the shoulder in both the horizontal and the vertical planes in a patient with combined loss of active elevation and external rotation. **A,** External rotation is restored by the latissimus dorsi (LD)/ teres major (TM) transfer, whereas active elevation is restored by the action of the deltoid with the reverse shoulder arthroplasty. Preoperative photographs demonstrate loss of active external rotation (**B**), maintained passive external rotation (**C**), and a positive hornblower sign (**D**). After a reverse shoulder arthroplasty and L'Episcopo transfer, the patient has improved active external rotation (**E**), a negative hornblower sign (**F**), and restored active elevation (**G**).

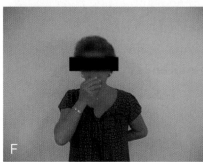
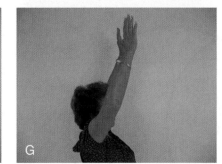

determine if it would be better to temporize or proceed with early surgical treatment. In these circumstances, CT or MRI studies can be helpful because they aid in determing the chronicity of the so-called massive rotator cuff tear (the presence of severe fatty infiltration and thin tendon ends). In such instances, the surgeon should not encourage the patient to elect surgical treatment but should begin conservative medical treatment and rehabilitation. Progressive recovery of active shoulder motion (new muscle balance) is commonly obtained, with a decrease in pain and the need for physical therapy. Conversely, if imaging studies show favorable prognostic factors, such as the absence of the early stages

of muscle fatty infiltration and thick tendon ends, repair should be performed without delay.

It has been shown that large defects in the rotator cuff are compatible with good function.[3,4,70] This finding challenges the validity of classifying rotator cuff tears by size only, and the concept that size correlates directly with the resulting functional deficit. Therefore, current management strategies for these lesions should be reevaluated. In degenerative lesions, nature has ample time to rearrange the mechanics of the shoulder joint to prevent the development of dysfunction. In a traumatic rupture, time for this natural mechanical rearrangement is lacking; thus, marked impairment of function can be

result. However, with time, the necessary natural alterations to restore function may occur.

Summary

Irreparability of the rotator cuff tear is indicated by a severe tendon retraction (Patte stage 3 or greater), an acromiohumeral distance of less than 7 mm, and fatty infiltration of muscle (Goutallier stage 3 or greater). In patients with symptomatic massive irreparable rotator cuff tears, the muscle balance can be conserved or lost in the vertical plane, the horizontal plane, or both planes. Assessment of the plane of shoulder muscle imbalance is a key feature in the decision-making process. Patients with an irreparable tear can be

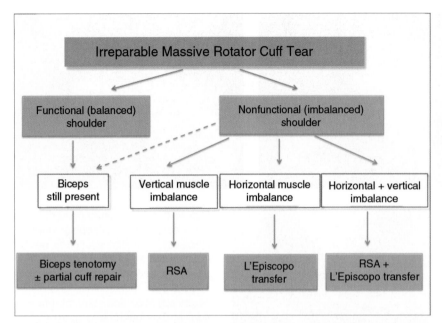

Figure 10 Algorithm for treating irreparable massive rotator cuff tears. RSA = reverse shoulder arthroplasty.

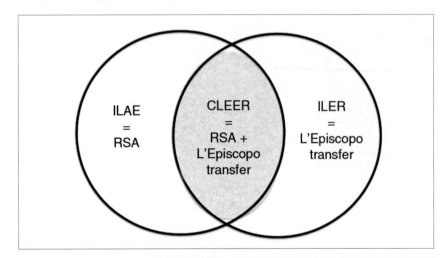

Figure 11 Illustration of the surgical treatment of a nonfunctional rotator cuff–deficient shoulder. ILAE = isolated loss of active elevation, RSA = reverse shoulder arthroplasty, CLEER = combined loss of active elevation and external rotation, ILER = isolated loss of active external rotation.

categorized into four groups: those with painful loss of active elevation, those with shoulder pseudoparalysis or isolated loss of active elevation, those with an isolated loss of active external rotation, and those with combined loss of active elevation and external rotation.

For patients in whom surgery is indicated, the best procedure is tailored to the patient's symptoms and the type of muscular imbalance. Patients with pain-limited active elevation have no real loss of vertical and horizontal muscle balance. Because their shoulder pain and dysfunction is mainly related to a pathologic biceps tendon and possible extension of the tear, they are best treated with an arthroscopic biceps tenotomy/tenodesis, with or without partial rotator cuff repair. Patients with shoulder pseudoparalysis have a definitive muscular imbalance in the vertical plane. Because their vertical muscle balance cannot be restored with rehabilitation or a rotator cuff repair, these patients are best treated with a reverse shoulder arthroplasty. Patients with isolated loss of active external rotation have a definitive muscular imbalance in the horizontal plane because of the absence of external rotator cuff muscles. These patients are best treated with an isolated latissimus dorsi and teres major transfer, with or without biceps tenotomy/tenodesis. In patients with combined loss of active elevation and external rotation, there is both vertical and horizontal muscle imbalance; these patients are best treated with a latissimus dorsi and teres major tendon transfer combined with a reverse shoulder arthroplasty.

References

1. Bedi A, Dines J, Warren RF, Dines DM: Massive tears of the rotator cuff. *J Bone Joint Surg Am* 2010;92(9):1894-1908.

2. Bokor DJ, Hawkins RJ, Huckell GH, Angelo RL, Schickendantz MS: Results of nonoperative management of full-thickness tears of the rotator cuff. *Clin Orthop Relat Res* 1993;294:103-110.

3. DePalma AF, White JB, Callery G: Degenerative lesions of the shoulder at various age groups are compatible with good function. *Instr Course Lect* 1950;7:168-180.

4. DePalma AF: Surgical anatomy of the rotator cuff and the natural history of degenerative periarthritis. *Surg Clin North Am* 1963;43:1507-1520.

5. Dines DM, Moynihan DP, Dines JS, McCann P: Irreparable rotator cuff tears: What to do and when to do it. The surgeon's dilemma. *Instr Course Lect* 2007;56:13-22.

6. Gerber C, Wirth SH, Farshad M: Treatment options for massive rotator cuff tears. *J Shoulder Elbow Surg* 2011;20(2):S20-S29.

7. Boileau P, Chuinard C, Roussanne Y, Neyton L, Trojani C: Modified latissimus dorsi and teres major transfer through a single delto-pectoral approach for external rotation deficit of the shoulder: As an isolated procedure or with a reverse arthroplasty. *J Shoulder Elbow Surg* 2007;16(6):671-682.

8. Colachis SC Jr, Strohm BR: Effect of suprascapular and axillary nerve blocks on muscle force in upper extremity. *Arch Phys Med Rehabil* 1971;52(1):22-29.

9. Favard L, Berhouet J, Colmar M, et al: Massive rotator cuff tears in patients younger than 65 years: What treatment options are available? *Orthop Traumatol Surg Res* 2009;95(4):S19-S26.

10. Howell SM, Imobersteg AM, Seger DH, Marone PJ: Clarification of the role of the supraspinatus muscle in shoulder function. *J Bone Joint Surg Am* 1986;68(3):398-404.

11. McMahon PJ, Debski RE, Thompson WO, Warner JJ, Fu FH, Woo SL: Shoulder muscle forces and tendon excursions during glenohumeral abduction in the scapular plane. *J Shoulder Elbow Surg* 1995;4(3):199-208.

12. Neer CS II, Craig EV, Fukuda H: Cuff-tear arthropathy. *J Bone Joint Surg Am* 1983;65(9):1232-1244.

13. Patte D: Classification of rotator cuff lesions. *Clin Orthop Relat Res* 1990;254:81-86.

14. Goutallier D, Postel JM, Bernageau J, Lavau L, Voisin MC: Fatty muscle degeneration in cuff ruptures: Pre- and postoperative evaluation by CT scan. *Clin Orthop Relat Res* 1994;304:78-83.

15. Goutallier D, Postel JM, Gleyze P, Leguilloux P, Van Driessche S: Influence of cuff muscle fatty degeneration on anatomic and functional outcomes after simple suture of full-thickness tears. *J Shoulder Elbow Surg* 2003;12(6):550-554.

16. Hamada K, Fukuda H, Mikasa M, Kobayashi Y: Roentgenographic findings in massive rotator cuff tears: A long-term observation. *Clin Orthop Relat Res* 1990;254:92-96.

17. Melis B, Nemoz C, Walch G: Muscle fatty infiltration in rotator cuff tears: Descriptive analysis of 1688 cases. *Orthop Traumatol Surg Res* 2009;95(5):319-324.

18. Nové-Josserand L, Lévigne C, Noël E, Walch G: The acromio-humeral interval: A study of the factors influencing its height. *Rev Chir Orthop Reparatrice Appar Mot* 1996;82(5):379-385.

19. Walch G, Maréchal E, Maupas J, Liotard JP: Surgical treatment of rotator cuff rupture: Prognostic factors. *Rev Chir Orthop Reparatrice Appar Mot* 1992;78(6):379-388.

20. Weiner DS, Macnab I: Superior migration of the humeral head: A radiological aid in the diagnosis of tears of the rotator cuff. *J Bone Joint Surg Br* 1970;52(3):524-527.

21. Boileau P, Ahrens PM, Hatzidakis AM: Entrapment of the long head of the biceps tendon: The hourglass biceps. A cause of pain and locking of the shoulder. *J Shoulder Elbow Surg* 2004;13(3):249-257.

22. Goldberg BA, Nowinski RJ, Matsen FA III: Outcome of nonoperative management of full-thickness rotator cuff tears. *Clin Orthop Relat Res* 2001;382:99-107.

23. Rockwood CA Jr, Williams GR Jr, Burkhead WZ Jr, irreparable lesions of the rotator cuff. *J Bone Joint Surg Am* 1995;77(6):857-866.

24. Yamaguchi K, Tetro AM, Blam O, Evanoff BA, Teefey SA, Middleton WD: Natural history of asymptomatic rotator cuff tears: A longitudinal analysis of asymptomatic tears detected sonographically. *J Shoulder Elbow Surg* 2001;10(3):199-203.

25. Zingg PO, Jost B, Sukthankar A, Buhler M, Pfirrmann CW, Gerber C: Clinical and structural outcomes of nonoperative management of massive rotator cuff tears. *J Bone Joint Surg Am* 2007;89(9):1928-1934.

26. Burkhart SS, Barth JR, Richards DP, Zlatkin MB, Larsen M: Arthroscopic repair of massive rotator cuff tears with stage 3 and 4 fatty degeneration. *Arthroscopy* 2007;23(4):347-354.

27. Galatz LM, Ball CM, Teefey SA, Middleton WD, Yamaguchi K: The outcome and repair integrity of completely arthroscopically repaired large and massive rotator cuff tears. *J Bone Joint Surg Am* 2004;86(2):219-224.

28. Visotsky JL, Basamania C, Seebauer L, Rockwood CA, Jensen KL: Cuff tear arthropathy: Pathogenesis, classification, and algorithm for treatment. *J Bone Joint Surg Am* 2004;86(suppl 2):35-40.

29. Burkhart SS: Fluoroscopic comparison of kinematic patterns in massive rotator cuff tears: A suspension bridge model. *Clin Orthop Relat Res* 1992;284:144-152.

30. Boileau P, Watkinson D, Hatzidakis AM, Hovorka I: The Grammont reverse shoulder prosthesis: Results in cuff tear arthritis, fracture sequelae, and revision arthroplasty. *J Shoulder Elbow Surg* 2006;15(5):527-540.

31. Kapandji IA. *The Physiology of the Joint: Upper Limb*, ed 5. London, England, Churchill Livingstone, 1983.

32. Walch G, Boulahia A, Calderone S, Robinson AH: The 'dropping' and 'hornblower's' signs in evaluation of rotator-cuff tears. *J Bone Joint Surg Br* 1998;80(4):624-628.

33. Boileau P, Rumian AP, Zumstein MA: Reversed shoulder arthroplasty with modified L'Episcopo for combined loss of active elevation and external rotation. *J Shoulder Elbow Surg* 2010;19(2): 20-30.

34. Thompson WO, Debski RE, Boardman ND III, et al: A biomechanical analysis of rotator cuff deficiency in a cadaveric model. *Am J Sports Med* 1996;24(3): 286-292.

35. Boileau P, Baqué F, Valerio L, Ahrens P, Chuinard C, Trojani C: Isolated arthroscopic biceps tenotomy or tenodesis improves symptoms in patients with massive irreparable rotator cuff tears. *J Bone Joint Surg Am* 2007;89(4): 747-757.

36. Szabó I, Boileau P, Walch G: The proximal biceps as a pain generator and results of tenotomy. *Sports Med Arthrosc* 2008;16(3): 180-186.

37. Walch G, Edwards TB, Boulahia A, Nové-Josserand L, Neyton L, Szabo I: Arthroscopic tenotomy of the long head of the biceps in the treatment of rotator cuff tears: Clinical and radiographic results of 307 cases. *J Shoulder Elbow Surg* 2005;14(3):238-246.

38. Walch G, Nové-Josserand L, Boileau P, Levigne C: Subluxations and dislocations of the tendon of the long head of the biceps. *J Shoulder Elbow Surg* 1998;7(2): 100-108.

39. Burkhart SS: Partial repair of massive rotator cuff tears: The evolution of a concept. *Orthop Clin North Am* 1997;28(1):125-132.

40. Duralde XA, Bair B: Massive rotator cuff tears: The result of partial rotator cuff repair. *J Shoulder Elbow Surg* 2005;14(2):121-127.

41. Klinger HM, Spahn G, Baums MH, Steckel H: Arthroscopic débridement of irreparable massive rotator cuff tears: A comparison of debridement alone and combined procedure with biceps tenotomy. *Acta Chir Belg* 2005; 105(3):297-301.

42. Boileau P, Gonzalez JF, Chuinard C, Bicknell R, Walch G: Reverse total shoulder arthroplasty after failed rotator cuff surgery. *J Shoulder Elbow Surg* 2009;18(4): 600-606.

43. Gartsman GM: Massive, irreparable tears of the rotator cuff: Results of operative debridement and subacromial decompression. *J Bone Joint Surg Am* 1997;79(5): 715-721.

44. Gerber C, Fuchs B, Hodler J: The results of repair of massive tears of the rotator cuff. *J Bone Joint Surg Am* 2000;82(4):505-515.

45. Jost B, Pfirrmann CW, Gerber C, Switzerland Z: Clinical outcome after structural failure of rotator cuff repairs. *J Bone Joint Surg Am* 2000;82(3):304-314.

46. Zumstein MA, Jost B, Hempel J, Hodler J, Gerber C: The clinical and structural long-term results of open repair of massive tears of the rotator cuff. *J Bone Joint Surg Am* 2008;90(11):2423-2431.

47. Cuff D, Pupello D, Virani N, Levy J, Frankle M: Reverse shoulder arthroplasty for the treatment of rotator cuff deficiency. *J Bone Joint Surg Am* 2008;90(6):1244-1251.

48. Molé D, Favard L: Excentered scapulohumeral osteoarthritis. *Rev Chir Orthop Reparatrice Appar Mot* 2007;93(6):37-94.

49. Sirveaux F, Favard L, Oudet D, Huquet D, Walch G, Molé D: Grammont inverted total shoulder arthroplasty in the treatment of glenohumeral osteoarthritis with massive rupture of the cuff: Results of a multicentre study of 80 shoulders. *J Bone Joint Surg Br* 2004;86(3):388-395.

50. Wall B, Nové-Josserand L, O'Connor DP, Edwards TB, Walch G: Reverse total shoulder arthroplasty: A review of results according to etiology. *J Bone Joint Surg Am* 2007;89(7):1476-1485.

51. Werner CM, Steinmann PA, Gilbart M, Gerber C: Treatment of painful pseudoparesis due to irreparable rotator cuff dysfunction with the Delta III reverse-ball-and-socket total shoulder prosthesis. *J Bone Joint Surg Am* 2005; 87(7):1476-1486.

52. Favard L, Lautmann S, Sirveaux F, Oudet D, Kerjean Y, Huguet D: Hemiarthroplasty versus reverse arthroplasty in the treatment of osteoarthritis with massive rotator cuff tear, in Walch G, Boileau P, Mole D, eds: *2000 Shoulder Prostheses: Two to Ten Year Follow-up.* Paris, France, Sauramps Medical, 2001, pp. 261-268.

53. Field LD, Dines DM, Zabinski SJ, Warren RF: Hemiarthroplasty of the shoulder for rotator cuff arthropathy. *J Shoulder Elbow Surg* 1997;6(1):18-23.

54. Goldberg SS, Bell JE, Kim HJ, Bak SF, Levine WN, Bigliani LU: Hemiarthroplasty for the rotator cuff-deficient shoulder. *J Bone Joint Surg Am* 2008;90(3): 554-559.

55. Warner JJ: Management of massive irreparable rotator cuff tears: The role of tendon transfer. *Instr Course Lect* 2001;50:63-71.

56. Williams GR Jr, Rockwood CA Jr: Hemiarthroplasty in rotator cuff-deficient shoulders. *J Shoulder Elbow Surg* 1996;5(5): 362-367.

57. Costouros JG, Espinosa N, Schmid MR, Gerber C: Teres minor integrity predicts outcome of latissimus dorsi tendon transfer for irreparable rotator cuff tears. *J Shoulder Elbow Surg* 2007;16(6): 727-734.

58. Gerber C, Vinh TS, Hertel R, Hess CW: Latissimus dorsi transfer for the treatment of massive tears of the rotator cuff: A prelim-

inary report. *Clin Orthop Relat Res* 1988;232:51-61.

59. Gerber C, Maquieira G, Espinosa N: Latissimus dorsi transfer for the treatment of irreparable rotator cuff tears. *J Bone Joint Surg Am* 2006;88(1):113-120.

60. Elhassan B, Ozbaydar M, Massimini D, Diller D, Higgins L, Warner JJ: Transfer of pectoralis major for the treatment of irreparable tears of subscapularis: Does it work? *J Bone Joint Surg Br* 2008;90(8):1059-1065.

61. Iannotti JP, Hennigan S, Herzog R, et al: Latissimus dorsi tendon transfer for irreparable posterosuperior rotator cuff tears: Factors affecting outcome. *J Bone Joint Surg Am* 2006;88(2):342-348.

62. Nové-Josserand L, Costa P, Liotard JP, Safar JF, Walch G, Zilber S: Results of latissimus dorsi tendon transfer for irreparable cuff tears. *Orthop Traumatol Surg Res* 2009;95(2):108-113.

63. Resch H, Povacz P, Ritter E, Matschi W: Transfer of the pectoralis major muscle for the treat-ment of irreparable rupture of the subscapularis tendon. *J Bone Joint Surg Am* 2000;82(3):372-382.

64. Warner JJ, Parsons IM IV: Latissimus dorsi tendon transfer: A comparative analysis of primary and salvage reconstruction of massive, irreparable rotator cuff tears. *J Shoulder Elbow Surg* 2001;10(6):514-521.

65. Boileau P, Rumian A, Alami GB, Melis B, McClelland WB Jr, in Boileau P, ed: *Shoulder Concepts 2012: Arthroscopy, Arthroplasty and Fractures.* Montpellier, France, Sauramps Médical, 2012.

66. Hertel R, Ballmer FT, Lombert SM, Gerber C: Lag signs in the diagnosis of rotator cuff rupture. *J Shoulder Elbow Surg* 1996;5(4):307-313.

67. L'Episcopo JB: Tendon transplantation in obstetrical paralysis. *Am J Surg* 1934;25:122-125.

68. Boileau P, Chuinard C, Roussanne Y, Bicknell RT, Rochet N, Trojani C: Reverse shoulder arthroplasty combined with a modified latissimus dorsi and teres major tendon transfer for shoulder pseudoparalysis associated with dropping arm. *Clin Orthop Relat Res* 2008;466(3):584-593.

69. Gerber C, Pennington SD, Lingenfelter EJ, Sukthankar A: Reverse Delta-III total shoulder replacement combined with latissimus dorsi transfer: A preliminary report. *J Bone Joint Surg Am* 2007;89(5):940-947.

70. DePalma AF: *Surgery of the Shoulder*, ed 3. Philadelphia, PA, JB Lippincott, 1983.

Video Reference

Chalmers PN, Frank RM, Gupta AK, et al: *All-Arthroscopic Patch Augmentation of a Massive Rotator Cuff Tear: Surgical Technique* [video]. Rosemont, IL, American Academy of Orthopaedic Surgeons, 2014. *Orthopaedic Video Theater 2.* http://orthoportal.aaos.org/emedia/singleVideoPlayer.aspx?resource=EMEDIA_OSVL_14_02. Accessed January 2, 2014.

8

What Went Wrong and What Was Done About It: Pitfalls in the Treatment of Common Shoulder Surgery

Brent B. Wiesel, MD
Gary M. Gartsman, MD
Cyrus M. Press, MD
Edwin E. Spencer Jr, MD
Brent J. Morris, MD
Joseph D. Zuckerman, MD
Reza Roghani, MD
Gerald R. Williams Jr, MD

Abstract

When performing revision shoulder surgery, it is important that the surgeon understands why the index procedure failed and has a clear plan to address problems in the revision procedure. The most common cause of failure after anterior instability shoulder surgery is a failure to treat the underlying glenoid bone loss. For most defects, a Latarjet transfer can effectively restore anterior glenoid bone stock and restore shoulder stability. Persistent anterior shoulder pain after rotator cuff surgery may be the result of missed biceps pathology. This can be effectively treated via a biceps tenodesis. The most difficult failures to treat after acromioclavicular joint reconstruction surgery are those involving fractures of either the coracoid or the clavicle. Clavicle hook plates can be used as supplemental fixation during the treatment of these fractures to help offload the fracture site and allow healing while restoring stability to the acromioclavicular articulation. A failed hemiarthroplasty for a proximal humeral fracture frequently results when the tuberosities fail to heal correctly. This complication can be avoided by paying close attention to the implant position and the tuberosity fixation. If hemiarthroplasty is unsuccessful, the patient is best treated with conversion to a reverse shoulder arthroplasty.

Inst Course Lect 2014;63:85-93.

Fortunately, most shoulder surgical procedures yield consistently good results. However, when a surgical procedure fails, identifying and eliminating the causative factors helps make the revision procedure successful. This chapter highlights common problems that can occur during surgery to treat shoulder instability, rotator cuff tears, acromioclavicular joint dislocations, and proximal humeral fractures and discusses techniques that can be used to address these problems during revision surgery.

Instability Surgery

There are multiple complications that can occur after surgery to treat glenohumeral instability, including recurrent instability, stiffness, arthritis, loose or prominent implants, nerve injury, and infection. The most common complication following an anterior soft-tissue repair is recurrent glenohumeral instability secondary to bone loss. The remainder of this section focuses on the evaluation and treatment of these patients. Burkhart and De Beer[1] reported a 4% incidence of recurrent instability after an arthroscopic Bankart repair in patients without substantial bone loss compared with a 67% rate of recurrence with anterior-glenoid bone loss or an engaging Hill-Sachs lesion.

A 33-year-old physician (case 1) underwent an arthroscopic Bankart repair for traumatic anterior glenohu-

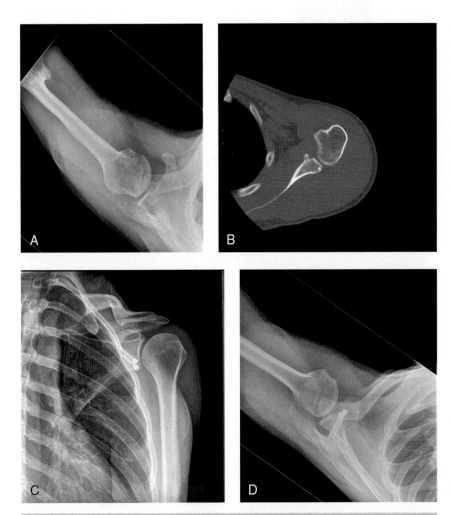

Figure 1 Case 1. A 30-year-old physician had previously undergone an arthroscopic Bankart repair for traumatic anterior glenohumeral instability. A redislocation occurred within 3 months after the original surgery, and the patient continued to have frequent dislocations with daily activities. Axillary radiographs (**A**) and an axial CT scan (**B**) show substantial anterior glenoid bone loss, which was treated with a Latarjet transfer (**C** and **D**).

ure 1, A). A CT scan with three-dimensional reconstructions and digital subtraction of the humeral head was obtained to further evaluate for potential osseous causes of instability. If the patient has had a prior open repair and there is concern on physical examination for the integrity of the subscapularis muscle, an MRI arthrogram or ultrasound can be added to the imaging evaluation. The CT scan of this patient demonstrated a large anteroinferior glenoid bone fragment (**Figure 1, B**). If the length of the anterior glenoid bone fragment is greater than the maximum radius of the glenoid, then the force required to dislocate the joint is reduced by at least 30%.[2]

A Latarjet transfer is the procedure of choice of this chapter's authors for treating most patients with anterior glenoid bone loss. In addition to providing an anterior bone block, this procedure reestablishes stability of the shoulder via a sling created anterior to the humeral head by the conjoint tendon and reinforcement of the anterior capsule with the stump of the coracoacromial ligament.[3] Several recently introduced commercial products make this procedure technically easier by aiding the surgeon in placing the coracoid fragment flush with the glenoid articular surface and correctly spacing the fixation screws so that they do not split the fragment. Walch and Boileau[4] reported a recurrence rate of 1% in a study of 160 patients, with more than 98% of the patients rating their results as good or excellent. More recently,

meral joint instability. He had a redislocation 3 months after the index procedure and continued to have frequent dislocations with daily activities. On physical examination, he had slightly reduced external rotation, a negative abdominal compression test, and substantial apprehension with apprehension testing. An axillary radiograph showed a concentrically reduced glenohumeral joint with irregularity of the anterior aspect of the glenoid (**Fig-**

Dr. Gartsman or an immediate family member is a member of a speakers' bureau or has made paid presentations on behalf of Tornier; serves as a paid consultant to Tornier; and has received research or institutional support from Tornier. Dr. Spencer or an immediate family member has received royalties from Tornier; serves as a paid consultant to Tornier; has stock or stock options held in Tornier; and has received research or institutional support from DePuy and Tornier. Dr. Zuckerman or an immediate family member has received royalties from Exactech; has stock or stock options held in Hip Innovation Technology and Neostem; has received nonincome support (such as equipment or services), commercially derived honoraria, or other non–research-related funding (such as paid travel) from Orthonet; and serves as a board member, owner, officer, or committee member of the American Orthopaedic Association. Dr. Williams or an immediate family member has received royalties from DePuy; is a member of a speakers' bureau or has made paid presentations on behalf of DePuy; serves as a paid consultant to DePuy; has stock or stock options held in In Vivo Therapeutics; has received research or institutional support from Tornier; and serves as a board member, owner, officer, or committee member of the American Shoulder and Elbow Surgeons, the Mid-Atlantic Shoulder and Elbow Society, and the Pennsylvania Orthopaedic Society. None of the following authors or any immediate family member has received anything of value from or has stock or stock options held in a commercial company or institution related directly or indirectly to the subject of this chapter: Dr. Wiesel, Dr. Press, Dr. Morris, and Dr. Roghani.

Shah et al[5] found a 25% complication rate, including a 10% rate of neurologic injury, with this surgery in the hands of an experienced, fellowship-trained shoulder surgeon. This patient had a Latarjet transfer performed through a subscapularis split (**Figure 1, C** and **D**) and had returned to all activities with no further instability at the time of the latest follow-up.

One area that has not been fully defined is the upper limit of size for which glenoid defects can be effectively treated with a coracoid transfer. For larger defects, Warner et al[6] reported good results with reconstruction of the anterior aspect of the glenoid using tricortical iliac crest autograft. Although this procedure does not allow for reinforcement of the osseous repair with a soft-tissue sling, it does have the advantage of preserving the normal anatomic relationships anterior to the glenohumeral joint, which facilitates later surgery. As an alternative to iliac crest autograft, Provencher et al[7] presented encouraging results using distal tibial allograft to reconstruct the anterior aspect of the glenoid. They noted that the distal tibial articular surface has a radius of curvature that closely approximates that of the anterior aspect of the glenoid. A concern with this procedure is the possibility of graft resorption, and no long-term follow-up data are available.

Although anterior glenoid deficiency tends to be more problematic, posterior humeral head defects can also contribute to recurrent instability. What constitutes a clinically important humeral head-sized defect remains another area of controversy. For large, engaging Hill-Sachs defects with no anterior glenoid bone loss, Boileau et al[8] recently reported excellent results in a prospective study combining an arthroscopic Bankart repair with imbrication of the infraspinatus tendon

into the humeral head defect using two suture anchors placed transtendinously. The authors referred to this as an arthroscopic remplissage and stated that this procedure is not appropriate if there is any glenoid bone loss. For small- to medium-sized Hill-Sachs defects combined with anterior glenoid bone loss, this chapter's authors typically perform a Latarjet transfer. For defects that are greater than 25% to 30% of the humeral articular surface, Miniaci and Gish[9] described filling the defect with a wedge of humeral head allograft secured with two countersunk screws. This can be combined with a procedure to restore anterior glenoid bone loss if needed.

Rotator Cuff Surgery

Although most patients treated with rotator cuff repair obtain pain relief and return of strength, some have suboptimal outcomes. There are many reasons for persistent pain after rotator cuff repair that may occur singularly or in combination. These include biceps tendon entrapment, biceps tears and/or degeneration, labral tears, postoperative stiffness, unrecognized preexisting adhesive capsulitis, failure of rotator cuff healing, retearing of the rotator cuff, acromioclavicular arthrosis, suprascapular nerve compression, cervical radiculopathy, and scapular dyskinesis. A failure to assess and recognize these issues during the preoperative and intraoperative evaluation increases the risk for persistent postoperative pain. A careful and thorough evaluation of these potential complicating factors is recommended before rotator cuff surgery.

Although each of these causes is a topic in itself, this discussion is limited to biceps pathology because this concomitant pathology is often undertreated during rotator cuff surgery, and a failure to address the biceps can lead to persistent pain. Biceps lesions com-

monly occur, are difficult to diagnose, and have multiple treatment options. There is no consensus about the optimal treatment. Management of the biceps tendon during rotator cuff repair continues to evolve, and controversy exists regarding the true function of the biceps. Some surgeons prefer to leave it intact during rotator cuff repair if an abnormality is not readily apparent. Some surgeons believe that with rotator cuff tears, the biceps acts as a secondary humeral head depressor and should be preserved even with some biceps degeneration.

In an illustrative example, a 62-year-old man (case 2) underwent an uncomplicated rotator cuff repair but continued to report anterior shoulder pain. A normal intra-articular biceps tendon was seen during surgery. Resisted forward flexion and the O'Brien test produced pain in the area of the biceps groove. An MRI scan showed rotator cuff healing. An ultrasound-guided injection of the biceps sheath resulted in partial pain relief. At the time of arthroscopic examination, flexion of the arm showed that the patient had the hourglass lesion as described by Boileau et al[10] (**Figure 2, A**). The arthroscope was inserted into the subacromial space, and the biceps sheath was opened distal to the transverse humeral ligament. Tendon degeneration was identified (**Figure 2, B**). The biceps was tenodesed in its groove with an interference screw midway between the transverse humeral ligament and the pectoralis major tendon insertion (**Figure 2, C**). The patient recovered uneventfully, gaining complete movement and pain relief.

After rotator cuff repair, an abnormal or normal biceps tendon may become a source of postoperative pain. Rotator cuff tears that involve the anterior portion of the supraspinatus, when repaired, are in direct contact with the biceps tendon. The repeated

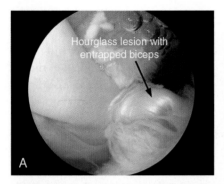 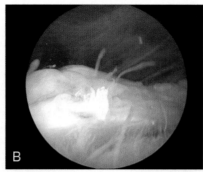 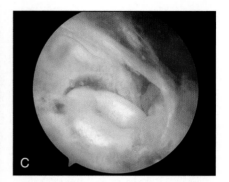

Figure 2 Case 2. A 62-year-old man was treated with an uncomplicated rotator cuff repair but continued to report anterior shoulder pain. **A,** An arthroscopic view showing the hourglass lesion (arrow), as described by Boileau et al.[10] **B,** Opening of the biceps tendon sheath distal to the transverse humeral ligament revealed fraying of the tendon. **C,** Screw tenodesis within the biceps groove successfully resolved the symptoms.

motion of even a healthy biceps tendon past an area characterized by inflammation and then fibrosis may be a pain generator. In addition, the biceps tendon may become involved in the healing rotator cuff repair, lose its gliding ability, and become entrapped.

On this basis, along with clinical experience, this chapter's authors routinely perform biceps tenodesis with rotator cuff repairs. It should be stressed that a normal-appearing intraarticular biceps, even one that is displaced into the joint with traction, may not reveal a source of biceps disease distal to the transverse humeral ligament. Advanced disease in the biceps tendon distal to the transverse humeral ligament can coexist with a completely normal intra-articular biceps tendon. For this reason, patients should be informed that concomitant pathology unrelated specifically to the rotator cuff tear (and appearing normal on MRI) may be present in the shoulder and may require surgical treatment. This chapter's authors prefer tenodesis over tenotomy because patients have reported biceps deformity and cramping pain after tenotomy.

The experience of this chapter's authors that a normal-appearing biceps tendon may be, in fact, pathologic, has basic science and clinical support. Basic science studies have demonstrated

neoangiogenesis and increased vascular endothelial growth factor expression (a marker for tendon degeneration) in biceps tendons associated with rotator cuff tears.[11] A study by Walch et al[12] reported that 70% of patients with impingement-type symptoms presented with biceps tendon abnormalities. Murthi et al[13] showed almost half of all patients with rotator cuff pathology had disease in the biceps tendon. Walch et al[14] demonstrated no acceleration of degenerative glenohumeral changes and minimal superior humeral head migration after biceps tenotomy with irreparable rotator cuff tears but noted improved pain scores.

This chapter's authors do not perform or advocate tenodesis in every rotator cuff repair. However, because we tenodese the biceps in all anterior supraspinatus tears, and because most of our practice is composed of these tears, biceps tenodesis is performed frequently.

Acromioclavicular Joint Reconstruction

Nonsurgical treatment is preferred for acute type I and II acromioclavicular joint injuries, whereas surgical stabilization is recommended for more severe injuries (types IV, V, and VI).[15-20] Treatment of type III dislocations of the acromioclavicular joint is less clear,

and reports are varied for surgical or nonsurgical treatment.

There is no consensus on which technique to use for acromioclavicular joint fixation or reconstruction; more than 60 techniques have been described.[21] Limited evidence is available to dictate the best strategy for surgical treatment, and even less evidence is available regarding complications and recommended treatment strategies for revision after failed fixation. Reported complications after surgical treatment of acromioclavicular joint dislocation include loss of reduction, implant failure, clavicular and coracoid fractures, graft tunnel widening and/or osteolysis, secondary acromioclavicular joint arthritis, infection, and acromial erosion.[22-28]

The most common postoperative complication after surgical fixation of acromioclavicular joint dislocation is loss of reduction, with failure rates reported to range between 15% and 44%.[23,29-31] Patients with minimal symptoms after loss of reduction may be successfully treated nonsurgically. Revision of a symptomatic failed reconstruction depends on the mode of failure. An intact coracoid and clavicle allow the coracoid to be used as a mooring to secure alternate fixation and grafts. Likewise, an intact clavicle provides a stable structure by which fixation and a graft can be secured. As an example, a failed modified Weaver-Dunn coracoacromial ligament transfer can be revised with semitendinosus autograft or allograft looped around the coracoid base and secured to the clavicle through bone tunnels and suture or screw augmentation.[32,33]

Implant failure and migration can be a devastating complication. Primary fixation of the acromioclavicular joint with smooth pin fixation has largely been abandoned because of potentially catastrophic complications of pin migration.[34-37] Primary coracoclavicular screw fixation provides high tensile strength and stiffness but requires eventual screw removal and has a high complication rate.[38] Mechanical coracoid button pullout also has been reported as a common method of failure.[39,40] Primary fixation of the acromioclavicular joint with hook-plate fixation has also been associated with complications, including implant failure, plate dislocation, acromial erosion, and infection.[22] Many complications can occur, and most are specific to the method of fixation except for loss of reduction, which is common to all. This chapter's authors attempt to minimize the complication rate by choosing a procedure that uses autologous tissue to reconstruct the joint with minimal effect on the local tissue (that is, with smaller holes in the coracoid and clavicle).

If the implant failure has resulted in a coracoid fracture, a decision must be made as to how to address the fracture or the insufficiency. If the distal fragment is large enough to accept a screw, open reduction and internal fixation with single-screw fixation from the tip of the coracoid into the scapula has been performed. If the coracoid fixation is strong enough, a graft can be passed under the coracoid and secured to the clavicle. This chapter's authors usually augment this revision con-

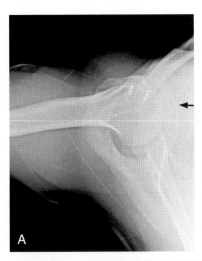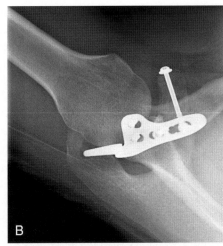

Figure 3 A coracoid fracture occurred in a patient after treatment of an acromioclavicular separation. **A,** Preoperative axillary radiograph of the coracoid fracture with a loose implant (arrow). **B,** The coracoid fracture was reduced with a screw, and the acromioclavicular separation was treated with a modified Weaver-Dunn procedure. A clavicle hook plate was used as supplemental fixation.

struct with a hook plate to decrease the load on the clavicle (**Figure 3**). A hook plate also can be used to stabilize the acromioclavicular joint if the coracoid fragment is too small for open reduction and internal fixation. This chapter's authors strongly believe this construct requires biologic fixation between the coracoid and the clavicle by securing graft to the remaining coracoid or using the coracoacromial ligament that is attached to the coracoid as local graft. Hook plates need to be removed by 3 months to prevent erosion of the hook through the acromion.

Clavicular fractures have been reported after acromioclavicular joint reconstruction.[25,41,42] Minimization of the clavicular tunnel diameter to allow at least 20 to 25 mm between clavicular tunnels and at least 10 to 15 mm between the lateral tunnel and the distal edge of the clavicle reduces the number of clavicular fractures.[43] Minimally displaced clavicular fractures noted after anatomic coracoclavicular reconstruction have been successfully

treated nonsurgically.[41] Clavicular tunnel widening has been noted with both synthetic materials and allograft and may lead to fractures.[44-46] This chapter's authors have treated displaced clavicular fractures via open reduction and internal fixation with a hook plate. These fractures often require bone grafting to prevent nonunion. For larger segments of bone loss, structural grafts with 5 to 7 cm of iliac crest have been used successfully.

Techniques using drill holes through the coracoid for graft placement and fixation as part of anatomic reconstruction of coracoclavicular ligaments introduce the potential for coracoid fracture and cutout.[40] Up to a 20% prevalence of coracoid fracture has been reported with coracoclavicular ligament reconstruction using coracoid tunneling.[25] Minimization of the tunnel diameter in the coracoid and appropriate visualization are recommended to help prevent coracoid fracture or cutout. Coracoid fractures are managed as previously described with hook-plate stabilization, with or with-

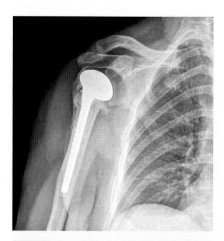

Figure 4 AP radiograph showing malunion of the tuberosities after hemiarthroplasty for a proximal humeral fracture.

out open reduction and internal fixation of the coracoid.

There are multiple modes of failure in acromioclavicular joint reconstructions. When choosing a method of initial stabilization, it is important that the surgeon consider the potential complications particular to the type of fixation. For primary surgery, this chapter's authors prefer an open modified Weaver-Dunn type of reconstruction with the osseous origin of the coracoacromial ligament transferred into the medullary canal of the distal end of the clavicle and concomitant suture fixation from the coracoid to the clavicle augmented with EndoButtons (Smith & Nephew). The complication rate is low with this procedure. When complications occur, the cause is usually loss of reduction, which, if symptomatic, can be more easily treated because the clavicle and coracoid are still intact, leaving multiple options. The rate of reduction loss has been markedly reduced by slower postoperative progression of physical therapy.

The literature regarding rotator cuff repairs has shown that slower rehabilitation leads to higher healing rates.[47] This information, coupled with the fact that acromioclavicular reconstruc-

tions are extra-articular, led this chapter's authors to adopt a slower course of rehabilitation. The patient is managed with immobilization in a sling for 6 weeks. No therapy is initiated for the first 2 weeks. At 2 weeks postoperatively, supine passive external rotation with a stick is initiated to prevent adhesions under the acromioclavicular reconstruction. At 4 weeks postoperatively, supine passive forward elevation is added. Active-assisted exercises are initiated at 6 weeks postoperatively, with active exercises starting at 8 weeks postoperatively. This protocol has resulted in less loss of reduction and no noticeable stiffness.

Hemiarthroplasty for Proximal Humeral Fractures

Although hemiarthroplasty has been a mainstay in the treatment of displaced proximal humeral fractures, its use has decreased because of improvements in open reduction and internal fixation and the development of reverse shoulder arthroplasty as a treatment option.[48-50] The unpredictable results after hemiarthroplasty, particularly with respect to shoulder motion and function, are another reason alternate treatments have been sought.[51-53] However, hemiarthroplasty continues to be an important treatment option, and, when selected, it is essential to use techniques that will minimize the risk of complications.[54-56]

The principles of hemiarthroplasty for proximal humeral fractures are as follows: (1) a deltopectoral approach should be used to preserve the deltoid origin; (2) humeral length and retroversion should be restored; and (3) secure fixation of the tuberosity to the shaft, the implant, and to each other should be attempted.

Successful achievement of these principles does not guarantee a successful outcome; however, if these goals are not achieved, a compromised

outcome often results. Use of a deltopectoral approach and preservation of the deltoid are easily achieved. Restoring humeral length and retroversion is essential, and different methods have been described. These include determining humeral length from radiographs of the contralateral humerus and maintaining the implant at a fixed position above the pectoralis major insertion.[57,58] Restoring the exact humeral length is not as important as avoiding lengthening or shortening of more 1 cm. Retroversion should be restored by one of two methods: (1) placement of the humeral component in the so-called average amount of retroversion, which is usually 20° to 30°,[59] or (2) alignment of the lateral flange of the implant just posterior to the remains of the bicipital groove, which also reproduces a reasonable range of retroversion.[60,61] It is important that the humeral length and retroversion be maintained during implantation of the prosthesis. Although some surgeons implant humeral components without cement, this chapter's authors prefer using cement to maintain proper length and rotation.[62]

Achieving secure tuberosity fixation and healing, and avoiding tuberosity displacement, malunion, and nonunion are a challenge with this procedure for several reasons (**Figure 4**). First, the bone of the tuberosity is generally osteopenic with compromised healing potential.[63] Second, the displacing forces of the rotator cuff tendons tend to distract the tuberosities and interfere with healing. Third, many implant designs place the tuberosity under excessive tension during rotation, which increases the risk of displacement.[56,59]

The probability of the tuberosity healing in a nearly anatomic position is enhanced by a variety of measures. First, the use of fracture-specific implants, including different implants for the right and left shoulders, is beneficial. These design modifications include a fenestration in the proximal portion of the implant to allow bone grafting between the tuberosities, specific suture attachment sites to enhance suture passage and fixation of the tuberosities, and adherence to the principles of tuberosity fixation using heavy nonabsorbable sutures. These principles include the following: (1) placing horizontal sutures through each tuberosity and through the implant, (2) placing vertical sutures through each tuberosity and to the shaft, (3) closing the rotator interval, and (4) using a cerclage suture around the entire construct and the implant to enhance tuberosity fixation in a reduced position.

All sutures should be passed through the tendon at the tendon-tuberosity junction because the tendon provides better fixation for the suture than the osteopenic bone of the tuberosity.[59] Cancellous bone graft from the humeral head should be placed between the tuberosities and between the tuberosities and the shaft to enhance healing.[64] When tuberosity fixation is completed, an intraoperative assessment should be performed to assess the stability of the construct and determine the parameters for postoperative rehabilitation.

Complications in hemiarthroplasty for fracture can result in a painful, stiff shoulder with compromised function.[63] The reverse shoulder arthroplasty has provided an important treatment option for patients in whom tuberosity displacement with associated pain, instability, and loss of shoulder motion and function develops.[65] Prior to the development of reverse shoulder arthroplasty, patients with pain after hemiarthroplasty after fracture had few, if any, reasonable treatment options. This is no longer the case, although revision of a hemiar-

throplasty to a reverse shoulder arthroplasty is a technically challenging procedure that is best performed by an experienced shoulder surgeon.[66]

Summary

Complications are an unavoidable consequence of surgery. The best treatment of complications is avoidance via meticulous preoperative planning and careful surgical technique. However, it is important to understand that, even with excellent planning and surgical technique, complications can be only minimized, not completely avoided in most cases. When contemplating revision surgery for the treatment of complications, it is important that the surgeon has a clear idea of what was done the first time and a clear plan about what to do differently the second time because simply repeating the same procedure the same way is unlikely to be successful.

References

1. Burkhart SS, De Beer JF: Traumatic glenohumeral bone defects and their relationship to failure of arthroscopic Bankart repairs: Significance of the inverted-pear glenoid and the humeral engaging Hill-Sachs lesion. *Arthroscopy* 2000;16(7):677-694.

2. Gerber C, Nyffeler RW: Classification of glenohumeral joint instability. *Clin Orthop Relat Res* 2002;400:65-76.

3. Lunn J, Castellanos-Ross J, Walch G: *Operative Techniques in Shoulder and Elbow Surgery*. Philadelphia, PA, Lippincott Williams & Wilkins, 2011, pp 59-65.

4. Walch G, Boileau P: Latarjet-Bristow procedure for recurrent anterior instability. *Tech Shoulder Elbow Surg* 2000;1(4):256-261.

5. Shah AA, Butler RB, Romanowski J, Goel D, Karadagli D, Warner JJ: Short-term complications of the Latarjet procedure. *J Bone*

Joint Surg Am 2012;94(6): 495-501.

6. Warner JJ, Gill TJ, O'Hollerhan JD, Pathare N, Millett PJ: Anatomical glenoid reconstruction for recurrent anterior glenohumeral instability with glenoid deficiency using an autogenous tricortical iliac crest bone graft. *Am J Sports Med* 2006;34(2):205-212.

7. Provencher MT, Ghodadra N, LeClere L, Solomon DJ, Romeo AA: Anatomic osteochondral glenoid reconstruction for recurrent glenohumeral instability with glenoid deficiency using a distal tibia allograft. *Arthroscopy* 2009;25(4): 446-452.

8. Boileau P, O'Shea K, Vargas P, Pinedo M, Old J, Zumstein M: Anatomical and functional results after arthroscopic Hill-Sachs remplissage. *J Bone Joint Surg Am* 2012;94(7):618-626.

9. Miniaci A, Gish MW: Management of anterior glenohumeral instability associated with large Hill-Sachs defects. *Tech Should Elbow* 2004;5(3):170-175.

10. Boileau P, Ahrens PM, Hatzidakis AM: Entrapment of the long head of the biceps tendon: The hourglass biceps. A cause of pain and locking of the shoulder. *J Shoulder Elbow Surg* 2004;13(3):249-257.

11. Lakemeier S, Reichelt JJ, Timmesfeld N, Fuchs-Winkelmann S, Paletta JR, Schofer MD: The relevance of long head biceps degeneration in the presence of rotator cuff tears. *BMC Musculoskelet Disord* 2010;11:191.

12. Walch G, Nove-Josserand L, Levigne C, Renaud E: Tears of the supraspinatus tendon associated with "hidden" lesions of the rotator interval. *J Shoulder Elbow Surg* 1994;3(6):353-360.

13. Murthi AM, Vosburgh CL, Neviaser TJ: The incidence of pathologic changes of the long head of the biceps tendon. *J Shoulder Elbow Surg* 2000;9(5):382-385.

14. Walch G, Edwards TB, Boulahia A, Nové-Josserand L, Neyton L, Szabo I: Arthroscopic tenotomy of the long head of the biceps in the treatment of rotator cuff tears: Clinical and radiographic results of 307 cases. *J Shoulder Elbow Surg* 2005;14(3):238-246.

15. Allman FL Jr: Fractures and ligamentous injuries of the clavicle and its articulation. *J Bone Joint Surg Am* 1967;49(4):774-784.

16. Bannister GC, Wallace WA, Stableforth PG, Hutson MA: A classification of acute acromioclavicular dislocation: A clinical, radiological and anatomical study. *Injury* 1992;23(3):194-196.

17. Bannister GC, Wallace WA, Stableforth PG, Hutson MA: The management of acute acromioclavicular dislocation: A randomised prospective controlled trial. *J Bone Joint Surg Br* 1989;71(5):848-850.

18. Rockwood CA, Williams GR, Young DC: *The Shoulder*. Philadelphia, PA, WB Saunders, 1998, pp 483-553.

19. Tossy JD, Mead NC, Sigmond HM: Acromioclavicular separations: Useful and practical classification for treatment. *Clin Orthop Relat Res* 1963;28:111-119.

20. Urist MR: The treatment of dislocations of the acromioclavicular joint: A survey of the past decade. *Am J Surg* 1959;98:423-431.

21. Mazzocca AD, Arciero RA, Bicos J: Evaluation and treatment of acromioclavicular joint injuries. *Am J Sports Med* 2007;35(2):316-329.

22. Sim E, Schwarz N, Höcker K, Berzlanovich A: Repair of complete acromioclavicular separations using the acromioclavicular-hook plate. *Clin Orthop Relat Res* 1995;314:134-142.

23. Salzmann GM, Walz L, Buchmann S, Glabgly P, Venjakob A, Imhoff AB: Arthroscopically assisted 2-bundle anatomical reduction of acute acromioclavicular joint separations. *Am J Sports Med* 2010;38(6):1179-1187.

24. Geaney LE, Miller MD, Ticker JB, et al: Causation and treatment. *Sports Med Arthrosc* 2010;18(3):167-172.

25. Milewski MD, Tompkins M, Giugale JM, Carson EW, Miller MD, Diduch DR: Complications related to anatomic reconstruction of the coracoclavicular ligaments. *Am J Sports Med* 2012;40(7):1628-1634.

26. Fleming RE, Tornberg DN, Kiernan H: An operative repair of acromioclavicular separation. *J Trauma* 1978;18(10):709-712.

27. Kappakas GS, McMaster JH: Repair of acromioclavicular separation using a Dacron prosthesis graft. *Clin Orthop Relat Res* 1978;131:247-251.

28. Park JP, Arnold JA, Coker TP, Harris WD, Becker DA: Treatment of acromioclavicular separations: A retrospective study. *Am J Sports Med* 1980;8(4):251-256.

29. Weinstein DM, McCann PD, McIlveen SJ, Flatow EL, Bigliani LU: Surgical treatment of complete acromioclavicular dislocations. *Am J Sports Med* 1995;23(3):324-331.

30. Yoo JC, Ahn JH, Yoon JR, Yang JH: Clinical results of single-tunnel coracoclavicular ligament reconstruction using autogenous semitendinosus tendon. *Am J Sports Med* 2010;38(5):950-957.

31. Stam L, Dawson I: Complete acromioclavicular dislocations: Treatment with a Dacron ligament. *Injury* 1991;22(3):173-176.

32. Jones HP, Lemos MJ, Schepsis AA: Salvage of failed acromioclavicular joint reconstruction using autogenous semitendinosus tendon from the knee: Surgical technique and case report. *Am J Sports Med* 2001;29(2):234-237.

33. Tauber M, Eppel M, Resch H: Acromioclavicular reconstruction using autogenous semitendinosus tendon graft: Results of revision surgery in chronic cases. *J Shoulder Elbow Surg* 2007;16(4):429-433.

34. Grauthoff H, Klammer HL: Complications due to migration of a Kirschner wire from the clavicle (author's transl) [in German]. *Rofo* 1978;128(5):591-594.

35. Lindsey RW, Gutowski WT: The migration of a broken pin following fixation of the acromioclavicular joint: A case report and review of the literature. *Orthopedics* 1986;9(3):413-416.

36. Norrell H Jr, Llewellyn RC: Migration of a threaded Steinmann pin from an acromioclavicular joint into the spinal canal: A case report. *J Bone Joint Surg Am* 1965;47:1024-1026.

37. Sethi GK, Scott SM: Subclavian artery laceration due to migration of a Hagie pin. *Surgery* 1976;80(5):644-646.

38. Jari R, Costic RS, Rodosky MW, Debski RE: Biomechanical function of surgical procedures for acromioclavicular joint dislocations. *Arthroscopy* 2004;20(3):237-245.

39. Thomas K, Litsky A, Jones G, Bishop JY: Biomechanical comparison of coracoclavicular reconstructive techniques. *Am J Sports Med* 2011;39(4):804-810.

40. Gerhardt DC, VanDerWerf JD, Rylander LS, McCarty EC: Postoperative coracoid fracture after transcoracoid acromioclavicular joint reconstruction. *J Shoulder Elbow Surg* 2011;20(5):e6-e10.

41. Turman KA, Miller CD, Miller MD: Clavicular fractures following coracoclavicular ligament reconstruction with tendon graft: A report of three cases. *J Bone Joint Surg Am* 2010;92(6):1526-1532.

42. Dust WN, Lenczner EM: Stress fracture of the clavicle leading to nonunion secondary to coracoclavicular reconstruction with

Dacron. *Am J Sports Med* 1989; 17(1):128-129.

43. Carofino BC, Mazzocca AD: The anatomic coracoclavicular ligament reconstruction: Surgical technique and indications. *J Shoulder Elbow Surg* 2010;19(2): 37-46.

44. Simovitch R, Sanders B, Ozbaydar M, Lavery K, Warner JJ: Acromioclavicular joint injuries: Diagnosis and management. *J Am Acad Orthop Surg* 2009;17(4):207-219.

45. Cook JB, Shaha JS, Rowles DJ, Bottoni CR, Shaha SH, Tokish JM: Early failures with single clavicular transosseous coracoclavicular ligament reconstruction. *J Shoulder Elbow Surg* 2012; 21(12):1746-1752.

46. Yoo JC, Choi NH, Kim SY, Lim TK: Distal clavicle tunnel widening after coracoclavicular ligament reconstruction with semitendinous tendon: A case report. *J Shoulder Elbow Surg* 2006;15(2): 256-259.

47. Millett PJ, Wilcox RB III, O'Holleran JD, Warner JJ: Rehabilitation of the rotator cuff: An evaluation-based approach. *J Am Acad Orthop Surg* 2006;14(11): 599-609.

48. Court-Brown CM, McQueen M: Open reduction and internal fixation of proximal humeral fractures with use of the locking proximal humerus plate. *J Bone Joint Surg Am* 2009;91(11):2771-2772.

49. Wall B, Nové-Josserand L, O'Connor DP, Edwards TB, Walch G: Reverse total shoulder arthroplasty: A review of results according to etiology. *J Bone Joint Surg Am* 2007;89(7):1476-1485.

50. Frankle MA, Chacon-Balados A, Cuff D: Reverse shoulder prosthesis for acute and chronic fractures, in Dines DM, Williams Jr. GR, Laurencin CT, eds: *Arthritis and Arthroplasty: The Shoulder.* Philadelphia, PA, Saunders, 2009, pp 218-231.

51. Kralinger F, Schwaiger R, Wambacher M, et al: A retrospective multicentre study of 167 patients. *J Bone Joint Surg Br* 2004;86(2): 217-219.

52. Becker R, Pap G, Machner A, Neumann WH: Strength and motion after hemiarthroplasty in displaced four-fragment fracture of the proximal humerus: 27 patients followed for 1-6 years. *Acta Orthop Scand* 2002;73(1):44-49.

53. Mighell MA, Kolm GP, Collinge CA, Frankle MA: Outcomes of hemiarthroplasty for fractures of the proximal humerus. *J Shoulder Elbow Surg* 2003;12(6):569-577.

54. Hettrich CM, Weldon E III, Boorman RS, Parsons IM IV, Matsen FA III: Preoperative factors associated with improvements in shoulder function after humeral hemiarthroplasty. *J Bone Joint Surg Am* 2004;86(7):1446-1451.

55. Prakash U, McGurty DW, Dent JA: Hemiarthroplasty for severe fractures of the proximal humerus. *J Shoulder Elbow Surg* 2002;11(5):428-430.

56. Zuckerman JD, Cuomo F, Koval KJ: Proximal humeral replacement for complex fractures: Indications and surgical technique. *Instr Course Lect* 1997;46:7-14.

57. Murachovsky J, Ikemoto RY, Nascimento LG, Fujiki EN, Milani C, Warner JJ: Pectoralis major tendon reference (PMT): A new method for accurate restoration of humeral length with hemiarthroplasty for fracture. *J Shoulder Elbow Surg* 2006;15(6):675-678.

58. Dines DM, Warren RF, Craig EV, Lee D, Dines JS: Intramedullary fracture positioning sleeve for proper placement of hemiarthroplasty in fractures of the proximal humerus. *Tech Shoulder Elbow Surg* 2007;8(2):69-74.

59. Boileau P, Walch G, Krishnan SG: Tuberosity osteosynthesis and hemiarthroplasty for four-part fractures of the proximal hu-

merus. *Tech Shoulder Elbow Surg* 2000;1:96-109.

60. Kummer FJ, Perkins R, Zuckerman JD: The use of the bicipital groove for alignment of the humeral stem in shoulder arthroplasty. *J Shoulder Elbow Surg* 1998;7(2):144-146.

61. Hempfing A, Leunig M, Ballmer FT, Hertel R: Surgical landmarks to determine humeral head retrotorsion for hemiarthroplasty in fractures. *J Shoulder Elbow Surg* 2001;10(5):460-463.

62. Hawkins RJ, Switlyk P: Acute prosthetic replacement for severe fractures of the proximal humerus. *Clin Orthop Relat Res* 1993;289:156-160.

63. Boileau P, Krishnan SG, Tinsi L, Walch G, Coste JS, Molé D: Tuberosity malposition and migration: Reasons for poor outcomes after hemiarthroplasty for displaced fractures of the proximal humerus. *J Shoulder Elbow Surg* 2002;11(5):401-412.

64. Abrutyn DA, Dines DM: Secure tuberosity fixation in shoulder arthroplasty for fractures. *Tech Shoulder Elbow Surg* 2004;5(4): 177-183.

65. Boileau P, Watkinson D, Hatzidakis AM, Hovorka I: The Grammont reverse shoulder prosthesis: Results in cuff tear arthritis, fracture sequelae, and revision arthroplasty. *J Shoulder Elbow Surg* 2006;15(5):527-540.

66. Parnes N, Rolf RH, Zimmer ZR, Higgins LD, Warner JJ: Management of failed hemiarthroplasty with reverse prosthesis. *Tech Shoulder Elbow Surg* 2008;9(4): 216-225.

Video Reference

Press CM, Gartsman GM, Wiesel BB, et al: Video. *Arthroscopic Biceps Tenodesis.* Woodbridge, VA, 2013.

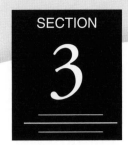

SECTION

3

Hand and Wrist

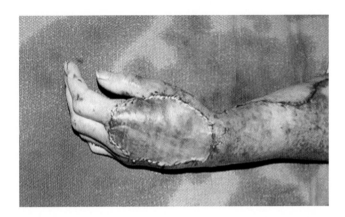

Complications of Common Hand and Wrist Surgery Procedures: Flexor and Extensor Tendon Surgery

Lauren H. Fischer, MD

Joshua M. Abzug, MD

A. Lee Osterman, MD

Peter J. Stern, MD

James Chang, MD

Abstract

Orthopaedic and hand surgeons frequently treat disorders of the flexor and extensor tendon systems. Common conditions, such as trigger finger, de Quervain tenosynovitis, extensor tendon injury, and zone II flexor tendon injury, can be challenging to treat. Complications that limit normal hand function still occur despite advances in surgical techniques and therapy protocols. It is helpful to be aware of the complications related to the treatment of these hand disorders and understand surgical techniques to minimize their frequency.

Instr Course Lect 2014;63:97-103.

Common disorders and injuries of the hand, including trigger finger, de Quervain tenosynovitis, extensor tendon injury, and zone II flexor tendon injury are frequently managed by orthopaedic and hand surgeons. This chapter will discuss these conditions and complications associated with their treatment. The preferred surgical treatment techniques of this chapter's authors are presented.

Trigger Finger Release

Stenosing flexor tenosynovitis, more commonly known as trigger finger, is a common condition seen by both primary care physicians and hand surgeons. The flexor tendons, composed mostly of type I collagen, glide through the synovial-lined sheath during normal digit flexion and extension. Pulleys hold the tendons in close proximity to the phalanges to facilitate optimal biomechanics. Five annular and three cruciate pulleys are spaced throughout the length of the digit (**Figure 1**). The thumb has a unique pulley system consisting of A1, oblique, and A2 pulleys. In trigger finger, tendons cannot glide freely under the most proximal A1 pulley because of tenosynovitis of the flexor tendons. Histologic studies comparing normal A1 pulleys to those of patients diagnosed with trigger finger suggest fibrocartilage metaplasia as a possible cause of the disease process.[1]

Patients report hearing clicking during flexion or extension of the finger or thumb. In more severe cases, the digit becomes locked in flexion and cannot be extended actively. Pain can be substantial and may limit normal hand function. Repetitive motion and systemic disease, most commonly diabetes mellitus, contribute to the disease process. The incidence of trigger

Dr. Osterman or an immediate family member has received royalties from Medartis and Biomet; is a member of a speakers' bureau or has made paid presentations on behalf of Auxilium, Medartis, Arthrex, and Synthes; serves as a paid consultant to Auxilium; has received research or institutional support from Auxilium and Skeletal Dynamics; and serves as a board member, owner, officer, or committee member of the American Association for Hand Surgery and the American Society for Surgery of the Hand. Dr. Chang or an immediate family member serves as a paid consultant to Zone II Surgical; has stock or stock options held in Zone II Surgical; and serves as a board member, owner, officer, or committee member of the American Board of Plastic Surgery and the American Society for Surgery of the Hand. None of the following authors nor any immediate family member has received anything of value from or owns stock in a commercial company or institution related directly or indirectly to the subject of this chapter: Dr. Fischer, Dr. Abzug, and Dr. Stern.

finger in the general population is reported to be from 1% to 3%, compared with 5% to 20% in patients with diabetes.[2] In children, trigger thumb frequently presents as fixed flexion at the interphalangeal joint rather than palpable clicking. Controversy exists regarding whether trigger thumb in children is congenital versus acquired, because some cases of the condition documented at 1 year or older were not present at birth.[3] Described treatment modalities in adults include a corticosteroid injection. If this treatment is not successful, percutaneous versus open release of the A1 pulley may be done. Unresolved trigger thumb in children usually requires surgical release. As with any surgery, complications can arise, including wrong-site surgery, incomplete release, and bowstringing of the flexor tendon.

Wrong-Site Surgery

The Joint Commission reports wrong-site surgery as one of the five most frequently occurring sentinel events.[4] Between 1995 and 2012, at total of 1,186 cases of surgeries involving the wrong patient, wrong site, or wrong procedure were investigated by the Joint Commission. Unlike other disease processes of the hand and upper extremity, no gross deformity exists in trigger finger, except for the occasionally palpable nodule near the A1 pulley. To prevent wrong-patient, wrong-site, and wrong-procedure events, the Joint Commission created a universal protocol for implementation by medical personnel, which includes preprocedural verification of the correct patient, procedure, and site by all members of the surgical team; marking of the surgical site by the surgeon with the patient awake; and a final verification to confirm the correct patient, procedure, and site. These measures, particularly marking of the surgical site by the surgeon with the patient awake,

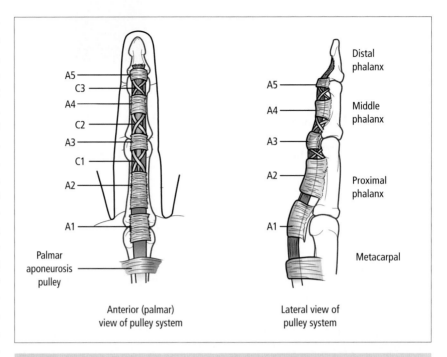

Figure 1   Illustrations of the anterior (left) and lateral (right) views of the digit pulley system anatomy. (Reproduced from Bindra R, Sinclair M: Trigger finger release, in Flatow E, Colvin AC, eds: *Atlas of Essential Orthopaedic Procedures.* Rosemont, IL, American Academy of Orthopaedic Surgeons, 2013, pp 253-258.)

will help the surgeon correctly identify the problematic digit. After induction of sedation or anesthesia, it is exceedingly difficult to identify the correct digit because it may not trigger with passive range of motion.

Incomplete Release

The overall complication rate of open trigger finger release in adults varies widely in the literature. In 2010, Will and Lubahn[5] described a 31% (3% major and 28% minor) complication rate for a single surgeon performing open release surgeries for trigger finger. A recent retrospective analysis of 1,598 open trigger finger releases over 10 years reported a 0.6% rate of persistent triggering at 6 weeks, and 0.3% rate of recurrent triggering between 9 and 60 months postoperatively. Important factors in recurrent triggering included young age and insulin-dependent diabetes.[6] In children, open A1 pulley release has a high rate of complete reso-

lution of triggering in the thumb; however, outcomes vary substantially in the fingers. In a series of 33 trigger fingers in 18 children, 8 patients had persistent triggering after open A1 pulley release; this complication was largely caused by unrecognized anatomic variations that contributed to triggering.[7] The key point to remember in open trigger finger release in children is the need to explore the flexor digitorum superficialis tendon for tendon nodules, a more proximal decussation, and/or an abnormal insertion into the flexor digitorum profundus tendon. Resection of a slip of the superficialis tendon may be necessary. A stenotic A3 pulley can also contribute to persistent triggering in children and will require release.

Bowstringing

Although incomplete release of the A1 pulley may result in persistent triggering, excessive release, including full re-

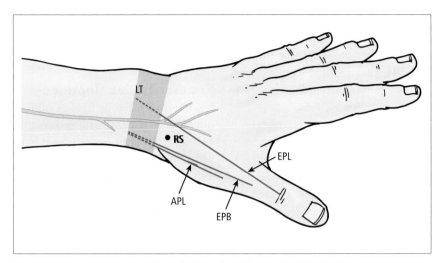

Figure 2 Illustration of the superficial branch of radial nerve in the distal forearm. APL = abductor pollicis longus, EPB = extensor pollicis brevis, EPL = extensor pollicis longus, LT = Lister tubercle, RS = radial styloid process. (Reproduced from Venouziou AI, Giannoulis FS, Sotcreanos DG: First dorsal extensor compartment release, in Flatow E, Colvin AC, eds: *Atlas of Essential Orthopaedic Procedures.* Rosemont, IL, American Academy of Orthopaedic Surgeons, 2013, pp 247-252.)

lease of the A2 pulley, may cause bowstringing of the tendon. When the pulley system no longer holds the tendon in close approximation with the metacarpophalangeal (MCP) joint, the moment arm (defined as the perpendicular distance from the line of force application to the axis of rotation) increases.[8] The work of finger flexion increases because the same amount of flexor tendon excursion results in a smaller arc of rotation of the MCP joint. In the rheumatoid hand, the annular pulleys are weak and must be preserved to prevent bowstringing and ulnar drift. Treating the inflamed synovium with tenosynovectomy, superficialis slip resection, or nodule resection allows the flexor tendon to glide more freely under the entire pulley system.

Technique of This Chapter's Authors

To prevent trigger finger complications, this chapter's authors prefer the following technique. An incision is made in a normal crease over the A1 pulley, approximately 1.5 cm in length. Ragnell retractors are used to spread the tissue until the A1 pulley is completely visualized. The A1 pulley is then sharply transected using a No. 15-blade scalpel blade or scissors. Complete visualization of the A1 pulley facilitates inadvertent transection of the A2 pulley. In patients with rheumatoid arthritis, extensive tenosynovectomy is performed rather than full release of the A1 pulley. In children with a trigger finger (other than the thumb), a Bruner skin incision proceeding distally to the proximal phalanx is performed to properly explore the flexor tendons for any abnormalities.

de Quervain Tenosynovitis

de Quervain tenosynovitis involves entrapment of the abductor pollicis longus and extensor pollicis brevis tendons in the first extensor compartment of the wrist, which overlies the radial styloid.[9] Repetitive pinching movements with radial and ulnar deviation of the wrist contribute to thickening of the fibro-osseous sheath and restricted movement of the tendons within the compartment.

Patients often present with radial-sided wrist pain and increased pain with thumb movement. Focal swelling may be appreciated over the radial styloid. The Finkelstein test, which involves placing the thumb within the palm and forcibly deviating the wrist ulnarly to place maximum stretch on the tendons within the first extensor compartment, can assist in the diagnosis.[10]

Conservative treatment includes steroid injection and splinting. Complications of open first extensor compartment release include radial sensory nerve injury; incomplete release of the first extensor compartment; and overrelease, resulting in tendon subluxation.

Radial Sensory Nerve Injury

The superficial branch of the radial nerve provides sensation to the dorsum of the first web space, the dorsal thumb, and the index and middle fingers. Injury to this nerve results in paresthesias or a painful neuroma. In a cadaver study, the superficial branch of the radial nerve was found to emerge from between the heads of the brachioradialis and the extensor carpi radialis longus an average of 8.3 cm proximal to the radial styloid process.[11] The first branch formed on average at 4.9 cm proximal to the radial styloid and travelled in a radial direction to provide sensation to the radial aspect of the thumb. The main trunk travels distally and radial to the dorsal tubercle of the radius. An additional three to five branches of the radial nerve continue off the main trunk and pass over the extensor pollicis longus tendon and arborize distal to the radial styloid. Because of the close proximity of its branches to the first extensor compartment, the superficial branch of the radial nerve is at risk for direct and/or traction injury during release

(**Figure 2**). Regardless of the type of incision (transverse, longitudinal, or oblique), direct visualization of the nerve and knowledge of the surrounding anatomy decreases the risk of inadvertent nerve damage during surgery.

Incomplete Release

Anatomic variations can contribute to incomplete release of the first extensor compartment. Several cadaver studies have reported variants, with two or more abductor pollicis longus slips (most commonly two), a single extensor pollicis brevis tendon, or septae within the fibro-osseous tunnel.[12] Failure to recognize septae within the compartment results in incomplete release of the compartment and persistent symptoms postoperatively.

Overrelease and Tendon Subluxation

Overzealous release of both volar and dorsal aspects of the tendon sheath can cause volar subluxation of the abductor pollicis longus and extensor pollicis brevis tendons. The tendons sublux, volarly causing pain because of the loss of the tendons' volar supportive shelf.[13] This complication often necessitates reconstruction of a new tendon sheath to prevent further subluxation and persistent pain. Commonly described techniques include a distally based brachioradialis tendon flap and an extensor retinaculum flap.[14]

Technique of This Chapter's Authors

Local anesthesia is administered to anesthetize the skin overlying the first extensor compartment. A transverse skin incision is made over the radial styloid. Dissection is used to identify the superficial branch of the radial nerve and its branches. A longitudinal (as dorsally as possible) or stair-step incision releases the fibro-osseous band. All tendons are identified and septae

are released. An extensor retinaculum flap can be created if needed to help prevent volar subluxation of the tendons. The hand is then splinted, and range of motion therapy is started early to help prevent adhesions.

Extensor Tendon Injury

The hand surgeon commonly encounters extensor tendon injuries because they are prone to laceration, given the thin overlying dorsal skin, rupture in the setting of fractures and rheumatoid arthritis, or exposure from skin loss after avulsion injuries or infection. Unlike flexor tendon injuries, proximal retraction of the extensor tendon is limited by intertendinous connections called juncturae tendinae.[10] Patients with an extensor tendon injury often present with extensor lag, although the deformity may be less obvious in the rheumatoid hand. Lag at the distal interphalangeal joint, as in mallet finger, can be treated with splinting; however, injury in other zones can cause greater functional impairment. Common scenarios of extensor tendon injury requiring surgical intervention include extensor tendon scarring, rupture, and tendon exposure from dorsal hand wounds.

Extensor Tendon Scarring

Peritendinous inflammation occurs after hand trauma or tendon repair and can promote scar formation with secondary limitations of tendon excursion. Tenolysis can lead to a vicious cycle of scar release, inflammation, and the redevelopment of scar tissue.[15] After extensor tendon repair, use of the Merritt relative motion splint may help prevent adhesions while allowing the patient to return to work as soon as 3 days postoperatively.[16] This splint is designed to keep the MCP joint of the lacerated extensor tendon extended 30° more than the MCP joints of the uninjured extensor tendons. When tenolysis is required, the patient should be awake during sur-

gery to facilitate participation and ensure that full, active extension of the digit is achieved in the operating room.[17]

Extensor Tendon Rupture

Spontaneous extensor tendon rupture can occur in patients with rheumatoid arthritis, osteoarthritis, and distal radius fractures. In patients with rheumatoid arthritis, the most common cause of tendon rupture at the wrist is attrition from dorsal protrusion of the head of the ulna (caput ulnae syndrome).[17] Distal radial ulnar joint instability and supination deformity of the carpus cause this dorsal protrusion. End-to-end primary or secondary repair is generally not possible in the rheumatoid hand. For extensor pollicis longus rupture with functional disability, extensor indicis proprius transfer is recommended because it has strength similar to the extensor pollicis longus and its sacrifice does not cause loss of independent index finger extension.[18-20] For extensor digitorum communis rupture to a single digit, end-to-side tenodesis to an adjacent extensor digitorum communis tendon or extensor indicis proprius tendon transfer can restore function.[18]

Dorsal Hand Wound With Extensor Tendon Exposure

Dorsal degloving injuries of the hand frequently can occur during trauma from the friction between the thin, pliable dorsal hand skin and a hard surface. Exposed tendons require urgent soft-tissue coverage to prevent desiccation and infection and facilitate tendon gliding for extension of the digits and wrist. Reconstruction is staged and involves skin coverage, silastic rod placement, tendon grafting and/or tendon transfers, and secondary tenolysis and/or capsulotomies.

There are many options for dorsal hand coverage, although the pros and cons of each should be weighed care-

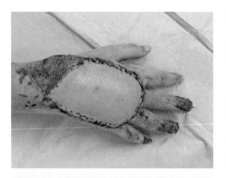

Figure 3 Clinical photograph of right dorsal hand reconstruction using a radial forearm fasciocutaneous flap. Note the dorsal hand bulk.

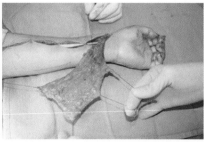

Figure 4 The radial forearm fascia-only flap is elevated and ready for rotation onto the dorsum of the hand. Note the donor site is approximated with staples because it will be closed primarily.

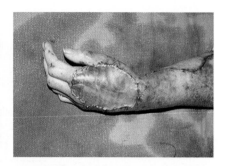

Figure 5 The radial forearm fascia-only flap is covered with skin graft over the dorsum of the left hand. Note the natural contour of the dorsal hand.

fully to most accurately restore form and function. The radial forearm fasciocutaneous flap, although easily accessible, has several drawbacks, including an obvious donor-site scar and a skin graft over the tendons of the forearm that is prone to wound healing complications. The reconstruction is bulky because the volar skin is considerably thicker than the dorsal skin (**Figure 3**).

Technique of This Chapter's Authors

For reconstruction of degloving injuries or other open dorsal hand wounds, this chapter's authors prefer the radial forearm fascia flap. A lazy S-shaped incision is made over the volar forearm overlying the radial artery. Dissection proceeds to elevate the skin from the fascia. The proximal radial artery is divided, and the fascia, pedicled to the distal radial artery, is transposed to cover the dorsum of the hand (**Figure 4**). The donor site can be closed primarily, and the fascia is covered with a split-thickness sheet graft (**Figure 5**). Although the radial artery is sacrificed, the flap is believed to be superior to the fasciocutaneous flap because the fascia-only flap allows for staged tendon reconstruction and substantially better dorsal hand contour.

Flexor Tendon Injury in Zone II

Flexor tendon injuries in zone II continue to challenge even the most skilled hand surgeons. Although advances have been made in repair techniques, suture materials, and therapy protocols, complications, including rupture, adhesions, and contracture still occur. Strickland[21] described the characteristics of an ideal flexor tendon repair, including easily placed sutures, secure knots, a smooth juncture between the tendon ends, minimal gapping, minimal interference with vascularity, and repair of sufficient strength to facilitate early motion. Despite efforts to adhere to these principles, the revision rate for flexor tendon repair is reported at 6%, with 91% of revision procedures occurring within the first year.[22]

Flexor Tendon Rupture

Factors contributing to tendon rupture include weak suture material, a poor repair technique with gapping, overly aggressive therapy, and patient noncompliance (such as splint removal or heavy lifting).[23] Repairs are weakest at 6 to 18 days after surgery, although rupture can occur at 6 to 7 weeks postoperatively.[24,25] Although patient compliance is a largely uncontrollable variable, the surgeon can optimize the

repair by selecting the appropriate suture material and repair technique (for example, 3-0 suture material increases fatigue strength two to three times compared with 4-0 suture, and the locking technique increases the tensile strength of a repair).[26,27] Independent of the suture caliber, the number of strands crossing the repair site affects fatigue strength. Specifically, repairs using four strands or more withstand more force before failure than two-strand repairs.[27]

Flexor Tendon Adhesions

Formation of scar tissue surrounding the flexor tendon limits tendon excursion. A recent meta-analysis indicates a 4% rate of adhesions for zone II flexor tendon repairs.[28] Although many factors cannot be controlled by the surgeon, implementing a hand therapy regimen is an important factor in improving outcomes. Early, controlled active range of motion when compared with passive range of motion produces overall better range of motion, smaller flexion contractures, and better patient satisfaction scores.[29] Current research efforts are investigating the relationship between various growth factors and adhesion formation and methods to regulate growth factor activity to decrease scarring.[30] In the future, the ability to upregulate production of

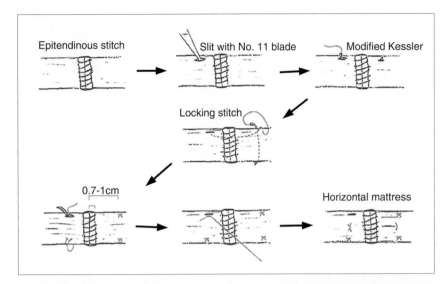

Figure 6 Illustration of this chapter's authors preferred technique for flexor tendon repair. Note the epitendinous repair is performed first. (Reproduced with permission from Bari AS, Woon CY, Pridgen B, Chang J: Overcoming the learning curve: A curriculum-based model for teaching zone ii flexor tendon repairs. *Plast Reconstr Surg* 2012;130(2):381-388.)

lubricating substances in vivo or synthesize similar substances that adhere to the tendon surface could contribute to overall improved hand function after flexor tendon repair.[31]

Flexor Tendon Contracture

Despite improvements in splinting and therapy protocols, the incidence of proximal interphalangeal and distal interphalangeal joint contractures is reported at 17%.[25] Correcting the deformity relies on accurately diagnosing the location of the problem. Joint contracture issues in any tissue layer can result from problems ranging from insufficient volar skin to bony abnormalities.

Primary Flexor Tendon Repair Technique of This Chapter's Authors

This chapter's authors prefer to start with the epitendinous repair using a 6-0 double-armed monofilament suture in a running fashion (**Figure 6**). A No. 11 scalpel blade is used to slit the tendon where the modified Kessler

locking stitch will begin. After the locking modified Kessler stitch is placed using a 3-0 braided suture, the four-strand repair is completed with a horizontal mattress suture, also using a 3-0 braided suture. Performing the epitendinous repair first allows the surgeon to establish the appropriate tension within the tendons so they neither overlap nor gap. The technique also minimizes knots on the volar aspect of the repair, which allows the tendon to glide more freely under the pulley mechanism because knots contribute to bulk and friction. An early active motion protocol is begun within 4 days of surgery.

Contracture Release Technique of This Chapter's Authors

To achieve optimal contracture release, this chapter's authors prefer to work volarly to dorsally, addressing each tissue layer in a stepwise fashion. After the volar skin is released, the fascia, tendon sheath, and flexor tendons are explored for adhesions. The volar plate (including check-rein ligaments) and

accessory and proper collateral ligaments are examined. Bony abnormalities, which lead to blocked motion within the joint, may be the final structures that require release before full extension is achieved.

Summary

Flexor and extensor tendon surgery requires a clear understanding of anatomy, wound healing, and scar formation. Technical precision is required because both overcorrection and undercorrection will result in abnormal tendon biomechanics. Understanding the problems associated with common hand and wrist surgery procedures will help orthopaedic and hand surgeons avoid these complications.

References

1. Sampson SP, Badalamente MA, Hurst LC, Seidman J: Pathobiology of the human A1 pulley in trigger finger. *J Hand Surg Am* 1991;16(4):714-721.

2. Vance MC, Tucker JJ, Harness NG: The association of hemoglobin A1c with the prevalence of stenosing flexor tenosynovitis. *J Hand Surg Am* 2012;37(9):1765-1769.

3. Kikuchi N, Ogino T: Incidence and development of trigger thumb in children. *J Hand Surg Am* 2006;31(4):541-543.

4. Sentinel event data: Event type by year: 1995 to 2012. Joint Commission website: http://www.jointcommission.org/assets/1/18/Event_Type_Year_1995_2Q2012.pdf. Accessed October 15, 2012.

5. Will R, Lubahn J: Complications of open trigger finger release. *J Hand Surg Am* 2010;35(4):594-596.

6. Bruijnzeel H, Neuhaus V, Fostvedt S, Jupiter JB, Mudgal CS, Ring DC: Adverse events of open A1 pulley release for idiopathic

trigger finger. *J Hand Surg Am* 2012;37(8):1650-1656.

7. Cardon LJ, Ezaki M, Carter PR: Trigger finger in children. *J Hand Surg Am* 1999;24(6):1156-1161.

8. Ryzewicz M, Wolf JM: Trigger digits: Principles, management, and complications. *J Hand Surg Am* 2006;31(1):135-146.

9. de Quervain F: On a form of chronic tendovaginitis by Dr. Fritz de Quervain in la Chaux-de-Fonds. 1895. *Am J Orthop (Belle Mead NJ)* 1997;26(9):641-644.

10. Pick RY: De Quervain's disease: A clinical triad. *Clin Orthop Relat Res* 1979;143:165-166.

11. Robson AJ, See MS, Ellis H: Applied anatomy of the superficial branch of the radial nerve. *Clin Anat* 2008;21(1):38-45.

12. Kulthanan T, Chareonwat B: Variations in abductor pollicis longus and extensor pollicis brevis tendons in the Quervain syndrome: A surgical and anatomical study. *Scand J Plast Reconstr Surg Hand Surg* 2007;41(1):36-38.

13. McMahon M, Craig SM, Posner MA: Tendon subluxation after de Quervain's release: Treatment by brachioradialis tendon flap. *J Hand Surg Am* 1991;16(1):30-32.

14. White GM, Weiland AJ: Symptomatic palmar tendon subluxation after surgical release for de Quervain's disease: A case report. *J Hand Surg Am* 1984;9(5):704-706.

15. Skoff HD: Extensor tenolysis: A modern version of an old approach. *Plast Reconstr Surg* 1994;93(5):1056-1060, discussion 1061.

16. Lalonde DH, Kozin S: Tendon disorders of the hand. *Plast Reconstr Surg* 2011;128(1):1e-14e.

17. Schindele SF, Herren DB, Simmen BR: Tendon reconstruction for the rheumatoid hand. *Hand Clin* 2011;27(1):105-113.

18. Nalebuff PG, Feldo LH: Millender: Rheumatoid arthritis in the hand and wrist, in Green DP, ed: *Operative Hand Surgery.* New York, NY, Churchhill Livingstone, 1988, pp 1667-1677.

19. Browne EZ Jr, Teague MA, Snyder CC: Prevention of extensor lag after indicis proprius tendon transfer. *J Hand Surg Am* 1979;4(2):168-172.

20. Moore JR, Weiland AJ, Valdata L: Independent index extension after extensor indicis proprius transfer. *J Hand Surg Am* 1987;12(2):232-236.

21. Strickland JW: Development of flexor tendon surgery: Twenty-five years of progress. *J Hand Surg Am* 2000;25(2):214-235.

22. Dy CJ, Daluiski A, Do HT, Hernandez-Soria A, Marx R, Lyman S: The epidemiology of reoperation after flexor tendon repair. *J Hand Surg Am* 2012;37(5):919-924.

23. Harris SB, Harris D, Foster AJ, Elliot D: The aetiology of acute rupture of flexor tendon repairs in zones 1 and 2 of the fingers during early mobilization. *J Hand Surg Br* 1999;24(3):275-280.

24. Zhao C, Amadio PC, Momose T, Couvreur P, Zobitz ME, An KN: Effect of synergistic wrist motion on adhesion formation after repair of partial flexor digitorum profundus tendon lacerations in a canine

model in vivo. *J Bone Joint Surg Am* 2002;84-A(1):78-84.

25. Taras JS, Gray RM, Culp RW: Complications of flexor tendon injuries. *Hand Clin* 1994;10(1):93-109.

26. Barrie KA, Tomak SL, Cholewicki J, Merrell GA, Wolfe SW: Effect of suture locking and suture caliber on fatigue strength of flexor tendon repairs. *J Hand Surg Am* 2001;26(2):340-346.

27. Hatanaka H, Zhang J, Manske PR: An in vivo study of locking and grasping techniques using a passive mobilization protocol in experimental animals. *J Hand Surg Am* 2000;25(2):260-269.

28. Dy CJ, Hernandez-Soria A, Ma Y, Roberts TR, Daluiski A: Complications after flexor tendon repair: A systematic review and meta-analysis. *J Hand Surg Am* 2012;37(3):543-551, e1.

29. Trumble TE, Vedder NB, Seiler JG III, Hanel DP, Diao E, Pettrone S: Zone-II flexor tendon repair: A randomized prospective trial of active place-and-hold therapy compared with passive motion therapy. *J Bone Joint Surg Am* 2010;92(6):1381-1389.

30. Derby BM, Reichensperger J, Chambers C, Bueno RA, Suchy H, Neumeister MW: Early growth response factor-1: Expression in a rabbit flexor tendon scar model. *Plast Reconstr Surg* 2012;129(3):435e-442e.

31. Kohrs RT, Zhao C, Sun YL, et al: Tendon fascicle gliding in wild type, heterozygous, and lubricin knockout mice. *J Orthop Res* 2011;29(3):384-389.

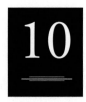

Iatrogenic Nerve Injuries in Common Upper Extremity Procedures

Matthew S. Zimmermann, MD
Joshua M. Abzug, MD
James Chang, MD
Peter J. Stern, MD
A. Lee Osterman, MD

Abstract

Iatrogenic nerve injuries frequently occur during procedures around the hand and wrist, although they are not always recognized at the time of injury or in the immediate postoperative period. Because preventing injuries is of paramount importance, extensive knowledge of the anatomy of the at-risk nerves is critical. Best results occur after immediate repair because a substantial delay before secondary surgery diminishes the chances for recovery from motor or sensory nerve dysfunction and relief from pain. It is helpful to review iatrogenic nerve injuries associated with common hand surgical procedures.

Instr Course Lect 2014;63:105-111.

Iatrogenic nerve injuries are common and occur secondary to several factors. The most frequent causes of these injuries include compression with a tourniquet, pressure from insufficient padding during procedures, injections, venipuncture, excessive direct or indirect retraction, and direct laceration of the nerve itself.[1,2] The true incidence of iatrogenic nerve injuries is difficult to ascertain because lesions are frequently undetected, not correctly identified, ignored, or not reported by the operating surgeon[2,3] (**Table 1**). Iatrogenic nerve injuries comprise 9.5% to 20% of surgical referrals to nerve centers.[4-6] Approximately 15% of iatrogenic nerve injuries occur because of hand surgery, with 50% of those injuries resulting from endoscopic procedures (**Table 2**).[2]

Carpal Tunnel Release

Overall, nerve injuries caused by open or endoscopic carpal tunnel release are quite rare. However, because these procedures are common, median nerve injuries after open or endoscopic carpal tunnel release accounted for 36% of all upper extremity nerve injuries treated at one upper extremity nerve center[2] (AL Osterman, MD, Philadelphia, PA, personal communication, 2003). Forty-one percent of these injuries are complete lesions. Benson et al[7] performed a meta-analysis of 22,327 endoscopic and 5,669 open carpal tunnel releases. The authors reported an incidence of transient neurapraxia in 1.45% of endoscopic releases and 0.25% of open releases. Major nerve injuries occurred in 0.13% of the endoscopic carpal tunnel releases and

Dr. Chang or an immediate family member serves as a paid consultant to or is an employee of Zone II Surgical; has stock or stock options held in Zone II Surgical; and serves as a board member, owner, officer, or committee member of the American Board of Plastic Surgery and the American Society for Surgery of the Hand. Dr. Osterman or an immediate family member has received royalties from Medartis and Biomet; is a member of a speakers' bureau or has made paid presentations on behalf of Auxilium, Medartis, Arthrex, and Synthes; serves as a paid consultant to or is an employee of Auxilium; has received research or institutional support from Auxilium and Skeletal Dynamics; and serves as a board member, owner, officer, or committee member of the American Association for Hand Surgery and the American Society for Surgery of the Hand. None of the following authors or any immediate family member has received anything of value from or has stock or stock options held in a commercial company or institution related directly or indirectly to the subject of this chapter: Dr. Zimmermann, Dr. Abzug, and Dr. Stern.

Table 1

Recognition of Iatrogenic Nerve Injuries in 85 Cases That Presented to an Upper Extremity Nerve Center

Nerve Injury	No. of Patients (%)
Recognized intraoperatively by the operating surgeon and referred for treatment.	30 (28%)
Recognized postoperatively by the original operating surgeon and referred for treatment.	59 (55%)
Never recognized by the operating surgeon. The patient was seen for a second opinion or referred by another physician, but without a diagnosis of a known nerve injury.	18 (17%)
Repaired by the operating surgeon during the index procedure and documented in the surgical report; the patient was informed.	22 (26%)
Recognized by the operating surgeon but not addressed during the index procedure. The wound was closed, and the patient was subsequently referred for treatment.	6 (7%)
Recognized by the operating surgeon during the index procedure and repaired silently, without mention in the surgical report; the patient was not informed.	2 (2%)

Table 2

Procedures Involved in 85 Iatrogenic Nerve Injuries That Presented to an Upper Extremity Nerve Center

Procedure	%
Carpal tunnel release	36%
Open	20%
Endoscopic	16%
Dupuytren release	11%
Volar ganglionectomy	7%
Open reduction and internal fixation and/or plate removal	5%
Trigger release	5%
Shoulder or elbow arthroscopy	5%
Benign tumor removal	5%
Palmaris longus graft harvest	3%

0.10% of the open releases, with digital nerve injuries found in 0.03% and 0.39%, respectively.[1]

Most injuries to the median nerve and its branches are caused by inappropriately placed incisions that result in poor exposure of the carpal canal and poor hemostasis.[8]

Incisions placed radial to the thenar crease or a transverse incision at the wrist crease can result in injury to the palmar cutaneous nerve, which is likely the most common nerve injury after open carpal tunnel release.[2,9-11] Laceration of the main trunk or terminal branches can lead to the development of a painful neuroma.[9] After a

trial of 4 to 6 months of conservative treatment with desensitization therapy, such neuromas should be resected if they are still symptomatic.[8]

Incisions placed too radially can result in a more devastating laceration of the recurrent motor branch of the median nerve because of the frequent variations in its course in the carpal tunnel.[12,13] Knowledge about the typical anatomy and the many variations of the branches of the median nerve is paramount for avoiding nerve injury.[11-14] Incisions placed too ulnarly can result in injury to the ulnar nerve or ulnar cutaneous branch of the median nerve.[8] Osterman reported

that ulnar nerve injuries after open and endoscopic carpal tunnel release accounted for nearly one third of all the ulnar nerve injuries that presented to an upper extremity nerve center (AL Osterman, MD, Philadelphia, PA, personal communication, 2003).

Early recognition and treatment of iatrogenic nerve injuries is crucial. If an injury to the main trunk or recurrent motor branch of the median nerve is identified within the first 12 months, a primary repair should be performed; otherwise an opposition transfer is indicated. Sensory nerve injuries can be treated with direct repair if found during the primary procedure or by excision of the neuroma and implantation in muscle or bone if identified later (AL Osterman, MD, Philadelphia, PA, personal communication, 2003).

Cubital Tunnel Release

Nerve injuries resulting from surgery around the cubital tunnel occur more often to the medial antebrachial cutaneous nerve than the ulnar nerve.[8,15-17] Trauma to the medial antebrachial cutaneous nerve can be an important cause of morbidity, and it has been reported to have occurred in as many as 90% of patients with persistent pain after cubital tunnel surgery.[18,19] Transection of the nerve leads to a painful neuroma or a bothersome anesthetic patch over the olecranon region (**Figure 1**). Pain can limit elbow extension and result in a worse outcome.[15,20] To minimize risk, careful dissection should be performed, especially at the distal end of the incision where terminal branches run from the posterior branch of the medial antebrachial cutaneous nerve.[15,21-23] Recognizing the injury at the time of surgery is of primary importance. Treatment includes resection of the proximal stump back to the subcutaneous tissue of the brachium, away from the elbow and any possible area of scar formation.[15]

Ulnar nerve injuries can occur as a result of direct injury to the nerve itself or secondary to the creation of a new compression point.[16,24] This most often results from a failure to resect the medial intermuscular septum, the arcade of Struthers, or deep flexor-pronator aponeurosis.[25] Because intraneural and extraneural circulation can be impaired in nerves that are separated from their mesoneurium for distances greater than 8 cm, diabetes is a relative contraindication for transposition because of a patient's compromised intraneural vascularity.[26-28] Direct nerve injuries occur most often during revision cubital tunnel surgery and account for 20% of iatrogenic ulnar nerve injuries about the elbow (AL Osterman, MD, Philadelphia, PA, personal communication, 2003). Injuries to the ulnar nerve secondary to endoscopic cubital tunnel release have not been reported.

Dupuytren Surgery

Damage to the cutaneous and digital nerves occur more often than suspected, with surgery for Dupuytren disease possibly having the highest predictable rate of neurovascular injury.[2] Osterman reported that 12 of 21 iatrogenic digital nerve injuries that pre-

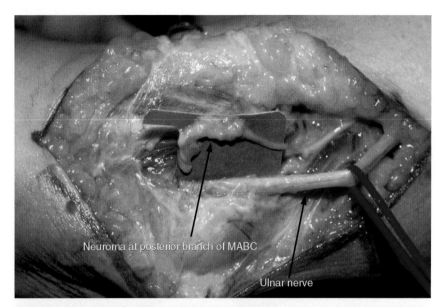

Figure 1 Intraoperative photograph of an intact ulnar nerve and a previously lacerated branch of the medial antebrachial cutaneous (MABC) nerve with a large neuroma. Treatment is by repair or resection and implantation of the stump in muscle or bone.

sented to a nerve center resulted from Dupuytren surgery (AL Osterman, MD, Philadelphia, PA, personal communication, 2003). Nerve injury rates vary by technique and are inconsistent across the literature. Partial fasciectomy rates range from 0% to 5% for primary surgery and up to 12% for revision surgery.[29-32] Percutaneous needle aponeurotomy has a lower reported rate of neurologic injuries, although the true incidence may be underestimated. Pess et al[33] reported temporary neurapraxia in 1.2% of patients and complete laceration in only 0.1% of 1,013 fingers treated with percutaneous needle aponeurotomy. Foucher et al[34] reported 3 neurapraxias and 1 nerve transection in 311 fingers treated with percutaneous needle aponeurotomy. Nerve injury is most often associated with spiral cords and severe contractures, especially with proximal interphalangeal joint contractures greater than 60°.[35] Limited literature is available regarding nerve injury associated with the use of injectable collagenase.

de Quervain Release

Injury (usually a neurapraxia) to the dorsal radial sensory nerve is common after release of the first dorsal extensor compartment[36,37] (**Figure 2**). Two of the four dorsal radial sensory nerve lesions seen at one nerve center occurred secondary to a de Quervain release (AL Osterman, MD, Philadelphia, PA, personal communication, 2003). Transverse skin incisions may predispose a patient to nerve injury.[38-41] There is also risk of a traction neuroma when attempting to obtain better exposure. Arons[39] reported five dorsal radial sensory nerve injuries secondary to de Quervain releases, two with neuroma formation and three secondary to scarring and adhesion. The author advocated using a gently curved modified Bruner incision.

Trigger Release

Injury to the digital nerves during a trigger release is common. Digital nerve injuries resulting from trigger release surgery comprised 7 of 21 iatrogenic digital nerve injuries that presented to one institution (AL Osterman, MD, Philadelphia, PA, personal communication, 2003). These injuries most often involve the radial digital nerve of the thumb or index finger secondary to their anatomy. The radial digital nerve to the thumb is most vulnerable to injury because it crosses ulnarly to radially across the A-1 pulley and runs superficially, averaging 1 to 2 mm deep to the dermis at the metacarpophalangeal joint flexion crease. It may be transected with a deep skin incision, especially when the nerve lies directly over the radial sesamoid.[36,42] In the digits, extra caution should be taken with a transverse incision to avoid nerve injury.[41] It is important that nerve injuries are recognized early and treated with microsurgical repair. Late recognition may require resection of a neuroma and implantation in muscle or bone.

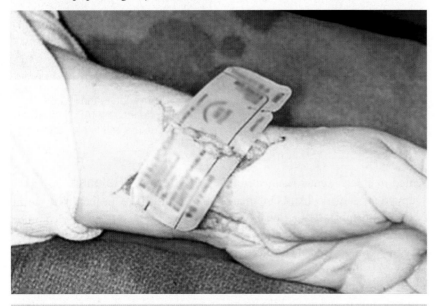

Figure 2 Photograph of a neuroma of the dorsal radial sensory nerve after a de Quervain release. The patient was treated with resection of the neuroma and implantation in a collagen tube.

Carpometacarpal Arthroplasty

Nerve trauma after thumb carpometacarpal arthroplasty most often involves an injury to a terminal branch of the dorsal radial sensory nerve secondary to retraction or laceration but may also involve the palmar cutaneous nerve or the median nerve proper.[43] The palmar cutaneous nerve is most vulnerable to injury during palmaris longus tendon harvest for ligament reconstruction with tendon interposition because of the transverse incision made at the wrist crease and the superficial course of the nerve. There also have been case reports of inadvertent median nerve excision in patients lacking palmaris longus tendons[44-48] (**Figure 3**). Davis et al[43] reported an incidence of dorsal radial sensory nerve injury and palmar cutaneous nerve injury in 18.5% and 6.6% of patients, respectively, treated with carpometacarpal arthroplasty. Residual numbness was present in 7% and 3.8%, respectively, at the 12-month follow-up. Scarred nerves are treated with neurolysis, and lacerated branches can be treated with direct repair if found early or implantation in muscle or bone if discovered or treated late.

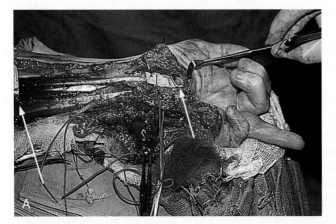
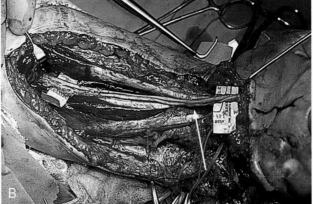

Figure 3 Intraoperative photographs during median nerve grafting after inadvertent median nerve harvest for a palmaris graft. **A,** The median nerve in the forearm has a 16-cm defect. Note the proximal stump of the mediam nerve (long arrow) and distal stump of the resected median nerve (short arrow). **B,** Cable grafting of the median nerve using sural nerve (arrow) interposition. A concomitant Huber opposition transfer was also performed.

Wrist Arthroscopy

Iatrogenic nerve injuries have been described after wrist arthroscopy. Nerve lacerations are described in higher frequency with the use of specific portals. Perhaps at highest risk is the dorsal sensory branch of the ulnar nerve during triangular fibrocartilage complex repair or when using the 6U portal.[49] The nerve may be damaged from strangulation by suture or by laceration with a scalpel or trocar.

McAdams and Hentz[50] reported inside-out sutures can be as close as 0.4 mm to the main trunk of the dorsal sensory branch of the ulnar nerve, suggesting that if the nerve is not visualized and protected, there is a 50% chance of nerve branch strangulation. Several studies on the arthroscopic excision of intra-articular dorsal ganglia have reported transient neurapraxias of the dorsal radial and ulnar sensory nerves that recovered by 6 months.[51-53] Injury to the posterior interosseous nerve has been described with use of the 3-4 portal.[54] A variety of safety procedures should be followed to minimize the incidence of iatrogenic nerve injury, including the use of a hypodermic needle to confirm portal placement, insufflation of the joint, the use of a longitudinal incision that penetrates only the dermis, and spreading the soft tissue with a hemostat to move aside important structures. The 6U portal should be avoided if possible.[49] Visualization of the dorsal sensory branch of the ulnar nerve during repair of the triangular fibrocartilage complex is critical.

Elbow Arthroscopy

Iatrogenic nerve injury during elbow arthroscopy is probably underreported in the literature.[17] All of the nerves that cross the elbow are at risk for iatrogenic nerve injury, with injuries reported in up to 14% of patients.[55-59] A Mayo Clinic study documented nerve palsies after elbow arthroscopy.[58] The authors reported transient nerve palsies in 2.5% of the patients, affecting the ulnar nerve (most often), the superficial radial nerve, the posterior interosseous nerve, the anterior interosseous nerve, and the medial antebrachial cutaneous nerve. The radial nerve is at risk during placement of the anterolateral portal, which typically lies within 2 to 10 mm of the nerve.[60-62] Flexion of the elbow to 90° will assist in displacing vital structures in the antecubital fossa away from the portals.

Contracture release has a particularly high risk of radial nerve injury.[56] Injuries should be identified and promptly repaired or grafted. Ulnar nerve injury has been documented, and special care should be taken if the patient had a prior transposition. Careful examination for subluxation of the ulnar nerve should be performed preoperatively in all patients. Injury to the median nerve also has been described because the anteromedial portal typically lies 7 to 20 mm away from the nerve.[60,61,63] Particular caution is warranted if resecting the tip of the coronoid because the median nerve is in especially close proximity.

Summary

Constant vigilance is needed to avoid iatrogenic nerve injury in upper extremity procedures. Extensive knowledge of the relevant anatomy is critical, including standard and common variations of the nerves at risk for injury. When preforming procedures around the wrist, particular attention is needed to avoid excessive retraction, especially of the dorsal radial sensory nerve. Arthroscopic incisions should be made through the dermis only, with blunt dissection to and through the capsule. Saline insufflation should be routinely used to move critical structures away from the joint. If a nerve injury occurs, early recognition and repair is critical for a favorable outcome. Cutaneous nerves can often be treated with excision of the neuroma and implantation into muscle or bone, repair, revision repair, nerve stripping, or nerve coaptation. Larger nerves may be grafted using a cable graft technique, with tendon transfers being reserved for late cases to maximize function. Before a surgical procedure, the patient should be counseled about the possibility of nerve injuries. If a nerve laceration occurs, it should be documented, and the patient should be advised.

References

1. Birch R, Bonney G, Dowell J, Hollingdale J: Iatrogenic injuries of peripheral nerves. *J Bone Joint Surg Br* 1991;73(2):280-282.

2. Kretschmer T, Heinen CW, Antoniadis G, Richter H-P, König RW: Iatrogenic nerve injuries. *Neurosurg Clin N Am* 2009;20(1):73-90, vii.

3. Khan R, Birch R: Latropathic injuries of peripheral nerves. *J Bone Joint Surg Br* 2001;83(8):1145-1148.

4. Hirasawa Y, Oda R, Nakatani K, Shikata Y, Makino T: Statistical study on peripheral nerve injury. *Nihon Geka Hokan* 1976;45(3):213-221.

5. Goth D: Iatrogenic nerve injuries of the arm. *Handchir Mikrochir Plast Chir* 1982;14(1):6-10.

6. Kretschmer T, Antoniadis G, Braun V, Rath SA, Richter HP: Evaluation of iatrogenic lesions in 722 surgically treated cases of peripheral nerve trauma. *J Neurosurg* 2001;94(6):905-912.

7. Benson LS, Bare AA, Nagle DJ, Harder VS, Williams CS, Visotsky JL: Complications of endoscopic and open carpal tunnel release. *Arthroscopy* 2006;22(9):919-924, e1-e2.

8. Hunt TR, Osterman AL: Complications of the treatment of carpal tunnel syndrome. *Hand Clin* 1994;10(1):63-71.

9. Taleisnik J: The palmar cutaneous branch of the median nerve and the approach to the carpal tunnel: An anatomical study. *J Bone Joint Surg Am* 1973;55(6):1212-1217.

10. MacDonald RI, Lichtman DM, Hanlon JJ, Wilson JN: Complications of surgical release for carpal tunnel syndrome. *J Hand Surg Am* 1978;3(1):70-76.

11. Beris AE, Lykissas MG, Kontogeorgakos VA, Vekris MD, Korompilias AV: Anatomic variations of the median nerve in carpal tunnel release. *Clin Anat* 2008;21(6):514-518.

12. Lanz U: Anatomical variations of the median nerve in the carpal tunnel. *J Hand Surg Am* 1977;2(1):44-53.

13. Siverhus SW, Kremchek TE, Smith WR, Basch TM, Drake RL: A cadaveric study of the anatomic variations of the recurrent motor branch of the median nerve. *Orthop Rev* 1989;18(3):315-320.

14. Amadio PC: Anatomic variations of the median nerve within the carpal tunnel. *Clin Anat* 1988;1(1):23-31.

15. Dellon AL, MacKinnon SE: Injury to the medial antebrachial cutaneous nerve during cubital tunnel surgery. *J Hand Surg Br* 1985;10(1):33-36.

16. Jackson LC, Hotchkiss RN: Cubital tunnel surgery: Complications and treatment of failures. *Hand Clin* 1996;12(2):449-456.

17. Adams JE, Steinmann SP: Nerve injuries about the elbow. *J Hand Surg Am* 2006;31(2):303-313.

18. Mackinnon SE, Dellon AL, Hudson AR, Hunter DA: A primate model for chronic nerve compression. *J Reconstr Microsurg* 1985;1(3):185-195.

19. Rogers MR, Bergfield TG, Aulicino PL: The failed ulnar nerve transposition: Etiology and treatment. *Clin Orthop Relat Res* 1991;269:193-200.

20. Sarris I, Göbel F, Gainer M, Vardakas DG, Vogt MT, Sotereanos DG: Medial brachial and antebrachial cutaneous nerve injuries: Effect on outcome in revision cubital tunnel surgery. *J Reconstr Microsurg* 2002;18(8):665-670.

21. Masear VR, Meyer RD, Pichora DR: Surgical anatomy of the medial antebrachial cutaneous nerve. *J Hand Surg Am* 1989;14(2, pt 1):267-271.

22. Race CM, Saldana MJ: Anatomic course of the medial cutaneous nerves of the arm. *J Hand Surg Am* 1991;16(1):48-52.

23. Patterson SD, Bain GI, Mehta JA: Surgical approaches to the elbow. *Clin Orthop Relat Res* 2000;370:19-33.

24. Bednar MS, Blair SJ, Light TR: Complications of the treatment of cubital tunnel syndrome. *Hand Clin* 1994;10(1):83-92.

25. Broudy AS, Leffert RD, Smith RJ: Technical problems with ulnar nerve transposition at the elbow: Findings and results of reoperation. *J Hand Surg Am* 1978;3(1):85-89.

26. Smith JW: Factors influencing nerve repair: II. Collateral circulation of peripheral nerves. *Arch Surg* 1966;93(3):433-437.

27. Ogata K, Manske PR, Lesker PA: The effect of surgical dissection on regional blood flow to the ulnar nerve in the cubital tunnel. *Clin Orthop Relat Res* 1985;193:195-198.

28. Osterman AL, Davis CA: Subcutaneous transposition of the ulnar nerve for treatment of cubital tunnel syndrome. *Hand Clin* 1996;12(2):421-433.

29. Mäkelä EA, Jaroma H, Harju A, Anttila S, Vainio J: Dupuytren's contracture: The long-term results after day surgery. *J Hand Surg Br* 1991;16(3):272-274.

30. Robins RH, Scott TD, Griffiths DP: Day care surgery for Dupuytren's contracture. *J Hand Surg Br* 1993;18(4):494-498.

31. Ebskov LB, Boeckstyns ME, Sørensen AI, Haugegaard M: Day care surgery for advanced Dupuytren's contracture. *J Hand Surg Br* 1997;22(2):191-192.

32. Coert JH, Nérin JP, Meek MF: Results of partial fasciectomy for Dupuytren disease in 261 consecutive patients. *Ann Plast Surg* 2006;57(1):13-17.

33. Pess GM, Pess RM, Pess RA: Results of needle aponeurotomy for Dupuytren contracture in over 1,000 fingers. *J Hand Surg Am* 2012;37(4):651-656.

34. Foucher G, Medina J, Navarro R: Percutaneous needle aponeurotomy: Complications and results. *J Hand Surg Br* 2003;28(5):427-431.

35. Bulstrode NW, Jemec B, Smith PJ: The complications of Dupuytren's contracture surgery. *J Hand Surg Am* 2005;30(5):1021-1025.

36. Ryzewicz M, Wolf JM: Trigger digits: Principles, management, and complications. *J Hand Surg Am* 2006;31(1):135-146.

37. Scheller A, Schuh R, Hönle W, Schuh A: Long-term results of surgical release of de Quervain's stenosing tenosynovitis. *Int Orthop* 2009;33(5):1301-1303.

38. Alegado RB, Meals RA: An unusual complication following surgical treatment of deQuervain's disease. *J Hand Surg Am* 1979;4(2):185-186.

39. Arons MS: de Quervain's release in working women: A report of failures, complications, and associated diagnoses. *J Hand Surg Am* 1987;12(4):540-544.

40. Savage R: *Plastic Surgery*. Philadelphia, PA, WB Saunders, 1990, pp 4725-4756.

41. Sampson SP, Wisch D, Badalamente MA: Complications of conservative and surgical treat-

ment of de Quervain's disease and trigger fingers. *Hand Clin* 1994; 10(1):73-82.

42. Carrozzella J, Stern PJ, Von Kuster LC: Transection of radial digital nerve of the thumb during trigger release. *J Hand Surg Am* 1989;14(2, pt 1):198-200.

43. Davis TR, Brady O, Dias JJ: Excision of the trapezium for osteoarthritis of the trapeziometacarpal joint: A study of the benefit of ligament reconstruction or tendon interposition. *J Hand Surg Am* 2004;29(6):1069-1077.

44. Kovácsy A: Removal of the median nerve instead of the palmaris longus tendon. *Magy Traumatol Orthop Helyreallito Seb* 1980; 23(2):156-158.

45. Vastamäki M: Median nerve as free tendon graft. *J Hand Surg Br* 1987;12(2):187-188.

46. Toros T, Vatansever A, Ada S: Accidental use of the median nerve as an interposition material in first carpometacarpal joint arthroplasty. *J Hand Surg Br* 2006; 31(5):574-575.

47. Weber RV, Mackinnon SE: Median nerve mistaken for palmaris longus tendon: Restoration of function with sensory nerve transfers. *Hand (NY)* 2007;2(1):1-4.

48. Gangopadhyay S, McKenna H, Burke FD, Davis TR: Five- to 18-year follow-up for treatment of trapeziometacarpal osteoarthritis: A prospective comparison of excision, tendon interposition, and ligament reconstruction and tendon interposition. *J Hand Surg Am* 2012;37(3):411-417.

49. Ahsan ZS, Yao J: Complications of wrist arthroscopy. *Arthroscopy* 2012;28(6):855-859.

50. McAdams TR, Hentz VR: Injury to the dorsal sensory branch of the ulnar nerve in the arthroscopic repair of ulnar-sided triangular fibrocartilage tears using an inside-out technique: A cadaver study. *J Hand Surg Am* 2002; 27(5):840-844.

51. Rocchi L, Canal A, Fanfani F, Catalano F: Articular ganglia of the volar aspect of the wrist: Arthroscopic resection compared with open excision. A prospective randomised study. *Scand J Plast Reconstr Surg Hand Surg* 2008; 42(5):253-259.

52. Chen AC, Lee W-C, Hsu K-Y, Chan Y-S, Yuan L-J, Chang C-H: Arthroscopic ganglionectomy through an intrafocal cystic portal for wrist ganglia. *Arthroscopy* 2010;26(5):617-622.

53. Gallego S, Mathoulin C: Arthroscopic resection of dorsal wrist ganglia: 114 cases with minimum follow-up of 2 years. *Arthroscopy* 2010;26(12):1675-1682.

54. del Piñal F, Herrero F, Cruz-Camara A, San Jose J: Complete avulsion of the distal posterior interosseous nerve during wrist arthroscopy: A possible cause of persistent pain after arthroscopy. *J Hand Surg Am* 1999;24(2): 240-242.

55. Jobe FW, Stark H, Lombardo SJ: Reconstruction of the ulnar collateral ligament in athletes. *J Bone Joint Surg Am* 1986;68(8):1158-1163.

56. Jones GS, Savoie FH III: Arthroscopic capsular release of flexion contractures (arthrofibrosis) of the elbow. *Arthroscopy* 1993;9(3): 277-283.

57. Schneider T, Hoffstetter I, Fink B, Jerosch J: Long-term results of elbow arthroscopy in 67 patients. *Acta Orthop Belg* 1994;60(4): 378-383.

58. Kelly EW, Morrey BF, O'Driscoll SW: Complications of elbow arthroscopy. *J Bone Joint Surg Am* 2001;83(1):25-34.

59. Maak TG, Osei D, Delos D, Taylor S, Warren RF, Weiland AJ: Peripheral nerve injuries in sports-related surgery: Presentation, evaluation, and management. *J Bone Joint Surg Am* 2012;94(16): e1211.

60. Lynch GJ, Meyers JF, Whipple TL, Caspari RB: Neurovascular anatomy and elbow arthroscopy: Inherent risks. *Arthroscopy* 1986; 2(3):190-197.

61. Verhaar J, van Mameren H, Brandsma A: Risks of neurovascular injury in elbow arthroscopy: Starting anteromedially or anterolaterally? *Arthroscopy* 1991;7(3): 287-290.

62. Adolfsson L: Arthroscopy of the elbow joint: A cadaveric study of portal placement. *J Shoulder Elbow Surg* 1994;3(2):53-61.

63. Marshall PD, Fairclough JA, Johnson SR, Evans EJ: Avoiding nerve damage during elbow arthroscopy. *J Bone Joint Surg Br* 1993;75(1):129-131.

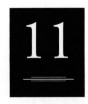

Complications of Distal Radial and Scaphoid Fracture Treatment

Carissa Meyer, MD
James Chang, MD
Peter J. Stern, MD
A. Lee Osterman, MD
Joshua M. Abzug, MD

Abstract

Fractures of the distal radius and the scaphoid are common injuries in adults. In recent years, surgical fixation of these types of fractures has increased in response to improved patient outcomes and evolving fixation techniques. Potential soft-tissue, neurovascular, or osseous complications, including tendon injuries, carpal tunnel syndrome, loss of fracture reduction, and osteonecrosis, can increase the time the patient requires immobilization and can lead to poor patient outcomes. Prompt recognition and diagnosis of these complications may improve patient outcomes and satisfaction.

Instr Course Lect 2014;63:113-122.

Fractures of the distal aspect of the radius and the scaphoid are common injuries in adults. Surgical fixation of both distal radial and scaphoid fractures has increased in recent years in response to improved patient outcomes and evolving fixation techniques. Potential soft-tissue, neurovascular, or osseous complications, including tendon injuries, carpal tunnel syndrome, loss of fracture reduction, and osteonecrosis, can increase immobilization time and the number of surgical procedures and can lead to poor patient outcomes. Prompt recognition and diagnosis of these complications may lead to improved patient outcomes and satisfaction.

Complications of Distal Radial Fractures

Fractures of the distal aspect of the radius are common orthopaedic injuries, comprising 10% to 25% of all fractures.[1] These fractures are prevalent in all age groups and occur after high- and low-energy trauma. More than 85,000 Medicare beneficiaries sustain a distal radial fracture each year, with a rising percentage being treated surgically.[2,3]

Shortening of the distal end of the radius by as little as 2.5 mm substantially increases the load transmitted across the distal end of the ulna and can lead to wrist pain, disordered wrist kinematics, and early arthritis formation.[4] It is important to understand the complications involved in the treatment of distal radial fractures and how to adequately address these complications.

Several treatment options exist for distal radial fractures, including immobilization with or without closed re-

Dr. Chang or an immediate family member serves as a paid consultant to or is an employee of Zone II Surgical; has stock or stock options held in Zone II Surgical; and serves as a board member, owner, officer, or committee member of the American Board of Plastic Surgery and the American Society for Surgery of the Hand. Dr. Osterman or an immediate family member has received royalties from Medartis and Biomet; is a member of a speakers' bureau or has made paid presentations on behalf of Auxilium, Medartis, Arthrex, and Synthes; serves as a paid consultant to or is an employee of Auxilium; has received research or institutional support from Auxilium and Skeletal Dynamics; and serves as a board member, owner, officer, or committee member of the American Association for Hand Surgery and the American Society for Surgery of the Hand. None of the following authors or any immediate family member has received anything of value from or has stock or stock options held in a commercial company or institution related directly or indirectly to the subject of this chapter: Dr. Meyer, Dr. Stern, and Dr. Abzug.

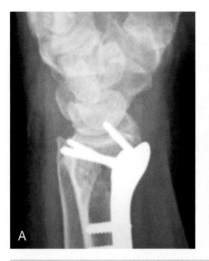
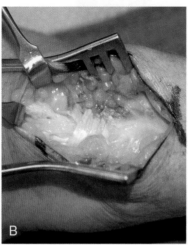
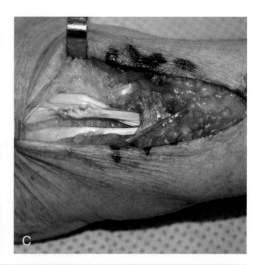

Figure 1   Tendon injury resulting from surgical treatment. **A,** Screw penetration through the dorsal cortex 9 months after volar plating. The patient noted increasing dorsal wrist pain and swelling. **B,** Extensor indicis proprius rupture. **C,** End-to-side transfer of the extensor indicis proprius to the extensor digitorum communis of the long finger. (Courtesy of Joshua M. Abzug, MD, Timonium, MD.)

duction, percutaneous pin fixation, external fixation, and open reduction and internal fixation (ORIF). Options for ORIF include dorsal plating, volar plating, and fragment-specific fixation. In 2010, the American Academy of Orthopaedic Surgeons (AAOS) published guidelines for the treatment of distal radial fractures, which included recommendations for surgical fixation of fractures using radiographic parameters.[5] Surgical fixation is recommended for fractures with postreduction radial shortening of more than 3 mm, dorsal tilt of more than 10°, or intra-articular displacement or step-off of more than 2 mm.[5] The authors of the guidelines, however, were unable to recommend for or against any specific surgical method.

Volar fixed-angle plating has become popular in recent years. Because it does not rely on a buttress effect, it can be used for fractures with either volar or dorsal tilt and those with intra-articular extension or comminution. The plate gains purchase in the subchondral bone and neutralizes the load across the fracture site. The locking construct does not require good quality bone, allowing for use in os-

teopenic bone or areas with comminution.

Soft-Tissue Complications

Tendon irritation and rupture are complications of both surgical and nonsurgical treatment of distal radial fractures. Although traditionally associated with dorsal plating, tendon irritation and rupture can occur with volar plating or cast treatment.[6]

The most common tendon ruptured is the extensor pollicis longus, with extensor tendons more commonly involved than flexor tendons. Tendon rupture, particularly of the extensor pollicis longus, may occur in as many as 3% of patients after nonsurgical treatment of a distal radial fracture.[7-9] This is believed to be the result of mechanical attrition and/or vascular insult. When treatment is surgical, tendon injury typically occurs because of drill-bit penetration or dorsal screw prominence with volar plating, and screw-head or plate prominence with dorsal plating (**Figure 1**).

Tendon rupture is usually predated by extensor tenosynovitis and wrist pain. The tendon rupture rate with volar plate fixation has been reported

to range from 0.8% to 12%, with higher percentages cited for earlier plate models.[10] Tendon irritation is even more common. In studies by Rozental et al[11] and Rozental and Blazar,[12] implant removal resulting from tendon irritation occurred in 10% of fractures treated with volar plates and 32% of fractures treated with dorsal plates. In studies of newer low-profile (1.2 to 1.5-mm) dorsal plates, nearly equal rates of tenosynovitis and tendon rupture occurred in the dorsal (6.7%) and volar (4.8%) plate groups.[13]

Extensor tendon complications can be avoided by careful surgical technique. This includes drilling to—but not through—the dorsal cortex for distal locking screws and obtaining a set with 1-mm screw increments to avoid screws that are too long. Careful attention should be paid to symptoms of extensor tendon irritation or pain, with early surgical intervention for removal of implants if tendon irritation is suspected.

Flexor tendon injuries are usually caused by distal placement of the volar locking plate. The watershed line is a transverse ridge along the distal volar surface of the radius lying between the pronator quadratus and volar radiocarpal ligaments (**Figure 2**). Plates positioned distal to the watershed line may place the plate and screw heads in direct contact with the deep flexor tendons.[14,15] Tendon irritation, especially of the deep flexor tendons, can occur from malreduced fractures with residual dorsal angulation. Tendon irritation and injury can occur from screw backout, if the screws are not fully engaged in the locking threads. The index finger flexor digitorum profundus and flexor pollicis longus are most at risk. Flexor pollicis longus rupture has been reported to occur from 4 to 68 months after placement of a volar plate,[16,17] with recent studies reporting a 2% to 12% rupture rate.[10,18] Reapproximation of the pronator quadratus muscle at the end of the procedure can provide a layer of soft-tissue protection between the plate and the flexor tendons. After an attritional flexor pollicis longus rupture, reconstruction can be accomplished with a palmaris longus tendon graft.[18] If the palmaris is not available, the plantaris or long toe extensor tendons may be used for intercalated graft.[19] If the flexor pollicis longus tendon is not suitable for grafting, the flexor digitorum superficialis of the ring finger may be used for tendon transfer.

The cases of three patients who had a flexor tendon rupture after the surgeon inadvertently failed to remove preplaced distal locking-hole drill guides have been reported.[20] Loosening of locked screws is another potential complication, and has been reported to occur in 1% to 2% of patients.[10,18]

Neurovascular Complications

Carpal tunnel syndrome may occur after a distal radial fracture regardless of treatment modality. Acute carpal tunnel syndrome may develop because of the initial injury, whereas subacute or late carpal tunnel syndrome may occur

because of fracture-healing or treatment. Carpal tunnel syndrome can cause long-term decreases in patient outcome scores: one series with 10-year follow-up showed that 62% of the patients with unsatisfactory outcomes after distal radial fracture had objective signs of carpal tunnel syndrome compared with a 6% rate of carpal tunnel syndrome in patients with satisfactory outcomes.[21]

The prevalence of carpal tunnel syndrome associated with a distal radial fracture remains unknown, as many patients may have symptoms of carpal tunnel syndrome before their injury, but it has been reported to range from 2% to 14%.[9,22-24] Some surgeons advocate release of the carpal tunnel on all surgically treated distal radial fractures.[22,23] Careful preoperative examination is essential to determine whether median nerve symptoms are present before closed reduction or surgical treatment. This chapter's authors prefer to perform carpal tunnel release at the time of distal radial fixation in all patients with acute onset of median nerve symptoms, as well as in patients who can accurately describe preexisting carpal tunnel syndrome symptoms.

Injury to the palmar cutaneous branch of the median nerve may occur with volar fixation of distal radial fractures. The palmar cutaneous nerve branches from the median nerve 5 cm proximal to the distal wrist crease and travels with the median nerve for 16 to 25 mm. It then runs radially and obliquely into the palm along the ulnar border of the flexor carpi radialis.[25] Injury to the nerve may occur if the initial incision is extended to include a carpal tunnel release. Therefore, a separate incision is recommended for carpal tunnel release to avoid injury to this nerve.[23] A mini-open carpal tunnel release performed through an incision that does not cross the wrist flexion crease is preferred.

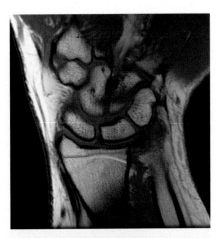

Figure 2 Coronal MRI scan of the distal aspect of the radius showing the watershed line (red line) and pronator quadratus (blue line) insertion. (Courtesy of Joshua M. Abzug, MD, Timonium, MD.)

Injury to the superficial branch of the radial nerve may occur during volar fixation of distal radial fractures. This injury is usually a neurapraxia caused by excessive retraction of the nerve during fracture reduction. Alternatively, injury may occur during percutaneous placement of Kirschner wires in the radial styloid for fracture fixation.[26]

Radial artery injury is a rare complication of distal radial fractures. Dao et al[27] reported a case of pseudoaneurysm formation 11 months after initial fixation with known delayed healing. Pseudoaneurysm formation was attributed to continued motion at the fracture site and design of the AO/ASIF (Association for the Study of Internal Fixation) low-profile volar distal radial plate.

Osseous Complications

Screw penetration through the distal radial articular cartilage may occur at the time of fracture fixation, from loss of fixation, or from fracture subsidence (**Figure 3**). The use of several radiographic views, as well as live fluoroscopy, during initial fixation helps in the assessment of the radiocarpal joint.

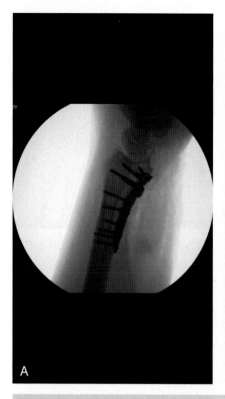
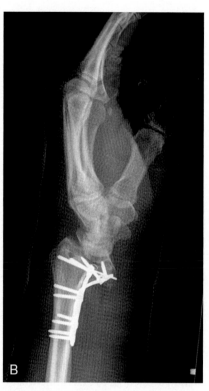

Figure 3   Initial fixation of an intra-articular fracture (**A**) and loss of fixation 2 weeks after surgery after the patient started immediate weight bearing (**B**). (Courtesy of Joshua M. Abzug, MD, Timonium, MD.)

Tilt views in the PA and lateral planes can increase surgeon accuracy in determining the presence of an intra-articular screw.[28] More ulnar screws are viewed with the beam tilted 23° from the plane of the surgical table on the lateral radiograph, whereas the radial styloid screw is best seen at a 30° tilt from the plane of the surgical table. The x-ray plate or fluoroscope remains flat while the patient's arm is tilted in the vertical axis with the forearm in a neutral position. A PA radiograph can be made in full pronation with the wrist tilted 11° from the plane of the surgical table off the imaging plate, again in the vertical plane. Dynamic fluoroscopy including evaluation of tilt views is more accurate for determining intra-articular screw placement than are static views alone.[29]

Poor fracture reduction may be a result of inadequate reduction at the time of the initial procedure or from fracture subsidence over time. Failure to initially achieve reduction is usually caused by inadequate exposure. The extended flexor carpi radialis exposure increases visualization of the radial and dorsal sides of the distal end of the radius.[23] The standard volar approach is extended distally and radially with release of the first extensor compartment, and the distal insertion of the brachioradialis is taken down to increase visibility of any radial styloid fragments and permit visualization of the dorsal aspect of the fracture. This chapter's authors use this extended exposure when extensive dorsal comminution is present because it allows for direct reduction of these fracture fragments.

Loss of reduction after surgical or closed reduction is the result of dorsal collapse or dorsal tilt, radial shortening, or loss of reduction of the lunate facet. Dorsal tilt is the most common mode of failure and can lead to decreased wrist motion and pain after fracture healing.[12] It may also lead to distal radioulnar joint arthritis, flexor tendon irritation, or tendon rupture. When a volar plate is used for fractures with extensive dorsal comminution, plates designed with two distal rows of locking screws provide more stable fixation.[23,30] Volar collapse, although less common, may occur with dorsal plating of complex intra-articular fractures.[23]

Radial shortening resulting from collapse across the fracture site can lead to abnormal distribution of forces across the wrist joint and increased load on the ulnocarpal articulation. To reduce the risk of collapse, the distal screws should be placed as close to the subchondral bone as possible.[10,23,31] Drobetz et al,[32] who compared distal radial fractures that had plates applied subchondrally and those that had plates applied more than 4.5 mm proximal to the subchondral zone, demonstrated that the placement of distal screws more than 4 mm proximal to the subchondral zone led to a 50% reduction in radial length.

The lunate facet can be difficult to reduce anatomically because of poor visualization, or it may be difficult to maintain reduction with an intra-articular distal radial fracture. Harness et al[33] reported on seven patients with intra-articular distal radial fractures involving a volar shear component. All seven patients initially had anatomic reduction of their fractures and volar plate fixation but subsequently lost reduction of the lunate facet fragment, requiring revision surgery in five patients.

Tangential lateral radiographs may be useful in evaluating adequate reduction and fixation of the lunate facet.[34] The same tilted radiograph used for determining intra-articular screw placement provides an accurate picture of the lunate facet and any residual articular step-off. When a standard volar plate does not adequately capture the lunate facet fragment, plates that may be placed more distally should be used.[30] Fixation may be augmented with dorsal plate fixation or postoperative immobilization to allow adequate fragment healing.[35]

Complex Regional Pain Syndrome

Complex regional pain syndrome of unknown cause is a complication of many orthopaedic injuries. It is a pain syndrome characterized by autonomic nerve dysfunction, trophic changes, and functional impairment. The prevalence after distal radial fracture has been reported to range from 8% to 35% in retrospective series and occurs with both surgical and nonsurgical treatment.[36-39] In a recent prospective study, complex regional pain syndrome developed in 10% of patients who sustained a fracture of the distal aspect of the radius.[40]

Diagnosis of complex regional pain syndrome is based on physical examination findings because no specific laboratory or radiographic abnormalities are pathognomonic. Symptoms include pain, diffuse edema, changes in skin color and temperature compared with the contralateral limb, and limited motion of the affected extremity. The bones may be osteopenic on radiographs with subchondral and periarticular resorption, although as many as 30% of patients will have normal findings on radiographs.[41] Technetium Tc-99m bone scanning is often used for diagnosis, with specificity between 75% and 98%; however, it is only 50% sensitive.[42]

Vitamin C may have a preventive effect on complex regional pain syndrome. In a double-blind prospective randomized study, 500 mg of vitamin C taken daily for 50 days after in-

jury lowered the risk of complex regional pain syndrome from 10% to 2.4%.[40] The study included patients treated both surgically and nonsurgically. The AAOS guidelines recommend the use of vitamin C to lower the risk of complex regional pain syndrome after a distal radial fracture.[5] Side effects of vitamin C are generally minimal but can include diarrhea, abdominal cramping, and kidney stone formation when taken at high doses. Narcotic medications are generally not effective for complex regional pain syndrome and should be avoided.[41]

This chapter's authors use both preventive and treatment strategies for patients with or at risk for the development of complex regional pain syndrome. Vitamin C is prescribed at the first clinic visit for all patients receiving nonsurgical treatment and at the time of surgery for all patients receiving surgical treatment. Range-of-motion exercises are encouraged at 2 to 4 weeks postoperatively or at 4 to 6 weeks for patients treated nonsurgically. Narcotic usage is limited to 1 to 2 weeks postoperatively. Formal physical therapy is essential for desensitization exercises and to encourage range of motion in all patients with complex regional pain syndrome.

Infection

Infection is an uncommon complication of surgically treated distal radial fractures. Although minor pin site infections may occur in up to 11.9% of patients treated primarily or secondarily with external fixation, the rate of infection after internal fixation has been reported to be between 0% and 0.8%.[43]

Complications of Scaphoid Fractures

Scaphoid fractures constitute 60% of all carpal fractures.[44] In adults, 70% to 80% of these occur at the waist, 10% to 20% at the proximal pole, and the

remainder at the distal pole.[45] The average age of a patient with an acute scaphoid fracture is 25 years, and the yearly incidence is 23 to 43 per 100,000 people.[44,46]

Scaphoid fractures often pose a diagnostic challenge, particularly for nondisplaced fractures. It may be difficult to assess fracture displacement or confirm union and adequate treatment.[47-49] Failure to treat occult fractures or to recognize fracture displacement can lead to altered carpal kinematics and the development of dorsal intercalated segment instability over time. This progressive deformity can lead to altered grip strength, decreased wrist motion, and early arthrosis.[50]

Radiographs often fail to show nondisplaced fractures of the scaphoid.[51] Therefore, when patients are suspected of having a scaphoid fracture without a radiographic abnormality, they are usually placed in a thumb spica cast.[52] Physical examination is sensitive, but specificity is low, ranging from 74% to 80%.[53,54] Bone scintigraphy has been reported to be 92% to 95% sensitive and 60% to 95% specific.[55] MRI is more consistent, with a specificity of 90% and a sensitivity of 90% to 100%.[56] This chapter's authors prefer to use MRI when a scaphoid fracture is suspected but not seen on radiographs because MRI is more routinely available. After an informed discussion with the patient, a 2-week trial of casting may be tried before obtaining an MRI.

Although most scaphoid fractures heal with nonsurgical treatment, this may require prolonged cast immobilization, leading to stiffness, possible cast complications, and loss of productivity.[57,58] For these reasons, surgical fixation has become increasingly common for the acute treatment of scaphoid fractures. Fixation may be performed with a percutaneous technique for nondisplaced fractures or via an open approach if open reduction is needed.

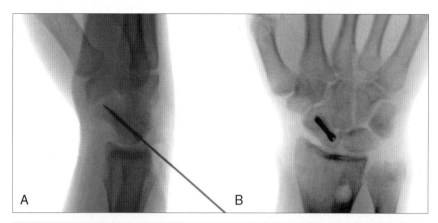

Figure 4 Methods to avoid complications related to screw length. **A,** At least 4 mm should be subtracted from the wire length to avoid intra-articular screw placement. **B,** Screw placement should be centered on PA and lateral radiographs (PA radiograph is shown). (Courtesy of Joshua M. Abzug, MD, Timonium, MD.)

Osteonecrosis

More than 80% of the scaphoid surface is covered with articular cartilage. The main blood supply is retrograde, with the more proximal 70% to 80% supplied by the dorsal scaphoid branches entering along the dorsal ridge. The remaining distal 20% to 30% receives its blood supply via the volar scaphoid branches entering at the distal tubercle.[59] This tenuous blood supply makes the scaphoid prone to osteonecrosis after injury, especially of the proximal pole, which has been reported to occur in 13% to 50% of such patients regardless of treatment. The prevalence is higher in fractures through the proximal pole.[60]

If osteonecrosis is present at the time of surgical fixation, a vascularized bone graft using the 1,2 intercompartmental supraretinacular artery is performed.[61] If this fails, the preferred salvage procedure for symptomatic osteonecrosis is four-corner arthrodesis or proximal row carpectomy.

Fracture Nonunion

Nonunion remains a frequent complication, particularly for displaced fractures. Factors associated with nonunion include fracture displacement of more than 1 mm, proximal pole fracture, osteonecrosis, vertical oblique fracture, and tobacco smoking.[62,63] Mack et al[64] found that over the course of 20 to 30 years, pancarpal arthritis develops in patients with scaphoid nonunion. Arthritis development is accelerated in patients with displaced fractures or dorsal intercalated segment instability patterns.

For nondisplaced scaphoid waist fractures treated with casting, nonunion rates have been reported to range from 5% to 12%.[65] In a prospective study of nondisplaced scaphoid fractures treated with short or long arm casting, only 2 of 51 fractures failed to heal.[66] Nonunion rates for displaced scaphoid fractures treated nonsurgically are higher, reaching 50%.[63] However, the difficulty remains in determining fracture displacement at the time of injury. Therefore, when displacement is unclear, this chapter's authors prefer to obtain a CT scan to determine the extent and plane of displacement.

Complications of Internal Fixation

The most common errors in surgical fixation are caused by screw length and screw placement. Controversy exists regarding screw placement. Some authors recommend screw placement centrally in the scaphoid,[67] whereas others advocate that the screw should be perpendicular to the fracture line.[68,69] Screws placed eccentrically decrease the strength of fixation and risk penetrating the scaphocapitate joint.[67] Chan and McAdams[68] found in an anatomic study that the dorsal approach resulted in a centered screw throughout the scaphoid, whereas screw placement via the volar approach was centered in the waist and proximal pole but not the distal pole. However, Jeon et al[69] reported no difference in functional outcome or healing between the volar and dorsal approaches. Recent evidence suggests that this has more to do with placement perpendicular to the fracture line than central screw placement.[70] Eccentric placement may be beneficial in some fracture patterns by increasing the osseous surface available for apposition at the fracture site.[71] This chapter's authors prefer to place the screw centrally in all fracture patterns because screw placement perpendicular to the fracture line is often difficult, given the limits of intraoperative fluoroscopy.

Complications related to screw length can be prevented by avoiding penetration of the far cortex with the guidewire and screw. Screw length should be shorter than the measured length of the guidewire. Bedi et al[72] advocate subtracting 4 mm from the measured screw length to avoid screw penetration (**Figure 4**). The dorsal approach, although technically simpler, has specific complications compared with the volar approach: guidewire placement is antegrade, and care should be taken to avoid screw penetration into the scaphotrapezial joint or screw prominence proximally into the radioscaphoid joint. Dorsal antegrade guidewire placement requires flexion of the wrist to 90°, which can be difficult to attain and risks bending the guidewire.[73] The percutaneous dorsal approach can place several structures at risk. In a cadaver study, guidewire placement was measured an average of 17.4 mm from the superficial branch of the radial nerve, 5.1 mm from the extensor pollicis longus, 2.2 mm from the posterior interosseous nerve, and 3.1 mm from the extensor indicis proprius. In a study of 12 wrists, the wire passed through the extensor indicis proprius in 2 wrists and it went through the extensor pollicis longus in another 2 wrists.[74]

Positioning of the wrist for placement of the guidewire and screw via a volar approach is technically less difficult. Guidewire placement is retrograde, and guidewire penetration into the radioscaphoid joint, as well as possible screw penetration into the joint, can lead to pain and early arthrosis. Percutaneous fixation may be accomplished safely with careful attention to positioning and protection of the radial artery. Fracture reduction may be accomplished using finger trap traction to pull the wrist into extension and ulnar deviation. After a small incision is made, a 14-gauge angiocatheter can be used to locate the point of desired screw placement and can be tapped into the starting point. The needle is then removed, and the angiocatheter sheath is used to protect the soft tissues during wire placement.[73] This is the preferred technique of this chapter's authors for all nondisplaced fractures.

If displacement is present, an open approach is preferred to avoid potential complications, as well as visualize the fracture site, joint surface, and reduction.[75] The radial artery, superficial branch of the radial nerve, and recurrent branch of the median nerve may be placed at risk if a percutaneous volar procedure is performed.

Summary

Surgical fixation of both distal radial and scaphoid fractures has become increasingly popular in the past decade. New evidence continues to support more indications for acute surgical intervention for displaced distal radial and scaphoid fractures. Several treatments are available for either fracture, each with its own set of risks and benefits. It is important to recognize and understand the complications that exist with each treatment option to continue to improve patient outcomes.

References

1. Letsch R, Infanger M, Schmidt J, Kock HJ: Surgical treatment of fractures of the distal radius with plates: A comparison of palmar and dorsal plate position. *Arch Orthop Trauma Surg* 2003; 123(7):333-339.

2. Shauver MJ, Clapham PJ, Chung KC: An economic analysis of outcomes and complications of treating distal radius fractures in the elderly. *J Hand Surg Am* 2011; 36(12):1912-1918, e1-e3.

3. Chung KC, Shauver MJ, Yin H, Kim HM, Baser O, Birkmeyer JD: Variations in the use of internal fixation for distal radial fracture in the United States Medicare population. *J Bone Joint Surg Am* 2011;93(23):2154-2162.

4. Graham TJ: Surgical correction of malunited fractures of the distal radius. *J Am Acad Orthop Surg* 1997;5(5):270-281.

5. Lichtman DM, Bindra RR, Boyer MI, et al: Treatment of distal radius fractures. *J Am Acad Orthop Surg* 2010;18(3):180-189.

6. Diaz-Garcia RJ, Oda T, Shauver MJ, Chung KC: A systematic review of outcomes and complications of treating unstable distal radius fractures in the elderly. *J Hand Surg Am* 2011;36(5):824-835, e2.

7. Bonatz E, Kramer TD, Masear VR: Rupture of the extensor pollicis longus tendon. *Am J Orthop (Belle Mead NJ)* 1996;25(2):118-122.

8. Skoff HD: Postfracture extensor pollicis longus tenosynovitis and tendon rupture: A scientific study and personal series. *Am J Orthop (Belle Mead NJ)* 2003;32(5):245-247.

9. White BD, Nydick JA, Karsky D, Williams BD, Hess AV, Stone JD: Incidence and clinical outcomes of tendon rupture following distal radius fracture. *J Hand Surg Am* 2012;37(10):2035-2040.

10. Drobetz H, Kutscha-Lissberg E: Osteosynthesis of distal radial fractures with a volar locking screw plate system. *Int Orthop* 2003;27(1):1-6.

11. Rozental TD, Beredjiklian PK, Bozentka DJ: Functional outcome and complications following two types of dorsal plating for unstable fractures of the distal part of the radius. *J Bone Joint Surg Am* 2003; 85(10):1956-1960.

12. Rozental TD, Blazar PE: Functional outcome and complications after volar plating for dorsally displaced, unstable fractures of the distal radius. *J Hand Surg Am* 2006;31(3):359-365.

13. Yu YR, Makhni MC, Tabrizi S, Rozental TD, Mundanthanam G, Day CS: Complications of low-profile dorsal versus volar locking plates in the distal radius: A comparative study. *J Hand Surg Am* 2011;36(7):1135-1141.

14. Orbay JL, Touhami A: Current concepts in volar fixed-angle fixation of unstable distal radius fractures. *Clin Orthop Relat Res* 2006; 445:58-67.

15. Orbay J: Volar plate fixation of distal radius fractures. *Hand Clin* 2005;21(3):347-354.

16. Bell JS, Wollstein R, Citron ND: Rupture of flexor pollicis longus tendon: A complication of volar

plating of the distal radius. *J Bone Joint Surg Br* 1998;80(2): 225-226.

17. Koo SC, Ho ST: Delayed rupture of flexor pollicis longus tendon after volar plating of the distal radius. *Hand Surg* 2006;11(1-2): 67-70.

18. Arora R, Lutz M, Hennerbichler A, Krappinger D, Espen D, Gabl M: Complications following internal fixation of unstable distal radius fracture with a palmar locking-plate. *J Orthop Trauma* 2007;21(5):316-322.

19. Taras JS, Kaufmann RA: Flexor tendon reconstruction, in Green DP, Hotchkiss RN, Pederson WC, Wolfe SC, eds: *Green's Operative Hand Surgery*, ed 5. WB Saunders, Philadelphia, PA, 2005, pp 241-276.

20. Bhattacharyya T, Wadgaonkar AD: Inadvertent retention of angled drill guides after volar locking plate fixation of distal radial fractures: A report of three cases. *J Bone Joint Surg Am* 2008;90(2): 401-403.

21. Warwick D, Field J, Prothero D, Gibson A, Bannister GC: Function ten years after Colles' fracture. *Clin Orthop Relat Res* 1993; 295:270-274.

22. Hove LM, Nilsen PT, Furnes O, Oulie HE, Solheim E, Mölster AO: Open reduction and internal fixation of displaced intraarticular fractures of the distal radius: 31 patients followed for 3-7 years. *Acta Orthop Scand* 1997;68(1): 59-63.

23. Orbay JL: The treatment of unstable distal radius fractures with volar fixation. *Hand Surg* 2000; 5(2):103-112.

24. Ruch DS, Papadonikolakis A: Volar versus dorsal plating in the management of intra-articular distal radius fractures. *J Hand Surg Am* 2006;31(1):9-16.

25. Taleisnik J: The palmar cutaneous branch of the median nerve and the approach to the carpal tunnel: An anatomical study. *J Bone Joint Surg Am* 1973;55(6):1212-1217.

26. Lee HC, Wong YS, Chan BK, Low CO: Fixation of distal radius fractures using AO titanium volar distal radius plate. *Hand Surg* 2003;8(1):7-15.

27. Dao KD, Venn-Watson E, Shin AY: Radial artery pseudoaneurysm complication from use of AO/ ASIF volar distal radius plate: A case report. *J Hand Surg Am* 2001;26(3):448-453.

28. Boyer MI, Korcek KJ, Gelberman RH, Gilula LA, Ditsios K, Evanoff BA: Anatomic tilt x-rays of the distal radius: An ex vivo analysis of surgical fixation. *J Hand Surg Am* 2004;29(1):116-122.

29. Tweet ML, Calfee RP, Stern PJ: Rotational fluoroscopy assists in detection of intra-articular screw penetration during volar plating of the distal radius. *J Hand Surg Am* 2010;35(4):619-627.

30. Buzzell JE, Weikert DR, Watson JT, Lee DH: Precontoured fixed-angle volar distal radius plates: A comparison of anatomic fit. *J Hand Surg Am* 2008;33(7): 1144-1152.

31. Orbay JL, Fernandez DL: Volar fixation for dorsally displaced fractures of the distal radius: A preliminary report. *J Hand Surg Am* 2002;27(2):205-215.

32. Drobetz H, Bryant AL, Pokorny T, Spitaler R, Leixnering M, Jupiter JB: Volar fixed-angle plating of distal radius extension fractures: Influence of plate position on secondary loss of reduction. A biomechanic study in a cadaveric model. *J Hand Surg Am* 2006; 31(4):615-622.

33. Harness NG, Jupiter JB, Orbay JL, Raskin KB, Fernandez DL: Loss of fixation of the volar lunate facet fragment in fractures of the distal part of the radius. *J Bone Joint Surg Am* 2004;86(9):1900-1908.

34. Lundy DW, Quisling SG, Lourie GM, Feiner CM, Lins RE: Tilted lateral radiographs in the evaluation of intra-articular distal radius fractures. *J Hand Surg Am* 1999; 24(2):249-256.

35. Lozano-Calderón SA, Souer S, Mudgal C, Jupiter JB, Ring D: Wrist mobilization following volar plate fixation of fractures of the distal part of the radius. *J Bone Joint Surg Am* 2008;90(6):1297-1304.

36. Atkins RM, Duckworth T, Kanis JA: Features of algodystrophy after Colles' fracture. *J Bone Joint Surg Br* 1990;72(1):105-110.

37. Field J, Protheroe DL, Atkins RM: Algodystrophy after Colles fractures is associated with secondary tightness of casts. *J Bone Joint Surg Br* 1994;76(6): 901-905.

38. Zollinger PE, Tuinebreijer WE, Kreis RW, Breederveld RS: Effect of vitamin C on frequency of reflex sympathetic dystrophy in wrist fractures: A randomised trial. *Lancet* 1999;354(9195): 2025-2028.

39. Atkins RM, Duckworth T, Kanis JA: Algodystrophy following Colles' fracture. *J Hand Surg Br* 1989; 14(2):161-164.

40. Zollinger PE, Tuinebreijer WE, Breederveld RS, Kreis RW: Can vitamin C prevent complex regional pain syndrome in patients with wrist fractures? A randomized, controlled, multicenter dose-response study. *J Bone Joint Surg Am* 2007;89(7):1424-1431.

41. Patterson RW, Li Z, Smith BP, Smith TL, Koman LA: Complex regional pain syndrome of the upper extremity. *J Hand Surg Am* 2011;36(9):1553-1562.

42. Teasdall RD, Smith BP, Koman LA: Complex regional pain syndrome (reflex sympathetic dystrophy). *Clin Sports Med* 2004;23(1): 145-155.

43. Margaliot Z, Haase SC, Kotsis SV, Kim HM, Chung KC: A meta-analysis of outcomes of external fixation versus plate osteosynthesis for unstable distal radius fractures. *J Hand Surg Am* 2005;30(6):1185-1199.

44. Hove LM: Epidemiology of scaphoid fractures in Bergen, Norway. *Scand J Plast Reconstr Surg Hand Surg* 1999;33(4):423-426.

45. Kozin SH: Incidence, mechanism, and natural history of scaphoid fractures. *Hand Clin* 2001;17(4):515-524.

46. Larsen CF, Brøndum V, Skov O: Epidemiology of scaphoid fractures in Odense, Denmark. *Acta Orthop Scand* 1992;63(2):216-218.

47. Gelberman RH, Wolock BS, Siegel DB: Fractures and non-unions of the carpal scaphoid. *J Bone Joint Surg Am* 1989;71(10):1560-1565.

48. Jacobsen S, Hassani G, Hansen D, Christensen O: Suspected scaphoid fractures: Can we avoid overkill? *Acta Orthop Belg* 1995;61(2):74-78.

49. Dias JJ, Taylor M, Thompson J, Brenkel IJ, Gregg PJ: Radiographic signs of union of scaphoid fractures: An analysis of interobserver agreement and reproducibility. *J Bone Joint Surg Br* 1988;70(2):299-301.

50. Lindström G, Nyström A: Natural history of scaphoid non-union, with special reference to "asymptomatic" cases. *J Hand Surg Br* 1992;17(6):697-700.

51. Gäbler CH, Kukla CH, Breitenseher MJ, Trattnig S, Vécsei V: Diagnosis of occult scaphoid fractures and other wrist injuries: Are repeated clinical examinations and plain radiographs still state of the art? *Langenbecks Arch Surg* 2001;386(2):150-154.

52. Kawamura K, Chung KC: Management of wrist injuries. *Plast Reconstr Surg* 2007;120(5):73e-89e.

53. Grover R: Clinical assessment of scaphoid injuries and the detection of fractures. *J Hand Surg Br* 1996;21(3):341-343.

54. Parvizi J, Wayman J, Kelly P, Moran CG: Combining the clinical signs improves diagnosis of scaphoid fractures: A prospective study with follow-up. *J Hand Surg Br* 1998;23(3):324-327.

55. Beeres FJ, Hogervorst M, Rhemrev SJ, den Hollander P, Jukema GN: A prospective comparison for suspected scaphoid fractures: Bone scintigraphy versus clinical outcome. *Injury* 2007;38(7):769-774.

56. Raby N: Magnetic resonance imaging of suspected scaphoid fractures using a low field dedicated extremity MR system. *Clin Radiol* 2001;56(4):316-320.

57. Skirven T, Trope J: Complications of immobilization. *Hand Clin* 1994;10(1):53-61.

58. O'Brien L, Herbert T: Internal fixation of acute scaphoid fractures: A new approach to treatment. *Aust N Z J Surg* 1985;55(4):387-389.

59. Gelberman RH, Menon J: The vascularity of the scaphoid bone. *J Hand Surg Am* 1980;5(5):508-513.

60. Steinmann SP, Adams JE: Scaphoid fractures and nonunions: Diagnosis and treatment. *J Orthop Sci* 2006;11(4):424-431.

61. Zaidemberg C, Siebert JW, Angrigiani C: A new vascularized bone graft for scaphoid nonunion. *J Hand Surg Am* 1991;16(3):474-478.

62. Cooney WP III, Linscheid RL: Nonunion of the scaphoid: Analysis of the results from bone grafting. *J Hand Surg Am* 1980;5(4):343-354.

63. Szabo RM, Manske D: Displaced fractures of the scaphoid. *Clin Orthop Relat Res* 1988;230:30-38.

64. Mack GR, Bosse MJ, Gelberman RH, Yu E: The natural history of scaphoid non-union. *J Bone Joint Surg Am* 1984;66(4):504-509.

65. Cooney WP, Dobyns JH, Linscheid RL: Fractures of the scaphoid: A rational approach to management. *Clin Orthop Relat Res* 1980;149:90-97.

66. Gellman H, Caputo RJ, Carter V, Aboulafia A, McKay M: Comparison of short and long thumb-spica casts for non-displaced fractures of the carpal scaphoid. *J Bone Joint Surg Am* 1989;71(3):354-357.

67. McCallister WV, Knight J, Kaliappan R, Trumble TE: Central placement of the screw in simulated fractures of the scaphoid waist: A biomechanical study. *J Bone Joint Surg Am* 2003;85(1):72-77.

68. Chan KW, McAdams TR: Central screw placement in percutaneous screw scaphoid fixation: A cadaveric comparison of proximal and distal techniques. *J Hand Surg Am* 2004;29(1):74-79.

69. Jeon IH, Micic ID, Oh CW, Park BC, Kim PT: Percutaneous screw fixation for scaphoid fracture: A comparison between the dorsal and the volar approaches. *J Hand Surg Am* 2009;34(2):228-236, e1.

70. Luria S, Hoch S, Liebergall M, Mosheiff R, Peleg E: Optimal fixation of acute scaphoid fractures: Finite element analysis. *J Hand Surg Am* 2010;35(8):1246-1250.

71. Hart A, Mansuri A, Harvey EJ, Martineau PA: Central versus eccentric internal fixation of acute scaphoid fractures. *J Hand Surg Am* 2013;38(1):66-71.

72. Bedi A, Jebson PJ, Hayden RJ, Jacobson JA, Martus JE: Internal fixation of acute, nondisplaced scaphoid waist fractures via a limited dorsal approach: An assess-

ment of radiographic and functional outcomes. *J Hand Surg Am* 2007;32(3):326-333.

73. Zlotolow DA, Knutsen E, Yao J: Optimization of volar percutaneous screw fixation for scaphoid waist fractures using traction, positioning, imaging, and an angiocatheter guide. *J Hand Surg Am* 2011;36(5):916-921.

74. Adamany DC, Mikola EA, Fraser BJ: Percutaneous fixation of the scaphoid through a dorsal approach: An anatomic study. *J Hand Surg Am* 2008;33(3): 327-331.

75. Kamineni S, Lavy CB: Percutaneous fixation of scaphoid fractures: An anatomical study. *J Hand Surg Br* 1999;24(1):85-88.

Complications Following Dislocations of the Proximal Interphalangeal Joint

John J. Mangelson, MD
Peter J. Stern, MD
Joshua M. Abzug, MD
James Chang, MD
A. Lee Osterman, MD

Abstract

Dorsal fracture-dislocations of the proximal interphalangeal joint are challenging injuries to treat and are associated with many complications. The determination of stability is crucial to appropriate management. Stable injuries can usually be treated nonsurgically, whereas unstable injuries typically require surgical stabilization. Many surgical techniques have been used, including extension block pinning, volar plate arthroplasty, open reduction and internal fixation, external fixation, and hemihamate autografting. Because stiffness and flexion contracture are frequent complications, every effort should be made to initiate early motion while maintaining concentric reduction. Other complications include redislocation, chronic swelling, swan neck and coronal plane deformities, and pin tract infections. Assessing injury characteristics, including chronicity, the percentage of articular surface fractured, and the degree of comminution, and understanding complications will help in determining the most appropriate treatment. Chronic dislocations and those injuries in which painful arthritis develops can be successfully treated with salvage procedures, including arthroplasty and arthrodesis.

Instr Course Lect 2014;63:123-130.

Dislocations of the proximal interphalangeal joint can be challenging injuries, both from a clinical decision-making and technical standpoint. Although the "jammed" finger is at times ignored by clinicians and coaches, failure to properly diagnose and treat these injuries can result in a permanently stiff, deformed, and painful finger. The proximal interphalangeal joint is susceptible to injury because of its long lever arm and the high level of congruity between the proximal and middle phalanges. This congruity provides stability and strength through a wide range of motion but is unforgiving to angular, axial, and rotational stress. Dorsal fracture-dislocation, the most common injury pattern, results from hyperextension and axial load.[1,2] This mechanism leads to either distal pull-off of the volar plate or fracture of the volar base of the middle phalanx. Loss of both the cup-shaped geometry of the articular surface and the ligamentous restraint of the volar plate can lead to an unstable joint. Even with timely and appropriate treatment, many complications can occur.

Dr. Chang or an immediate family member serves as a paid consultant to or is an employee of Zone II Surgical; has stock or stock options held in Zone II Surgical; and serves as a board member, owner, officer, or committee member of the American Board of Plastic Surgery and the American Society for Surgery of the Hand. Dr. Osterman or an immediate family member has received royalties from Medartis and Biomet; is a member of a speakers' bureau or has made paid presentations on behalf of Auxilium, Medartis, Arthrex, and Synthes; serves as a paid consultant to or is an employee of Auxilium; has received research or institutional support from Auxilium and Skeletal Dynamics; and serves as a board member, owner, officer, or committee member of the American Association for Hand Surgery and the American Society for Surgery of the Hand. None of the following authors or any immediate family member has received anything of value from or has stock or stock options held in a commercial company or institution related directly or indirectly to the subject of this chapter: Dr. Mangelson, Dr. Stern, and Dr. Abzug.

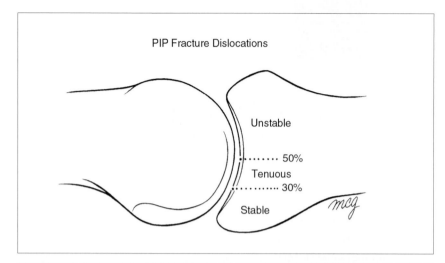

Figure 1 Radiographic classification of palmar lip fractures. Fractures involving less than 30% of the middle phalanx base are generally stable, 30% to 50% are tenuous, and more than 50% represent unstable injuries. The stability of injuries that fall in the tenuous range can further be determined by functional testing. PIP = proximal interphalangeal joint. (Reproduced with permission of Clayton A. Peimer, MD, FACS, Marquette, MI.)

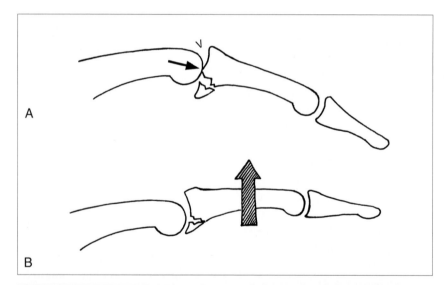

Figure 2 Radiographic signs of instability and malreduction. **A,** The dorsal V sign, indicating hinging at the fracture site (arrow) as opposed to gliding motion. Hinging leads to high contact stresses at the site of contact. **B,** Loss of collinearity of the dorsal cortices of the proximal and middle phalanx, indicating dorsal subluxation of the middle phalanx (arrow).

Treatment Principles

Although the treatments of proximal interphalangeal joint dislocations are diverse, several principles have repeatedly been shown to be important. Obtaining and maintaining a concentric reduction while allowing early motion is the key to successful treatment of proximal interphalangeal joint injuries. The appropriate balance between stability and motion can be difficult to determine and requires judgment on the part of the treating physician. Early motion at the proximal interphalan-

geal joint must be physiologic gliding, rather than hinging, at the fracture site. Edema control is also important to reduce stiffness and contracture. Although accomplishing a perfect reduction of displaced articular bone might seem critical, it seems to be less important than maintaining reduction of the dislocation and reproducing gliding motion.[1]

Classification According to Stability

Determining the stability of the joint is an essential first step in avoiding complications. Stability is determined both by radiographic parameters and functional evaluation.[1,2] The most important radiographic determinant is the percentage of middle phalanx articular surface that has been fractured (**Figure 1**). Generally, fractures at the proximal interphalangeal joint involving less than 30% of the middle phalanx articular surface are stable. Those involving 30% to 50% are considered borderline or tenuous and require further functional evaluation to determine stability. Finally, fractures involving more than 50% are unstable. Other radiographic signs of instability include the dorsal V sign and loss of collinearity of the dorsal cortices of the proximal and middle phalanges[3] (**Figure 2**).

Functional evaluation is also important to determine stability, especially for the injuries classified as "tenuous" radiographically. Functional stability is tested by fluoroscopically evaluating the proximal interphalangeal joint while the patient actively flexes and extends the finger (a metacarpal anesthetic block is usually necessary). If the middle phalanx subluxates dorsally during terminal extension of the proximal interphalangeal joint, the dislocation is deemed tenuous. If it subluxates in more than 30° of flexion of the proximal interphalangeal joint, it is

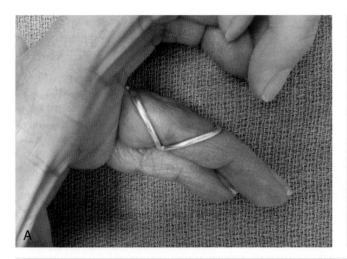
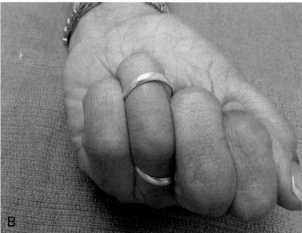

Figure 3   **A** and **B,** Two views of a figure-of-8 splint that allows for range of motion while providing a 10° extension block and radioulnar stability.

considered unstable. The dislocations that remain reduced even in full extension are stable.

Treatment

If the dislocation is stable, proceed with nonsurgical treatment. A figure-of-8 splint with a 10° extension block is usually adequate (**Figure 3**). This splint allows sufficient immediate active range of motion and provides radioulnar stability. Alternatively, buddy taping can be used. Dislocations that are tenuously stable (subluxate only near full extension) may be treated with a figure-of-8 splint as well, but only if the joint remains reduced in the splint as confirmed by a lateral radiograph. Weekly clinical and radiographic monitoring is essential to detect redislocation or inadequate rehabilitation.

Most unstable fracture-dislocations of the proximal interphalangeal joint are treated surgically. There are many surgical options, including extension block pinning, volar plate arthroplasty, open reduction and internal fixation (ORIF), various forms of external fixation, and hemihamate autografting. There are no definite guidelines for which option to choose. Understanding the common and procedure-

specific complications, however, helps in selecting the best treatment of each situation.

Common Complications
Stiffness and Flexion Contracture

The most common and problematic complications of dislocations of the proximal interphalangeal joint are stiffness and flexion contracture. Several factors make the proximal interphalangeal joint particularly susceptible to stiffness. Although the proper collateral ligaments have a relatively stable tension in extension and flexion, the accessory collateral ligaments are lax in flexion, which may partially explain why stiffness and contracture result from prolonged immobilization in flexion.[4] Other contributing factors include lack of extensor power from central slip attenuation, flexor tendon adhesion, and articular incongruity. Posttraumatic hemarthrosis may also contribute to flexion contracture because the joint is preferentially held in 30° to 40° of flexion to maximize joint volume.[5] Poor compliance with hand therapy and poor control of edema can contribute to stiffness. Distal interphalangeal joint stiffness is another com-

mon complication, which usually results from concomitant splinting of the distal interphalangeal joint with the proximal interphalangeal joint.

In general, preventing stiffness and flexion contracture is easier than treating it. Immobilization for more than 3 to 4 weeks should be avoided. Early supervised active range of motion as permitted by stability is recommended. Edema should be controlled with an elastic tape or garment. Loss of motion is minimized with these measures.

The literature indicates that successful surgical management typically results in an average arc of motion of the proximal interphalangeal joint between 65° and 90°, with flexion contracture ranging from only a few degrees to nearly 25°.[6-15] These reported results do not include the poorest outcomes, which required salvage procedures before follow-up.

Although most patients tolerate a 15° to 20° flexion contracture and experience no functional deficit, more severe contractures may require treatment. The initial treatment of an established flexion contracture is nonsurgical with serial casting or static or dynamic splinting. An average

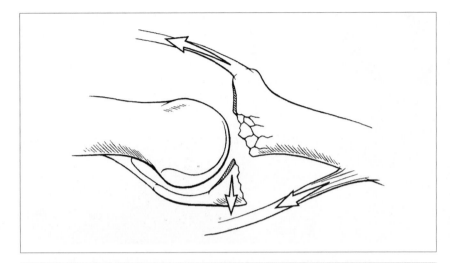

Figure 4 Forces leading to dislocation of the proximal interphalangeal joint after palmar lip fractures. The central slip pulls the base of the middle phalanx dorsally and proximally, whereas the more distal attachment of flexor digitorum superficialis creates a lever arm that accentuates dorsal displacement. The head of the proximal phalanx falls into the sloped fracture defect. Stabilizing forces from the volar plate and the osseous volar lip are lost in the injury. (Reproduced with permission of Clayton A. Peimer, MD, FACS, Marquette, MI.)

improvement of 16° to 18° with splinting is anticipated, with approximately 50% of the total correction obtained in the first 2 weeks of treatment.[16,17] If nonsurgical treatment fails, surgical release can help to decrease the flexion contracture. Hogan and Nunley[5] reviewed and summarized the results of surgical release and noted that most protocols recommend sequentially releasing the accessory collateral ligaments, volar plate, proper collateral ligaments, and flexor tendon adhesions until adequate extension is obtained. Open release typically restored 25° to 30° of extension while reducing flexion, resulting in an overall effect of shifting the arc of motion into a more functional range.

Chronic Swelling

Chronic swelling is difficult to treat and is bothersome to patients because it limits the proximal interphalangeal joint arc of motion. In the experience of this chapter's authors, swelling slowly diminishes over 6 to 9 months, although frequently it never completely resolves. Patient expectations should be managed with counseling about the chronic nature of swelling with proximal interphalangeal joint dislocations. Coban wraps (3M Corporation) or an elastic sleeve worn for 6 months are recommended. There is no surgical treatment of this problem.

Swan Neck Deformity

Volar plate incompetence following inappropriate treatment of a proximal interphalangeal joint dislocation can lead to chronic proximal interphalangeal joint hyperextension, either in isolation or with associated flexion of the distal interphalangeal joint (swan neck deformity), with painful snapping as the lateral bands displace over the condyles when the patient flexes the hyperextended joint. If the deformity is supple, the use of a figure-of-8 splint for 6 to 8 weeks usually restores stability by inducing a small flexion contracture of the proximal interphalangeal joint. If deformity persists or the pa-

tient does not tolerate a splint, volar plate advancement and reattachment or flexor digitorum superficialis tenodesis can be performed. Catalano et al[18] reported complete correction of chronic traumatic hyperextension of the proximal interphalangeal joint in 83% of patients treated with flexor digitorum superficialis tenodesis. Correction of the distal interphalangeal joint contracture in the patients with swan neck deformity was variable. Melone et al[19] demonstrated that volar plate repair can lead to satisfactory outcomes even in the chronic deformity. If left untreated, supple hyperextension deformity of the proximal interphalangeal joint can become fixed, requiring open release or an arthrodesis of the proximal interphalangeal joint.

Redislocation and Subluxation

Although most commonly seen after volar plate arthroplasty, dorsal subluxation or redislocation can occur with any treatment method. The forces that contribute to the tendency for these injuries to dislocate, even after appropriate reduction, are shown in **Figure 4**. This chapter's authors recommend follow-up serial radiographic evaluation every 7 to 10 days for 4 weeks. This is particularly important if a tenuously stable dislocation is treated nonsurgically in a figure-of-8 splint. Rates of redislocation reported in the literature have ranged from 0% to 31%, with volar plate arthroplasty having the highest rates.[6-15] When redislocation occurs, the cause must be treated, which may include fixation failure, inadequate extension block, insufficient reconstitution of the cup-shaped contour of the base of the middle phalanx, overly aggressive therapy, or incorrect classification of stability. Subluxation or redislocation usually requires revision or a surgical salvage procedure.

Treatment-Specific Complications

Extension Block Pinning

First described by Viegas[6] in 1992, extension block pinning is done by placing a pin dorsally through the head of the proximal phalanx with the joint flexed. The free end of the pin (which protrudes from the dorsal head of the proximal phalanx) is a mechanical extension block. This technique allows active and passive motion at the proximal interphalangeal joint, but only within the range allowed by the extension block pin. As with any percutaneous technique, pin tract infection and loosening are potential complications. Despite leaving pins in place for 4 to 6 weeks, there were no pin tract infections or other complications in an initial series of three patients described by Viegas.[6] More recently, Waris and Alanen[7] used extension block pinning in conjunction with intramedullary fracture reduction. Pins were removed after 3 weeks, and only one rotational deformity occurred, with no infections or redislocations.

Volar Plate Arthroplasty

Volar plate arthroplasty, as described by Eaton and Malerich,[8] is a partial resurfacing of the proximal interphalangeal joint by advancing the avulsed volar plate to the remaining intact articular surface of the middle phalanx. Redislocation is a devastating complication, and it often occurs after removing the transarticular pin. Several authors have noted that the head of the proximal phalanx sinks into the osseous defect at the volar base of the middle phalanx, rather than the advanced volar plate failing.[9,10] Reported redislocation rates have varied widely, and variable surgical indications make comparison difficult. Deitch et al[10] treated 23 patients with volar plate arthroplasty; redislocation occurred in 3 patients, even though all had a trans-

articular pin for 3 weeks after surgery. Others have reported dislocation rates after volar plate arthroplasty that were as low as 4% (1 of 24 patients) and as high as 33% (2 of 6 patients).[8,9] Because the risk of redislocation with this procedure is unacceptable when more than 50% to 60% of the base of the middle phalanx is fractured, volar plate arthroplasty is not recommended for such injuries.

Another potential complication of volar plate arthroplasty is coronal plane angulation. This has been attributed to a failure to recognize asymmetry in coronal impaction on preoperative radiographs or creating a trough for the volar plate that is not perpendicular to the long axis of the digit.[8-10] Dionysian and Eaton[11] reported the outcome at long-term follow-up (mean, 11.5 years) after volar plate arthroplasty in 17 patients, including 2 patients who had coronal deformities of more than 10° requiring corrective osteotomy. Deitch et al[10] reported that approximately one third of their patients had coronal deformities of more than 10° at the time of long-term follow-up.

Open Reduction and Internal Fixation

With the introduction of smaller implants, ORIF has become a more frequent choice for surgical treatment and should be considered when the volar lip bone fragment is displaced more than 2 mm, is not comminuted, and is large enough to accommodate mini-screws.[12] Secure internal fixation of the volar fragment allows the patient to initiate active motion immediately. Restoration of the articular surface potentially decreases the rate of degenerative arthritis, although this has not been definitively demonstrated. ORIF is technically demanding and must be done well to benefit the patient. Redislocation is a relatively common complication but is nearly al-

ways associated with implant failure. Intra-articular implants, whether by inadvertent placement at the time of surgery or because of failed fixation, accelerate degeneration of the articular cartilage.

In a series of 33 dislocations of the proximal interphalangeal joint treated with ORIF,[10] there were 3 recurrent dislocations, all of which occurred after removal of a transarticular pin. Fixation failure was the cause in all cases. The authors retrospectively noted that these fractures may have been better served by another procedure, which highlights the importance of careful procedure selection. More recently, Hamilton et al[12] reported nine fracture-dislocations treated with ORIF with the use of mini-screws through a volar approach. Protected motion was begun within the first week after surgery. One dorsal subluxation occurred with associated failure of fixation with an intra-articular screw. Few patients had degenerative changes or pain at the time of follow-up. Lee and Teoh[13] performed ORIF from a dorsal approach on injuries with a single large volar fragment. Postoperatively, the proximal interphalangeal joint was further stabilized with a splint in full extension for 6 weeks. During that time, they allowed temporary splint removal for an immediate and aggressive range-of-motion protocol. No malunions or redislocations were reported. Studies have indicated that patient selection is a key determinant of complications after ORIF. Injuries with substantial comminution are better treated with an alternative procedure.

External Fixation and Dynamic Traction

External fixation of various kinds has been used alone or in conjunction with other procedures to treat unstable proximal interphalangeal joint injuries. Regardless of the specific type of external fixation, multiple percutaneous pins increase the prevalence of pin tract infections, loosening, and the resultant loss of stability. Two studies using external fixation reported pin tract infections in 1 of 8 patients and in 8 of 34 patients.[14,15] All infections were treated successfully with oral antibiotics and did not progress to osteomyelitis. None of the infections required early removal of the fixator.

Dynamic traction is a simple and ingenious form of external fixation designed to reduce fracture fragments through ligamentotaxis while simultaneously allowing for range of motion.[15] These systems have been particularly helpful in injuries with considerable comminution precluding ORIF. Dynamic traction requires rotation about a pin in the head of the proximal phalanx. Failure to place this pin in the center of the head can lead to cam-type hinging of the joint, with pin loosening and joint subluxation. Even with appropriate placement of this pin, osteolysis in the head of the proximal phalanx has been seen and has been attributed to frame translation about the center of rotation. Radiographic resolution was seen after fixator removal.

Despite excellent fracture healing and maintenance of reduction with dynamic traction, intra-articular step-off may persist, and radiographic evidence of arthritis may occur. Ellis et al[14] reported step-off or joint space narrowing in five of eight patients treated with dynamic traction. Ruland et al[15] also reported no improvement in intra-articular step-off. Most of these patients were pain free at the time of the latest follow-up, despite the high prevalence of these radiographic findings.

Hemihamate Autograft
Originally described in 1999, hemihamate autografting has been success-

fully used to treat unstable fracture-dislocations when ORIF and volar plate arthroplasty are not feasible or advisable (H. Hastings, MD, et al, Boston, MA, unpublished material presented at the American Society for Surgery of the Hand annual meeting, 1999). The dorsal distal osteoarticular surface of the hamate is used as autograft to re-create the palmar lip of the middle phalanx and is held in place with screws. This procedure has been particularly useful in injuries involving more than 50% of the articular surface of the middle phalanx or in chronic injuries.

Williams et al,[20] in a study of 13 patients who had dislocations treated with hemihamate autografting, reported 2 patients who had recurrent subluxations. Many authors believe that adequate restoration of the concavity of the middle phalangeal base provides sufficient osseous stability to prevent dorsal subluxation, and that volar plate repair and extension block splinting is rarely necessary.[21,22] Those authors emphasized that placing the articular surface of the graft too vertically fails to re-create the cup-shaped contour of the palmar lip and leads to instability. Two recent long-term follow-up studies on a total of 30 patients who had hemihamate grafts found no subluxations or dislocations.[22,23] Donor site pain was infrequent, and graft collapse generally did not occur. Like other techniques, many patients showed radiographic evidence of degeneration at the time of the latest follow-up, despite being pain free.

Chronic Injuries and Salvage Procedures
Even with efforts to appropriately diagnose and treat proximal interphalangeal joint dislocations, some patients have a chronic dislocation, malunion or nonunion, stiffness, and pain. Op-

tions include accepting the deformity and disability with symptomatic management, open reduction and stabilization (for example, hemihamate autografting), or salvage procedures (arthrodesis or implant arthroplasty). For any open reduction to be successful, three criteria must be fulfilled: reduction must be achievable, stability must be restored, and the remaining cartilage must be in reasonable condition. When these conditions are met, hemihamate grafting has shown reasonable results, with improvements in range of motion, pain, and stability, even in chronic injuries.[20,22] Salvage procedures should be considered if the three criteria for open reduction cannot be met or the joint is reduced but symptomatic arthritis has developed.

Resection arthroplasty with silicone spacer interposition eliminates pain and deformity while maintaining range of motion and stability. First described in 1954 as simple joint resection, the procedure evolved to include interposition of biologic or synthetic materials, the most common being the hinged silicone spacer.[24] Recently, Takigawa et al,[25] in a study of silicone implant arthroplasties with a mean follow-up of 6.5 years, reported no change in range of motion but a decrease or elimination of pain in 70% of the patients. Unfortunately, long-term follow-up of silicone arthroplasty in this and other studies has also demonstrated important complications, including implant fracture, synovitis, and deformity.[26]

Limitations of silicone implant arthroplasty have fueled the development of surface replacement arthroplasty to restore the anatomy of the proximal interphalangeal joint, leading to more physiologic biomechanics and potentially longer implant survival. Nunley et al,[27] however, reported unsatisfactory outcomes after pyrocarbon resurfacing for posttraumatic arthritis.

They attributed these results to poor bone and soft-tissue quality and advised against the use of resurfacing for traumatized joints. More recently, satisfactory outcomes using pyrocarbon arthroplasty have been reported in two studies with a minimum follow-up of 2 years.[28,29] The patients with posttraumatic arthritis (approximately 20% of the joints) did as well as patients with other conditions. Regardless of indication, resurfacing arthroplasty typically provides improvement with regard to pain and strength but not motion.[28-30]

Arthrodesis eliminates pain and improves hand function. It should be considered if other measures to preserve painless effective motion have failed or if there is insufficient bone stock or stability to support an implant. Many fixation methods have been described, with rates of successful fusion ranging from less than 50% to 100% of the arthrodeses.[31] Although it is seen as a reliable procedure, complications are common.[32] Jones et al[33] reported on arthrodesis as a salvage for failed proximal interphalangeal joint arthroplasty. Eight of 13 joints fused at an average of 5.8 months after arthrodesis, and there was a particularly high rate of hardware removal. The low fusion rate and prolonged time to union after arthrodesis for failed arthroplasty should be considered when choosing a salvage procedure.

Summary

Dorsal fracture-dislocations of the proximal interphalangeal joint are challenging injuries to treat. The determination of stability both functionally and radiographically is crucial in avoiding complications. There are many techniques for treating unstable injuries, but clinical judgment is needed in procedure selection based on the percentage of the articular surface that is fractured, the amount of

comminution, chronicity, and surgeon comfort. Stiffness and flexion contracture are common complications, and every effort should be made to initiate early motion while maintaining concentric reduction. Even with appropriate care, complications such as redislocation, chronic swelling, swan neck and coronal deformities, and pin tract infections can occur. Chronic dislocations and the injuries in which painful arthritis develops can be successfully treated with salvage procedures, including arthroplasty and arthrodesis.

References

1. Kiefhaber TR, Stern PJ: Fracture dislocations of the proximal interphalangeal joint. *J Hand Surg Am* 1998;23(3):368-380.

2. Calfee RP, Sommerkamp TG: Fracture-dislocation about the finger joints. *J Hand Surg Am* 2009;34(6):1140-1147.

3. Light TR: Buttress pinning techniques. *Orthop Rev* 1981;10: 49-55.

4. Leibovic SJ, Bowers WH: Anatomy of the proximal interphalangeal joint. *Hand Clin* 1994;10(2): 169-178.

5. Hogan CJ, Nunley JA: Posttraumatic proximal interphalangeal joint flexion contractures. *J Am Acad Orthop Surg* 2006;14(9): 524-533.

6. Viegas SF: Extension block pinning for proximal interphalangeal joint fracture dislocations: Preliminary report of a new technique. *J Hand Surg Am* 1992;17(5): 896-901.

7. Waris E, Alanen V: Percutaneous, intramedullary fracture reduction and extension block pinning for dorsal proximal interphalangeal fracture-dislocations. *J Hand Surg Am* 2010;35(12):2046-2052.

8. Eaton RG, Malerich MM: Volar plate arthroplasty of the proximal

interphalangeal joint: A review of ten years' experience. *J Hand Surg Am* 1980;5(3):260-268.

9. Hastings H II, Carroll C IV: Treatment of closed articular fractures of the metacarpophalangeal and proximal interphalangeal joints. *Hand Clin* 1988;4(3): 503-527.

10. Deitch MA, Kiefhaber TR, Comisar BR, Stern PJ: Dorsal fracture dislocations of the proximal interphalangeal joint: Surgical complications and long-term results. *J Hand Surg Am* 1999; 24(5):914-923.

11. Dionysian E, Eaton RG: The long-term outcome of volar plate arthroplasty of the proximal interphalangeal joint. *J Hand Surg Am* 2000;25(3):429-437.

12. Hamilton SC, Stern PJ, Fassler PR, Kiefhaber TR: Mini-screw fixation for the treatment of proximal interphalangeal joint dorsal fracture-dislocations. *J Hand Surg Am* 2006;31(8):1349-1354.

13. Lee JY, Teoh LC: Dorsal fracture dislocations of the proximal interphalangeal joint treated by open reduction and interfragmentary screw fixation: Indications, approaches and results. *J Hand Surg Br* 2006;31(2):138-146.

14. Ellis SJ, Cheng R, Prokopis P, et al: Treatment of proximal interphalangeal dorsal fracture-dislocation injuries with dynamic external fixation: A pins and rubber band system. *J Hand Surg Am* 2007;32(8):1242-1250.

15. Ruland RT, Hogan CJ, Cannon DL, Slade JF: Use of dynamic distraction external fixation for unstable fracture-dislocations of the proximal interphalangeal joint. *J Hand Surg Am* 2008; 33(1):19-25.

16. Prosser R: Splinting in the management of proximal interphalangeal joint flexion contracture. *J Hand Ther* 1996;9(4):378-386.

17. Hunter E, Laverty J, Pollock R, Birch R: Nonoperative treatment of fixed flexion deformity of the proximal interphalangeal joint. *J Hand Surg Br* 1999;24(3): 281-283.

18. Catalano LW III, Skarparis AC, Glickel SZ, et al: Treatment of chronic, traumatic hyperextension deformities of the proximal interphalangeal joint with flexor digitorum superficialis tenodesis. *J Hand Surg Am* 2003;28(3): 448-452.

19. Melone CP Jr, Polatsch DB, Beldner S, Khorsandi M: Volar plate repair for posttraumatic hyperextension deformity of the proximal interphalangeal joint. *Am J Orthop (Belle Mead NJ)* 2010;39(4): 190-194.

20. Williams RM, Kiefhaber TR, Sommerkamp TG, Stern PJ: Treatment of unstable dorsal proximal interphalangeal fracture/dislocations using a hemi-hamate autograft. *J Hand Surg Am* 2003; 28(5):856-865.

21. McAuliffe JA: Hemi-hamate autograft for the treatment of unstable dorsal fracture dislocation of the proximal interphalangeal joint. *J Hand Surg Am* 2009; 34(10):1890-1894.

22. Calfee RP, Kiefhaber TR, Sommerkamp TG, Stern PJ: Hemi-hamate arthroplasty provides functional reconstruction of acute and chronic proximal interphalangeal fracture-dislocations. *J Hand Surg Am* 2009;34(7):1232-1241.

23. Afendras G, Abramo A, Mrkonjic A, Geijer M, Kopylov P, Tägil M: Hemi-hamate osteochondral transplantation in proximal interphalangeal dorsal fracture dislocations: A minimum 4 year follow-up in eight patients. *J Hand Surg Eur Vol* 2010;35(8): 627-631.

24. Carroll RE, Taber TH: Digital arthroplasty of the proximal interphalangeal joint. *J Bone Joint Surg Am* 1954;36(5):912-920.

25. Takigawa S, Meletiou S, Sauerbier M, Cooney WP: Long-term assessment of Swanson implant arthroplasty in the proximal interphalangeal joint of the hand. *J Hand Surg Am* 2004;29(5): 785-795.

26. Rizzo M, Beckenbaugh RD: Proximal interphalangeal joint arthroplasty. *J Am Acad Orthop Surg* 2007;15(3):189-197.

27. Nunley RM, Boyer MI, Goldfarb CA: Pyrolytic carbon arthroplasty for posttraumatic arthritis of the proximal interphalangeal joint. *J Hand Surg Am* 2006;31(9): 1468-1474.

28. Bravo CJ, Rizzo M, Hormel KB, Beckenbaugh RD: Pyrolytic carbon proximal interphalangeal joint arthroplasty: Results with minimum two-year follow-up evaluation. *J Hand Surg Am* 2007; 32(1):1-11.

29. Watts AC, Hearnden AJ, Trail IA, Hayton MJ, Nuttall D, Stanley JK: Pyrocarbon proximal interphalangeal joint arthroplasty: Minimum two-year follow-up. *J Hand Surg Am* 2012;37(5): 882-888.

30. Jennings CD, Livingstone DP: Surface replacement arthroplasty of the proximal interphalangeal joint using the PIP-SRA implant: Results, complications, and revisions. *J Hand Surg Am* 2008; 33(9):e1-e11.

31. Amadio PC, Shin AY: Arthrodesis and arthroplasty of small joints in the hand, in Wolfe SW, Pederson WC, Hotchkiss RN, Kozin MD, eds: *Green's Operative Hand Surgery*. Philadelphia, PA, Churchill Livingstone, 2011, pp 389-404.

32. Stern PJ, Fulton DB: Distal interphalangeal joint arthrodesis: An analysis of complications. *J Hand Surg Am* 1992;17(6):1139-1145.

33. Jones DB Jr, Ackerman DB, Sammer DM, Rizzo M: Arthrodesis as a salvage for failed proximal interphalangeal joint arthroplasty. *J Hand Surg Am* 2011;36(2): 259-264.

13

Contemporary Management of Dupuytren Contracture

Marco Rizzo, MD
Peter J. Stern, MD
Prosper Benhaim, MD
Lawrence C. Hurst, MD

Abstract

Dupuytren contracture is a condition that affects the palmar fascia. It most commonly affects men of northern European ancestry and initially presents at middle age. The diseased fascia may form cords that extend into the digits, resulting in limited motion and function. Treatment is aimed at either releasing or removing the diseased cord so that the finger can extend fully. Common interventions include surgery, needle aponeurotomy, and collagenase injection. Surgery remains the gold standard in treatment and most commonly includes a limited fasciectomy. Although often successful, surgery carries inherent risks and may involve a lengthy recovery with extensive therapy. Needle aponeurotomy and collagenase injections are office-based alternatives that aim to weaken the cord and release the contracture. Needle aponeurotomy involves repeated needling along the cord in intervals and collagenase injections to dissolve a portion of the cord. Despite being less invasive, problems such as nerve and/or tendon injury, skin tears, and autoimmune reactions have been reported. Regardless of treatment, recurrence remains a concern.

Instr Course Lect 2014;63:131-142.

Dupuytren contracture is a disease of the palmar fascia. It typically affects people of northern European ancestry and men more often than women. In 1613, Felix Platt, a Swiss physician, provided one of the earliest descriptions of Dupuytren contracture when he described it as stonemason's hand and attributed the disorder to a tendon contracture.[1] Although Guillaume Dupuytren, a French surgeon, is credited with the name of this condition, prior investigators, such as Henry Cline and Sir Astley Cooper, identified the palmar fascia as the source of the contracture and recommended treatments such as fasciotomy.[1] Dupuytren contracture is a benign condition that can result in a progressive contracture of the fingers and palm, secondary to the formation of nodules and cords.

Epidemiology

The prevalence of Dupuytren contracture ranges from 2% to 42% and is influenced by multiple factors, including age, sex, geography, and ethnicity.[2] Most patients present with Dupuytren contracture in middle age, between the fourth and sixth decades of life. Men are more often affected than women. Geographically, it is more prevalent in northern European countries such as Scandinavia and Scotland; is common in the United Kingdom, Australia, Ireland, and North America; is uncommon in Southern Europe, South America, and Central Asia; and is rare in Africa and East Asia. Ethnicity patterns reflect the geographic demographics. It is very common in decedents of the Celts and Caucasians of Northern Europe; common in Caucasians of North America; and

Dr. Rizzo or an immediate family member has received research or institutional support from SBI and TriMed and serves as a board member, owner, officer, or committee member of the American Academy of Orthopaedic Surgeons, the American Association for Hand Surgery, and the American Society for Surgery of the Hand. Dr. Hurst or an immediate family member has received royalties from Biospecifics Technologies Corporation; serves as a paid consultant to or is an employee of Auxilium Pharmaceuticals, Pfizer, and AsahiKASEI Pharma Corporation; and has received research or institutional support from AsahiKASEI Pharma Corporation. Dr. Benhaim or an immediate family member is a member of a speakers' bureau or has made paid presentations on behalf of Auxilium Pharmaceuticals and has stock or stock options held in Cytori. Neither Dr. Stern nor any immediate family member has received anything of value from or has stock or stock options held in a commercial company or institution related directly or indirectly to the subject of this chapter.

uncommon in African descendants, Native Americans, and Asians.

Associated Conditions and Predisposing Factors

Diabetes mellitus has a well-established link to Dupuytren contracture, with prevalence rates ranging from 13% to 67% in that population.[3-6] Smoking and alcohol consumption also have been associated with Dupuytren contracture.[6] Brenner et al[7] showed that the disease is more severe in these population groups. Hypercholesterolemia and elevated serum lipid levels have been associated with the disease.[8] Because hypercholesterolemia is more prevalent in individuals who consume alcohol and persons with diabetes, this may help to explain the increased incidence of these conditions in patients with Dupuytren contracture. Epilepsy also has been associated with the disease;[9] however, in a comparison of 821 patients with Dupuytren contracture and 1,642 control individuals, Geoghegan et al[10] reported that diabetes was associated with Dupuytren contracture, but no significant relationship with epilepsy was found. Not all reports of risk factors for Dupuytren contracture have been consistent. In a 50-year retrospective analysis of patients surgically treated for Dupuytren contracture, Loos et al[11] reported that the cohort in general had a slightly higher prevalence of the described risk factors compared with the general population; however, the authors could not confirm a statistically significant link between the disease and smoking, diabetes, epilepsy, or alcohol consumption.

An autosomal dominant inheritance with incomplete penetrance was identified as a factor in Dupuytren contracture.[12] However, more recent analyses suggest a more complicated genetic basis, including a rarely recessive autosomal penetrance that implied a mitochondrial heredity.[13,14] A link with chromosomal abnormalities has been suggested through cytogenetic analysis of cell cultures.[15] Bonnici et al[15] found that clones of cells trisomic for chromosome 8 were encountered along with abnormalities in the Y chromosome in cells from diseased fascia.

Etiology

Multiple etiologies have been proposed in the pathogenesis of Dupuytren contracture, including inflammatory, traumatic, neoplastic, genetic, and autoimmune mechanisms; however, no clear understanding of the underlying disease process has been established. Dupuytren contracture is commonly considered a neoplastic process characterized as fibromatosis. It is believed to be modulated by multiple growth factors (such as fibroblastic growth factor, platelet-derived growth factor, epidermal growth factor, and transforming growth factor). Modern histochemical analysis suggests a benign monoclonal tumor.[16,17] The diseased fascia has an increased ratio of type III to type I collagen. In contrast, Chansky et al[18] proposed that the disease is a reactive process rather than a neoplastic process based on the polyclonal versus monoclonal nature of the diseased fascia.

There is substantial controversy regarding a traumatic etiology. It has been proposed that Dupuytren contracture is two to five times more likely in workers exposed to repetitive handling tasks or vibration when compared with those not exposed to such trauma.[19] Pathologic analysis of Dupuytren nodules and cords has shown striking similarities to wound healing tissues, including myofibroblasts, fibronectin, collagen, and growth factors.[20,21] However, in a review of nearly 100,000 consecutive miners, Burke et al[6] found no link between occupational exposure or trauma and Dupuytren contracture. Evidence to support an autoimmune mechanism has been proposed and investigated by Baird et al.[22] An analysis of diseased fascia revealed evidence of CD3-positive lymphocytes and the expression of major histocompatibility complex class II proteins, suggesting the possibility of a T cell–mediated autoimmune etiology that may contribute to the pathogenesis of the disease.

Pathoanatomy

Normal palmar fascia has several functions, including retaining the flexor tendons, stabilizing the metacarpals, and supporting and anchoring the palmar skin. Anatomically, central, radial, and ulnar aponeuroses have been defined. The radial aponeurosis lies over the thenar fascia. Its primary components consist of a distal and proximal commissural ligament and a less important pretendinous band to the thumb. The ulnar aponeurosis overlies the hypothenar muscles. It is bound radially by the pretendinous band of the small finger. Ulnarly, the abductor digiti minimi also has an overlying confluence of fascial strands. The central aponeurosis comprises the largest portion of the palmar fascia. It is partially composed of the extension of the palmaris longus as it extends into the palm. However, it has a thick, three-dimensional orientation with longitudinally oriented fibers; transverse fibers, including the natatory ligament and the superficial transverse palmar ligament; and deep vertical fibers, including the septa of Legueu and Juvara, McGrouther fibers of the deep layer of the split pretendinous band, and small vertical bands that occupy the deep plane beneath the fascia.

Of the transversely oriented fibers, only the natatory ligaments are involved in Dupuytren contracture; the superficial transverse palmar ligament is typically spared. In the first web-space between the thumb and index finger, the proximal and distal commissural bands can be involved in Dupuytren contracture, which clinically manifests as the proximal and distal commissural cords, respectively. The palmodigital fascia is an extension of the natatory ligament and extends side to side at the web spaces. The digital fascia consists of the Grayson ligament and the lateral digital sheet volarly, the Cleland ligament dorsally, and the retrovascular fascia distally.

Pathophysiology

Dupuytren contracture affects normal fascial structures, typically beginning as a nodule and evolving into cords. The cords can shorten as they develop and extend into the fingers, commonly resulting in joint and soft-tissue contractures. Normal structures, such as the pretendinous band, lateral digital sheet, natatory ligament, and Grayson ligament, are commonly affected.

A variety of pathologic structures are defined in association with the diseased fascia. Dupuytren nodules are typically seen in the palm and are fixed to the aponeurosis and adherent to the skin. Central cords are common and develop from the pretendinous band. They are responsible for metacarpophalangeal (MCP) joint contractures and do not typically affect the neurovascular anatomy. The palmodigital cords extend into the fingers and include spiral, lateral, central, and natatory cords. The spiral cords are composed of four components: the pretendinous band, the spiral band, the lateral digital sheet, and the Grayson ligament. The cord can displace neurovascular structures medially, volarly, and proximally. The presence or absence of a spiral cord is difficult to predict from the clinical examination of the hand alone. The natatory cords arise from diseased natatory ligaments.

The typical U-shaped web space morphs into a V shape as the cords extend to the dorsolateral aspect of the adjacent digit. Although they do not affect neurovascular displacement, finger abduction is limited by the natatory cords. Central cords arise and extend from the pretendinous bands and course midline into the finger. The cord is fairly superficial and does not displace the neurovascular structures. Lateral cords arise from the lateral digital sheet and are associated with the natatory cord. They may attach to the skin or flexor tendon sheath and result in proximal and distal interphalangeal joint contractures. The abductor digiti minimi cord arises from the muscle and inserts into the ulnar side of the small finger. It courses superficial to the neurovascular bundle, which can be spiraled by this cord, and the dorsal ulnar sensory nerve, which supplies important ulnar border sensation, can be adjacent to this cord. The thumbs may have cords associated with their respective bands, including distal and proximal commissural cords, a pretendinous cord, and a thenar fascia cord.

Clinical Presentation

Patients typically present with a painless, palpable nodule in the hand. In rare instances, patients will have painful nodules, which are believed to be caused by local nerve compression from the proliferating fascia.[23] It is unclear why the nodular pain often ceases over time, even though the nodule remains. The nodules may evolve into cords, which can lead to progressive finger contractures of the MCP and interphalangeal joints. The cords tend to involve the ulnar digits, with the small finger most affected. The index finger is least commonly diseased.

Dupuytren diathesis is a more aggressive form of the disease. It typically affects patients at a younger age, more commonly involves both hands and

multiple digits, tends to progress more rapidly, and is more likely to recur. Proliferation of diseased fascia (Garrod or knuckle pads) over the dorsal aspect of the proximal interphalangeal (PIP) joints is more commonly seen in patients with diathesis. These patients will more likely have diseased fascia elsewhere in the body, such as the fascia of the penis (Peyronie disease) and plantar surface of the foot (Ledderhose disease).

Reilly et al[24] investigated the rates of progression from nodule to cord and contracture. Forty-nine patients who initially presented with nodules were retrospectively reviewed at an average clinical follow-up evaluation of nearly 9 years. Cords developed in 30 patients (60%), and 5 patients had contractures significant enough to satisfy the surgical criteria of at least 30° of contracture of the MCP joint or any PIP joint. Interestingly, regression of the disease occurred in seven patients.

The differential diagnoses for Dupuytren nodules include ganglia, inclusion cysts, stenosing tenosynovitis, callus formation, benign or malignant soft-tissue neoplasms, and rheumatoid nodules. In patients with cord development and contractures, the differential diagnoses will also include camptodactyly, traumatic scars, neuropathy (such as ulnar neuropathy with clawing), intrinsic muscle weakness, joint disease, Volkmann ischemic contracture, PIP joint capsular contracture, spastic contracture, locked chronic neglected stenosing tenosynovitis, and contracture after a cerebral vascular insult.

Treatment

Unfortunately, no demonstrable benefit from therapy or splinting in the management of early Dupuytren contracture has been proven, either in terms of reversing the contracture or curbing the progression. Steroid injections may

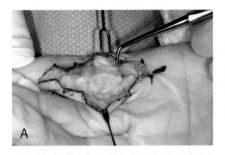
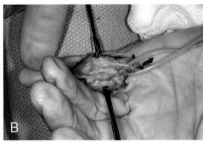

Figure 1 **A,** Intraoperative photograph of a limited fasciectomy for a small finger contracture and a cord. Note that the spiral cord has displaced the radial neurovascular bundle centrally, proximally, and superficially. **B,** After cord removal, the course of the displaced neurovascular bundle can be appreciated.

relieve the discomfort of painful nodules; one study reported incomplete temporary resolution of nodules with multiple steroid injections.[25] Currently, the most common treatments for Dupuytren contracture include surgery, percutaneous needle aponeurotomy, and collagenase injection.

Indications for treatment are varied and depend in large part on the patient's disability or preference. Hueston[26] described a tabletop test as a gauge of when to consider surgery. If a patient cannot lay the palm flat on a table, he or she may be considered a candidate for surgical treatment. Additional criteria for surgical intervention include symptoms that cause functional limitations, MCP joint contractures of 30° or greater, PIP joint contractures of 15° or greater, adduction contractures, or skin breakdown.[27] Flexion contractures that are progressing, especially in the PIP joint and to greater than 20°, would be considered a treatment indication by many physicians. Additional indications include recurrent disease, digital nerve deficit, diathesis, thumb involvement, and matted disease (especially in patients with diabetes).

Traditionally, surgery has been the gold standard for the treatment of Dupuytren contracture. Treatment options include fasciotomy, limited (regional) fasciectomy (**Figure 1**), total fasciectomy (removal of all diseased and nondiseased fasciae), dermofasciectomy, and the McCash[28] open palm technique. For the most part, surgical fasciotomy has been replaced by needle aponeurotomy (also known as percutaneous needle fasciotomy).

Fasciectomy

When compared with less invasive and office-based procedures, fasciectomy is advantageous because diseased fasciae are removed. Surgical treatment affords excellent exposure and visualization of the anatomy. Disadvantages of fasciectomy include all of the risks associated with surgery and anesthesia, including skin necrosis, wound dehiscence, nerve injury, hematoma, prolonged recovery, and limited finger range of motion (especially flexion). Although visualization is better, transient neurapraxia or nerve injury can occur. In complex, recurrent, and severe cases, finger necrosis and digit loss are possible. Although recurrence seems less likely with surgery, the effect of postoperative scar tissue on the hand after a recurrence increases the complexity of subsequent treatments when compared with recurrence after needle aponeurotomy and collagenase injection. The outcomes of further treatment(s) may be negatively affected.

Technique

Fasciectomy is typically performed through a Bruner, a V-Y, or a longitudinal incision with subsequent Z-plasty closure. This helps afford the appropriate exposure of the diseased fascia and allows lengthening of the skin (if necessary) for closure. Thick skin flaps help preserve the viability of the flaps. A prospective study comparing longitudinal incision with Z-plasties and Bruner incisions found no statistically significant differences in complications, outcomes, or recurrence rates between the groups.[29] The neurovascular structures then can be identified and protected while meticulously removing the diseased fascia. Typically, this procedure is best performed in a proximal-to-distal fashion because it is generally easier to identify the nerves and vessels in relationship to the cord in the palm than in the fingers. In difficult cases, a supplemental distal-to-proximal approach can be helpful in safely identifying the neurovascular structures because the surgeon approaches the most difficult area of dissection at the proximal or middle phalanx level. Displacement of the neurovascular structures by the cords in the digits may be present. The finger contracture will improve with cord release and removal, and any residual joint contractures can be released by palmar plate or check-rein ligament release. If a Bruner incision is used, the surgeon can defer the flap design in the finger until the contracture is partially released in the palm, because the partially corrected flexion contracture may allow for a more accurate flap design distally.

Prior to skin closure, the tourniquet is released, and meticulous hemostasis is obtained. Liberal use of drains can minimize the risk of a postoperative hematoma. The skin flaps should be visualized with the tourniquet released to assess viability. Tight closure, as indicated by white skin flaps, will lead to skin necrosis. In such instances, skin tension must be released by suture removal. Transverse incisions may be left open and will heal by secondary intention over 2 to 3 weeks. Dermal defects may be closed with full-thickness skin grafts, which can be harvested from the ipsilateral hypothenar eminence, volar wrist, medial arm, or groin.

Postoperative Care

Therapy after surgery includes edema control with an elastic garment, active-passive finger range-of-motion exercises, the use of a nighttime extension splint, and the intermittent use of a daytime extension splint. In patients with more severe disease, a continuous dynamic extension device has been advocated.[30] After the wound has healed, scar massage and desensitization can be added to the therapy regimen. Nighttime splinting is advocated for 3 months. Care should be taken to ensure that the patient works on both flexion and extension of the fingers because loss of flexion after surgery can occur.[31]

Outcomes

Outcomes of limited fasciectomy have been variable. Correction of deformity is generally achievable, but recurrence is common over time, and the complication rates are substantial. Recurrence following limited fasciectomy at various follow-up intervals has ranged from 0% to 66%.[29,32-38] Mavrogenis et al[34] reported the outcomes of 196 patients with Dupuytren contracture treated with partial fasciectomy at an average follow-up of 6.6 years. All of the patients had a minimum contracture of the PIP joint of 20°, and 93 patients had a concomitant 30° or more contracture of the MCP joint. After partial fasciectomy, 72.5% of the patients had complete range of motion of both the MCP and PIP joints. The authors also reported that 20.2% of the patients had 5° to 10° of extension deficit, and 7.3% of the patients had recurrence with greater than 20° con-

tracture of the PIP joint and underwent revision surgery. Complications included neurovascular compromise (5%), complex regional pain syndrome (10%), and wound healing problems (15%) such as infection.

Lerclercq and Tubiana[38] reported on an average 10-year follow-up of 50 patients treated with fasciectomy. Although full extension was initially restored in all of the patients, the recurrence rate was 66%, and loss of extension was reported in 46% of the patients. Twenty-four percent of the patients did not have at least 45° of PIP extension. A second surgery was needed in 16% of the patients.

Rombouts et al[36] proposed that histologic staging of diseased fasciae after fasciectomy could help predict recurrence. The authors defined type I lesions as having high cellular proliferation, type II as fibrocellular fasciae with a reticulin network, and type III lesions as those with a predominantly fibrous histology and few cells. They reported an overall recurrence rate of 39% in 77 hands treated by fasciectomy, with 70% of the recurrences in type I lesions versus only 18% in type III lesions. In a 2009 study, Balaguer et al[32] echoed these results. The authors reviewed 139 hands treated over a 7-year period and found recurrence rates that differed substantially based on the histologic type.

Misra et al[35] examined the reasons for recurrence and failure after a Dupuytren fasciectomony. They evaluated 37 patients (49 digits), with a primary focus on factors associated with recurrence. They found that severe preoperative deformity (> 60° at the PIP joint), incomplete surgical correction of the contracture, and poor patient compliance with the postoperative therapy regimen correlated with recurrence of the contracture. At an average follow-up of 7.3 years, Coert et al[39] reviewed the outcomes of 558 consecu-

tive patients treated with limited fasciectomy. The authors attempted to determine possible factors related to revisions and complications. They reported that patient age (younger than 45 years) was associated with revision surgery. A higher incidence of complications and poorer results occurred in patients who underwent revision surgery or had PIP joint contractures.

To evaluate complications associated with fasciectomy, Denkler[40] performed a meta-analysis on 41 articles published over a 20-year period that met certain inclusion criteria. The complication rates were quite variable, ranging between 3.6% and 39.1%. Major complications accounted for 15.7% of the complications, with complex regional pain syndrome being the most common (5.5%); other complications included digital nerve injury (3.4%), infection (2.4%), hematoma (2.1%), and arterial injury (2%). Wound healing problems (22.9%) were the most common minor complication. Patients undergoing revision surgery were 10 times more likely to have nerve or artery complications compared with those undergoing treatment for primary disease (20% versus 2%, respectively).

Dermofasciectomy and Full-Thickness Skin Grafting

Dermofasciectomy and full-thickness skin grafting are considered useful in treating Dupuytren contracture, especially in minimizing the rate of recurrence. Ketchum and Hixson[41] reviewed a 16-year experience of 68 patients treated with dermofasciectomy and full-thickness skin grafting. Although the study evaluated only 36 hands (24 patients), the authors reported no recurrence of disease beneath the areas that underwent skin grafting (average follow-up, 3.9 years). Extension beyond the grafts was seen in 8% of the hands. Armstrong et al[42] reported an overall recurrence rate of 11.6% in 103 patients (143 digits) with Dupuytren contracture who were treated with dermofasciectomy (average follow-up, 5.8 years). The authors concluded that dermofasciectomy is a better method of disease control when compared with limited fasciectomy. However, a more recent prospective randomized trial by Ullah et al[37] did not find similar results. The authors randomized 79 patients to treatment with fasciectomy (40 patients) versus dermofasciectomy and skin grafting (39 patients) and followed them for 3 years. The overall recurrence rate was 12.2%; no significant difference was found between the groups.

Open Palm Method

Technique and Postoperative Care

The open palm technique of Mc-Cash[28] is performed by making multiple transverse incisions in the palm and fingers. The diseased cord and fascia are removed beneath the intervening skin bridges. After removing the cord, the wound is left open and allowed to heal by secondary intention. Advantages of the open palm technique include no hematoma, no skin necrosis, and less postoperative pain. It also can be combined with a Bruner incision or other methods and can be an alternative to skin grafting, which will allow for early range of motion. The disadvantages include poor visualization of the neurovascular structures, prolonged wound healing time (3 to 4 weeks), the inconvenience of daily wound care until fully healed, and the increased risk of infection. Postoperatively, in addition to early therapy and extension splinting, the patient is instructed on wound care and edema control.

Outcomes

Shaw et al[43] reported on the outcomes of 39 digits treated with an open palm technique, with an average 9.6-year follow-up. All of the wounds healed within 3 to 5 weeks. The average preoperative MCP joint contracture was 41°, and PIP extension contracture was 56°. Postoperatively, the average MCP contracture improved to 1°, and the average PIP extension contracture to 9°. Complications included one digital nerve injury and one patient with pain and stiffness.

Bulstrode et al[33] reported on the complications of 253 patients treated with fasciectomy with the modified Skoog[44] technique, leaving palmar wounds open. The authors reported complications in 46 patients (18%); 35 patients had 1 complication, and more than 1 complication occurred in 11 patients. Complications included infection (9.6%), complex regional pain syndrome (2.4%), skin loss (2.4%), nerve injury (2%), hematoma (2%), and arterial injury (0.8%). Recurrence was noted in 31% of the patients (23 of 75) at an average 9.4-year follow-up period.

Needle Aponeurotomy

Indications, Advantages, and Disadvantages

Needle aponeurotomy has gained popularity in the past 15 years as an attractive alternative to surgery for many patients. It is an office-based procedure that requires only local anesthetic. Eaton[45] indicated the procedure for treating a contracture caused by a palpable cord lying beneath redundant skin in a cooperative patient. These specific indications have been expanded to a wider range of patients as surgeons have gained experience with this technique. The advantages of needle aponeurotomy include faster recovery, fewer wound healing complications, less postprocedural pain, earlier return to work and activities, the need for local anesthetic only, and lower costs compared with surgery or en-

zyme injection. The disadvantages are that it is a blind procedure, which can increase the risk of nerve, artery, and tendon injuries; it has limited efficacy for severe contractures; cords and nodules cannot be resected; there is the possibility of open skin tears; it has a higher recurrence rate; and there is a steep learning curve for the surgeon.

Technique

Needle aponeurotomy is performed using a sterile technique in a clinic or room for minor procedures (**Figure 2**). Evenly spaced intervals along the cord are marked to allow for effective severing of the cord at each interval. Local anesthetic, lidocaine with or without epinephrine, is injected into the epidermis and the superficial dermis at the proposed needle sites through a 30- or 27-gauge needle. Needle aponeurotomy takes advantage of the fact that the Dupuytren cords have no sensory nerve fibers and are insensate. Only the overlying skin needs to be anesthetized to allow for insertion of the needle. The depth of the anesthetic injection is only a fraction of a millimeter at each interval. Care should be taken to inject only the skin because the deeper digital nerves must not be anesthetized to allow for possible Tinel sign feedback during the needling procedure. The surgeon should carefully monitor the patient to ensure that the needle does not elicit a Tinel sign, which would indicate that the needle was in too close proximity to the nearby digital nerve. If a Tinel's sign is encountered, the needle should be immediately withdrawn and redirected to avoid injuring the digital nerve.

The needle procedure can be done with a 25-, 22-, 20- or 18-gauge needle. After the injection of local anesthetic, the percutaneous needle fasciotomy can be initiated. Sequential needling of the cord in either a sweeping (radial to ulnar direction) or sew-

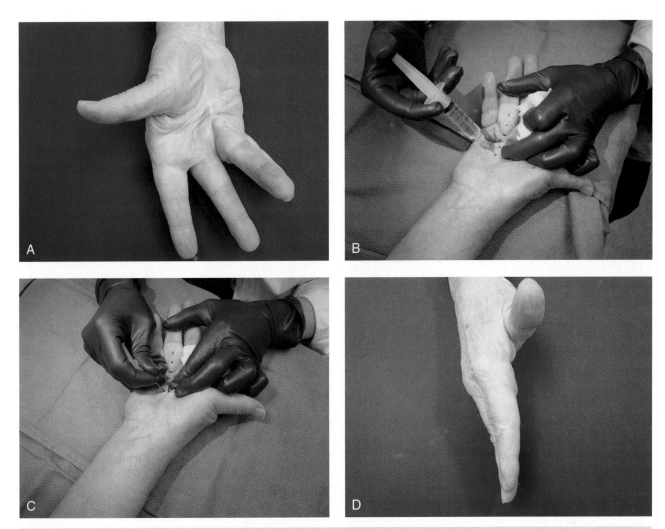

Figure 2   **A,** Clinical photograph of the hand of a patient with ring finger contracture and a Dupuytren cord. **B,** The skin overlying the cord is anesthetized in evenly spaced intervals along the cord. **C,** Sequential needling is performed at each site. After release, manipulation, and correction of the flexion contracture, soft dressings are applied. **D,** Photograph of the hand after needle aponeurotomy.

ing machine (repeated up and down direction) fashion is then performed. The smaller caliber needles (25- or 22-gauge) rely more on a repetitive perforating technique, whereas the larger caliber (18- or 20-gauge) needles use more of a slicing approach through the cords. The surgeon can proceed from proximal to distal or vice versa. Extending the finger during the needling procedure will help keep the cord taut and prominent, although caution must be exercised with using a needle at the MCP joint level with the joint in hyperextension because this position places the flexor tendons relatively

close to the skin and at risk for injury. In general, care must be taken to remain central on the cord in the palm to avoid injury to the adjacent common digital neurovascular bundles and going too deeply with the needle to avoid injury to the underlying tendons. A gristle-like feel and sound should be appreciated as the cord is severed. This process is repeated for each interval until the cord is weakened to the point that it can be released with a forceful finger extension maneuver at the end of the procedure.

To minimize the risk of nerve injury, patients are queried repeatedly

during the procedure to inform the surgeon of the possible feeling of a "zinger" or electrical shock sensation (Tinel sign), which would indicate that the needle may be near or on the digital nerve or neurovascular bundle. Sensation at the tip of the finger is repeatedly assessed to ensure that the nerve is functional. After release, finger flexion is assessed to ensure that all individual flexor digitorum superficialis and flexor digitorum profundus tendons are intact, functional, and without triggering or clicking. Hemostasis is obtained with pressure, and a soft dressing or bandages are applied. If skin tears are encountered, an antibiotic ointment is applied to minimize the risk of infection and wound desication. Nighttime static extension splinting can help maintain extension, and daytime dynamic splinting can help stretch residual joint contractures.

Complications

Complications associated with needle aponeurotomy include skin tears; infection; nerve, artery, and tendon injuries; complex regional pain syndrome, and persistent swelling. During the release, skin tears may occur and can affect the postprocedure regimen. Most skin tears heal via secondary intention and daily dressing changes. The acknowledgment of the Tinel sign associated with needling will help avoid nerve injury. Staying superficial and avoiding hyperextension of the digit while needling should minimize the risk of tendon injury. Although reported, the risk of complex regional syndrome and Dupuytren flare is much lower than for open surgical techniques.

Outcomes

Published reports of outcomes after needle aponeurotomy have underscored the convenience and relative ease of use of this procedure. Foucher et al[46] retrospectively reviewed outcomes of needle aponeurotomy in 211 patients (311 palms/fingers); the first 100 patients had a minimum 3-year follow-up. The procedure was performed in the palm of 165 patients, in the palm and finger of 111 patients, and in the finger only of 35 patients. The correction rate for MCP contractures was 79% and 65% for PIP contractures. The overall revision rate was 24%; however, it was 59% among the first 100 patients. Complications were rare, with no tendon injury or infection; one nerve injury occurred. The authors concluded that elderly patients

with MCP joint contracture were ideal candidates for needle aponeurotomy.

Beaudreuil et al[47] reported on a general review (most were retrospective studies) of outcomes with needle aponeurotomy. Better results were typically seen in patients with early disease. Overall rates of good structural results were 80% in the short term and 69% at 5 years. Patient satisfaction was generally excellent. The most common complications were skin tears (8%), transient dysesthesia (3%), infection (0.7%), and tendon rupture (0.2%). In 2008, Lellouche[48] concluded that based on convenience of use and outcomes, needle aponeurotomy should be used as the first treatment option for patients with Dupuytren contracture.

A study by van Rijssen and Werker[49] of 74 needle aponeurotomies generally showed excellent results, with immediate improvement after the procedure. With recurrence defined as 30° or more of extension lag compared with the immediate postprocedural range of motion, the recurrence rate in 55 patients at 32 months was 65%. Complications included two digits with slightly limited sensibility. The authors concluded that needle aponeurotomy is effective in the short term and may have a role in delaying fasciectomy.

In a prospective comparison of outcomes of needle aponeurotomy and limited fasciectomy, van Rijssen et al[50] reported on 115 hands at a follow-up of 6 weeks. They found that limited fasciectomy afforded a 79% improvement in extension; whereas needle aponeurotomy corrected 62% of the extension. The surgical treatment resulted in greater discomfort and lower patient satisfaction compared with needle aponeurotomy. van Rijssen et al[51] reported on this same series of patients at 5-year follow-up. The recurrence rate was substantially higher in the needle aponeurotomy group

(85%) versus the limited fasciectomy group (21%). The only patient parameter associated with recurrence was age; older age at the time of treatment was associated with lower recurrence rates. Interestingly, in this series, patient satisfaction was higher in the surgically treated group; however, more than 50% of the patients with recurrence preferred treatment with needle aponeurotomy. The authors concluded that needle aponeurotomy may be preferable to surgery in elderly patients and those willing to accept early disease recurrence.

Pess et al[52] reported better overall results using a more aggressive needle approach. The cohort of patients included 474 patients and 1,013 fingers, with an average of 35° of MCP joint contracture and 50° of PIP contracture. Immediately after the procedure, the degree of correction was 99% at the MCP joints and 89% at the PIP joints. At a minimum 3-year follow-up, the maintained correction was 72% for the MCP joints and 31% for the PIP joints. As with other studies, MCP joints fared better than PIP joints, and older patients maintained a greater degree of correction than younger patients.

Collagenase Injection

In 2010, the FDA approved *Clostridium histolyticum* collagenase for the treatment of Dupuytren contracture in patients with a palpable cord. The treatment aims to dissolve a portion of the cord, effectively weakening it enough to allow for release (**Figure 3**). The collagenase commercially available in the United States (Xiaflex; Auxilium Pharmaceuticals) is a mixture of types I and II collagenase, which are derived from clostridia. These two types of collagenase work synergistically to rapidly degrade collagen, and they work much more efficiently and faster than native human collagenase.

Technique

Clostridial collagenase is administered via percutaneous injection directly into the Dupuytren contracture cords. It requires mixing the lyophilized crystalline form of collagenase with sterile diluent (normal saline with calcium chloride) to prepare the medication. The recommended dilution amount depends on whether the injection is being performed for release of an MCP or a PIP joint contracture. A total of 0.58 mg of collagenase is used regardless of the location of the cord; however, the amount of fluid injected is 0.2 mL for PIP joint contractures and 0.24 mL for MCP joint contractures. The hand is prepped in a standard sterile fashion. The cord is injected at the location of maximal prominence and separation from the underlying flexor tendons. Approximately one third of the injection is placed at the initial location. Subsequent injections 2 to 3 mm proximal and distal to the initial injection site are then performed. The injections are placed directly into the cord, with care taken to avoid too deep an injection because this may lead to enzymatic degradation of the underlying tendon. Resistance to the injection should be felt by the clinician, indicating that the needle is appropriately placed in the cord itself. The desired effect is to weaken a portion of the cord to allow release. The medication is then allowed 18 to 24 hours to hydrolyze the cord. The patient returns the next day for release of the cord through forceful manipulation of the involved digit. The hand will typically appear bruised and swollen at the injection sites. On the postinjection visit, the hand/finger can be anesthetized to minimize the pain of forcefully manipulating the finger into extension. The cord is released in a methodic and controlled fashion. Care should be taken to intermittently assess finger flexion after releasing the

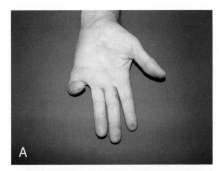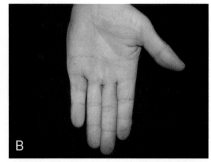

Figure 3 **A,** Clinical photograph showing the degree of Dupuytren contracture of the small finger prior to collagenase injection. **B,** Four weeks after the collagenase injection, the small finger has excellent extension, and the injection site is fully healed.

weakened cord to ensure that the tendons are intact. After release, a soft bulky dressing or bandages are applied. Edema control measures and splinting may also be used.

Complications

Potential complications associated with collagenase injection include allergic reaction; skin tears; tendon, pulley, nerve, and artery injuries; ecchymosis; pain or tenderness at the injection sites; edema; regional lymphadenopathy; complex regional pain syndrome; and skin discoloration. Although no cases of anaphylaxis have been reported to date, it is imperative that the facility where the injections are being performed has code carts and epinephrine pens readily available. As with needle aponeurotomy, the risk of complex regional syndrome and Dupuytren flare is much lower with collagenase treatment compared with open surgical techniques.

Outcomes

The original reports on the use of collagenase injections, published in 2000 and 2007, helped to lay the groundwork for future investigations.[53,54] Hurst et al[55] reported on a large, prospective, placebo-blinded, multicenter study of 308 patients. Patients receiving collagenase were injected with a

0.58-mg dose using the technique previously described in this chapter. All fingers were manipulated and released the following day (without anesthesia). With the primary end point being correction to within 5° of full extension, fingers injected with collagenase had a substantially higher success rate compared with placebo (64% versus 6.8%, respectively). In addition, there was a substantially higher overall arc of motion of both MCP and PIP joint motion in the fingers treated with collagenase. Complications included two tendon ruptures and one case of complex regional pain syndrome. Initial investigations did not include thumb contractures. The use of collagenase for thumb and first web space contractures has now been reported, and it appears that it is effective and safe in the short term for this group of patients.[56]

Bainbridge et al[57] investigated the efficacy of collagenase injections to treat hands and fingers previously treated with surgery. The authors reviewed 12 clinical trials that included more than 1,000 patients, of whom 39% had previous surgery. They found that MCP joint correction in the previously operated digits was comparable with those that were not previously operated on (75% and 80%, respectively). For the PIP joints, the results were comparable, with correction of

52% for the previously operated hands and 50% for the previously nonoperated hands. Some complications were higher in the previously surgically treated groups, but they did not appear to be clinically relevant. The authors concluded that collagenase injection can be used safely and effectively in patients who had previous surgery for Dupuytren contracture.

Rozen et al[58] investigated longer-term outcomes focusing on complications and adverse events associated with the use of collagenase. Twelve patients, originally included in a prospective study, were assessed at 12 months after collagenase injection. Two of the patients reported painful triggering that necessitated surgical intervention. Intraoperative findings suggested that extensive scarring and adhesions were the likely cause of the painful triggering.

Watt et al[59] reported on 8-year follow-up evaluations in patients who participated in the initial phase II trials of collagenase injections. Eight patients completed the 8-year follow-up evaluation. Six patients were treated for isolated MCP contracture and two for PIP contractures. Four of the six patients in the MCP group had recurrence of Dupuytren contracture at 8 years after the injection. In the entire MCP group, the average MCP contracture before injection was 57° versus 23° at 8-year follow-up. Both patients in the PIP group had recurrence. The average preinjection contracture was 45° versus 60° at the 8-year follow-up. Overall patient satisfaction was high, and 88% would again choose collagenase injection to treat recurrent or progressive disease.

Summary

Dupuytren contracture is a disease that affects the palmar fascia and leads to a characteristic thickening and cord formation that may limit finger extension.

It has a genetic preponderance and tends to primarily affect men of northern European ancestry in the fourth to sixth decades of life. There is no known cure. Treatment is usually reserved for patients with functional limitations. Current treatments may be surgical or nonsurgical. Surgery remains the gold standard for treating Dupuytren contracture, with limited fasciectomy the most common procedure. Needle aponeurotomy and collagenase injections are more convenient, office-based interventions aimed at weakening the cords to allow release and effective correction of the contracture. Although generally safe and effective, recurrence rates may be higher in nonsurgically treated patients. Level I prospective randomized studies are needed to help better define indications and treatment options.

References

1. Elliot D: The early history of contracture of the palmar fascia: Part 1. The origin of the disease: The curse of the MacCrimmons. The hand of benediction: Cline's contracture. *J Hand Surg Br* 1988;13(3):246-253.

2. Ross DC: Epidemiology of Dupuytren's disease. *Hand Clin* 1999;15(1):53-62, vi.

3. Ramchurn N, Mashamba C, Leitch E, et al: Upper limb musculoskeletal abnormalities and poor metabolic control in diabetes. *Eur J Intern Med* 2009;20(7):718-721.

4. Arkkila PE, Kantola IM, Viikari JS: Dupuytren's disease: Association with chronic diabetic complications. *J Rheumatol* 1997;24(1):153-159.

5. Al-Homood IA: Rheumatic conditions in patients with diabetes mellitus. *Clin Rheumatol* 2013;32(5):527-533.

6. Burke FD, Proud G, Lawson IJ, McGeoch KL, Miles JN: An assessment of the effects of exposure to vibration, smoking, alcohol and diabetes on the prevalence of Dupuytren's disease in 97,537 miners. *J Hand Surg Eur Vol* 2007;32(4):400-406.

7. Brenner P, Krause-Bergmann A, Van VH: [Dupuytren contracture in North Germany. Epidemiological study of 500 cases]. *Unfallchirurg* 2001;104(4):303-311.

8. Sanderson PL, Morris MA, Stanley JK, Fahmy NR: Lipids and Dupuytren's disease. *J Bone Joint Surg Br* 1992;74(6):923-927.

9. Critchley EM, Vakil SD, Hayward HW, Owen VM: Dupuytren's disease in epilepsy: Result of prolonged administration of anticonvulsants. *J Neurol Neurosurg Psychiatry* 1976;39(5):498-503.

10. Geoghegan JM, Forbes J, Clark DI, Smith C, Hubbard R: Dupuytren's disease risk factors. *J Hand Surg Br* 2004;29(5):423-426.

11. Loos B, Puschkin V, Horch RE: 50 years experience with Dupuytren's contracture in the Erlangen University Hospital: A retrospective analysis of 2919 operated hands from 1956 to 2006. *BMC Musculoskelet Disord* 2007;8:60.

12. Burge P: Genetics of Dupuytren's disease. *Hand Clin* 1999;15(1):63-71.

13. Michou L, Lermusiaux JL, Teyssedou JP, Bardin T, Beaudreuil J, Petit-Teixeira E: Genetics of Dupuytren's disease. *Joint Bone Spine* 2012;79(1):7-12.

14. Shih BB, Tassabehji M, Watson JS, McGrouther AD, Bayat A: Genome-wide high-resolution screening in Dupuytren's disease reveals common regions of DNA copy number alterations. *J Hand Surg Am* 2010;35(7):1172-1183, e7.

15. Bonnici AV, Birjandi F, Spencer JD, Fox SP, Berry AC: Chromosomal abnormalities in Dupuy-

tren's contracture and carpal tunnel syndrome. *J Hand Surg Br* 1992;17(3):349-355.

16. Picardo NE, Khan WS: Advances in the understanding of the aetiology of Dupuytren's disease. *Surgeon* 2012;10(3):151-158.

17. Al-Qattan MM: Factors in the pathogenesis of Dupuytren's contracture. *J Hand Surg Am* 2006; 31(9):1527-1534.

18. Chansky HA, Trumble TE, Conrad EU III, Murray LW, Raskind WH: Evidence for a polyclonal etiology of palmar fibromatosis. *J Hand Surg Am* 1999;24(2): 339-344.

19. Liss GM, Stock SR: Can Dupuytren's contracture be work-related? Review of the evidence. *Am J Ind Med* 1996;29(5): 521-532.

20. Baird KS, Crossan JF, Ralston SH: Abnormal growth factor and cytokine expression in Dupuytren's contracture. *J Clin Pathol* 1993;46(5):425-428.

21. Tomasek J, Rayan GM: Correlation of alpha-smooth muscle actin expression and contraction in Dupuytren's disease fibroblasts. *J Hand Surg Am* 1995;20(3): 450-455.

22. Baird KS, Alwan WH, Crossan JF, Wojciak B: T-cell-mediated response in Dupuytren's disease. *Lancet* 1993;341(8861):1622-1623.

23. von Campe A, Mende K, Omaren H, Meuli-Simmen C: Painful nodules and cords in Dupuytren disease. *J Hand Surg Am* 2012;37(7):1313-1318.

24. Reilly RM, Stern PJ, Goldfarb CA: A retrospective review of the management of Dupuytren's nodules. *J Hand Surg Am* 2005;30(5): 1014-1018.

25. Ketchum LD, Donahue TK: The injection of nodules of Dupuytren's disease with triamcinolone acetonide. *J Hand Surg Am* 2000; 25(6):1157-1162.

26. Hueston JT: Current state of treatment of Dupuytren's disease. *Ann Chir Main* 1984;3(1):81-92.

27. McFarlane RM: Dupuytren's disease. *J Hand Surg Br* 1996;21(4): 566-567.

28. McCash CR: The open palm technique in Dupuytren's contracture. *Br J Plast Surg* 1964;17: 271-280.

29. Citron ND, Nunez V: Recurrence after surgery for Dupuytren's disease: A randomized trial of two skin incisions. *J Hand Surg Br* 2005;30(6):563-566.

30. Bailey AJ, Tarlton JF, Van der Stappen J, Sims TJ, Messina A: The continuous elongation technique for severe Dupuytren's disease: A biochemical mechanism. *J Hand Surg Br* 1994;19(4): 22-527.

31. Schneider LH, Hankin FM, Eisenberg T: Surgery of Dupuytren's disease: A review of the open palm method. *J Hand Surg Am* 1986;11(1):23-27.

32. Balaguer T, David S, Ihrai T, Cardot N, Daideri G, Lebreton E: Histological staging and Dupuytren's disease recurrence or extension after surgical treatment: A retrospective study of 124 patients. *J Hand Surg Eur Vol* 2009; 34(4):493-496.

33. Bulstrode NW, Jemec B, Smith PJ: The complications of Dupuytren's contracture surgery. *J Hand Surg Am* 2005;30(5): 1021-1025.

34. Mavrogenis AF, Spyridonos SG, Ignatiadis IA, Antonopoulos D, Papagelopoulos PJ: Partial fasciectomy for Dupuytren's contractures. *J Surg Orthop Adv* 2009; 18(2):106-110.

35. Misra A, Jain A, Ghazanfar R, Johnston T, Nanchahal J: Predicting the outcome of surgery for the proximal interphalangeal joint in Dupuytren's disease. *J Hand Surg Am* 2007;32(2): 240-245.

36. Rombouts JJ, Noël H, Legrain Y, Munting E: Prediction of recurrence in the treatment of Dupuytren's disease: Evaluation of a histologic classification. *J Hand Surg Am* 1989;14(4):644-652.

37. Ullah AS, Dias JJ, Bhowal B: Does a 'firebreak' full-thickness skin graft prevent recurrence after surgery for Dupuytren's contracture? A prospective, randomised trial. *J Bone Joint Surg Br* 2009; 91(3):374-378.

38. Leclercq C, Tubiana R: [Long-term results of aponeurectomy for Dupuytren's disease]. *Chirurgie* 1986;112(3):194-197.

39. Coert JH, Nérin JP, Meek MF: Results of partial fasciectomy for Dupuytren disease in 261 consecutive patients. *Ann Plast Surg* 2006;57(1):13-17.

40. Denkler K: Surgical complications associated with fasciectomy for Dupuytren's disease: A 20-year review of the English literature. *Eplasty* 2010;10:e15.

41. Ketchum LD, Hixson FP: Dermofasciectomy and full-thickness grafts in the treatment of Dupuytren's contracture. *J Hand Surg Am* 1987;12(5, pt 1):659-664.

42. Armstrong JR, Hurren JS, Logan AM: Dermofasciectomy in the management of Dupuytren's disease. *J Bone Joint Surg Br* 2000; 82(1):90-94.

43. Shaw DL, Wise DI, Holms W: Dupuytren's disease treated by palmar fasciectomy and an open palm technique. *J Bone Joint Surg Br* 1996;21(4):484-485.

44. Skoog T: Dupuytren's contracture: Pathogenesis and surgical treatment. *Surg Clin North Am* 1967;47(2):433-444.

45. Eaton C: Percutaneous fasciotomy for Dupuytren's contracture. *J Hand Surg Am* 2011;36(5): 910-915.

46. Foucher G, Medina J, Navarro R: Percutaneous needle aponeurotomy: Complications and re-

sults. *J Hand Surg Br* 2003;28(5): 427-431.

47. Beaudreuil J, Lellouche H, Orcel P, Bardin T: Needle aponeurotomy in Dupuytren's disease. *Joint Bone Spine* 2012;79(1): 13-16.

48. Lellouche H: [Dupuytren's contracture: Surgery is no longer necessary]. *Presse Med* 2008;37(12): 1779-1781.

49. van Rijssen AL, Werker PM: Percutaneous needle fasciotomy in Dupuytren's disease. *J Hand Surg Br* 2006;31(5):498-501.

50. van Rijssen AL, Gerbrandy FS, Ter Linden H, Klip H, Werker PM: A comparison of the direct outcomes of percutaneous needle fasciotomy and limited fasciectomy for Dupuytren's disease: A 6-week follow-up study. *J Hand Surg Am* 2006;31(5):717-725.

51. van Rijssen AL, ter Linden H, Werker PM: Five-year results of a randomized clinical trial on treatment in Dupuytren's disease: Percutaneous needle fasciotomy versus limited fasciectomy. *Plast Reconstr Surg* 2012;129(2): 469-477.

52. Pess GM, Pess RM, Pess RA: Results of needle aponeurotomy for Dupuytren contracture in over 1,000 fingers. *J Hand Surg Am* 2012;37(4):651-656.

53. Badalamente MA, Hurst LC: Enzyme injection as nonsurgical treatment of Dupuytren's disease. *J Hand Surg Am* 2000;25(4): 629-636.

54. Badalamente MA, Hurst LC: Efficacy and safety of injectable mixed collagenase subtypes in the treatment of Dupuytren's contracture. *J Hand Surg Am* 2007;32(6): 767-774.

55. Hurst LC, Badalamente MA, Hentz VR, et al: Injectable collagenase clostridium histolyticum for Dupuytren's contracture. *N Engl J Med* 2009;361(10): 968-979.

56. Bendon CL, Giele HP: Collagenase for Dupuytren's disease of the thumb. *J Bone Joint Surg Br* 2012; 94(10):1390-1392.

57. Bainbridge C, Gerber RA, Szczypa PP, et al: Efficacy of collagenase in patients who did and did not have previous hand surgery for Dupuytren's contracture. *J Plast Surg Hand Surg* 2012; 46(3-4):177-183.

58. Rozen WM, Edirisinghe Y, Crock J: Late complications of clinical clostridium histolyticum collagenase use in Dupuytren's disease. *PLoS One* 2012;7(8):e43406.

59. Watt AJ, Curtin CM, Hentz VR: Collagenase injection as nonsurgical treatment of Dupuytren's disease: 8-year follow-up. *J Hand Surg Am* 2010;35(4):534-539, e1.

Video Reference

Birman MV: Video. *Dupuytren Contracture Manipulation.* Arlington Heights, IL, 2013.

Venturing Into the Overlap Between Pediatric Orthopaedics and Hand Surgery

Scott H. Kozin, MD
Dan A. Zlotolow, MD
Joshua A. Ratner, MD

Abstract

There is an overlap between pediatric orthopaedic surgery and hand surgery. A pediatric orthopaedic surgeon is accustomed to the intricacies of the immature skeleton, whereas a hand surgeon is more familiar with the regional anatomy and finer surgical techniques. Many hand diagnoses and surgical techniques are appropriate for the pediatric orthopaedic surgeon, including straightforward duplicated thumb reconstruction of a trigger thumb. Many pediatric diagnoses are more suitable for treatment by a hand surgeon, including simple syndactyly release and complex duplicated thumb reconstruction. Other procedures, such as pollicization, cleft hand reconstruction, synpolydactyly release, and macrodactyly management, require more advanced expertise for successful treatment. It is helpful for pediatric orthopaedic surgeons and hand surgeons to be familiar with the indications, surgical techniques, outcomes, and complications of pediatric hand surgery.

Instr Course Lect 2014;63:143-156.

There is an overlap between pediatric orthopaedic surgery and hand surgery. A pediatric orthopaedic surgeon is familiar with the nuances of the immature skeleton, whereas a hand surgeon is more familiar with the regional anatomy and surgical techniques. Many hand diagnoses and surgical techniques are appropriate for the pediatric orthopaedic surgeon, whereas other pediatric diagnoses are more suitable for treatment by a hand surgeon. Some procedures require additional familiarity, expertise, and experience to achieve the best possible outcomes (**Table 1**).

Thumb Duplication (Preaxial Polydactyly)

Thumb duplication, which is more accurately described as split thumb deformity, is a congenital anomaly of the hand. Occurring sporadically, thumb duplication occurs when the tissues genetically present in the thumb position develop a cleft, yielding two distinct portions of thumb tissue. The deformity is seen unilaterally, has a reported incidence of 1 in 1,000 to 10,000 births, and occurs more frequently in Caucasians.[1]

The morphology of the individual thumbs is variable, but each is typically smaller than the contralateral thumb. Split thumb deformity has been classified by Wassel.[2] The Wassel classification system can be simplified by counting the number of abnormal bones seen on plain radiographs of the affected thumb, including the phalangeal bones and the metacarpal. The exception to the rule is a type VII or triphalangeal thumb. Type IV thumb deformities are the most common.

Surgical Techniques for Reconstruction

Surgical reconstruction is usually

Dr. Kozin or an immediate family member serves as a board member, owner, officer, or committee member of the American Society for Surgery of the Hand. Dr. Zlotolow or an immediate family member serves as a paid consultant to Osteomed and Arthrex; serves as an unpaid consultant to Arthrex and Osteomed; has received research or institutional support from Arthrex and Osteomed; and has received nonincome support (such as equipment or services), commercially derived honoraria, or other non–research-related funding (such as paid travel) from Osteomed and Arthrex. Dr. Ratner or an immediate family member is a member of a speakers' bureau or has made paid presentations on behalf of Axogen and serves as a paid consultant to Axogen.

Table 1

Procedures Rated by Expertise and Experience[a]

Procedure	Pediatric Orthopaedist	General Hand Surgeon	Pediatric Hand Surgeon
Simple syndactyly	×	×	×
Complex syndactyly	*	*	×
Complicated syndactyly			*
Postaxial polydactyly type A	×	×	×
Postaxial polydactyly type B	×	×	×
Preaxial polydactyly, simple	×	×	×
Preaxial polydactyly, complex			*
Trigger thumb	×	×	×
Trigger finger		*	×
Type II thumb hypoplasia		*	×
Pollicization		*	×
Mirror hand			*
Cleft hand		*	×
Macrodactyly			*

[a]Procedures that are suitable to each specialty are identified with a (×). Specialized training required is marked with a (*).

indicated for cosmesis in subtle type I thumbs or functional enhancement in other types. The timing of reconstruction varies with the degree of the deformity. A polydactylous thumb with a small rudimentary skin tag may be excised early (before 1 year of age). More complex deformities requiring osteotomy and tendon transfers should be delayed until the surgeon believes that corrective procedures can be performed safely on structures of a given size.

Types I and II Polydactyly of the Thumb

Baek et al[3] modified the original Bilhaut-Cloquet procedure for polydactyly of the thumb to allow consolidation of the bifid distal phalanx while maintaining most of the distal phalanx and nail elements of the ulnar thumb. A smaller radial osteoperiosteal flap allows the scar to be positioned away from the midline and avoids the common nail deformity of the traditional approach. This is a particularly challenging procedure and should be performed by a congenital hand surgeon.

Types III Through VI Polydactyly of the Thumb

An organized preoperative plan is the key to successful reconstruction of types III through VI split thumb deformities. Anatomic variation must be considered and may include a pollex abductus (an anomalous connection between the flexor pollicis longus and extensor pollicis longus that tethers the interphalangeal joint into abduction and requires release), aberrant neurovascular structures, and anomalous tendon insertions. In planning reconstruction, the anatomic elements of the thumb that are vital to thumb function must be considered, including maintaining the thumb-index web

space, the stability of the carpometacarpal joint, the integrity of the ulnar collateral ligaments of the metacarpophalangeal (MCP) joint, and the overall linear alignment.

A thumb that is larger and more skeletally developed (often the ulnar thumb) is usually retained (**Figure 1**). Given the need for stable pinch, the ulnar thumb, with competent ulnar collaterals, is best maintained. Elements of the extra digit, which may include the extra flexor pollicis longus, the extensor pollicis longus, and intrinsic tissue, should be harvested and used to enhance the form and function of the reconstructed thumb. In patients with a bifid proximal phalanx or metacarpal, a thick capsuloperiosteal sleeve, inclusive of the abductor pollicis brevis and the radial collateral ligament insertions on the radial-sided proximal phalanx, is raised and transferred to the ulnar-sided thumb (**Figure 1, C**). In rare instances in which the radial thumb is preserved, the adductor insertion from the ulnar thumb must be similarly transferred using a capsuloperiosteal sleeve.

Osteotomy for angular correction or narrowing of a broad, two-facet metacarpal or proximal phalanx head is easily done with a beaver blade and can be fixed with small gauge (0.028 to 0.035 inch) Kirschner wires (**Figure 1, D**). Surgeons who are comfortable with hand anatomy are capable of straightforward reconstruction of types III through VI duplications. Unusual duplications are best performed by a pediatric hand surgeon because complications are more common.

Type VII (Triphalangeal Thumb)

Reconstruction of a triphalangeal thumb requires reduction of the number of bones in the thumb by partial excision or complete resection of the frequently delta-shaped middle phalanx. When a thumb is split and one of

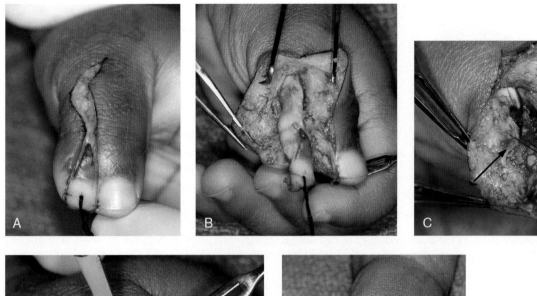

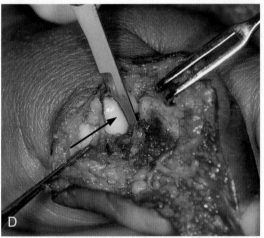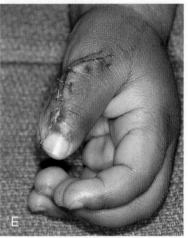

Figure 1   Photographs showing reconstruction of a Wassel type IV right thumb duplication in a 1-year-old child. **A,** A skin incision is made for deletion of the radial component and reconstruction of the ulnar thumb. **B,** The radial component skeleton is isolated with preservation of important soft-tissue structures. **C,** The preserved osteoperiosteal sleeve held by suture (arrow) is raised from the deleted thumb with the collateral ligament and abductor pollicis brevis. **D,** A scalpel is used to remove the radial facet from the metacarpal head (arrow). **E,** The thumb after final reconstruction has good alignment, stability, and bulk. (Courtesy of Shriners Hospitals for Children, Philadelphia, PA.)

the two components is itself triphalangeal, the decision on which component to retain depends on the size, the intrinsic and extrinsic tendon function, and joint stability. These complex reconstructions are best done by surgeons experienced in treating congenital hand disorders.

Complications

The viability of the postoperative thumb is of principal importance. Arterial and venous structures must be protected during surgery and should not be sacrificed, if possible. It is imperative that the reconstructed polydactylous thumb be stable, straight, and of appropriate size.[4] A zig-zag deformity can result from joint malalignment, ligament laxity, and/or aberrant tendon insertions. Although avoiding complications is challenging because of the need to consider the anatomy of multiple structures, correcting complications is more difficult. It should not be assumed that bony deformities will grow out and remodel. Osteotomies for angular correction are needed. Tendon reinsertion (transfer) should be

considered when anatomic variation is encountered.

Syndactyly

Syndactyly, which is the most common congenital difference in the upper limb, can range in severity from a slightly distal web to a rosebud hand, as seen with Apert syndrome. Most parents choose to have their child's fingers separated, and many wish to have this surgery performed soon after the child's birth. For nonborder digits (ring-long and long-index) syndactyly, there is no medical reason for early

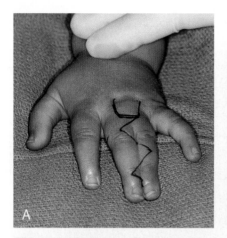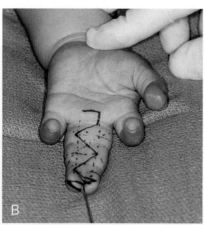

Figure 2 Photographs showing the basic principles of flap design for syndactyly reconstruction. The tenets include no longitudinal scars, commissure reconstruction without grafting, and reconstructing the lateral nail folds. **A,** The dimples over the dorsum of the MCP joint are marked, and a tapering open box is drawn extending two thirds the distance to the proximal interphalangeal joint. **B,** A transverse line of the same width as the distal end of the dorsal commissure flap is drawn on the palm. Dotted lines are drawn along the central axis of each digit, and a dot is used to mark where each interphalangeal crease meets the midpoint of the syndactyly. To avoid grafting the ring finger, a line is drawn from the docking line to the MCP joint crease, and zigzag lines are then drawn at 45° to the axis of the fingers and extended to the midaxis of each digit and ended at the whirl of one of the digits. (Courtesy of Shriners Hospitals for Children, Philadelphia, PA.)

digital separation and reconstruction. If the border digits are involved or there is a progressive deformity of the digits because of tethering of one digit by the other, surgery may be performed as soon as the child can safely undergo general anesthesia. The goal of early surgery is to limit the flexion contractures and the rotational deformities that occur if a smaller digit tethers its larger neighbor.

Ideally, syndactyly reconstruction should be delayed until a child is at least 18 months old. Because the hand doubles in size in the first 2 years of life, delaying surgery results in a technically simpler surgical procedure with more predictable results. In most patients, only one of any digit should be surgically treated at a time. Surgery on both sides of a finger can compromise the neurovascular bundles and risks digital loss. Compromised vascularity also can lead to necrosis of skin flaps

and poor healing of skin grafts. After 3 months, the finger usually has recovered sufficiently and can be safely separated from the opposite side.

For surgeons who see a limited number of patients with syndactyly, first gaining experience with incomplete syndactylies is recommended. Web spaces proximal to the proximal interphalangeal joint can be reconstructed using a myriad of flap designs.[5] More distal web spaces require more complicated flaps and, in most instances, the use of full-thickness skin grafting. The dorsal V-to-Y advancement flap can be used in select patients to avoid skin grafting, but it has limited indications. The results are best if the syndactyly is incomplete and the skin and soft tissue between the digits is less than 2 mm in thickness.[6] The flap also leaves a prominent scar on the dorsal hand.

Complete or Nearly Complete Syndactyly

The most versatile surgical technique for complete or nearly complete syndactyly reconstruction is a combination of flaps and grafts. This chapter's authors prefer a modification of the flaps, with a large trapezoidal dorsal flap to reconstruct the commissure and multiple small zigzag-type flaps for the finger. Full-thickness skin grafting is used to fill in the inevitable gaps near the commissure. The surgeon should not be tempted to avoid skin grafting because the circumference of two independent digits is 22% larger than two conjoined digits. Primary closure without skin grafting can lead to web creep and digital necrosis.[7]

The flap design begins with marking the dimples over the dorsum of the MCP joint (**Figure 2, A**). A tapering open box is then drawn, extending two thirds the distance to the proximal interphalangeal joint. A transverse line matching the distal end of the dorsal commissure flap is then drawn on the palm, nearly as proximal to the joint crease as the line is wide. The volar line should not be drawn directly over the MCP joint crease because this will result in a transverse incision at the web space and lead to web creep. The hand should be turned back and forth to ensure that the dorsal flap will reach the transverse line. If this has not been achieved, the size of the dorsal flap or the location of the volar docking line should be adjusted.

Beginning on the volar side, dotted lines are drawn along the central axis of each digit, and a dot is used to mark where each interphalangeal crease meets the midpoint of the syndactyly. To avoid grafting the ring finger, a line is drawn from the docking line to the MCP joint crease, and zigzag lines are then drawn at 45° to the axis of the fingers and extended to the midaxis of

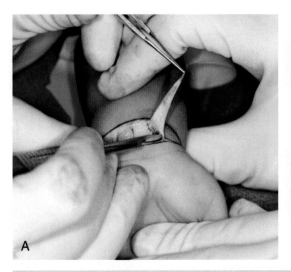
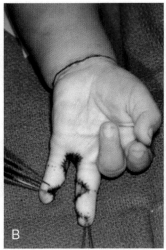
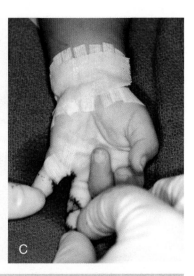

Figure 3 Photographs showing skin graft harvest and closure in syndactyly reconstruction. **A,** An elliptical graft centered over the proximal wrist crease is harvested sharply superficial to the small cutaneous veins. **B,** If dissected at the correct level, the graft does not have to be defatted, and the bed does not bleed. Closure typically results in a thin scar concealed within the skin crease. **C,** Within the fingers, the graft recipient site is shielded from shear and compressed by petroleum dressing and gauze held down by noncircumferential adhesive strips. (Courtesy of Shriners Hospitals for Children, Philadelphia, PA.)

each digit and ended at the whirl of one of the digits (**Figure 2, B**). For complete syndactylies, tighter zigzag lines are drawn over the tip of the finger to avoid the need for a composite graft. The distal zigzag lines should extend beyond the midaxis of each digit and will serve to reconstruct the lateral nail fold. The identical pattern should be drawn on the dorsal side of the hand to the level of the distal interphalangeal joint. The most distal angular flap is extended to the midline of the syndactyly and continued along the midline to connect with the volar flaps. The surgeon should ensure that the eponychial folds are not compromised by the flap design.

A tourniquet should be used to improve intraoperative hemostasis. The dorsal commissure flap is raised as a full-thickness flap. If there is any question about the status of the neurovascular bundles, the bundles can be located by dissecting between the digits from dorsal to volar. Next, the thick distal flaps are raised if the syndactyly was complete. The remainder of the dorsal flaps are raised, and the volar

neurovascular bundles are identified. It is easiest and safest to defat the dorsal flaps at this point. Because the blood supply to the tip of the flap is contained in the subcutaneous fat, only as much fat as necessary should be removed to obtain primary closure of the flaps.

The volar flaps are incised and are gently spread dorsally to volarly between the neurovascular bundles to separate the volar flaps. This chapter's authors find it easier to separate the digits distally first and then progress proximally. The proximal limit of the dissection is marked either by the branch point of the proper digital arteries from the common digital ligament or the intervolar plate ligament (whichever is encountered first). If the digital nerves branch distal to the arteries, the fascicles are separated (as if splitting string cheese) back to the arterial branch point.

The commissure flap is closed first, followed by the distal nail fold flaps and the remainder of the flaps. Only absorbable suture should be used, but fast-absorbing gut should be avoided.

This chapter's authors prefer 5-0 plain gut, but other options are acceptable. Remaining deficits not covered by the flaps should be filled in with full-thickness skin graft. After trying various graft-harvest sites, this chapter's authors prefer the proximal wrist crease because the skin is usually a perfect match in terms of color and thickness and is hairless (**Figure 3, A and B**). The scar is also more cosmetically acceptable than antecubital or forearm harvest sites. To optimize harvesting of the graft, the tissue bed should be well vascularized, but meticulous hemostasis should be maintained. The postoperative dressing is crucial for limiting shear between the graft and the tissue bed and for providing compression. An alternative is to use a piece of petroleum dressing and gauze cut to the size of the graft and applied on top of the graft with noncircumferential adherent strips (**Figure 3, C**). Because the early oxygen and nutrient supplies occur via imbibition, hematoma, seroma, or purulent collection can lead to early graft loss. If the tissue bed is poor or there is shear be-

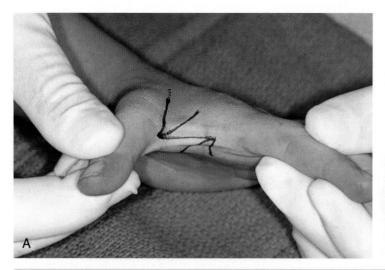
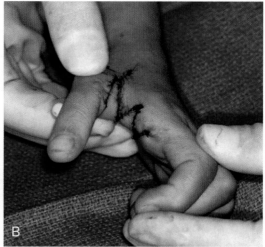

Figure 4   A narrowed thumb-index web space is treated with four-flap Z-plasty. **A,** Markings show the skin design for ample web deepening. **B,** Photograph of the hand after web widening and flap closure. (Courtesy of Shriners Hospitals for Children, Philadelphia, PA.)

tween the graft and the tissue bed, the process of angiogenesis (primary inosculation) cannot proceed, and the graft fails within the first 3 to 7 days. After 3 weeks, secondary inosculation begins, and the graft is sufficiently robust to survive outside the postoperative dressing.

Reconstruction of the Thumb-Index Web Space

Reconstruction of the first web space is more challenging than reconstruction of nonborder digits and requires a different set of flaps and grafts. For mild web space narrowing with no flexion contracture of the thumb, this chapter's authors prefer the classic four flap Z-plasty (**Figure 4**). The skin flaps allow excellent access to the adductor and the first dorsal interosseous muscles. Release of the fascia overlying the muscles and fibrous interconnections between the muscles yields greater radial and palmar abduction without compromising muscle function.

Patients with a tight first web space and an MCP joint flexion contracture of the thumb (clasp thumb) are ideal candidates for the index rotation flap (known as the stiletto flap).[8] Redun-

dant skin on the radial aspect of the index finger is rotated into the area of the MCP joint crease, expanding both the skin of the volar thumb and the skin of the first web space (**Figure 5**). To ensure a smooth flap contour after it is rotated, the more ulnar limb of the flap should be more distal than the radial limb.

If the first web space syndactyly is complete or nearly complete, the best flap option is the modified dorsal rotation advancement flap described by Ghani.[9] Although this flap typically requires adjunctive skin grafting, it provides for deepening and widening of the web space. This flap has dramatically improved outcomes (**Figure 6**).

Trigger Thumb

Trigger thumb has not been found in newborns, despite screening of more than 14,500 newborns.[10-13] By age 1 year, approximately 3 in 1,000 children will have a trigger thumb. Up to 60% of these trigger thumbs resolve spontaneously by the age of 5 years.[14] As the child grows, the Notta nodule on the flexor pollicis longus is believed to gradually dilate the pulley system and resolve the triggering in some chil-

dren. The outcome in the 40% of children with unresolved trigger thumbs is unclear.

Because of the low morbidity and low risks of surgical release, most parents choose not to wait for spontaneous resolution and opt for a release. This chapter's authors prefer to use a shallow transverse incision in the joint flexion crease of the thumb. Because the skin is very supple in this area, it is easy to make a deeper cut than intended. Great care should be taken not to hyperextend the thumb during the incision because this puts the volar neurovascular bundles at additional risk by tenting them against the skin. The neurovascular bundles should be identified and retracted out of the way. The radial bundle crosses the flexor tendon sheath and is at greatest risk during proximal release. Division of the entire first annular pulley is usually sufficient to allow the interphalangeal joint to extend. Closure is accomplished with an absorbable suture. A soft dressing is used for up to 2 weeks if it stays on for that length of time. No further follow-up is usually required.

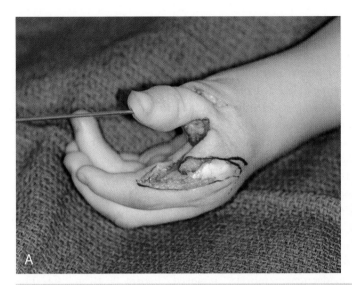
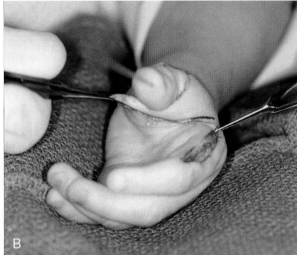

Figure 5 A narrowed thumb-index web space in both the coronal and the sagittal planes is treated with a stiletto flap. **A,** The stiletto flap is elevated from the radial side of the index finger. **B,** The flap is mobilized to widen the web space and cover the volar aspect of the thumb. (Courtesy of Shriners Hospitals for Children, Philadelphia, PA.)

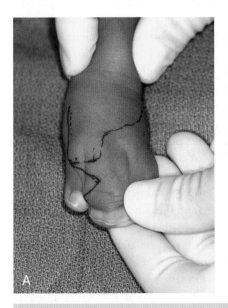
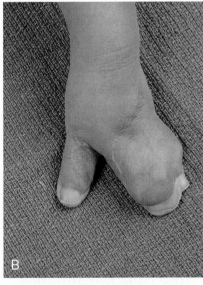

Figure 6 Photographs of a 1-year-old child with a nearly complete thumb-index web space syndactyly. **A,** A Ghani flap is drawn on the dorsum of the hand. **B,** The healed flap shows ample first web space. (Courtesy of Shriners Hospitals for Children, Philadelphia, PA)

Conditions That Require Specialized Training

Certain procedures are best managed by a surgeon experienced in pediatric upper extremity surgery. The complexity of the problem and the intricacies of the procedure(s) require consider-able familiarity in congenital hand differences.

Pollicization

Pollicization is a complex procedure that requires the advanced skill of the surgeon and the brain plasticity of the patient. A functioning finger (usually the index finger) is substituted for a deficient or absent thumb. The most common congenital reason for pollicization is thumb hypoplasia, with absence or instability of the carpometacarpal joint.[15-17] Some parents may not agree with the concept of thumb ablation and index finger pollicization. Parents may want the child to keep a deficient thumb; however, the surgeon should avoid surgery to reconstruct a thumb with carpometacarpal joint instability (type IIB hypoplastic thumb) because of the superior results of index finger pollicization.[18]

Brain plasticity and motor relearning play a crucial role in function after pollicization. There is normally a large region of the sensorimotor cortex (SMC) homunculus dedicated to the hand. Giraux et al[19] showed that after hand transplantation, the original SMC map for hand activation is restored. The transplantation actually reverses the SMC loss after the initial hand amputation. Similarly, successful toe transfer produces temporal activation within the SMC consistent with cortical plasticity.[20] The effects of pollicization have yet to be studied, but essential changes occur in the SMC as the index finger converts into a thumb.

Technique

Many surgical steps and nuances are necessary to achieve optimum outcomes in pollicization procedures. A stepwise approach is used to avoid missing a crucial step in this multiple-step procedure.[21-24] The skin incision is designed to allow transposition of the index finger and creation of an adequate thumb-index web space. The palmar skin is incised first, and the neurovascular bundles are isolated (**Figure 7**). The proper digital artery to the long finger is ligated to allow tension-free index finger pollicization vascularized by both the radial and common digital arteries (**Figure 7, B**). The first annular pulley of the index finger is incised to prevent buckling of the flexor tendons after pollicization. The intermetacarpal ligament is divided. The dorsal incision is then sharply elevated, with preservation of as many dorsal veins as possible. The first dorsal and palmar interossei muscles are traced to their attachments into the extensor hood and released in preparation of the transfer.

The index finger is shortened by removing the metacarpal bone from its base to the epiphysis. Physeal ablation (epiphysiodesis) prevents unwanted growth of the index finger pollicization. The index MCP joint is fixed into hyperextension prior to pollicization to prevent unwanted MCP joint hyperextension. Using a wire driver, a Kirschner wire is passed antegrade from the metacarpal epiphysis into the proximal phalanx and out of the proximal interphalangeal joint. The Kirschner wire is used as a joystick to carefully position the index finger into the thumb position. The Kirschner wire is drilled retrograde across the metacarpal base to maintain its posi-

tion. Additional stability is obtained via tendon transfer of the first dorsal interosseous muscle to the radial lateral band and the first palmar interosseous muscle to the ulnar lateral band (**Figure 7, C**). The skin is carefully inset with absorbable sutures (**Figure 7, D**). Any redundant skin is excised. The tourniquet is deflated, and the constructed thumb is observed for 5 minutes. Postoperative dressings are critical. A long-arm soft cast made of Scotchcast Soft Cast Casting Tape (3M Corporation) is applied with the elbow flexed to more than 100° to decrease the chance of inadvertent removal. The patient remains in the hospital overnight, and the arm is elevated to promote venous drainage.

Outcome

A variety of factors affect the outcome after surgery. The principal influence is the preoperative status of the index digit and the presence of adequate musculotendinous units.[15,16,21,23,24] A mobile index finger with robust extrinsic and intrinsic musculotendinous units has the potential to become an excellent thumb that can participate in grasp and has mobility for pinch. In contrast, an index finger with limited active and passive motion may provide stability for gross grasp but is less likely to be incorporated into pinch.

Mirror Hand Reconstruction

Mirror hand is a rare congenital anomaly characterized by duplication of the limb in the midline (**Figure 8, A**). Typically, there is a central digit with three digits on each side that represent the middle, ring, and small digits in mirrored symmetry.[25] Although the hand has seven digits, the thumb is always absent. Within the forearm, there are two ulnae and no radius (also known as ulnar dimelia).[26] The soft-tissue anatomy is bizarre, complicated, and unpredictable. Surgical recon-

struction requires specialized skill in pediatric hand surgery.

The treatment strategy is to reconstruct the hand by reducing the number of digits to four and constructing a thumb from the deleted digits. The procedure is similar to pollicization; however, the large number of digits complicates the design of the skin incision and making a thumb.[27] The principles of pollicization and the use of parts from the deleted digits are the tenets of reconstruction. The most mobile radial digit is selected for pollicization, and the stiffer radial digits are removed (**Figure 8, B** and **C**). The skin from the ablated digits is used to augment the first web space (**Figure 8, D**). Surgery is challenging because the redundant musculotendinous units and bony elements frequently obstruct positioning of the selected digit for pollicization. The rarity of this condition necessitates treatment by an experienced pediatric hand surgeon because the outcome is directly related to the surgical technique.

Macrodactyly Reconstruction

Macrodactyly is one of the most challenging conditions for a child, the family, and the hand surgeon. The diagnosis is usually straightforward and is often evident at birth or within the first 3 years of life.[28,29] In contrast, the treatment algorithm is complicated, and the outcome is often disappointing. Macrodactyly can be divided into two distinct growth patterns—progressive or static.[28] In the progressive form, the digital growth is disproportionate to the uninvolved digits. In the static form, the growth pattern is consistent with the rest of the hand. Macrodactyly also usually involves more than one digit within a territory innervated by a single proximal nerve (also known as nerve territory–oriented macrodactyly).[29] When two digits are involved, they usually deviate away

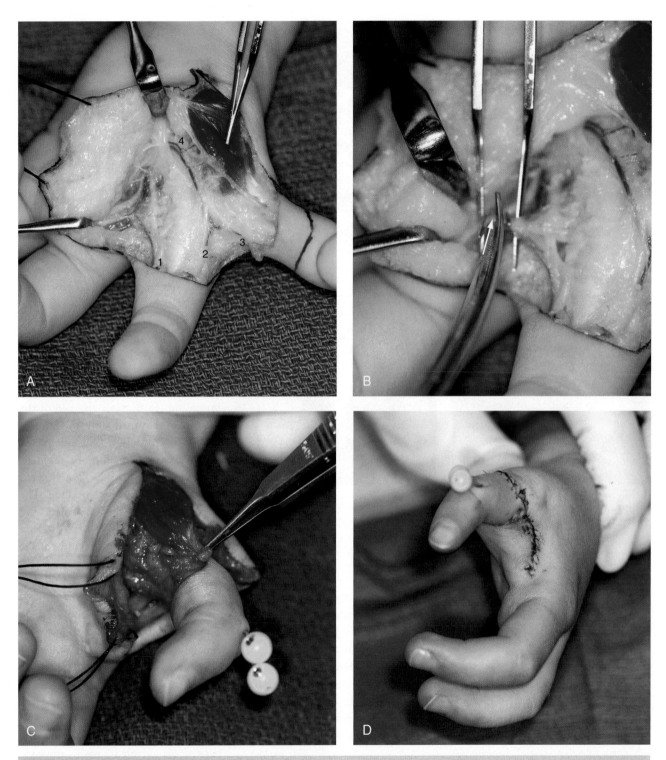

Figure 7   Photographs of the pollicization procedure in the left hypoplastic thumb of a 3-year-old girl. **A,** A volar skin incision is made, and the neurovascular bundles are isolated: (1) ulnar digital artery to the index finger; (2) radial digital artery to the index finger; (3) ulnar digital artery to the thumb; (4) superficial arch. **B,** The radial digital artery (arrow) to the long finger is ligated. **C,** Tendon transfer is performed for intrinsic muscle reconstruction. **D,** After skin closure, there is ample thumb-index web space and good thumb position. (Courtesy of Shriners Hospitals for Children, Philadelphia, PA.)

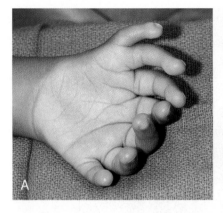
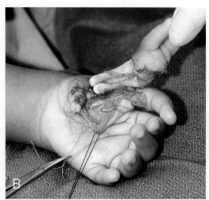
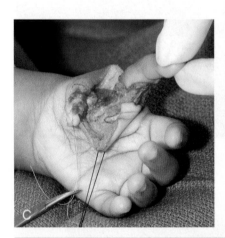
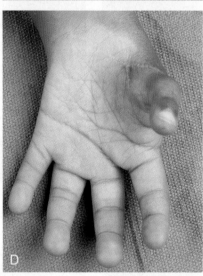

Figure 8   **A,** Preoperative photograph of the hand of a 3-year-old girl with mirror hand and seven fingers. **B,** The two less mobile radial digits are ablated. **C,** Pollicization of the most mobile radial digit. **D,** Clinical appearance of the hand after pollicization. (Courtesy of Shriners Hospitals for Children, Philadelphia, PA.)

from each other. The bony growth continues unabated until skeletal maturity, and the digits stiffen over time.

Management

The first decision in the management of a child with macrodactyly is whether the digit(s) are salvageable. Strategic factors include the form of macrodactyly (progressive or static), the digit(s) involved, and the functional outlook. For progressive macrodactyly, early amputation avoids repeat surgeries that often results in an unsatisfactory digit that interferes with hand function and causes social embarrassment. This option should be discussed with a

pediatric hand surgeon who routinely treats children with macrodactyly. The child's parents are often skeptical and need to be comfortable with the expertise and advice from the surgeon. Digital retention is reserved for thumb involvement, static macrodactyly, and parents who are willing to accept multiple surgeries for their child.

Surgery

Many surgical procedures have been described to treat macrodactyly.[30-33] There are sophisticated and complicated drawings of procedures to restore alignment, contour, and appearance to the disfigured digit; however, none of

these surgical procedures will restore normal form and function. Prudent surgical options include amputation, epiphysiodesis to limit longitudinal growth, debulking to reduce the size of the digit, and osteotomy to correct bony angulation. Epiphysiodesis stops longitudinal growth but does not prevent the relentless appositional growth and subsequent stiffness.

Amputation follows similar surgical principles as ray amputation in adults (**Figure 9**). Long or ring finger amputation may require concomitant transposition of the index or small finger, respectively, to prevent a gap between the retained digits. Epiphysiodesis is performed when the digit reaches the matching length of the parent of the same sex. Mild digital deviation can be corrected with a closing wedge resection of the physis. Serial debulking procedures to decrease the size of the digit are performed only in static or thumb macrodactyly. One side of the digit is debulked at a time via a midlateral approach, with skin flaps elevated to the volar and dorsal midline. The neurovascular bundle is isolated, and excessive fat and skin is excised. Osseous reduction is difficult and can be achieved by either narrowing the enlarged bone or removing a central portion of bone.

Outcomes after digit-preserving surgery are often disappointing and ultimately result in a scarred, stiff digit that rarely participates in grasp.[30,31] In contrast, ray amputation is a valuable procedure and should be considered early in progressive macrodactyly and single-digit involvement, before the patient is treated with multiple surgical procedures to salvage a misshapen digit that has little function (**Figure 9, C**).

Cleft Hand Reconstruction

Central deficiency of the hand or cleft hand is another complicated congeni-

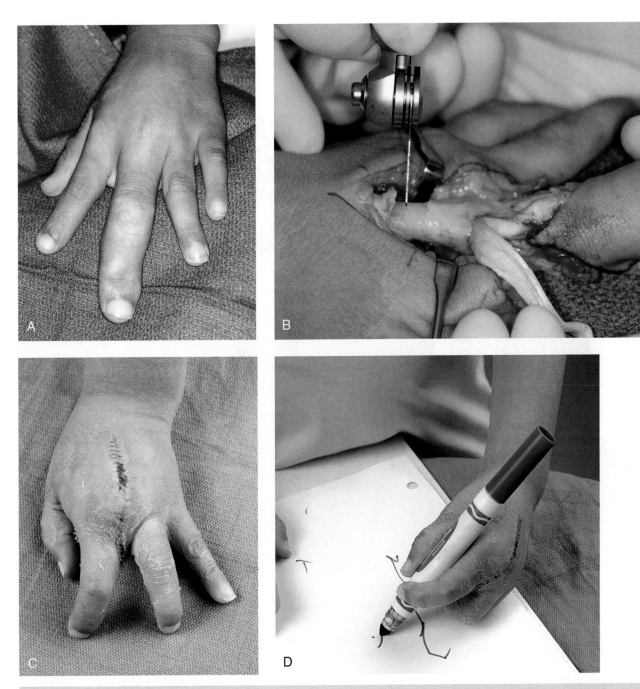

Figure 9   **A,** Preoperative dorsal view of the hand of a 4-year-old boy with isolated left long finger macrodactyly. **B,** Early ray amputation was performed on the long finger. **C,** Postoperative dorsal view of the hand after index finger transposition. **D,** Postoperative view of the hand shows good thumb index web space and cleft closure activity. (Courtesy of Shriners Hospitals for Children, Philadelphia, PA.)

tal difference that is best treated by an experienced pediatric hand surgeon. Cleft hand can occur as an isolated difference, but more commonly is associated with a number of syndromes, particularly split-hand/split-foot and ectrodactyly–ectodermal dysplasia–

cleft lip/palate syndromes.[34,35] There are a variety of phenotypes, but the trademark is a V-shaped cleft in the center of the hand with variable narrowing of the thumb-index web space (**Figure 10, A**). In severe cases, the hand may contain a single digit

(monodactyly), and the thumb may be completely absent.

The counseling and management of children with cleft hands require patience and experience. A cleft hand with a functioning thumb has been described as a "functional triumph, but a

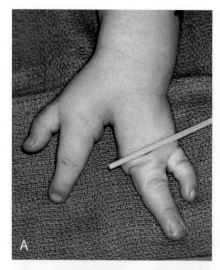

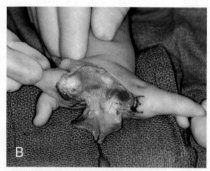

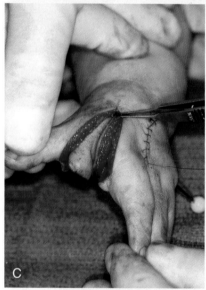

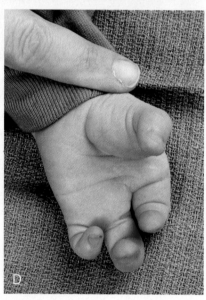

Figure 10   **A,** Preoperative dorsal view of the cleft hand and narrowed thumb index web space in a 16-month-old boy. **B,** A flap is elevated from the cleft. **C,** Intraoperative dorsal view of the hand with the flap reduced. **D,** Postoperative view shows good thumb index web space and cleft closure activity. (Courtesy of Shriners Hospitals for Children, Philadelphia, PA.)

dure, which was elaborated on by Flatt.[36] The ultimate thumb-index skin web space is designed from the cleft skin that is removed for cleft closure. This skin is raised as a palmar-based random flap, although a digital artery may be isolated and included with the flap to transform its blood supply from random to axial (**Figure 10, B**).

The index finger is relocated in a more ulnar direction to facilitate widening of the thumb-index web space and ease cleft closure. There are a variety of techniques to achieve index finger relocation, including formal transposition, metacarpal osteotomy, or carpal wedge osteotomy. Index finger relocation to the base of the third metacarpal widens the first web space and decreases the amount of flap transposition. The index finger must be carefully positioned to prevent malrotation and scissoring during finger flexion. After the cleft has been closed, attention is directed toward thumb-index web space reconstruction. The thumb-index space is opened by releasing constricting structures and investing fascia. The cleft commissure flap is inset with subtle tailoring of the flap. Supplementary skin grafts may be necessary to cover bare areas (**Figure 10, C**).

An acceptable outcome can be reliably achieved by adhering to the principles of adequate first web release, resurfacing with pliable tissue (avoiding skin graft within the commissure), transposition of the index finger, and restoration of an adequate commissure within the cleft[38] (**Figure 10, D**).

Summary

Surgery on the upper extremity of children combines the sensibilities of a pediatric orthopaedic surgeon with the anatomic and procedural expertise of a hand surgeon. Many procedures, such as simple syndactylies and polydactyl-

social disaster."[36] These hands function exceedingly well but are a frequent source of embarrassment and teasing. A family with one or more generations of cleft hands may not pursue surgery for their children because they recognize that function trumps aesthetic improvement. Such families must be carefully counseled when surgical indications are outlined. In contrast, families without affected members (spontaneous mutation) are

more likely to request surgery in an attempt to reconstruct the hand to a normal appearance.

The simultaneous closure of the cleft and reconstruction of the narrowed thumb-index web space require the expertise of a pediatric hand surgeon. This complex procedure requires transposition of the skin from the cleft into the thumb-index web space and closure of the cleft. Snow and Littler[37] initially described the surgical proce-

ies, are ideal gateways for the pediatric orthopaedist and the hand surgeon to venture into the overlap between the two specialties. For surgeons who have a specific interest in this patient population, specialized training can bring some of the most rewarding and challenging procedures, such as pollicization, within their field of expertise.

References

1. Flatt A: *The Care of Congenital Hand Anomalies*. St Louis, MO, Quality Medical Publishing, 1994, pp 228-275.

2. Wassel HD: The results of surgery for polydactyly of the thumb: A review. *Clin Orthop Relat Res* 1969;64:175-193.

3. Baek GH, Gong HS, Chung MS, Oh JH, Lee YH, Lee SK: Modified Bilhaut-Cloquet procedure for Wassel type-II and III polydactyly of the thumb. *J Bone Joint Surg Am* 2007;89(3):534-541.

4. Ogino T, Ishii S, Takahata S, Kato H: Long-term results of surgical treatment of thumb polydactyly. *J Hand Surg Am* 1996;21(3): 478-486.

5. Ostrowski DM, Feagin CA, Gould JS: A three-flap web-plasty for release of short congenital syndactyly and dorsal adduction contracture. *J Hand Surg Am* 1991; 16(4):634-641.

6. Hsu VM, Smartt JM Jr, Chang B: The modified V-Y dorsal metacarpal flap for repair of syndactyly without skin graft. *Plast Reconstr Surg* 2010;125(1):225-232.

7. Eaton CJ, Lister GD: Syndactyly. *Hand Clin* 1990;6(4):555-575.

8. Ezaki M, Oishi SN: Index rotation flap for palmar thumb release in arthrogryposis. *Tech Hand Up Extrem Surg* 2010;14(1):38-40.

9. Ghani HA: Modified dorsal rotation advancement flap for release of the thumb web space. *J Hand Surg Br* 2006;31(2):226-229.

10. Moon WN, Suh SW, Kim IC: Trigger digits in children. *J Hand Surg Br* 2001;26(1):11-12.

11. Slakey JB, Hennrikus WL: Acquired thumb flexion contracture in children: Congenital trigger thumb. *J Bone Joint Surg Br* 1996; 78(3):481-483.

12. Kikuchi N, Ogino T: Incidence and development of trigger thumb in children. *J Hand Surg Am* 2006;31(4):541-543.

13. Rodgers WB, Waters PM: Incidence of trigger digits in newborns. *J Hand Surg Am* 1994; 19(3):364-368.

14. Baek GH, Kim JH, Chung MS, Kang SB, Lee YH, Gong HS: The natural history of pediatric trigger thumb. *J Bone Joint Surg Am* 2008;90(5):980-985.

15. Manske PR, McCaroll HR Jr: Index finger pollicization for a congenitally absent or nonfunctioning thumb. *J Hand Surg Am* 1985;10(5):606-613.

16. Kozin SH, Weiss AA, Webber JB, Betz RR, Clancy M, Steel HH: Index finger pollicization for congenital aplasia or hypoplasia of the thumb. *J Hand Surg Am* 1992; 17(5):880-884.

17. Lister G: Reconstruction of the hypoplastic thumb. *Clin Orthop Relat Res* 1985;195:52-65.

18. Foucher G, Medina J, Navarro R: Microsurgical reconstruction of the hypoplastic thumb, type IIIB. *J Reconstr Microsurg* 2001;17(1): 9-15.

19. Giraux P, Sirigu A, Schneider F, Dubernard JM: Cortical reorganization in motor cortex after graft of both hands. *Nat Neurosci* 2001; 4(7):691-692.

20. Manduch M, Bezuhly M, Anastakis DJ, Crawley AP, Mikulis DJ: Serial fMRI of adaptive changes in primary sensorimotor cortex following thumb reconstruction. *Neurology* 2002;59(8):1278-1281.

21. Buck-Gramcko D: Pollicization of the index finger: Method and results in aplasia and hypoplasia of the thumb. *J Bone Joint Surg Am* 1971;53(8):1605-1617.

22. Littler JW: On making a thumb: One hundred years of surgical effort. *J Hand Surg Am* 1976;1(1): 35-51.

23. McCarroll HR: Congenital anomalies: A 25-year overview. *J Hand Surg Am* 2000;25(6):1007-1037.

24. Kozin SH: *Green's Operative Hand Surgery*, ed 6. Philadelphia, PA, Elsevier Churchill Livingstone, 2010, pp 1371-1404.

25. Al-Qattan MM, Al-Thunayan A, De Cordier M, Nandagopal N, Pitkanen J: Classification of the mirror hand-multiple hand spectrum. *J Hand Surg Br* 1998;23(4): 534-536.

26. Barton NJ, Buck-Gramcko D, Evans DM: Soft-tissue anatomy of mirror hand. *J Hand Surg Br* 1986;11(3):307-319.

27. Barton NJ, Buck-Gramcko D, Evans DM, Kleinert H, Semple C, Ulson H: Mirror hand treated by true pollicization. *J Hand Surg Br* 1986;11(3):320-336.

28. Barsky AJ: Macrodactyly. *J Bone Joint Surg Am* 1967;49(7):1255-1266.

29. Al-Qattan MM: Lipofibromatous hamartoma of the median nerve and its associated conditions. *J Hand Surg Br* 2001;26(4): 368-372.

30. Akinci M, Ay S, Erçetin O: Surgical treatment of macrodactyly in older children and adults. *J Hand Surg Am* 2004;29(6):1010-1019.

31. Ogino T: *Congenital Malformations of the Hand and Forearm*. London, England, Churchill Livingstone, 1998, pp 183-197.

32. Tsuge K: Treatment of macrodactyly. *J Hand Surg Am* 1985; 10(6 pt 2):968-969.

33. Tsuge K: Treatment of macrodactyly. *Plast Reconstr Surg* 1967; 39(6):590-599.

34. Bystrom EB, Sanger RG, Stewart R: The syndrome of ectrodactyly, ectodermal dysplasia, and clefting (EEC). *J Oral Surg* 1975; 33(3):192-198.

35. Gül D, Oktenli C: Evidence for autosomal recessive inheritance of split hand/split foot malformation: A report of nine cases. *Clin Dysmorphol* 2002;11(3):183-186.

36. Flatt A: *The Care of Congenital Hand Anomalies*. St. Louis, MO, Quality Medical Publishing, 1994, pp 296-306.

37. Snow J, Littler J: Surgical treatment of cleft hand, in *Transactions of the Society of Plastic and Reconstructive Surgery: 4th Congress in Rome*. Amsterdam, The Netherlands, Excerpta Medica Foundation, 1967, pp 888-893.

38. Rider MA, Grindel SI, Tonkin MA, Wood VE: An experience of the Snow-Littler procedure. *J Hand Surg Br* 2000;25(4): 376-381.

Adult Reconstruction: Hip and Knee

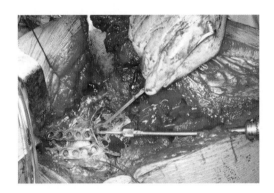

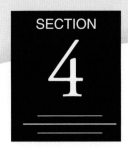

15

Hip Pain in the Young, Active Patient: Surgical Strategies

Michael R. Bloomfield, MD
Jill A. Erickson, PA-C
Joseph C. McCarthy, MD
Michael A. Mont, MD
Patrick Mulkey, MD
Christopher L. Peters, MD
Robert Pivec, MD
Matthew S. Austin, MD

Abstract

Hip disorders in young patients likely exist as a spectrum of prearthritic and arthritic conditions. With the increasing recognition of these disorders, surgical options are being popularized and more patients are being treated at a younger age. Hip surgeons must develop a careful set of evidenced-based indications and follow surgical outcomes in a rigorous, scientific manner.

Hip arthroscopy can be used to successfully treat some hip disorders, including labral tears, with or without femoroacetabular impingement, resulting in mechanical symptoms. Long-term outcomes after arthroscopy are determined by the condition of the cartilage at the time of surgery. Patients with preoperative radiographic evidence of moderate to severe arthritis have poor outcomes when treated with arthroscopy. Open joint preservation procedures (including periacetabular osteotomy and surgical hip dislocation with osteochondroplasty) can be done in the absence of substantial arthritis to treat hip dysplasia, femoroacetabular impingement, and related conditions. The results of these procedures are good in appropriately selected patients at short-term to midterm follow-ups.

In the presence of severe arthritis, joint replacement is the treatment of choice. Total hip arthroplasty using uncemented acetabular and femoral fixation provides reliable osseointegration; however, long-term results in young patients have historically been compromised by bearing surface wear, osteolysis, and component loosening. Contemporary, highly cross-linked polyethylene and ceramic-on-ceramic bearings have durable results, low complication rates, and offer the potential of long-term survivorship in this high-demand population. In general, metal-on-metal implants have higher complication rates versus other bearing surface options and should be avoided. The best results of hip resurfacing are seen in men younger than 55 years with large femoral head sizes. Although implant survivorship is comparable to that of total hip arthroplasty, the sequelae of metal wear debris continue to cause concern.

Instr Course Lect 2014;63:159-176.

Hip disorders in young patients have become increasingly recognized over the past decade. Because there is an established connection between variations in hip morphology and the development of osteoarthritis, many investigators now believe that these entities likely exist as a spectrum of pathology.[1-3]

Historically, treatment options for young patients with hip pathology have been limited; however, during the past decade, two trends have emerged. The identification of anatomic variants and the development and popularization of joint preservation procedures to address these morphologies have led to treatment at an earlier stage of hip disease, with the goal of relieving pain and preventing or delaying end-stage arthritis. At the same time, arthroplasty has been increasingly performed in younger patients because of promising results achieved with contemporary implants and bearing surfaces. Despite these successes, the rapid and widespread adoption of new techniques and technology by the orthopaedic community may prove problematic unless strict indications, careful patient selection, and outcomes are carefully scrutinized. This chapter outlines the spectrum of hip preservation and reconstructive options available for young patients and provides evidence regarding the appropriate indications and expected outcomes for selected procedures.

The Prearthritic Hip: Pathology and Treatment

In recent years, there has been an increasing appreciation of the contribution of hip dysplasia and femoroacetabular impingement (FAI) to the development of hip pain, dysfunction, and osteoarthritis. Arthroplasty remains the preferred treatment for hip arthritis; however, for hips that are prearthritic or at risk for arthritis because of anatomic abnormality, joint preservation surgery is gaining preference. As the understanding of the

many anatomic and physiologic factors leading to early-onset arthritis increases, multiple treatment approaches have been developed, including pelvic osteotomies to reorient the acetabulum, surgical dislocation and osteochondroplasty, labral repair or débridement, and the increasing use of hip arthroscopy.

The goals of joint preservation surgery are to correct underlying structural abnormalities that are damaging the hip, restore the normal biomechanical relationship of the proximal femur and acetabulum, débride or repair damage to the labrum or the cartilage, and extend the lifespan of the joint to the extent possible.

Hip Dysplasia

Hip dysplasia can be defined in the simplest terms as the lack of adequate coverage of the femoral head by the acetabulum, secondary to an anatomic abnormality. Classic acetabular dysplasia is characterized by the deficiency of anterior and lateral femoral head coverage. However, because dysplasia is a three-dimensional process, posterior deficiency (retroversion) can occur with or without lateral deficiency. Hip dysplasia causes pathologic point loading of the femoral head and early wear; it has traditionally been treated with redirectional acetabular osteotomy. A

variety of pelvic osteotomies are performed, including Bernese periacetabular osteotomy (PAO) and rotational acetabular osteotomy, which is commonly performed in Asia. In North America and Europe, PAO has become the surgical procedure of choice for maintaining the posterior column and the stability of the acetabular fragment. The presence of hip dysplasia alters the normal biomechanics of the hip joint and is well recognized as the most common cause of secondary hip osteoarthritis.[4,5]

Indications and Contraindications for PAO

Before PAO is performed, it should be determined that instability or subluxation and symptoms of groin pain or impingement pain with flexion are refractory to conservative treatment. The patient should have preserved range of motion and, at the most, only mild to moderate (Tönnis grade 2 or less) osteoarthritis. Radiographic evidence of dysplasia includes an upwardly sloping sourcil on an AP pelvic radiograph, a lateral and/or anterior center-edge angle of less than 25°, and congruency of the joint on an abduction/internal rotation view (**Figure 1**). In a younger patient, acetabular retroversion (identified by a positive crossover sign on the AP pelvic radiograph) with preservation of acetabular and femoral cartilage should be discernible. Patient selection is an often overlooked element that is crucial to success. It should be determined that the patient is compliant and rational and has realistic expectations before performing major reconstructive surgery. There is some controversy regarding the appropriate patient age criteria for PAO in the setting of hip dysplasia. In the United States and Europe, it is uncommon for a PAO to be performed on a patient older than 50 years, whereas the upper age limit is higher in Asia.

Dr. McCarthy or an immediate family member has received royalties from Arthrex, Innomed, and Stryker; has received nonincome support (such as equipment or services), commercially derived honoraria, or other non-research–related funding (such as paid travel) from Arthrex, Innomed, and Stryker; and serves as a board member, owner, officer, or committee member of the International Society of Hip Arthroscopists. Dr. Mont or an immediate family member has received royalties from Stryker and Wright Medical Technology; serves as a paid consultant to or is an employee of Biocomposites, DJ Orthopaedics, Janssen, Joint Active Systems, Medtronic, Sage Products, Stryker, TissueGene, and Wright Medical Technology; has received research or institutional support from DJ Orthopaedics, Joint Active Systems, National Institutes of Health (NIAMS & NICHD), Sage Products, Stryker, TissueGene, and Wright Medical Technology; and serves as a board member, owner, officer, or committee member of the American Academy of Orthopaedic Surgeons. Dr. Peters or an immediate family member has received royalties from Biomet; is a member of a speakers' bureau or has made paid presentations on behalf of Biomet; serves as a paid consultant to or is an employee of Biomet; and serves as a board member, owner, officer, or committee member of the American Academy of Orthopaedic Surgeons and the American Association of Hip and Knee Surgeons. Dr. Austin or an immediate family member has received royalties from Zimmer; is a member of a speakers' bureau or has made paid presentations on behalf of Zimmer; serves as a paid consultant to or is an employee of Zimmer and Biomet; and serves as a board member, owner, officer, or committee member of the American Association of Hip and Knee Surgeons. None of the following authors or any immediate family member has received anything of value from or has stock or stock options held in a commercial company or institution related directly or indirectly to the subject of this chapter: Dr. Bloomfield, Ms. Erickson, Dr. Mulkey, and Dr. Pivec.

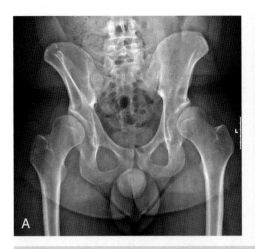

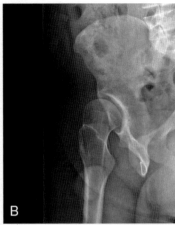

Figure 1 AP (**A**) and false-profile (**B**) radiographic views showing the classic appearance of a dysplastic hip, with upwardly sloping sourcil, a diminished center-edge angle, and minimal coverage of the femoral head by the acetabulum.

Moderate to severe osteoarthritis (Tönnis grade 3 or more), poor range of motion, a lack of joint congruency, and severe subluxation are contraindications for PAO. An older patient with any of these contraindications is not a candidate for hip preservation surgery and will be better served with a total joint replacement.

Proximal Femoral Osteotomy and PAO

In some instances of complex combined femoral and acetabular deformity, it is necessary to treat the femur in conjunction with a PAO to achieve a congruent and impingement-free hip. Indications for a combined procedure require that the previously discussed criteria for PAO be met. Proximal femoral dysplasia exists with a valgus neck-shaft angle greater than 150° (normal, 125° to 135°) and increased femoral anteversion on clinical examination (as evidenced by greater internal rotation versus external rotation). If the amount of valgus correction desired is less than 25°, a purely varus-producing femoral osteotomy can be considered; however, for larger amounts of anteversion, a varus derotational osteotomy is needed.

Outcomes of PAO

In a study of 73 patients (18 males and 55 females) treated with 83 PAOs for developmental dysplasia of the hip, 7 of the females had bilateral PAOs versus 3 bilateral PAOs in the males.[6] The mean age at the time of surgery was 28.5 years. At a mean follow-up of 46 months (range, 24 to 88 months), the postoperative Harris Hip score averaged 87 compared with 54 preoperatively. The average blood loss was approximately 650 mL, and complications included four hematomas requiring irrigation and débridement and two infections. Conversion to a total hip arthroplasty (THA) occured in three patients at an average of 3 years, and there was one revision PAO and one ischial and pubic nonunion that required revision. In total, 70 of 73 patients retained their native hip joint, and the mean Harris hip score improved significantly ($P < 0.001$) from the preoperative score at a mean follow-up of 46 months. Through the year 2010, the series had grown to 191 PAOs and included only seven additional conversions to THA.[7]

It is challenging to predict which hips will remain preserved and which will go on to require arthroplasty after PAO. In a single-surgeon series of 109 consecutive patients (135 hips) treated with PAO for acetabular dysplasia, 102 hips remained preserved at an average of 9 years after surgery.[8] Seventeen hips underwent arthroplasty at an average 6.1 years postoperatively. Univariate predictors of failure included age older than 35 years at the time of surgery, less than 2 mm of joint space, preoperative joint incongruency (indicating a mismatch in the radii of curvature, with at least partial loss of joint space), and a higher Tönnis grade (indicating more advanced osteoarthritis). Multivariate predictors of failure included increased age and decreased preoperative joint congruency. Patients with no predictors of failure had a 14% probability for failure, those with one predictor had a 36% probability rate, and those with two predictors had a 95% rate.

Complications and Risks of PAO

As with any major reconstructive surgery, there are inherent risks associated with PAO. Acute risks include nerve injury, infection, and hematoma. Delayed risks include nonunion with the need for additional surgery, persistent pain, and the progression of joint degeneration despite acetabular repositioning. A study by Matheney et al[8] evaluated 135 hips treated with Bernese PAO. The authors reported 20 complications, including transient peroneal nerve palsy and wound hematoma requiring surgical drainage. Two hips had asymptomatic nonunion at the site of the superior pubic ramus osteotomy, Brooker class 3 heterotopic ossification developed in two, and an intrapelvic abscess requiring surgical drainage developed in one patient at 2 months after surgery.

Femoroacetabular Impingement

FAI is a bony morphologic variant that

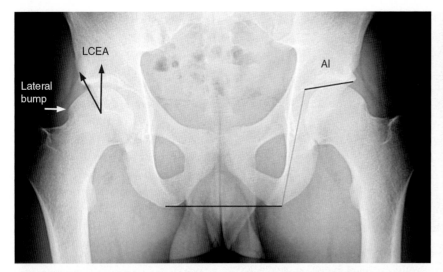

Figure 2 Radiograph showing common measurements, including the lateral center-edge angle (LCEA) and acetabular index (AI), determined on an AP pelvic radiograph. The femora show cam lesions with a lateral bump and loss of sphericity.

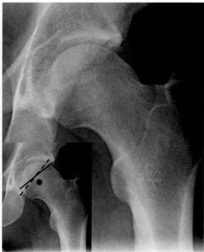

Figure 3 When the anterior wall (solid line) crosses over the posterior wall (dashed line) of the acetabulum, a positive crossover sign is seen, indicating acetabular retroversion. Deficient posterior wall coverage is indicated by a positive posterior wall sign, when the posterior wall lies medial to the center of the femoral head (circle).

predisposes the joint to intra-articular pathology, which can become symptomatic.[9] FAI may be caused by a combination of factors. There is evidence of a genetic link in the development of the abnormal anatomy leading to impingement.[10,11] It also has been theorized that physeal stresses, such as trauma or participation in rigorous sports, can contribute to the development of FAI.[12,13] Patients with coxa profunda, protrusio acetabula, asphericity of the femoral head, a large femoral neck or head, or reduced femoral head-neck offset are at risk for FAI. Acetabular retroversion (whether global or localized) can increase the risk of impingement. At its most basic, FAI is caused by two mechanisms (either alone or in combination): abnormal morphology of the femoral neck/head (a cam lesion) or overcoverage of the proximal femur by the acetabulum (a pincer lesion).[14] Based on their observations from 600 surgical dislocations, Ganz et al[15] suggested that FAI could be the causative factor in the development of osteoarthritis of the hip in the absence of acetabular dysplasia.

Radiographic Analysis

The center-edge angle is a measure of the shallowness of the acetabulum. It is measured on an AP radiograph as the angle between a vertical line drawn intersecting the middle of the femoral head and a line drawn between the center of the femoral head and the lateralmost aspect of the acetabulum[14] (**Figure 2**). When drawing the line to the lateral acetabulum, care must be taken not to include the osteophyte or calcified labrum because this will artificially increase the measurement of the center-edge angle; only the lateralmost aspect of the sourcil should be included.[16] A measurement of greater than 20° is generally accepted as a normal value (the acetabulum is not too shallow). Acetabular retroversion also can be identified on the AP radiograph by the presence of the crossover sign, which results from the proximal anterior rim of the acetabulum running lateral to the posterior rim (**Figure 3**). The alpha angle is used to quantitate the sphericity of the femoral head and the femoral head-neck offset.[14] The alpha angle is measured between a line

drawn parallel to the axis of the femoral neck and a line drawn from the center of the femoral head to the point at which the neck departs from the spherical contour of the head. In general, an alpha angle of less than 50° is considered normal.[14]

Cam Impingement

Anatomic abnormality of the femur is the primary causative factor for cam impingement. This type of impingement may occur with an aspheric femoral head, a reduced head-neck offset, or a combination of the two. Femoral retroversion, whether developmental or posttraumatic, also can contribute to impingement because of the prominent anterior border of the femoral neck. More severe forms of cam impingement are usually related to the sequelae of pediatric hip diseases such as Legg-Calvé-Perthes disease or slipped capital femoral epiphysis (SCFE).

With flexion and internal rotation

of the femur, the aspheric portion of the anterolateral femoral head enters the acetabulum. Initially, the outer or capsular margin of the acetabular labrum is pushed away by the deformity and, thus, is usually preserved until late in the disease process. As the disease progresses, the abnormally shaped femoral head abuts and pressurizes the acetabular chondrolabral junction at the margin of the acetabulum, leading to labrum and hyaline cartilage damage. A secondary or contrecoup insult can occur when the femoral head levers in a posteroinferior direction on acetabular cartilage, causing posteroinferior joint damage.

A patient with cam-type impingement is typically young (14 to 45 years), active, and male more often than female. The clinical presentation includes anterior groin pain, limited internal rotation, a positive impingement sign, and characteristic radiographic findings consistent with a cam deformity.

Pincer Impingement

Pincer impingement is characterized by overcoverage of the femoral head by the acetabulum. In acetabular retroversion, there is focal overcoverage anteriorly, with resulting impingement in flexion. In a patient with coxa profunda or protrusio, the depth of the socket in relation to the size of the femoral head leads to global overcoverage and impingement in multiple planes of motion. Spinopelvic malalignment also can lead to anterior overcoverage; supraphysiologic motion, which occurs in dancers and gymnasts, likely contributes to the malalignment.

With flexion and internal rotation of the femur, the femoral head-neck junction abuts the prominent anterior or anterolateral acetabular rim. The direct compression or pinching of the capsular margin of the acetabular labrum results in outer surface labral

damage. Over time, this impingement causes the development of a groove or cleft at the femoral head-neck junction that is visible on plain radiographs. There is also the possibility of a posteroinferior acetabular contrecoup lesion, which is caused by levering of the femoral head in that direction with the pincer impingement; this affects the posterior and inferior acetabulum. Hyaline cartilage within the acetabulum tends to be preserved.

A patient with pincer impingement is more likely female and presents with anterior groin pain, a positive impingement sign, and has characteristic radiographic findings consistent with pincer deformity (**Figure 4**). Pincer impingement has a bimodal age distribution, with the first group composed of very young patients and the second group made up of patients in their late 20s to their 40s.

Combined Cam and Pincer Impingement

Peters et al[17] found that 59% of the patients in their study with FAI had both cam and pincer components, compared with 45% in the ANCHOR report.[18] Multiple permutations and clinical presentations exist for combined cam and pincer FAI. For example, cam deformity with relative acetabular coverage may promote more severe chondrolabral damage because the aspheric head can more thoroughly enter the acetabulum. Conversely, acetabular overcoverage may provide a barrier for cam deformity leading to a presentation with labral damage of the inner and outer surfaces.

Surgical Treatment Indications in Patients With FAI

When considering surgical treatment for FAI, the primary concern is the effect on the patient's daily functioning. In situations in which conservative

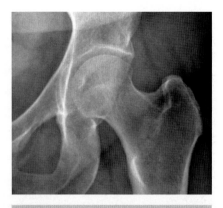

Figure 4 Radiograph showing overcoverage of the femoral head by the acetabulum, leading to pincer-type impingement as occurs with coxa profunda.

treatment options have been unsuccessful and hip or groin pain interferes with the activities of daily living, such as increased pain with flexion activities (such as squatting) or pain with prolonged sitting, a discussion with the patient about surgical intervention is warranted. Patients should be skeletally mature, with documented closure of growth plates. Adult patients should be physiologically young enough to be considered inappropriate candidates for THA or other reconstructive hip procedures. The patient's symptoms should be supported and re-created by a positive impingement test on clinical examination and radiographic evidence of cam impingement (an alpha angle > 50°), pincer impingement (acetabular retroversion or coxa profunda), or both. A prerequisite to hip preservation surgery is the absence of advanced osteoarthritis (Tönnis grade 2 or 3) or severe chondral damage (Outerbridge grade III or IV).

Surgical Dislocation and Osteochondroplasty Versus Mini-Open Versus Arthroscopy

Relative advantages and disadvantages of the various techniques for treating FAI are listed in **Table 1**. Regardless of the method chosen, the goals of treat-

Table 1

Advantages and Disadvantages of Open and Arthroscopic Approaches to FAI Treatment

	Advantages	Disadvantages
Open surgical dislocation	Good visualization of joint 360° joint access Enables treatment of all pathologies Ability to use templates to ensure sphericity	Major operation Soft-tissue damage Trochanteric osteotomy: risk of nonunion and painful hardware Sacrifice of ligamentum teres Increased blood loss Longer rehabilitation
Arthroscopic surgery	Minimally invasive Outpatient surgery Minor soft-tissue damage Faster rehabilitation Easy approach to peripheral compartment and soft tissues	Traction complications: genital and perineal injury, pudendal neurapraxia Difficult to access ligamentum teres and inferior portion of the joint Lateral femoral cutaneous nerve neurapraxia (portal injury) Abdominal compartment syndrome
Combined approach	Easy visualization of the femoral neck No dislocation or trochanteric osteotomy	Difficult to visualize intra-articular or superior parts of femoral neck Cannot use spheric templates Blood loss and scar associated with open surgery

(Reproduced from Botser IB, Smith TW, Nasser R, Domb BG: Open surgical dislocation versus arthroscopy for femoroacetabular impingement: A comparison of clinical outcomes. *Arthroscopy* 2011;27(2):270-278.)

ment include restoration of normal femoral head-neck offset, treatment of chondrolabral damage with either repair or resection, and (potentially) refixation of a separated labrum to the acetabular rim. Damage to hyaline cartilage is treated with either resection or reattachment of delaminated tissue.

In pincer impingement without a posterior wall deficiency, acetabular retroversion exists with normal coverage of the posterior wall. Treatment involves resecting an appropriate amount of the anterior wall to provide femoral neck clearance through a functional range of motion and refixation of the labrum. The femoral head-neck offset should be evaluated and a resection performed to improve this relationship if necessary. If the acetabulum is retroverted and there is deficient posterior wall coverage, a PAO with femoral osteochondroplasty can be considered, depending on patient factors such as age, activity level, and the degree of chondrolabral damage. In mild cases, anterior wall trimming combined with improvement of the

head-neck offset through osteochondroplasty may be an acceptable treatment.

In a large systematic review of 26 articles with data on 1,409 patients, arthroscopy was the most common surgical method (62%) for treating FAI. Labral repairs were performed more often in open or combined approaches compared with arthroscopy. Mean improvement in the Harris hip score was 26.4 points for arthroscopy versus 20.5 points for open surgical dislocation, versus 12.3 points for combined approaches.[19]

Combination of Dysplasia and FAI

The treatment of patients with acetabular dysplasia and overlying FAI is complex. For treating a large femoral head, some authors choose surgical dislocation and osteochondroplasty or a large delamination with posterior extension. Another option is a single procedure PAO with traction and arthrotomy.[20]

Impingement as a Sequela of Pediatric Hip Disease

The sequelae of congenital pediatric disease can lead to more profound and disabling forms of FAI. In the wake of Legg-Calvé-Perthes disease, the resultant femoral head is often large and aspheric, and the acetabulum is dysplastic.[21] In a patient with SCFE, the proximal femoral metaphysis is displaced anteriorly and cranially leading to relative posteroinferior positioning of the femoral head. Both of these deformities can lead to impingement.[22]

The typical clinical presentation in symptomatic FAI secondary to Legg-Calvé-Perthes disease includes coxa magna, coxa brevis, negative articulotrochanteric distance, mild to moderate acetabular dysplasia, and symptoms consistent with impingement or instability. The preferred treatment is relative femoral neck lengthening, with repair of damaged chondrolabral tissue via surgical dislocation.[23] The advantages of this treatment are a reduction in femoral head volume with the opportunity to reshape the overall contour of the femoral head as well as trochanteric distalization and lateralization to improve hip biomechanics and the function of the abductors. There is also the option of repair or resection of the chondrolabral complex, because labral detachment and hyaline cartilage delamination are common. In select patients, a staged PAO is necessary to fully correct the acetabular dysplasia component of the hip deformity.

Posterior translation and angulation of the capital epiphysis is the characteristic deformity in SCFE. The resulting translation of the head and loss of head-neck offset allows the anterior metaphysis to impinge on the anterior acetabulum, resulting in profound labral and hyaline cartilage injury and compensatory extension and external rotation deformity of the limb. Treatment of the impingement caused by SCFE depends on the degree of the slip and the resulting deformity. A slip angle of less than 35° is treated with osteochondroplasty with treatment of chondrolabral damage. Large slip angles ranging from 35° to 45° and greater are best treated with a subcapital correction osteotomy performed via a surgical dislocation, with treatment of chondrolabral damage at that time.[24]

Outcomes
Results of Surgical Dislocation and Osteochondroplasty
Overall, surgical dislocation and osteochondroplasty has resulted in excellent functional outcomes and midterm hip survivorship in patients with no or minimal osteoarthritis. In a study by Murphy et al,[25] 15 of 24 hips had significant improvement at a minimum follow-up of 2 years. In a study by Beaulé et al,[26] significant improvements in postoperative Western Ontario and McMaster Universities Osteoarthritis Index (WOMAC) scores

were reported at an average follow-up of 3.1 years after surgical dislocation. In a large series of 96 hips, Peters et al[17] reported significant improvement in postoperative Harris hip scores at an average follow-up of 24 months after surgical dislocation for FAI. A substantial challenge remains in managing severe (Outerbridge grade IV) cartilage delamination.

In 22 professional male athletes (including 14 ice hockey players) treated with open surgical hip dislocation for FAI, 21 athletes (96%) were still competing professionally (19 at their previous level and 2 in the minor leagues) at a mean follow-up of 45 months. Eighty-two percent of the patients were satisfied with the open hip surgery, and 86% were satisfied with their resultant athletic ability.[27] These findings tend to counter the argument that improvements in pain and motion are the result of activity modification rather than the surgical intervention. An additional important finding in this study was that 8 of the 22 athletes later had the contralateral hip treated with surgical dislocation, and 7 of 8 were satisfied with their resultant athletic ability.

As a caveat to these encouraging findings, moderate to severe arthritic changes found at the time of surgical dislocation or existing acetabular dysplasia that remains untreated results in a high likelihood of early failure or conversion to THA. Peters et al[17] found that 4 of 6 failures occurred in hips with severe acetabular cartilage damage (Outerbridge grade IV) at the time of surgery, and 5 of 6 of failures occurred in the initial 30 patients treated with surgical dislocation. Better selection criteria for patients and improved surgeon experience may decrease the risk of failure.

Acetabular cartilage damage is a frequent finding at the time of surgical dislocation. In an analysis of 302 hips,

Beck et al[3] found acetabular cartilage damage in all 26 study patients with pure cam-type pathology, with 10 of the patients having frank cartilage delamination. Similarly, Anderson et al[28] reported that 44% of patients treated with surgical dislocation and osteochondroplasty had acetabular cartilage delamination associated with cam impingement, with an odds ratio of 11.9. This finding is in concert with other reports.[3]

The treatment of delaminated acetabular cartilage lesions is evolving. One option is to excise the delaminated cartilage, with trimming of the acetabular rim and reattachment of the labrum to the new perimeter. Other options include reattachment of the delamination with fibrin glue or microfracture to stimulate fibrocartilage production. Further study is needed before any particular method can be recommended.

Acetabular labral damage is also a frequent finding at the time of surgical dislocation and osteochondroplasty. In a study of 19 patients, Beck et al[29] found that all 19 of the patients had labral tears, and 18 of 19 had cartilage lesions adjacent to the labral tear. All of the lesions were located in the anterosuperior quadrant of the acetabulum, which corresponds to the region of impact between the femoral neck and acetabular rim. Similarly, Peters et al[17] reported labral abnormalities in 82 of 96 hips, with 44 labral detachments, 15 tears, 9 degenerative labra, 10 calcified labra, and 4 absent labra because of previous surgery. Graves and Mast[30] evaluated 48 hips during surgical dislocation and osteochondroplasty: 14 had undersurface tears, 20 had base tears, 11 had labral ossification, and 4 had thickened labra. Espinosa et al[31] compared the functional results of 20 patients who underwent labral resection with 32 patients who were treated with labral repair after acetabuloplasty.

They found improved clinical outcomes in the patients treated with labral refixation compared with those treated with labral débridement.

Results of Mini-Open Procedures

A case series evaluated 234 patients (257 hips) treated with osteochondroplasty through a mini-open approach (a 4-cm incision, modified Smith-Peterson approach with no muscle detachment).[32] At an average follow-up of 22 months, the Harris hip, the Medical Outcomes Study 36-Item Short Form, and the WOMAC scores significantly improved for the cohort. Of the 44 patients with more than 1-year follow-up, 55% were able to return to their preoperative sporting activity. In a case series of 293 hips in 265 patients treated with direct anterior mini-open femoroacetabular osteoplasty, Parvizi et al[33] reported significantly improved Medical Outcomes Study 36-Item Short Form, WOMAC, University of California Los Angeles, Harris hip, and Super Simple Hip scores.

Clohisy et al[34] reported on hip arthroscopy combined with limited open osteochondroplasty for anterior FAI. Of 35 patients with cam impingement, 83% had at least a 10 point improvement in the Harris hip score. Two patients had progression of osteoarthritis from Tönnis grade 0 to grade 1; however, at a follow-up of more than 2 years, there had been no conversions to THA.

Results of Arthroscopic Procedures

In a case series of the first 100 patients with FAI to reach 2-year follow-up after arthroscopic treatment, Byrd and Jones[35] reported a median improvement of 21.5 points in the Harris hip score over a preoperative average of 65 points. The improvement in patients

with both femoral and acetabular damage was not statistically different from those with only acetabular damage. No patient in the study underwent conversion to THA, but six patients had a subsequent arthroscopic procedure for recurrent or persistent symptoms.

Similar to the results of open surgical dislocation and osteochondroplasty, Larson et al[36] found that labral refixation rather than arthroscopic débridement/focal excision was significantly associated with improved Harris hip and Medical Outcomes Study 12-Item Short Form scores and visual analog scale pain scores at a mean 3.5-year follow-up. The results of arthroscopy are similar to open procedures when bony abnormalities are identified. When arthroscopic débridement and reattachment is performed without osteochondroplasty in hips later identified with cam-type impingement, results are uniformly poorer.

Philippon et al[37] recognized a correlation between preexisting osteoarthritis and the failure of arthroscopic femoroplasty. Failure was directly correlated with the intraoperative discovery of cartilage damage in older patients. It has become clear that proper patient selection is critical to a good outcome, especially in regards to preexisting osteoarthritis. This realization has driven the development of improved preoperative imaging protocols to evaluate cartilage integrity and an effort to be more selective in offering hip preservation surgery only to appropriate patients.

Complications

Many studies have reported a low complication rate for surgical dislocation of the hip and osteochondroplasty.[17,26,35,38] Despite its relative safety, patients should be counseled on the risks of osteonecrosis of the femoral head, sciatic neuropathy, the devel-

opment of heterotopic ossification, femoral neck fracture, and nonunion of the greater trochanter.

Ganz et al[38] reported on complications from surgical hip dislocation in 213 hips over a 7-year period. The authors found 2 sciatic neurapraxias, which completely resolved; 3 failures of trochanteric fixation requiring reoperation; and 79 hips with heterotopic ossification (grade I, 68; grade II, 9; grade III, 2). The rate of heterotopic ossification decreased with surgeon experience; heterotopic ossification is not a commonly reported complication in more recent series. In a study by Byrd and Jones,[35] the first 100 patients with FAI treated with arthroscopic management had 2 transient neurapraxias (pudendal and lateral femoral cutaneous nerves) and 1 mild case of heterotopic ossification. In 96 hips treated with surgical dislocation for FAI, Peters et al[17] reported 2 failures of trochanteric fixation (1 early failure of fixation in a female patient caused by failure to acquire cortical screw purchase distally and 1 nonunion in a male patient). There were no instances of osteonecrosis, infection, femoral neck fracture, or sciatic compromise. In a study of 37 patients treated with osteochondroplasty of the femoral head-neck junction, Beaulé et al[26] reported 1 failure of trochanteric fixation, which required reoperation; 1 patient with heterotopic ossification, which required excision; and 9 patients requiring hardware removal for bursal irritation caused by the trochanteric screws. All of these complications had trochanteric-related issues. Patients should be counseled concerning the small risk of nonunion or the need for hardware removal.

Interestingly, fracture of the femoral neck after femoroplasty has been reported in arthroscopy studies, but not in the reviewed series using open surgical dislocation and osteochondroplasty.[39] Mardones et al[40] determined that up to 30% of the anterolateral neck could be removed before the risk of fracture increased, but the usual amount of resection is much less than 30%. Most surgeons recommend only partial weight bearing for 6 weeks to prevent femoral neck fracture.

Osteonecrosis of the femoral head remains a theoretic complication because no reports have been published in the literature involving either arthroscopic or open surgical dislocation with osteochondroplasty. Despite the lack of reported complications, it is critical to protect the medial circumflex femoral artery during the approach and hip dislocation.

Other Indications for Hip Arthroscopy

Labral tears can occur traumatically in addition to being associated with dysplasia and FAI. Sudden twisting or pivoting motions are the usual mechanism of injury for labral tears. Even minor trauma without dislocation can result in labral tears with mechanical symptoms (catching, locking, or giving way). Labral tears can contribute to or occur in association with articular cartilage lesions.[41-43]

Symptoms of more than 5-years' duration are more often associated with full-thickness chondral lesions.[41,44] Early-stage chondral lesions can be treated with chondroplasty. Full-thickness chondral lesions are treated with microfracture to facilitate fibrocartilage formation. The most frequently observed chondral lesion is the watershed lesion (separation of the labrum from the articular surface at the labrocartilage junction).[45] Watershed lesions tend to progress from the peripheral rim to the central fossa and are often full-thickness lesions. Lesions at the labrochondral junction (watershed zone) do not have the ability to heal.[45] These lesions subject subchon-

dral bone to fluid pressure resulting in the formation of subchondral cysts, which lead to further delamination and accelerated joint wear.[46] The extent or thickness of the cartilage injury is the most decisive predictor of surgical outcome.[41,42,44]

Loose bodies may occur as an isolated fragment or there may be multiple fragments (2 to 300) as seen in synovial chondromatosis. In this disorder, the loose bodies typically aggregate together in grape-like clusters and often adhere to the synovium about the fossa. Mechanical symptoms, such as locking or catching, can corroborate clinical suspicion of synovial chondromatosis. Arthroscopy establishes the diagnosis and provides simultaneous treatment using a minimally invasive technique.[47]

Arthroscopy also can be used for synovial biopsy and to evaluate the extent of the synovitis. Arthroscopic synovectomy can be useful in managing inflammatory conditions, including rheumatoid arthritis, gout, and pseudogout.[48] Labral and chondral articular surfaces can be simultaneously evaluated and treated when there is a history of mechanical symptoms.

Arthroplasty for the Young Patient

Several factors must be considered when treating a young patient with hip pain when arthroplasty is indicated. One of the most important considerations is the difference between a patient's life expectancy and the implant's longevity. Other secondary, but still critical factors, include the timing of surgery, the choice of arthroplasty (hip resurfacing versus conventional THA), and the type of stem design (long diaphyseal loading, standard metadiaphyseal loading, and short neck-preserving).

Historically, THA has demonstrated poor results at midterm follow-

up for patients younger than 50 years, with reported revision rates of 15% to 34% at a mean follow-up of less than 10 years usually caused by high rates of bearing surface wear and aseptic loosening of cemented implants.[49-51] Newer implant designs, including more wear resistant bearings, have led to markedly improved results, with recent reports of implant survivorship rates of 99% at less than 10-year and 94% at 10- to 15-year follow-ups.[52-54]

When to Perform THA
The economic effect of delaying THA is sometimes more costly than early intervention if there is clear evidence of disease. Young, employed patients who have severe arthritis and are unable to work to a full extent have been reported to lose a mean of $17,000 in annual productivity.[55] However, after THA, 90% of patients who were previously unable to work returned to their pre-disability type of employment.[56] For young patients with unequivocal findings of severe disability and pain, earlier surgical intervention may be considered.

Fixation and Stem Choices
Current fixation options include cemented and cementless designs. Currently, there are multiple cementless stem designs on the market, all with excellent long-term stem survivorship (> 99%).[57] In the United States, 90% of stems are cementless, whereas more than 90% of stems in many European countries are cemented. However, there appears to be a trend toward using cementless components in Europe and Canada, with Denmark and Canada now reporting more than 50% and 75% use of cementless stems, respectively.[58]

The stem choice depends on the femoral anatomy of the patient. Multiple stem designs are currently available, including proximally coated versus fully coated stems (metaphyseal versus diaphyseal fixation), anatomic stems, and newer short-stem designs. Although there are limited data on short stems, these designs, which preferentially load the femoral neck and calcar, may be better suited to avoiding the stress shielding and thigh pain observed with some traditional stem designs. Long-term studies are needed to demonstrate the benefit of short stems over current conventional stem designs.[59]

Hip Resurfacing

Successful outcomes with hip surface replacement require proper patient selection. Patients with the best outcomes after resurfacing are men who have native femoral head sizes greater than 48 mm and a primary diagnosis of osteoarthritis. Less optimal outcomes are seen in women and patients with small femoral heads, multiple femoral head cysts, or rheumatoid arthritis.[60]

Patient activity levels, especially in younger patients, should be assessed. Mont et al[61] reported improved gait dynamics, increased abductor and extensor moments, and better walking speed with hip resurfacing compared with standard THA. A recent study by Costa et al[62] reported that patients treated with resurfacing had a better quality of life compared with those treated with standard THA. In a matched comparison of 73 resurfacings to standard THAs at a mean 52-month follow-up, the Harris hip scores were greater than 90 points for both groups, and there were an equal number of revisions (one in each group), but patients treated with hip resurfacing had higher weighted activity scores.

Complications after resurfacing most commonly include femoral neck fracture, component loosening, and adverse local tissue reactions secondary to bearing surface wear. Of greater concern is the considerable learning curve for surgeons performing hip resurfacing.[63] Complications can be minimized with proper patient selection and good surgical technique (proper exposure, accurate head measurement, the use of intraoperative fluoroscopy, osteophyte removal, and avoiding femoral neck notching and varus placement of the femoral component).

Bearing Surface Choices

Although THA is one of the most successful orthopaedic surgical procedures, concerns exist regarding the durability of the bearing surface in young, active patients. Data from the Finnish Arthroplasty Registry indicate that bearing surface issues, rather than implant fixation, is the primary long-term mode of failure in young patients with an uncemented THA.[64] With the projected exponential increase of THAs in patients younger than 65 years over the next 20 years,[65] selection of a bearing couple with excellent durability and a low complication rate will continue to be of substantial importance. A number of alternate bearing surfaces have been popularized over the past decade in an attempt to limit osteolysis. It is important to review the current evidence for selecting an appropriate bearing surface for the young, high-demand patient.

Multiple randomized clinical trials have shown improved wear rates at short-term and midterm follow-ups with highly cross-linked polyethylene (HXLPE) compared with conventional polyethylene.[66-68] Results in young patients have been similarly promising. In a randomized trial of 45 patients, radiostereometric analysis determined that an HXLPE liner had 55% lower femoral head penetration than a conventional liner at 2-year follow-up.[69] Another study found substantially lower total and annual wear rates with an HXLPE liner versus a conventional polyethylene liner.[70] Significant reductions in osteolysis (24% versus 2%) detectable with CT have been reported with an HXLPE liner versus a conventional polyethylene liner at 5- to 10-year follow-ups.[71] Further improvements were seen at 5-year follow-up in a study evaluating a second-generation annealed HXLPE, which showed a 58% lower wear rate compared with a first-generation cross-linked polyethylene.[72]

Some authors have indicated that the reduced mechanical properties of HXLPE may have clinical consequences. A retrieval study comparing conventional polyethylene liners with HXLPE liners found similar patterns of wear damage and rates of creep; however, the HXLPE liners had a substantially higher (15%) rate of rim cracking or fracture.[73] This pattern has been confirmed in other retrieval analyses, and case reports have shown polyethylene rim fractures to be a clinical concern.[74-76] Rim damage and fractures are likely more common with thin liners and malpositioned acetabular components.

The femoral head is also an important factor influencing the volumetric wear rate of the bearing couple. In a study of HXLPE, it was found that linear wear rates did not differ between femoral head sizes, but volumetric wear rates were substantially higher when 36- or 40-mm diameter heads were used compared with 28- or 32-mm heads.[77] Biolox Delta ceramic (CeramTec AG) and oxidized zirconium femoral heads have been advocated over cobalt-chromium heads for young patients based on promising hip simulator data showing reduced in vitro wear.[78,79] Preliminary clinical evidence has been good; however, there are no high-level studies that prove a clinical benefit for these materials.[80-82]

Additionally, several studies report surface damage to oxidized zirconium heads after dislocation, which can potentially lead to increased wear.[83-85]

Ceramic-on-ceramic THA components have been advocated for young patients because of very low wear rates and the reduced potential for osteolysis compared with conventional polyethylene bearings. These advantages result from the tribologic properties of low surface roughness and high hardness and wettability, leading to a low-friction couple. Alumina ceramics have a better track record than zirconia because of their thermostability and consistently low wear rates.[86] The recently developed Delta ceramic implant is a composite of an alumina matrix impregnated with zirconia particles for increased hardness and fracture resistance.

Outcomes of current-generation alumina ceramic-on-ceramic bearings have been excellent, with reported 10-year survival rates from 92% to 99%.[87-89] Multiple studies have reported no cases of osteolysis at mid-term to long-term follow-ups.[90-93] Although not approved for use in the United States, Delta ceramic-on-ceramic bearings are available internationally. A prospective randomized investigational device exemption study evaluated this couple against a Delta ceramic-on-HXLPE couple. Similar short-term functional outcome scores and implant survivorship were reported, but ceramic liner chipping or fracture occurred in two patients and three intraoperative liner problems occurred in the Delta ceramic-on-ceramic group.[94]

Squeaking after ceramic-on-ceramic THA can be a substantial problem requiring revision.[95] The cause of squeaking appears to be multifactorial. Elevated rim liner designs have a substantially higher incidence of squeaking than nonelevated liners.[96,97] Squeaking hips also have been associated with taller and heavier patients.[98] Acetabular malpositioning causing edge loading and stripe wear has been postulated as a cause of squeaking, although the data are somewhat conflicting.[98,99] In one large prospective observational study, squeaking occurred in 6% of patients beginning at a mean of 20 months after surgery and was persistent in 70% of the patients.[100] Retrial analysis showed significantly higher wear rates in bearings that squeak versus nonsqueaking bearings.[101] Fracture, including chipping or fragmentation, is a rare complication of ceramic bearings.[102] The results of revision surgery for ceramic fracture have been reported as poor. This complication requires complete synovectomy and selection of another ceramic-on-ceramic bearing or a ceramic head with a polyethylene liner to avoid third-body wear damage to a metal femoral head. If there is damage to the trunnion or shell or if the components are malpositioned, revision of the femoral and/or acetabular components is required. Some evidence indicates that component revision rather than isolated bearing surface exchange may be beneficial after ceramic head fracture because revision allows more complete removal of ceramic debris.

At the present time, there is no role for metal-on-metal standard THA. Previously reported potential advantages of metal-on-metal THA included reduced wear and the benefits of a large diameter femoral head, which increases stability and decreases dislocation rates. However, several well-published concerns have arisen regarding complications with metal bearings, including earlier failure of these devices compared with metal-on-polyethylene or ceramic bearings.[103,104] Women younger than 40 years and patients with femoral heads larger than 52 mm (men) or 46 mm (women) are at the greatest risk for revision. A recent consensus management algorithm recommends that patients with metal-on-metal THAs who have hip pain but no evidence of loosening or other radiographic failure have regular follow-up examinations, with monitoring of serum ion levels (current cutoff of 7 parts per billion) and particular attention to changes compared with prior baseline levels.[105]

Other concerns with metal components are the possibility of the development of cystic or solid soft-tissue masses. Adverse local tissue reaction is a broad term used to encompass several observed sequelae of metal hips, including metallosis, aseptic lymphocytic vasculitis-associated lesions, pseudotumor formation, and elevated serum metal ion levels. Although soft-tissue reactions have been reported after THA using nonmetal-on-metal bearings, metal-on-metal implants clearly have a higher incidence of these complications.[106,107] Taper corrosion at the junction of the head and neck contribute to this problem along with wear at the primary bearing surface.[108] The incidence of pseudotumors may be as high as 10%.[106] However, the clinical relevance of these lesions, particularly if they are found incidentally, continues to be debated.[109]

Outcomes

Prior studies reported poor outcomes of hip arthroplasty in young patients, but many of these studies used conventional polyethylene components, small femoral head sizes, and first-generation cemented components.[50,51] Recent studies have demonstrated improved survivorship with modern implant designs in patients with varying etiologies of arthritis. In a recent review of 127 ceramic-on-ceramic THAs performed in patients younger than 30 years, Kim et al[110] observed excellent

Table 2

Total Hip Arthroplasty Implant Survivorship

Study (Year)	No. of Hips	Mean Age at Surgery (Years)	Follow-up (Years)	Survivorship (%)
Polyethylene Bearings				
Faldini et al[112] (2011)	34	47	12	100
Almeida et al[113] (2010)	75	38	10	88
Clohisy et al[114] (2010)	102	< 25	4	98
Liang et al[115] (2010)	81	< 50	6	95
Kang et al[116] (2010)	45	< 45	12	89
Jialiang et al[117] (2009)	67	< 50	6	100
Wangen et al[118] (2008)	49	< 30	13	51
Mont et al[119] (2006)	104	38	2	97
Archibeck et al[120] (2006)	100	39	9	87
McAuley et al[121] (2004)	256	< 40	15	54
Bessette et al[122] (2003)	16	16	13.5	68
Ceramic Bearings				
Kim et al[110] (2012)	127	< 30	15	99.2
Byun et al[123] (2012)	56	< 30	6	100
Finkbone et al[92] (2012)	24	16	5.5	96
Kamath et al[124] (2012)	21	18	4	95
Kim et al[125] (2011)	73	45	8.5	100
Kim et al[111] (2010)	93	< 45	10	100
Baek and Kim[126] (2008)	71	39	7	100
Nizard et al[127] (2008)	132	23	15	72
Ha et al[128] (2007)	74	37	6	100
Yoo et al[129] (2006)	72	30	5	100
Pignatti et al[130] (2003)	123	32	5	96

clinical outcomes at a mean follow-up of 10 years. The authors reported no incidence of thigh pain during the follow-up period, and implant survivorship for this cohort was 99% at a mean 10-year follow-up, with no stem failures and only one cup failure. Similar outcomes have been observed in other studies at midterm to long-term follow-ups[92,110-130] (**Table 2**). These outcomes show marked improvement over early reports of THA in young patients.[64,110,111]

Summary

Hip pain in the young active patient is an increasingly common clinical problem that has garnered substantial at-

tention in the orthopaedic community in recent years. Historically, surgical treatments have been limited; however, an explosion of new techniques, innovations, and research has increased options for these patients. When choosing between the many types of joint preservation and arthroplasty procedures available, careful attention to indications and surgical technique and the judicious use of new technology are critical in optimizing patient outcomes.

References

1. Murray RO: The aetiology of primary osteoarthritis of the hip.

Br J Radiol 1965;38(455):810-824.

2. Stulberg SD, Harris WH, Ramsey PL: Unrecognized childhood hip disease: A major cause of idiopathic osteoarthritis of the hip. *The Hip: Proceedings of the Third Open Scientific Meeting of the Hip Society*, 1975.

3. Beck M, Kalhor M, Leunig M, Ganz R: Hip morphology influences the pattern of damage to the acetabular cartilage: Femoroacetabular impingement as a cause of early osteoarthritis of the hip. *J Bone Joint Surg Br* 2005;87(7): 1012-1018.

4. Bombelli R, Santore RF, Poss R: Mechanics of the normal and os-

teoarthritic hip: A new perspective. *Clin Orthop Relat Res* 1984; 182:69-78.

5. Aronson J: Osteoarthritis of the young adult hip: Etiology and treatment. *Instr Course Lect* 1986; 35:119-128.

6. Peters CL, Erickson JA, Hines JL: Early results of the Bernese periacetabular osteotomy: The learning curve at an academic medical center. *J Bone Joint Surg Am* 2006; 88(9):1920-1926.

7. Ginnetti JG, Pelt CE, Erickson JA, Van Dine C, Peters CL: Prevalence and treatment of intraarticular pathology recognized at the time of periacetabular osteotomy for the dysplastic hip. *Clin Orthop Relat Res* 2013;471(2):498-503.

8. Matheney T, Kim YJ, Zurakowski D, Matero C, Millis M: Intermediate to long-term results following the Bernese periacetabular osteotomy and predictors of clinical outcome. *J Bone Joint Surg Am* 2009;91(9):2113-2123.

9. Byrd JW, Jones KS: Arthroscopic femoroplasty in the management of cam-type femoroacetabular impingement. *Clin Orthop Relat Res* 2009;467(3):739-746.

10. Pollard TC, Villar RN, Norton MR, et al: A sibling study. *J Bone Joint Surg Br* 2010;92(2): 209-216.

11. Hogervorst T, Eilander W, Fikkers JT, Meulenbelt I: Hip ontogenesis: How evolution, genes, and load history shape hip morphotype and cartilotype. *Clin Orthop Relat Res* 2012;470(12): 3284-3296.

12. Agricola R, Bessems JH, Ginai AZ, et al: The development of Cam-type deformity in adolescent and young male soccer players. *Am J Sports Med* 2012;40(5): 1099-1106.

13. Siebenrock KA, Ferner F, Noble PC, Santore RF, Werlen S, Mamisch TC: The cam-type deformity of the proximal femur

arises in childhood in response to vigorous sporting activity. *Clin Orthop Relat Res* 2011;469(11): 3229-3240.

14. Martin DE, Tashman S: The biomechanics of femoroacetabular impingement. *Oper Tech Orthop* 2010;20(4):248-254.

15. Ganz R, Parvizi J, Beck M, Leunig M, Nötzli H, Siebenrock KA: Femoroacetabular impingement: A cause for osteoarthritis of the hip. *Clin Orthop Relat Res* 2003; 417:112-120.

16. Anderson LA, Gililland J, Pelt C, Linford S, Stoddard GJ, Peters CL: Center edge angle measurement for hip preservation surgery: Technique and caveats. *Orthopedics* 2011;34(2):86.

17. Peters CL, Schabel K, Anderson L, Erickson J: Open treatment of femoroacetabular impingement is associated with clinical improvement and low complication rate at short-term followup. *Clin Orthop Relat Res* 2010;468(2):504-510.

18. Clohisy JC, Baca G, Beaulé PE, et al: Descriptive epidemiology of femoroacetabular impingement: A North American cohort of patients undergoing surgery. *Am J Sports Med* 2013;41(6):1348-1356.

19. Botser IB, Smith TW Jr, Nasser R, Domb BG: Open surgical dislocation versus arthroscopy for femoroacetabular impingement: A comparison of clinical outcomes. *Arthroscopy* 2011;27(2):270-278.

20. Anderson LA, Crofoot CD, Erickson JA, Peters CL: Staged surgical dislocation and redirectional periacetabular osteotomy: A report of five cases. *J Bone Joint Surg Am* 2009;91(10):2469-2476.

21. Clohisy JC, Ross JR, North JD, Nepple JJ, Schoenecker PL: What are the factors associated with acetabular correction in Perthes-like hip deformities? *Clin Orthop Relat Res* 2012;470(12):3439-3445.

22. Mamisch TC, Kim YJ, Richolt JA, Millis MB, Kordelle J: Femoral morphology due to impingement influences the range of motion in slipped capital femoral epiphysis. *Clin Orthop Relat Res* 2009;467(3):692-698.

23. Anderson LA, Erickson JA, Severson EP, Peters CL: Sequelae of Perthes disease: Treatment with surgical hip dislocation and relative femoral neck lengthening. *J Pediatr Orthop* 2010;30(8): 758-766.

24. Ziebarth K, Zilkens C, Spencer S, Leunig M, Ganz R, Kim YJ: Capital realignment for moderate and severe SCFE using a modified Dunn procedure. *Clin Orthop Relat Res* 2009;467(3):704-716.

25. Murphy S, Tannast M, Kim YJ, Buly R, Millis MB: Debridement of the adult hip for femoroacetabular impingement: Indications and preliminary clinical results. *Clin Orthop Relat Res* 2004; 429:178-181.

26. Beaulé PE, Le Duff MJ, Zaragoza E: Quality of life following femoral head-neck osteochondroplasty for femoroacetabular impingement. *J Bone Joint Surg Am* 2007; 89(4):773-779.

27. Naal FD, Miozzari HH, Wyss TF, Nötzli HP: Surgical hip dislocation for the treatment of femoroacetabular impingement in high-level athletes. *Am J Sports Med* 2011;39(3):544-550.

28. Anderson LA, Peters CL, Park BB, Stoddard GJ, Erickson JA, Crim JR: Acetabular cartilage delamination in femoroacetabular impingement: Risk factors and magnetic resonance imaging diagnosis. *J Bone Joint Surg Am* 2009;91(2): 305-313.

29. Beck M, Leunig M, Parvizi J, Boutier V, Wyss D, Ganz R: Anterior femoroacetabular impingement: Part II. Midterm results of surgical treatment. *Clin Orthop Relat Res* 2004;418:67-73.

30. Graves ML, Mast JW: Femoroacetabular impingement: Do outcomes reliably improve with surgical dislocations? *Clin Orthop Relat Res* 2009;467(3):717-723.

31. Espinosa N, Rothenfluh DA, Beck M, Ganz R, Leunig M: Treatment of femoro-acetabular impingement: Preliminary results of labral refixation. *J Bone Joint Surg Am* 2006;88(5):925-935.

32. Cohen SB, Huang R, Ciccotti MG, Dodson CC, Parvizi J: Treatment of femoroacetabular impingement in athletes using a mini-direct anterior approach. *Am J Sports Med* 2012;40(7): 1620-1627.

33. Parvizi J, Huang R, Diaz-Ledezma C, Og B: Mini-open femoroacetabular osteoplasty: How do these patients do? *J Arthroplasty* 2012;27(8):122-125.

34. Clohisy JC, Zebala LP, Nepple JJ, Pashos G: Combined hip arthroscopy and limited open osteochondroplasty for anterior femoroacetabular impingement. *J Bone Joint Surg Am* 2010;92(8):1697-1706.

35. Byrd JW, Jones KS: Arthroscopic management of femoroacetabular impingement: Minimum 2-year follow-up. *Arthroscopy* 2011; 27(10):1379-1388.

36. Larson CM, Giveans MR, Stone RM: Arthroscopic debridement versus refixation of the acetabular labrum associated with femoroacetabular impingement: Mean 3.5-year follow-up. *Am J Sports Med* 2012;40(5):1015-1021.

37. Philippon MJ, Schroder E Souza BG, Briggs KK: Hip arthroscopy for femoroacetabular impingement in patients aged 50 years or older. *Arthroscopy* 2012;28(1): 59-65.

38. Ganz R, Gill TJ, Gautier E, Ganz K, Krügel N, Berlemann U: Surgical dislocation of the adult hip: A technique with full access to the femoral head and acetabulum

without the risk of avascular necrosis. *J Bone Joint Surg Br* 2001; 83(8):1119-1124.

39. Sampson TG: Complications of hip arthroscopy. *Clin Sports Med* 2001;20(4):831-835.

40. Mardones RM, Gonzalez C, Chen Q, Zobitz M, Kaufman KR, Trousdale RT: Surgical treatment of femoroacetabular impingement: Evaluation of the effect of the size of the resection. Surgical technique. *J Bone Joint Surg Am* 2006;88(suppl 1 pt 1):84-91.

41. McCarthy JC, Lee JA: Arthroscopic intervention in early hip disease. *Clin Orthop Relat Res* 2004;429:157-162.

42. Byrd JW, Jones KS: Prospective analysis of hip arthroscopy with 10-year followup. *Clin Orthop Relat Res* 2010;468(3):741-746.

43. Farjo LA, Glick JM, Sampson TG: Hip arthroscopy for acetabular labral tears. *Arthroscopy* 1999; 15(2):132-137.

44. McCarthy JC, Lee JA: Hip arthroscopy: Indications, outcomes, and complications. *Instr Course Lect* 2006;55:301-308.

45. McCarthy JC, Noble PC, Schuck MR, Wright J, Lee J: The role of labral lesions to development of early degenerative hip disease. *Clin Orthop Relat Res* 2001;393: 25-37.

46. McCarthy JC, Noble PC, Schuck MR, Wright J, Lee J: The watershed labral lesion: Its relationship to early arthritis of the hip. *J Arthroplasty* 2001;16(8):81-87.

47. Marchie A, Glassner PJ, Panuncialman I, McCarthy JC: Technical pearls for hip arthroscopy in the management of synovial chondromatosis. *Am J Orthop (Belle Mead NJ)* 2012;41(6):284-287.

48. Krebs VE: The role of hip arthroscopy in the treatment of synovial disorders and loose bodies. *Clin Orthop Relat Res* 2003;406:48-59.

49. Bleasel JF, York JR, Korber J, Tyer HD: Total hip arthroplasty in the young arthritic patient. *Aust N Z J Med* 1994;24(3):296-300.

50. White SH: The fate of cemented total hip arthroplasty in young patients. *Clin Orthop Relat Res* 1988;231:29-34.

51. Gustilo RB, Burnham WH: Long-term results of total hip arthroplasty in young patients. *Hip* 1982;27-33.

52. Streit MR, Schröder K, Körber M, et al: High survival in young patients using a second generation uncemented total hip replacement. *Int Orthop* 2012;36(6): 1129-1136.

53. Springer BD, Connelly SE, Odum SM, et al: Review and meta-analysis of total hip arthroplasty and hip resurfacing. *J Arthroplasty* 2009;24(6):2-8.

54. Polkowski GG, Callaghan JJ, Mont MA, Clohisy JC: Total hip arthroplasty in the very young patient. *J Am Acad Orthop Surg* 2012;20(8):487-497.

55. Sadosky AB, Bushmakin AG, Cappelleri JC, Lionberger DR: Relationship between patient-reported disease severity in osteoarthritis and self-reported pain, function and work productivity. *Arthritis Res Ther* 2010;12(4): R162.

56. Nunley RM, Ruh EL, Zhang Q, et al: Do patients return to work after hip arthroplasty surgery? *J Arthroplasty* 2011;26(6):92-98.

57. Emerson RH Jr, Head WC, Emerson CB, Rosenfeldt W, Higgins LL: A comparison of cemented and cementless titanium femoral components used for primary total hip arthroplasty: A radiographic and survivorship study. *J Arthroplasty* 2002;17(5): 584-591.

58. Dunbar MJ: Cemented femoral fixation: The North Atlantic divide. *Orthopedics* 2009;32(9).

59. Molli RG, Lombardi AV Jr, Berend KR, Adams JB, Sneller MA: A short tapered stem reduces intraoperative complications in primary total hip arthroplasty. *Clin Orthop Relat Res* 2012; 470(2):450-461.

60. Johnson AJ, Zywiel MG, Hooper H, Mont MA: Narrowed indications improve outcomes for hip resurfacing arthroplasty. *Bull NYU Hosp Jt Dis* 2011;69(suppl 1): S27-S29.

61. Mont MA, Seyler TM, Ragland PS, Starr R, Erhart J, Bhave A: Gait analysis of patients with resurfacing hip arthroplasty compared with hip osteoarthritis and standard total hip arthroplasty. *J Arthroplasty* 2007;22(1):100-108.

62. Costa CR, Johnson AJ, Naziri Q, Mont MA: The outcomes of Cormet hip resurfacing compared to standard primary total hip arthroplasty. *Bull NYU Hosp Jt Dis* 2011;69(suppl 1):S12-S15.

63. Johnson AJ, Costa CR, Naziri Q, Mont MA: Is there a new learning curve with transition to a new resurfacing system? *Bull NYU Hosp Jt Dis* 2011;69(suppl 1): S16-S19.

64. Eskelinen A, Remes V, Helenius I, Pulkkinen P, Nevalainen J, Paavolainen P: Uncemented total hip arthroplasty for primary osteoarthritis in young patients: A mid-to long-term follow-up study from the Finnish Arthroplasty Register. *Acta Orthop* 2006;77(1): 57-70.

65. Kurtz S, Ong K, Lau E, Mowat F, Halpern M: Projections of primary and revision hip and knee arthroplasty in the United States from 2005 to 2030. *J Bone Joint Surg Am* 2007;89(4):780-785.

66. Thomas GE, Simpson DJ, Mehmood S, et al: A double-blind, randomized controlled trial using radiostereometric analysis. *J Bone Joint Surg Am* 2011;93(8): 716-722.

67. McCalden RW, MacDonald SJ, Rorabeck CH, Bourne RB, Chess DG, Charron KD: Wear rate of highly cross-linked polyethylene in total hip arthroplasty: A randomized controlled trial. *J Bone Joint Surg Am* 2009;91(4):773-782.

68. Mu Z, Tian J, Wu T, Yang J, Pei F: A systematic review of radiological outcomes of highly cross-linked polyethylene versus conventional polyethylene in total hip arthroplasty. *Int Orthop* 2009; 33(3):599-604.

69. Ayers DC, Hays PL, Drew JM, Eskander MS, Osuch D, Bragdon CR: Two-year radiostereometric analysis evaluation of femoral head penetration in a challenging population of young total hip arthroplasty patients. *J Arthroplasty* 2009;24(6):9-14.

70. Beksaç B, Salas A, González Della Valle A, Salvati EA: Wear is reduced in THA performed with highly cross-linked polyethylene. *Clin Orthop Relat Res* 2009; 467(7):1765-1772.

71. Mall NA, Nunley RM, Zhu JJ, Maloney WJ, Barrack RL, Clohisy JC: The incidence of acetabular osteolysis in young patients with conventional versus highly cross-linked polyethylene. *Clin Orthop Relat Res* 2011;469(2):372-381.

72. D'Antonio JA, Capello WN, Ramakrishnan R: Second-generation annealed highly cross-linked polyethylene exhibits low wear. *Clin Orthop Relat Res* 2012; 470(6):1696-1704.

73. Schroder DT, Kelly NH, Wright TM, Parks ML: Retrieved highly crosslinked UHMWPE acetabular liners have similar wear damage as conventional UHMWPE. *Clin Orthop Relat Res* 2011; 469(2):387-394.

74. Furmanski J, Kraay MJ, Rimnac CM: Crack initiation in retrieved cross-linked highly cross-linked ultrahigh-molecular-weight polyethylene acetabular liners: An in-

vestigation of 9 cases. *J Arthroplasty* 2011;26(5):796-801.

75. Tower SS, Currier JH, Currier BH, Lyford KA, Van Citters DW, Mayor MB: Rim cracking of the cross-linked longevity polyethylene acetabular liner after total hip arthroplasty. *J Bone Joint Surg Am* 2007;89(10):2212-2217.

76. Waewsawangwong W, Goodman SB: Unexpected failure of highly cross-linked polyethylene acetabular liner. *J Arthroplasty* 2012; 27(2):e321-e324.

77. Lachiewicz PF, Heckman DS, Soileau ES, Mangla J, Martell JM: Femoral head size and wear of highly cross-linked polyethylene at 5 to 8 years. *Clin Orthop Relat Res* 2009;467(12):3290-3296.

78. Galvin AL, Jennings LM, Tipper JL, Ingham E, Fisher J: Wear and creep of highly crosslinked polyethylene against cobalt chrome and ceramic femoral heads. *Proc Inst Mech Eng H* 2010; 224(10):1175-1183.

79. Good V, Ries M, Barrack RL, Widding K, Hunter G, Heuer D: Reduced wear with oxidized zirconium femoral heads. *J Bone Joint Surg Am* 2003;85(suppl 4):105-110.

80. Meftah M, Ebrahimpour PB, He C, Ranawat AS, Ranawat CS: Preliminary clinical and radiographic results of large ceramic heads on highly cross-linked polyethylene. *Orthopedics* 2011;34(6): 133.

81. Garvin KL, Hartman CW, Mangla J, Murdoch N, Martell JM: Wear analysis in THA utilizing oxidized zirconium and cross-linked polyethylene. *Clin Orthop Relat Res* 2009;467(1):141-145.

82. Lewis PM, Moore CA, Olsen M, Schemitsch EH, Waddell JP: Comparison of mid-term clinical outcomes after primary total hip arthroplasty with Oxinium vs cobalt chrome femoral heads. *Orthopedics* 2008;31(12):ii.

83. Kop AM, Whitewood C, Johnston DJ: Damage of Oxinium femoral heads subsequent to hip arthroplasty dislocation three retrieval case studies. *J Arthroplasty* 2007;22(5):775-779.

84. Jaffe WL, Strauss EJ, Cardinale M, Herrera L, Kummer FJ: Surface oxidized zirconium total hip arthroplasty head damage due to closed reduction effects on polyethylene wear. *J Arthroplasty* 2009; 24(6):898-902.

85. Evangelista GT, Fulkerson E, Kummer F, Di Cesare PE: Surface damage to an Oxinium femoral head prosthesis after dislocation. *J Bone Joint Surg Br* 2007;89(4): 535-537.

86. Hernigou P, Bahrami T: Zirconia and alumina ceramics in comparison with stainless-steel heads: Polyethylene wear after a minimum ten-year follow-up. *J Bone Joint Surg Br* 2003;85(4):504-509.

87. Zywiel MG, Sayeed SA, Johnson AJ, Schmalzried TP, Mont MA: Survival of hard-on-hard bearings in total hip arthroplasty: A systematic review. *Clin Orthop Relat Res* 2011;469(6):1536-1546.

88. D'Antonio JA, Capello WN, Naughton M: Ceramic bearings for total hip arthroplasty have high survivorship at 10 years. *Clin Orthop Relat Res* 2012; 470(2):373-381.

89. Gallo J, Goodman SB, Lostak J, Janout M: Advantages and disadvantages of ceramic on ceramic total hip arthroplasty: A review. *Biomed Pap Med Fac Univ Palacky Olomouc Czech Repub* 2012; 156(3):204-212.

90. Yeung E, Bott PT, Chana R, et al: Mid-term results of third-generation alumina-on-alumina ceramic bearings in cementless total hip arthroplasty: A ten-year minimum follow-up. *J Bone Joint Surg Am* 2012;94(2):138-144.

91. Sugano N, Takao M, Sakai T, Nishii T, Miki H, Ohzono K: Eleven- to 14-year follow-up results of cementless total hip arthroplasty using a third-generation alumina ceramic-on-ceramic bearing. *J Arthroplasty* 2012;27(5):736-741.

92. Finkbone PR, Severson EP, Cabanela ME, Trousdale RT: Ceramic-on-ceramic total hip arthroplasty in patients younger than 20 years. *J Arthroplasty* 2012; 27(2):213-219.

93. Tseng WS, Tao KT, Hsu J, Qiu JH, Li B, Goebert D: Longitudinal analysis of development among single and nonsingle children in Nanjing, China: Ten-year follow-up study. *J Nerv Ment Dis* 2000;188(10):701-707.

94. Hamilton WG, McAuley JP, Dennis DA, Murphy JA, Blumenfeld TJ, Politi J: THA with Delta ceramic on ceramic: Results of a multicenter investigational device exemption trial. *Clin Orthop Relat Res* 2010;468(2): 358-366.

95. Porat M, Parvizi J, Sharkey PF, Berend KR, Lombardi AV Jr, Barrack RL: Causes of failure of ceramic-on-ceramic and metal-on-metal hip arthroplasties. *Clin Orthop Relat Res* 2012; 470(2):382-387.

96. Parvizi J, Adeli B, Wong JC, Restrepo C, Rothman RH: A squeaky reputation: The problem may be design-dependent. *Clin Orthop Relat Res* 2011;469(6): 1598-1605.

97. Swanson TV, Peterson DJ, Seethala R, Bliss RL, Spellmon CA: Influence of prosthetic design on squeaking after ceramic-on-ceramic total hip arthroplasty. *J Arthroplasty* 2010;25(6):36-42.

98. Sexton SA, Yeung E, Jackson MP, et al: The role of patient factors and implant position in squeaking of ceramic-on-ceramic total hip replacements. *J Bone Joint Surg Br* 2011;93(4):439-442.

99. Restrepo C, Parvizi J, Kurtz SM, Sharkey PF, Hozack WJ, Rothman RH: The noisy ceramic hip: Is component malpositioning the cause? *J Arthroplasty* 2008;23(5): 643-649.

100. Restrepo C, Matar WY, Parvizi J, Rothman RH, Hozack WJ: Natural history of squeaking after total hip arthroplasty. *Clin Orthop Relat Res* 2010;468(9):2340-2345.

101. Walter WL, Kurtz SM, Esposito C, et al: Retrieval analysis of squeaking alumina ceramic-on-ceramic bearings. *J Bone Joint Surg Br* 2011;93(12):1597-1601.

102. Traina F, Tassinari E, De Fine M, Bordini B, Toni A: Revision of ceramic hip replacements for fracture of a ceramic component: AAOS exhibit selection. *J Bone Joint Surg Am* 2011;93(24):e147.

103. Smith AJ, Dieppe P, Vernon K, Porter M, Blom AW; National Joint Registry of England and Wales: Failure rates of stemmed metal-on-metal hip replacements: Analysis of data from the National Joint Registry of England and Wales. *Lancet* 2012;379(9822): 1199-1204.

104. Smith AJ, Dieppe P, Howard PW, Blom AW; National Joint Registry for England and Wales: Failure rates of metal-on-metal hip resurfacings: Analysis of data from the National Joint Registry for England and Wales. *Lancet* 2012; 380(9855):1759-1766.

105. Lombardi AV Jr, Barrack RL, Berend KR, et al: Algorithmic approach to diagnosis and management of metal-on-metal arthroplasty. *J Bone Joint Surg Br* 2012;94(11):14-18.

106. Williams DH, Greidanus NV, Masri BA, Duncan CP, Garbuz DS: Prevalence of pseudotumor in asymptomatic patients after metal-on-metal hip arthroplasty. *J Bone Joint Surg Am* 2011; 93(23):2164-2171.

107. Cooper HJ, Della Valle CJ, Berger RA, et al: The Hip Society: Algorithmic approach to diagnosis and management of metal-on-metal hip arhtroplasty. *J Bone Joint Surg Am* 2012;94(18):1655-1661.

108. Fricka KB, Ho H, Peace WJ, Engh CA Jr: Metal-on-metal local tissue reaction is associated with corrosion of the head taper junction. *J Arthroplasty* 2012;27(8)26-31.

109. Amstutz HC, Le Duff MJ, Campbell PA, Wisk LE, Takamura KM: Complications after metal-on-metal hip resurfacing arthroplasty. *Orthop Clin North Am* 2011;42(2):207-230.

110. Kim YH, Park JW, Kim JS: Cementless metaphyseal fitting anatomic total hip arthroplasty with a ceramic-on-ceramic bearing in patients thirty years of age or younger. *J Bone Joint Surg Am* 2012;94(17):1570-1575.

111. Kim YH, Choi Y, Kim JS: Cementless total hip arthroplasty with ceramic-on-ceramic bearing in patients younger than 45 years with femoral-head osteonecrosis. *Int Orthop* 2010;34(8):1123-1127.

112. Faldini C, Miscione MT, Chehrassan M, et al: Congenital hip dysplasia treated by total hip arthroplasty using cementless tapered stem in patients younger than 50 years old: Results after 12-years follow-up. *J Orthop Traumatol* 2011;12(4):213-218.

113. Almeida F, Pino L, Silvestre A, Gomar F: Mid- to long-term outcome of cementless total hip arthroplasty in younger patients. *J Orthop Surg* 2010;18(2):172-178.

114. Clohisy JC, Oryhon JM, Seyler TM, et al: Function and fixation of total hip arthroplasty in patients 25 years of age or younger. *Clin Orthop Relat Res* 2010;468(12):3207-3213.

115. Liang TJ, You MZ, Xing PF, Bin S, Ke ZZ, Jing Y: Uncemented total hip arthroplasty in patients younger than 50 years: A 6- to 10-year follow-up study. [published online ahead of print April 16. *Orthopedics* 2010;33(4): doi 103928/01477477-2010025-18.

116. Kang JS, Moon KH, Park SR, Choi SW: Long-term results of total hip arthroplasty with an extensively porous coated stem in patients younger than 45 years old. *Yonsei Med J* 2010;51(1):100-103.

117. Jialiang T, Zhongyou M, Fuxing P, Zongke Z, Bin S, Jing Y: Primary total hip arthroplasty with Duraloc cup in patients younger than 50 years: A 5- to 7-year follow-up study. *J Arthroplasty* 2009;24(8):1184-1187.

118. Wangen H, Lereim P, Holm I, Gunderson R, Reikeras O: Hip arthroplasty in patients younger than 30 years: Excellent ten to 16-year follow-up results with a HA-coated stem. *Int Orthop* 2008;32(2):203-208.

119. Mont MA, Seyler TM, Plate JF, Delanois RE, Parvizi J: Uncemented total hip arthroplasty in young adults with osteonecrosis of the femoral head: A comparative study. *J Bone Joint Surg Am* 2006;88(suppl 3):104-109.

120. Archibeck MJ, Surdam JW, Schultz SC Jr, Junick DW, White RE: Cementless total hip arthroplasty in patients 50 years or younger. *J Arthroplasty* 2006;21(4):476-483.

121. McAuley JP, Szuszczewicz ES, Young A, Engh CA Sr: Total hip arthroplasty in patients 50 years and younger. *Clin Orthop Relat Res* 2004;418:119-125.

122. Bessette BJ, Fassier F, Tanzer M, Brooks CE: Total hip arthroplasty in patients younger than 21 years: A minimum, 10-year follow-up. *Can J Surg* 2003;46(4):257-262.

123. Byun JW, Yoon TR, Park KS, Seon JK: Third-generation ceramic-on-ceramic total hip arthroplasty in patients younger than 30 years with osteonecrosis of femoral head. *J Arthroplasty* 2012;27(7):1337-1343.

124. Kamath AF, Sheth NP, Hosalkar HH, Babatunde OM, Lee GC, Nelson CL: Modern total hip arthroplasty in patients younger than 21 years. *J Arthroplasty* 2012;27(3):402-408.

125. Kim YH, Choi Y, Kim JS: Cementless total hip arthroplasty with alumina-on-highly cross-linked polyethylene bearing in young patients with femoral head osteonecrosis. *J Arthroplasty* 2011;26(2):218-223.

126. Baek SH, Kim SY: Cementless total hip arthroplasty with alumina bearings in patients younger than fifty with femoral head osteonecrosis. *J Bone Joint Surg Am* 2008;90(6):1314-1320.

127. Nizard R, Pourreyron D, Raould A, Hannouche D, Sedel L: Alumina-on-alumina hip arthroplasty in patients younger than 30 years old. *Clin Orthop Relat Res* 2008;466(2):317-323.

128. Ha YC, Koo KH, Jeong ST, et al: Cementless alumina-on-alumina total hip arthroplasty in patients younger than 50 years: A 5-year minimum follow-up study. *J Arthroplasty* 2007;22(2):184-188.

129. Yoo JJ, Kim YM, Yoon KS, et al: Contemporary alumina-on-alumina total hip arthroplasty performed in patients younger than forty years: A 5-year minimum follow-up study. *J Biomed Mater Res B Appl Biomater* 2006;78(1):70-75.

130. Pignatti G, Stagni C, Fravisini M, Giunti A: Ceramic-ceramic coupling: Total hip arthroplasty in young patients. *Chir Organi Mov* 2003;88(4):369-375.

Video Reference

Peters CL, Austin MS, Mulkey P, Erickson JA: Video. *Femoral Acetabular Impingement.* Salt Lake City, UT, 2013.

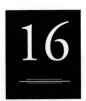

Advances in Acetabular Osteolysis: Biomarkers, Imaging, and Pharmacologic Management

Kenneth D. Illingworth, MD
Nathan Wachter, BS
William J. Maloney, MD
Wayne G. Paprosky, MD
Michael D. Ries, MD
Khaled J. Saleh, BSc, MD, MSc, FRCS(C), MHCM

Abstract

Acetabular osteolysis can be difficult to diagnose because patients often have no clinical symptoms even when there is substantial bone loss. Ideally, early detection would lead to early interventions. Imaging continues to be the frontline modality for the early detection of acetabular osteolysis. Although plain radiography is the current imaging modality most commonly used in routine follow-up examinations, its low sensitivity limits its usefulness. CT and MRI have proven to be better imaging modalities for the early detection of osteolysis; however, their use is limited by cost, radiation exposure, and time. Biomarkers hold promise for the early detection of osteolysis; however, their efficacy requires more rigorous research for validation. Early diagnosis and treatment of osteolysis may lead to better outcomes for patients.

Instr Course Lect 2014;63:177-186.

Dr. Maloney or an immediate family member serves as a board member, owner, officer, or committee member of the American Joint Replacement Registry, The Knee Society, and the Western Orthopaedic Association; has received royalties from Wright Medical Technology; serves as a paid consultant to Pipeline Orthopaedics; and has stock or stock options held in Abbott, Gillead, ISTO Technologies, Johnson and Johnson, Merck, Maximed, Pfizer, Pipeline Orthopaedics, and TJO. Dr. Paprosky or an immediate family member serves as a board member, owner, officer, or committee member of The Hip Society; has received royalties from Wright Medical Technology and Zimmer; is a member of a speakers' bureau or has made paid presentations on behalf of Zimmer; serves as a paid consultant to Biomet and Zimmer. Dr. Ries or an immediate family member serves as a board member, owner, officer, or committee member of the Foundation for the Advancement of Research in Medicine; has received royalties from Smith and Nephew; serves as a paid consultant to Smith and Nephew and Stryker; has stock or stock options held in OrthAlign. Dr. Saleh or an immediate family member serves as a board member, owner, officer, or committee member of the American Orthopaedic Association, and the Orthopaedic Research and Education Foundation; has received royalties from Aesculap/B. Braun; is a member of a speakers' bureau or has made paid presentations on behalf of Carefusion; serves as a paid consultant to Aesculap, the Memorial Medical Center Co-Management Orthopaedic Board and the Blue Cross Blue Shield Blue Ribbon Panel; has received research or institutional support from Smith & Nephew, the Orthopaedic Research and Education Foundation, and the National Institutes of Health/National Institute of Arthritis and Musculoskeletal Skin Diseases (R0-1). Neither of the following authors nor any immediate family member has received anything of value from or owns stock in a commercial company or institution related directly or indirectly to the subject of this chapter: Dr. Illingworth and Dr. Wachter.

Periprosthetic osteolysis contributes to nearly 10% of total hip arthroplasty (THA) revisions, accounting for approximately 9,700 revisions annually. Another 40% of all revision procedures are attributed to mechanical loosening, which in some cases occurs secondary to progressive osteolysis.[1,2] Revision THA is more challenging than primary THA because it often requires longer surgical times and is associated with greater blood loss and a higher risk of postoperative morbidity and mortality (particularly in elderly patients).[3] Revision THA also requires more expensive implants and the potential need for bone grafting of acetabular defects.[4,5]

It is currently believed that periprosthetic osteolysis is caused by a combination of environmental and genetic factors. Environmental factors include the bearing material, the fixation surfaces of the implanted components, the implant design, the component orientation, and the patient's activity level.[6,7] Genetic factors can increase susceptibility to osteolysis

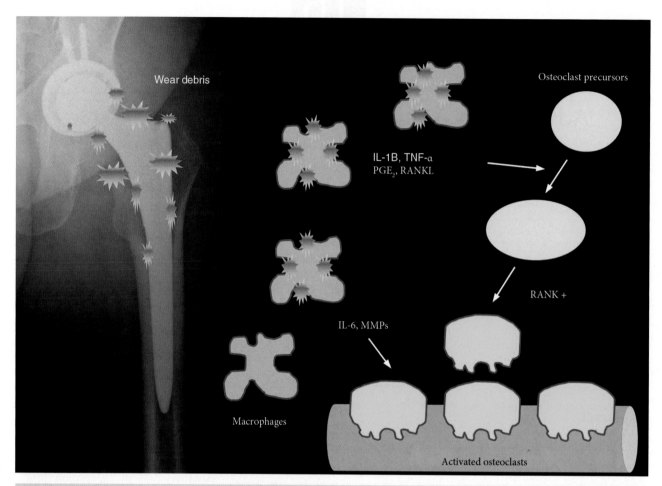

Figure 1 Illustration of the pathogenesis of osteolysis involving the phagocytosis of wear debris from monocytes and macrophages that activate cytokine release promoting a proinflammatory state. This shifts the homeostasis of bone maintenance toward an osteolytic destructive state caused by the activation of osteoclasts. TNF-α = tumor necrosis factor-α, PGE$_2$ = prostaglandin E$_2$, RANK= receptor activator of nuclear factor-κ B, RANKL = receptor activator of nuclear factor-κ B ligand, MMPs = matrix metalloproteinases.

because of a patient's unique response to the wear debris encountered.[1] Osteolysis involves the phagocytosis of wear debris from monocytes and macrophages that activate cytokine release, which promotes a proinflammatory state.[8,9] This activation shifts the homeostasis of bone maintenance toward an osteolytic destructive state secondary to the activation of osteoclasts[10] (**Figure 1**). This osteolytic destructive state can remain undetected for years, resulting in substantial bone loss.

Osteolysis often can be difficult to detect because patients have no clinical symptoms and remain completely asymptomatic even when substantial

bone loss has occurred.[3-5,11] Biomarkers hold promise because they are objective indicators and have the potential for detecting osteolysis in the early stages of the disease process. Imaging continues to be the frontline modality for early detection of osteolysis. Although plain radiography is the current imaging modality most commonly used in routine follow-up examinations, CT and MRI are also used in diagnosing osteolysis and monitoring its progression.

Ideally, patients with wear-induced osteolysis would be identified early and medical and/or pharmacologic management would prolong the lon-

gevity of the implant and delay the need for often complex revision surgery. This chapter focuses on the diagnosis of wear-induced acetabular osteolysis and subsequent aseptic implant loosening, with an emphasis on biomarkers, imaging, and potential pharmacologic interventions to treat acetabular osteolysis.

Biomarkers

Biomarkers are objective indicators of biologic and pathologic processes and pharmaceutic responses to therapeutic interventions.[12] Biomarkers hold promise in THA as a potential monitoring tool for the early detection of osteolysis. Telopeptides have been researched as a biomarker of bone turnover in osteolysis. Several studies have shown higher levels of urinary cross-linked N-telopeptides of type I collagen in patients with loose implants and in those with osteolysis compared with control groups.[13-15] Schneider et al[14] and Wilkinson et al[16] reported substantially increased levels of urinary cross-linked N-telopeptides of type I collagen in patients with loose THAs when compared with levels in those with stable hip arthroplasties. Serum C-terminal telopeptides of type I collagen also has been studied. Arabmotlagh et al[17] found that the presence of an increased level of serum C-terminal telopeptides of type I collagen 3 weeks after a cemented THA procedure was significantly correlated ($P = 0.003$) with bone loss at 1-year follow-up.

Several cytokines have been studied as potential biomarkers in the detection of osteolysis. Interleukin (IL)-6 acts as both a proinflammatory and anti-inflammatory cytokine, and osteoblasts secrete IL-6 to stimulate osteoclast formation. Hernigou et al[18] found that IL-6 levels are substantially increased in patients with osteolysis when compared with a control group.

IL-11 is a multifunctional cytokine and is a key regulator of multiple events in hematopoiesis, including the stimulation of megakaryocyte maturation. Fiorito el al[19] found IL-11 levels to be substantially lower in patients with osteolysis. Several other cytokines have been researched as potential biomarkers (IL-1β, transforming growth factor-β, and tumor necrosis factor-α); however, a significant association with osteolysis could not be identified.[18,19]

Wu et al[20] researched the use of peripheral blood levels of CD14+CD16+ monocytes as biomarkers and found them to be sensitive markers of aseptic loosening. Periprosthetic tissues also have been shown to have nonactive

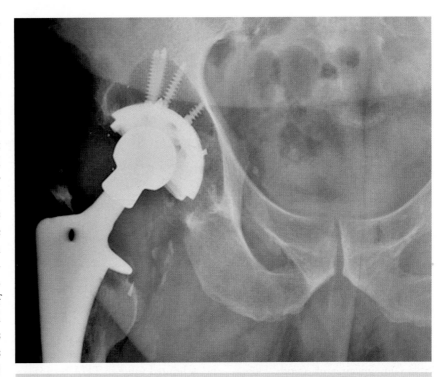

Figure 2   AP radiograph of the hip of a 56-year-old man 12 years after THA. Osteolytic acetabular lesions and well-demarcated, scalloped regions of bone loss (area highlighted in green) can be seen.

CD4 T cells, which may result from early stages of periprosthetic osteolysis in which T cells promoting osteoclastogenesis cause osteoclasts to activate FoxP3/CD8 T cells that inhibit CD4 T cells.[21] Tartrate-resistant acid phosphatase 5b, which is associated with resorbing multinucleated cells, has been shown to be a reliable biomarker for detecting late loosening in THA.[22] Bone alkaline phosphatase, osteocalcin, C-reactive protein, prostaglandin E_2, and matrix metalloproteinase-1 have been studied; no important link to osteolysis has been found.[17-19,23]

Biomarkers have the potential to become an easy and objective diagnostic and prognostic test for osteolysis after THA. At this time, however, evidence is lacking to support most biomarkers as viable indicators for osteolysis or aseptic loosening after THA.[23] Future research is needed to identify new biomarkers in osteolysis and further explore the role of promising biomarkers.

Imaging

Plain Radiography

After THA, patients are followed with physical examinations and radiographic evaluations with the intent of appropriate surgical intervention if there is evidence of component loosening or substantial bone loss from osteolysis.[9,24] Current radiographic evaluations yield limited information and commonly underestimate the degree of bone loss.[10,25,26] Osteolytic acetabular lesions often appear as well-demarcated scalloped regions of bone loss[27] (**Figure 2**). Early stages of acetabular bone loss secondary to osteolysis often cannot be seen on plain radiographs, or the magnitude of bone loss is underestimated because of the two-dimensional nature of plain radiographs and the complex three-dimensional anatomy of the acetabulum. However, plain radiography remains the current standard of care

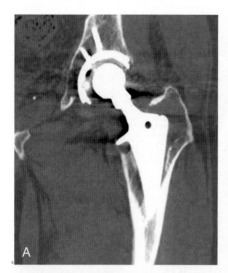
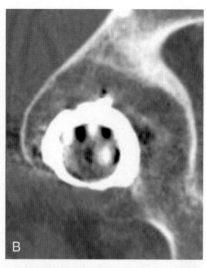

Figure 3   Acetabular osteolysis after THA is seen on sagittal (**A**) and coronal helical (**B**) CT scans.

for the initial evaluation and routine follow-up imaging of aseptic loosening.

Claus et al[28] evaluated cadaver specimens with varying sizes of pelvic defects to assess the diagnostic sensitivity and specificity of plain radiography. The overall sensitivity for the detection of osteolysis on a single radiograph was 41.5%, and the overall specificity was 93.0%. Sensitivity was dependent on the location and size of the lesions but not on the radiographic view. The addition of 45°–obturator-oblique and iliac-oblique projection views has been shown to increase the accuracy of detecting acetabular bony defects.[29]

CT and MRI

Several imaging modalities have the potential to become the new standard for evaluating periprosthetic osteolysis. CT and MRI can aid in quantifying bone loss compared with plain radiography. With recent improvements in metal-suppression artifact reduction software and protocols, diagnostic MRI and CT have gained considerable momentum in accurately quantifying osteolysis and the progression of lytic lesions.[25,30-32]

Traditional CT has been shown to be of limited value in THA because of the beam-hardening artifact generated by the severe attenuation of the radiographic beam.[33] Beam-hardening artifact presents as alternating high and low attenuation lines radiating from the prosthesis.[30] However, recent studies have concluded that helical CT is superior to plain radiography when evaluating the degree of osteolysis immediately adjacent to an implanted construct.[33-35] Osteolysis appears on CT images as a lucent area devoid of osseous trabeculae and is typically in contact with the prosthesis[30,34] (**Figure 3**). Leung et al[36] reported that CT detected 87% of osteolytic lesions, whereas plain radiography only identified 52% of lesions (as determined at the time of surgery). Howie et al[31] described the value of three-dimensional CT in quantifying the size of an acetabular osteolytic lesion. Schwarz et al[37] reported that volumetric three-dimensional CT can be used to accurately monitor the progression of osteolysis. Although CT has some benefits over plain radiography, the cost-effectiveness and radiation exposure associated with CT is a drawback

to its implementation as the standard imaging test for diagnosing osteolysis.[10]

A limitation of both plain radiography and CT is the lack of soft-tissue imaging. Particle-induced osteolysis first causes a synovial reaction. MRI offers superior soft-tissue contrast and does not produce ionizing radiation, which makes it a potential alternative to CT and plain radiography.[38] MRI has been shown to be the most accurate imaging technique for evaluating periprosthetic osteolysis and synovitis.[39-41] MRI techniques and usage have been limited because of its susceptibility to metal artifact from the prosthesis, which results in image distortion.[33] Optimal parameters for MRI use in THA have been published to aid in dealing with this limitation[40] (**Table 1**). Osteolysis manifests as well-marginated intraosseous lesions that contrast with the intramedullary fat, with a characteristic line of low signal intensity surrounding the area of focal marrow replacement[38] (**Figure 4**). MRI has been shown to be more effective in detecting the location and severity of periacetabular bone loss, with a higher sensitivity for lesion detection compared with CT and plain radiography.[33,39,42] The superior soft-tissue contrast of MRI allows the diagnosis of intracapsular particle disease before bone resorption occurs.[33]

Advanced Techniques

Multiacquisition variable-resonance image combination (MAVRIC) and fast spin-echo techniques can help visualize the hip after THA, with fewer artifacts from the metallic hardware than traditional MRI and are useful in detecting periprosthetic osteolysis. MAVRIC can detect more damage from osteolysis than fast spin-echo sequences[43] (**Figure 5**). Wear debris after THA will cause a soft-tissue synovial reaction before it progresses to

Table 1

Hospital for Special Surgery Recommended Protocol for MRI of THA[a]

Timing Parameters	Axial FSE Whole-Body Mode; Body Coil	Coronal FIR Whole-Body Mode; Body Coil	Coronal FSE; Surface Coil	Axial FSE; Surface Coil	Sagittal FSE; Surface Coil
Repetition time (msec)	4,500-5,500	4,500	4,500-5,800	4,500-5,500	5,500- 6,500
Echo time (msec effective)	21.4-32.0	18	24-30	24-30	24-30
Inversion time (msec)	–	150	–	–	–
Echo train length	20	9	18	20	20
Receiver bandwidth (kHz over entire frequency range)[b]	83-100	83-100	62-100	83-100	83-100
Field of view (cm)	32-36	34-36	18	17-19	18-20
Matrix	512 × 256	256 × 192	512 × 352	512 × 256-288	512 × 352
Slice thickness (mm)	5	5	4	4	2.5-3
Interslice gap (mm)	0	0	0	0	0
Number of excitations	4	2	4-5	4-5	4-5
Tailored radiofrequency	Yes	Yes	Yes	Yes	Yes
No phase wrap	Yes	Yes	No	Yes	Yes
Swap phase and frequency	Yes	Yes	Yes	Yes	Yes
Variable bandwidth	Yes	Yes	Yes	Yes	Yes
Frequency direction	Anterior to posterior	Right to left	Right to left	Anterior to posterior	Anterior to posterior

[a]Coil: Initial body coil (whole-body mode), followed by surface coil (two-part, four-channel shoulder phased-array coil).

[b]For General Electric systems, the receiver bandwidth is reported as half-bandwidth (maximum frequency), so reported receiver bandwidth of 62.5 kHz is actually acquired at 125 kHz over the entire frequency range. To convert to Hz/pixel, use the following formula:

Hz/pixel = [(General Electric receiver bandwidth) (2,000)] / matrix in frequency direction.

FIR = fast inversion recovery, FSE = fast spin-echo.

(Reproduced with permission from Malchau H, Potter HG; Implant Wear Symposium 2007 Clinical Work Group: How are wear-related problems diagnosed and what forms of surveillance are necessary? *J Am Acad Orthop Surg* 2008;(16 suppl 1):S14-S19.)

wear-induced osteolysis and acetabular bony defects. Hayter et al[38] showed that the presence of intermediate and low signal debris on MRI correlated with the debris characteristics found at the time of histologic analysis. MRI after THA can potentially be used to make an early diagnosis of osteolysis, which will allow earlier treatment. Cost, feasibility, and metal artifact remain barriers to the clinical applicability of MRI for evaluating aseptic loosening; however, the superior soft-tissue imaging of MRI makes it the most likely choice for increasing use in future imaging protocols.

Radionuclide imaging has also shown promise for assessing osteolysis. Technetium Tc-99 methylene diphosphonate bone scans are sensitive but lack specificity for prosthetic loosening and are only useful when plain radiographs show no signs of loosening.[44,45] Positron emission tomography has shown merit in evaluating polyethylene and metal wear-induced chronic inflammation and periprosthetic osteolysis and may be helpful in differentiating the former from infection.[46]

Aside from radiographic imaging studies that seek to qualify and quantify the presence of aseptic loosening with image analysis, other methods have emerged that may prove beneficial when attempting to evaluate the progression of debris-induced bone resorption. These methods include dual-energy x-ray absorptiometry (DEXA), morphometric grid analysis of lytic lesion advancement, and radiographic texture analysis of trabecular bone patterns.[47-50]

Monitoring Polyethylene Wear Progression

Along with radiographic detection of osteolysis, accurate methods of determining and quantifying wear progression are important in identifying patients at increased risk for THA failure because of advanced osteolysis. With more active and younger patients being treated with THA, the monitoring of implant wear will become increasingly important.[51] Accelerated polyethylene wear results in increased debris, placing the patient at increased risk of wear-induced osteolysis and potentially placing the patient at risk for a complex revision procedure. It has

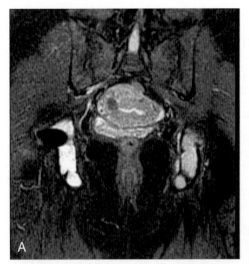
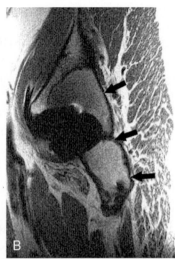

Figure 4   Bilateral THAs in a 52-year-old woman were performed 9 years prior on the right hip and 7 years prior on the left hip. **A,** Coronal body coil fast inversion recovery image showing fluid signal material replacing the ischia bilaterally, compatible with severe osteolysis. **B,** Sagittal fast spin-echo image of the right hip showing fluid signal material with a well-defined low signal rim involving the ischium and posterior column (arrows). (Reproduced from Malchau H, Potter HG; Implant Wear Symposium 2007 Clinical Work Group: How are wear-related problems diagnosed and what forms of surveillance are necessary? *J Am Acad Orthop Surg* 2008;(16 suppl 1):S14-S19.)

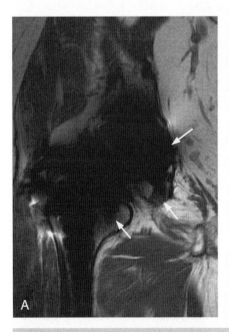
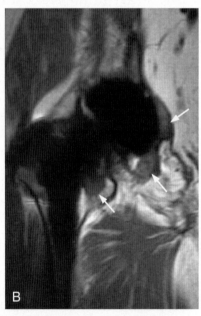

Figure 5   A 44-year-old man presented with pain 11 years after revision THA on the right hip. Corresponding fast spin-echo (**A**) and MAVRIC (**B**) images show improved depiction of the periacetabular and proximal femoral osteolysis (arrows) using the MAVRIC technique. (Reproduced with permission from Hayter CL, Koff MF, Shah P, Koch KM, Miller TT, Potter HG: MRI after arthroplasty: Comparison of MAVRIC and conventional fast spin-echo techniques. *AJR Am J Roentgenol* 2011;197(3):W405-411.)

been suggested that wear rates greater than 0.1 mm per year result in an increased risk of osteolysis.[52]

Methods to evaluate polyethylene wear progression include plain radiography, radiostereometric analysis, and CT.[53,54] Plain radiography is the most widely used method because of its ease of use and place in standard clinical follow-up evaluations. Measurement techniques include manual two-dimensional, computer-assisted three-dimensional (including edge detection and vector wear analysis), and computer-assisted three-dimensional methods. Radiostereometric analysis is considered the most accurate method of measuring wear rates in THA because of its high precision in measuring skeletal micromotion, with a calculated accuracy as low as 0.065 mm and a precision of 0.067 mm.[55] The need for specialized, costly equipment and the placement of tantalum beads during the primary arthroplasty procedure limit its use predominantly to research trials.

As previously mentioned, CT has the advantage over plain radiographic techniques because it is a more sensitive and accurate method for detecting osteolytic lesions and monitoring their progression. CT also has been used in detecting polyethylene wear while providing a true three-dimensional view for determining directional vector wear in all directions.[51] Because wear vectors can be perpendicular to the normal axis of the cup, plain radiographic measurements cannot account for this directional variation.[56,57] CT methods of determining wear have shown accuracy and precision values as low as 0.55 mm and 0.4 mm, respectively.[57] CT also has an advantage over two-dimensional imaging modalities because it allows the measurements of acetabular anteversion and inclination and the determination of linear and volumetric wear. Although a direct correlation between wear rates and the development of acetabular osteolysis has not been fully appreciated, advances in imaging modalities and future studies will help better predict and identify patients who are at risk for wear-induced osteolysis.

Pharmacologic Treatment

Bisphosphonates inhibit osteoclastic bone resorption and are the most widely studied of the pharmacologic treatments for periprosthetic osteolysis. A meta-analysis by Bhandari et al[58] showed that bisphosphonates have a beneficial effect in maintaining periprosthetic bone mineral density compared with a control group. Freidl et al[59] reported that patients receiving a single dose of zoledronic acid had a significantly decreased risk of acetabular subsidence (P = < 0.05) and a trend toward less femoral subsidence. However, bisphosphonates have not gained favor in off-label use for periprosthetic osteolysis. Prolonged use of bisphosphonates, most notably alendronate, has been linked to atypical subtrochanteric femoral fractures or diaphyseal femoral fractures, although a definitive pathophysiologic mechanism for these fractures has not been proven.[60-64] Theories suggest that long-term use of bisphosphonates induces long-term suppression of bone remodeling, which in turn can result in the accumulation of microdamage and subsequent stress fracture formation. Initial signs of this condition are diffuse cortical thickening, followed by fracture line propagation and, eventually, complete fracture.[65-67] More long-term quality studies are needed to fully understand the risks and potential benefits of bisphosphonates in treating osteolysis.

Cytokine inhibitors, including IL-1β, have been intimately linked to osteolysis to the extent that they are used as a secondary measure of periprosthetic bone resorption. IL-1β inhibitors have been proposed as a potential pharmacologic treatment. IL-1Ra is an anti-inflammatory immune modulator with promising prospective applications in mitigating wear-debris osteolysis.[68] Many cytokines and inflammatory mediators are critical participants in the biochemical pathway of wear-induced osteolysis and may represent prime targets for pharmacologic intervention, with tumor necrosis factor-α playing a central role in the pathophysiologic cascade. Tumor necrosis factor-α antagonists, such as etanercept, have displayed promising results in patients with rheumatoid and psoriatic arthritis, suggesting that they may offer a potential therapeutic option for patients with periprosthetic osteolysis.[9,37,69] However, concerns regarding their potential adverse side effects, including immunosuppression, have limited their use.

Perhaps one of the most promising candidates for the pharmacologic intervention of osteolysis, primarily because of its specificity, is a receptor activator of nuclear factor-κ B ligand (RANKL) antibody/antagonist, such as denosumab.[69-71] Pharmacologic treatment seems attractive, but there is no proven or approved drug therapy to prevent or inhibit periprosthetic osteolysis.[10]

Preferred Technique of This Chapter's Authors

Patients presenting for follow-up after THA are evaluated with close observation for radiographic and clinical signs of osteolysis. AP and lateral plain radiographs are obtained every year after THA for approximately 5 years and then every 2 to 3 years thereafter. At each follow-up evaluation, standard AP and lateral radiographs are closely examined for any signs of acetabular bone loss. Because bone lesions caused by osteolysis may be similar to those caused by infection, it is important to rule out infection in symptomatic and asymptomatic patients who have possible osteolysis-induced clinical and radiographic symptoms.[27] If an acetabular bony lesion is identified, additional imaging studies and testing are suggested. The first step is obtaining 45°–obturator-oblique and iliac-oblique projection views to better evaluate the three-dimensional nature of the acetabulum.[29] CT with three-dimensional reconstructions is obtained if there is substantial bone loss, the need for more accurate lesion detection, and for preoperative planning when revision THA is indicated. CT may be used to quantify the progression of an osteolytic lesion; however, the risks and benefits of the additional radiation exposure compared with plain radiography and/or MRI must be assessed. MRI may be added to the imaging protocol to better evaluate soft-tissue and synovial reactions if osteolysis is suspected without identifiable lesions on plain radiographs or as an adjunctive modality for detecting lesions. A lower threshold for advanced imaging for detecting and monitoring the progression of acetabular lesions is appropriate in high-risk patients, such as young patients and those with a high activity level.

Summary

Despite advances in THA, periprosthetic wear debris-induced acetabular osteolysis and aseptic loosening continue to be factors in prosthetic joint longevity. Routine follow-up evaluations and patient education are critical for diagnosing early aseptic loosening of prosthetic components and osteolysis. Early radiographic changes suggestive of osteolysis should be thoroughly investigated using plain radiography, and there should be a low threshold for ordering advanced imaging studies such as helical CT or MRI. Any suspicion of wear-induced synovitis should be thoroughly evaluated with MRI with metal artifact suppression techniques, with the goals of early detection and treatment. The initial evaluation of polyethylene wear progression should be made with standard plain radiographs, with concerns regarding accelerated wear being further investigated with CT. Efforts to reduce periprosthetic osteolysis with early detection and nonsurgical management will maximize the efficiency and cost-effectiveness of primary THA.

References

1. Beck RT, Illingworth KD, Saleh KJ: Review of periprosthetic osteolysis in total joint arthroplasty: An emphasis on host factors and future directions. *J Orthop Res* 2012;30(4):541-546.

2. Harris WH: The problem is osteolysis. *Clin Orthop Relat Res* 1995;311:46-53.

3. Strehle J, DelNotaro C, Orler R, Isler B: The outcome of revision hip arthroplasty in patients older than age 80 years: Complications and social outcome of different risk groups. *J Arthroplasty* 2000; 15(6):690-697.

4. Marshall A, Ries MD, Paprosky W; Implant Wear Symposium 2007 Clinical Work Group: How prevalent are implant wear and osteolysis, and how has the scope of osteolysis changed since 2000? *J Am Acad Orthop Surg* 2008; 16(suppl 1):S1-S6.

5. Baker PN, McMurtry IA, Chuter G, Port A, Anderson J: THA with the ABG I prosthesis at 15 years: Excellent survival with minimal osteolysis. *Clin Orthop Relat Res* 2010;468(7):1855-1861.

6. Gallo J, Kamínek P, Tichá V, Riháková P, Ditmar R: Particle disease: A comprehensive theory of periprosthetic osteolysis: A review. *Biomed Pap Med Fac Univ Palacky Olomouc Czech Repub* 2002;146(2):21-28.

7. Jacobs CA, Christensen CP, Berend ME: Sport activity after total hip arthroplasty: Changes in surgical technique, implant design, and rehabilitation. *J Sport Rehabil* 2009;18(1):47-59.

8. Tashjian RZ, Lin C, Aswad B, Terek RM: 11beta-hydroxysteroid dehydrogenase type 1 expression in periprosthetic osteolysis. *Orthopedics* 2008;31(6):545.

9. Talmo CT, Shanbhag AS, Rubash HE: Nonsurgical management of osteolysis: Challenges and opportunities. *Clin Orthop Relat Res* 2006;453:254-264.

10. Saleh KJ, Thongtrangan I, Schwarz EM: Osteolysis: Medical and surgical approaches. *Clin Orthop Relat Res* 2004;427:138-147.

11. Desai MA, Bancroft LW: The case: Diagnosis. Periprosthetic osteolysis. *Orthopedics* 2008; 31(6):518, 615-618.

12. Biomarkers Definitions Working Group: Biomarkers and surrogate endpoints: Preferred definitions and conceptual framework. *Clin Pharmacol Ther* 2001;69(3): 89-95.

13. Antoniou J, Huk O, Zukor D, Eyre D, Alini M: Collagen cross-linked N-telopeptides as markers for evaluating particulate osteolysis: A preliminary study. *J Orthop Res* 2000;18(1):64-67.

14. Schneider U, Breusch SJ, Termath S, et al: Increased urinary cross-link levels in aseptic loosening of total hip arthroplasty. *J Arthroplasty* 1998;13(6):687-692.

15. von Schewelov T, Carlsson A, Dahlberg L: Cross-linked N-telopeptide of type I collagen (NTx) in urine as a predictor of periprosthetic osteolysis. *J Orthop Res* 2006;24(7):1342-1348.

16. Wilkinson JM, Hamer AJ, Rogers A, Stockley I, Eastell R: Bone mineral density and biochemical markers of bone turnover in aseptic loosening after total hip arthroplasty. *J Orthop Res* 2003; 21(4):691-696.

17. Arabmotlagh M, Sabljic R, Rittmeister M: Changes of the biochemical markers of bone turnover and periprosthetic bone remodeling after cemented hip arthroplasty. *J Arthroplasty* 2006; 21(1):129-134.

18. Hernigou P, Intrator L, Bahrami T, Bensussan A, Farcet JP: Interleukin-6 in the blood of patients with total hip arthroplasty without loosening. *Clin Orthop Relat Res* 1999;366:147-154.

19. Fiorito S, Magrini L, Goalard C: Pro-inflammatory and anti-inflammatory circulating cytokines and periprosthetic osteolysis. *J Bone Joint Surg Br* 2003;85(8): 1202-1206.

20. Wu W, Zhang X, Zhang C, Tang T, Ren W, Dai K: Expansion of CD14+CD16+ peripheral monocytes among patients with aseptic loosening. *Inflamm Res* 2009; 58(9):561-570.

21. Roato I, Caldo D, D'Amico L, et al: Osteoclastogenesis in peripheral blood mononuclear cell cultures of periprosthetic osteolysis patients and the phenotype of T cells localized in periprosthetic tissues. *Biomaterials* 2010;31(29): 7519-7525.

22. Savarino L, Avnet S, Greco M, Giunti A, Baldini N: Potential role of tartrate-resistant acid phosphatase 5b (TRACP 5b) as a surrogate marker of late loosening in patients with total hip arthroplasty: A cohort study. *J Orthop Res* 2010;28(7):887-892.

23. Mertens MT, Singh JA: Biomarkers in arthroplasty: A systematic review. *Open Orthop J* 2011;5:92-105.

24. Stulberg BN, Della Valle AG; Implant Wear Symposium 2007 Clinical Work Group: What are the guidelines for the surgical and nonsurgical treatment of peripros-

thetic osteolysis? *J Am Acad Orthop Surg* 2008;16(suppl 1):S20-S25.

25. Vessely MB, Frick MA, Oakes D, Wenger DE, Berry DJ: Magnetic resonance imaging with metal suppression for evaluation of periprosthetic osteolysis after total knee arthroplasty. *J Arthroplasty* 2006;21(6):826-831.

26. Chiang PP, Burke DW, Freiberg AA, Rubash HE: Osteolysis of the pelvis: Evaluation and treatment. *Clin Orthop Relat Res* 2003;417:164-174.

27. Ries MD, Link TM: Monitoring and risk of progression of osteolysis after total hip arthroplasty. *J Bone Joint Surg Am* 2012;94(22):2097-2105.

28. Claus AM, Engh CA Jr, Xenos JS, Orishimo KF, Engh CA Sr: Radiographic definition of pelvic osteolysis following total hip arthroplasty. *J Bone Joint Surg Am* 2003;85(8):1519-1526.

29. Southwell DG, Bechtold JE, Lew WD, Schmidt AH: Improving the detection of acetabular osteolysis using oblique radiographs. *J Bone Joint Surg Br* 1999;81(2):289-295.

30. Cahir JG, Toms AP, Marshall TJ, Wimhurst J, Nolan J: CT and MRI of hip arthroplasty. *Clin Radiol* 2007;62(12):1163-1173.

31. Howie DW, Neale SD, Stamenkov R, McGee MA, Taylor DJ, Findlay DM: Progression of acetabular periprosthetic osteolytic lesions measured with computed tomography. *J Bone Joint Surg Am* 2007;89(8):1818-1825.

32. Kress AM, Schmidt R, Vogel T, Nowak TE, Forst R, Mueller LA: Quantitative computed tomography-assisted osteodensitometry of the pelvis after press-fit cup fixation: A prospective ten-year follow-up. *J Bone Joint Surg Am* 2011;93(12):1152-1157.

33. Malchau H, Potter HG; Implant Wear Symposium 2007 Clinical Work Group: How are wear-related problems diagnosed and what forms of surveillance are necessary? *J Am Acad Orthop Surg* 2008;16(suppl 1):S14-S19.

34. Puri L, Wixson RL, Stern SH, Kohli J, Hendrix RW, Stulberg SD: Use of helical computed tomography for the assessment of acetabular osteolysis after total hip arthroplasty. *J Bone Joint Surg Am* 2002;84(4):609-614.

35. Cook SD, Patron LP, Salkeld SL, Smith KE, Whiting B, Barrack RL: Correlation of computed tomography with histology in the assessment of periprosthetic defect healing. *Clin Orthop Relat Res* 2009;467(12):3213-3220.

36. Leung S, Naudie D, Kitamura N, Walde T, Engh CA: Computed tomography in the assessment of periacetabular osteolysis. *J Bone Joint Surg Am* 2005;87(3):592-597.

37. Schwarz EM, Campbell D, Totterman S, Boyd A, O'Keefe RJ, Looney RJ: Use of volumetric computerized tomography as a primary outcome measure to evaluate drug efficacy in the prevention of peri-prosthetic osteolysis: A 1-year clinical pilot of etanercept vs. placebo. *J Orthop Res* 2003;21(6):1049-1055.

38. Hayter CL, Koff MF, Potter HG: Magnetic resonance imaging of the postoperative hip. *J Magn Reson Imaging* 2012;35(5):1013-1025.

39. Walde TA, Weiland DE, Leung SB, et al: A cadaveric study. *Clin Orthop Relat Res* 2005;437:138-144.

40. Potter HG, Foo LF: Magnetic resonance imaging of joint arthroplasty. *Orthop Clin North Am* 2006;37(3):361-373, vi-vii.

41. Weiland DE, Walde TA, Leung SB, et al: Magnetic resonance imaging in the evaluation of periprosthetic acetabular osteolysis: A cadaveric study. *J Orthop Res* 2005;23(4):713-719.

42. Potter HG, Nestor BJ, Sofka CM, Ho ST, Peters LE, Salvati EA: Magnetic resonance imaging after total hip arthroplasty: Evaluation of periprosthetic soft tissue. *J Bone Joint Surg Am* 2004;86-A(9):1947-1954.

43. Hayter CL, Koff MF, Shah P, Koch KM, Miller TT, Potter HG: MRI after arthroplasty: Comparison of MAVRIC and conventional fast spin-echo techniques. *AJR Am J Roentgenol* 2011;197(3):W405-411.

44. Lieberman JR, Huo MH, Schneider R, Salvati EA, Rodi S: Evaluation of painful hip arthroplasties: Are technetium bone scans necessary? *J Bone Joint Surg Br* 1993;75(3):475-478.

45. Geerdink CH, Grimm B, Rahmy AI, Vencken W, Heyligers IC, Tonino AJ: Correlation of Technetium-99m scintigraphy, progressive acetabular osteolysis and acetabular component loosening in total hip arthroplasty. *Hip Int* 2010;20(4):460-465.

46. Mumme T, Reinartz P, Alfer J, Müller-Rath R, Buell U, Wirtz DC: Diagnostic values of positron emission tomography versus triple-phase bone scan in hip arthroplasty loosening. *Arch Orthop Trauma Surg* 2005;125(5):322-329.

47. Nixon M, Taylor G, Sheldon P, Iqbal SJ, Harper W: Does bone quality predict loosening of cemented total hip replacements? *J Bone Joint Surg Br* 2007;89(10):1303-1308.

48. Wilkie JR, Giger ML, Chinander MR, Engh CA, Hopper RH Jr, Martell JM: Temporal radiographic texture analysis in the detection of periprosthetic osteolysis. *Med Phys* 2008;35(1):377-387.

49. Smith LK, Cramp F, Palmer S, Coghill N, Spencer RF: Use of morphometry to quantify osteolysis after total hip arthroplasty. *Clin Orthop Relat Res* 2010;468(11):3077-3083.

50. Wilkie JR, Giger ML, Engh CA Sr, Martell JM: Radiographic texture analysis in the characterization of trabecular patterns in periprosthetic osteolysis. *Acad Radiol* 2008;15(2):176-185.

51. Rahman L, Cobb J, Muirhead-Allwood S: Radiographic methods of wear analysis in total hip arthroplasty. *J Am Acad Orthop Surg* 2012;20(12):735-743.

52. Dumbleton JH, Manley MT, Edidin AA: A literature review of the association between wear rate and osteolysis in total hip arthroplasty. *J Arthroplasty* 2002;17(5):649-661.

53. Charnley J, Halley DK: Rate of wear in total hip replacement. *Clin Orthop Relat Res* 1975;112:170-179.

54. Charnley J, Cupic Z: The nine and ten year results of the low-friction arthroplasty of the hip. *Clin Orthop Relat Res* 1973;95:9-25.

55. Selvik G: Roentgen stereophotogrammetry: A method for the study of the kinematics of the skeletal system. *Acta Orthop Scand Suppl* 1989;232:1-51.

56. Olivecrona L, Jedenmalm A, Aspelin P, et al: An ex vivo study. *Acta Radiol* 2005;46(8):852-857.

57. Jedenmalm A, Noz ME, Olivecrona H, Olivecrona L, Stark A: A new approach for assessment of wear in metal-backed acetabular cups using computed tomography: A phantom study with retrievals. *Acta Orthop* 2008;79(2):218-224.

58. Bhandari M, Bajammal S, Guyatt GH, et al: Effect of bisphosphonates on periprosthetic bone mineral density after total joint arthroplasty: A meta-analysis. *J Bone Joint Surg Am* 2005;87(2):293-301.

59. Friedl G, Radl R, Stihsen C, Rehak P, Aigner R, Windhager R: The effect of a single infusion of zoledronic acid on early implant migration in total hip arthroplasty: A randomized, double-blind, controlled trial. *J Bone Joint Surg Am* 2009;91(2):274-281.

60. Goh SK, Yang KY, Koh JS, et al: A caution. *J Bone Joint Surg Br* 2007;89(3):349-353.

61. Kwek EB, Goh SK, Koh JS, Png MA, Howe TS: An emerging pattern of subtrochanteric stress fractures: A long-term complication of alendronate therapy? *Injury* 2008;39(2):224-231.

62. Lenart BA, Neviaser AS, Lyman S, et al: A case control study. *Osteoporos Int* 2009;20(8):1353-1362.

63. Neviaser AS, Lane JM, Lenart BA, Edobor-Osula F, Lorich DG: Low-energy femoral shaft fractures associated with alendronate use. *J Orthop Trauma* 2008;22(5):346-350.

64. Odvina CV, Zerwekh JE, Rao DS, Maalouf N, Gottschalk FA, Pak CY: Severely suppressed bone turnover: A potential complication of alendronate therapy. *J Clin Endocrinol Metab* 2005;90(3):1294-1301.

65. Burr DB, Forwood MR, Fyhrie DP, Martin RB, Schaffler MB, Turner CH: Review: Bone microdamage and skeletal fragility in osteoporotic and stress fractures. *J Bone Miner Res* 1997;12(1):6-15.

66. Martin BR: The role of bone remodeling in preventing or promoting stress fractures, in Burr DB, Milgrom C, eds: *Musculoskeletal Fatigue and Stress Fractures.* Boca Raton, FL, CRC Press, 2001, pp 183-202.

67. Schaffler MB: Bone fatigue and remodeling in the development of stress fractures, in Burr DB, Milgrom C, eds: *Musculoskeletal Fatigue and Stress Fractures.* Boca Raton, FL, CRC Press, 2001, pp 161-182.

68. St Pierre CA, Chan M, Iwakura Y, Ayers DC, Kurt-Jones EA, Finberg RW: Periprosthetic osteolysis: Characterizing the innate immune response to titanium wear-particles. *J Orthop Res* 2010;28(11):1418-1424.

69. Schwarz EM; Implant Wear Symposium 2007 Biologic Work Group: What potential biologic treatments are available for osteolysis? *J Am Acad Orthop Surg* 2008;16(suppl 1):S72-S75.

70. Schwarz EM, Ritchlin CT: Clinical development of anti-RANKL therapy. *Arthritis Res Ther* 2007;9(suppl 1):S7.

71. Abu-Amer Y, Darwech I, Clohisy JC: Aseptic loosening of total joint replacements: Mechanisms underlying osteolysis and potential therapies. *Arthritis Res Ther* 2007;9(suppl 1):S6.

17

Maximizing Function and Outcomes in Acetabular Reconstruction: Segmental Bony Defects and Pelvic Discontinuity

David Pope, MD
Stuart Blankenship, MD
GaToya Jones, BS
Brooke S. Robinson, MPH
William J. Maloney, MD
Wayne G. Paprosky, MD
Michael D. Ries, MD
Khaled J. Saleh, BSc, MD, MSc, FRCS(C), MHCM

Abstract

Acetabular reconstruction in revision total hip arthroplasty can be complicated by acetabular bone loss. In patients with severe acetabular bone deficiency with segmental bone defects or pelvic discontinuity, obtaining a stable, well-fixed acetabular component can be challenging. Although porous-coated, uncemented hemispheric cups can be used in most acetabular revisions, as the severity of acetabular deficiency increases, more complex alternatives are needed. Antiprotrusio cages have traditionally been used in the presence of acetabular columnar deficits, but higher failure rates and complications necessitated the development of alternative treatments. More recently, porous-coated acetabular augments have become an attractive alternative to structural allograft and oblong components when segmental bone loss is present. In the setting of severe bone loss or pelvic discontinuity, multiple reconstructive options are available. Depending on individual patient characteristics, plating of the pelvic discontinuity along with structural allografts, custom components, and modular or standard reconstructive cages can be used to obtain a stable acetabular component.

Instr Course Lect 2014;63:187-197.

Approximately 36,000 revision total hip arthroplasties (THAs) were performed in the United States in 2005, and that number is estimated to increase to 96,700 per year by 2030.[1]

Acetabular revision is one of the most challenging procedures in orthopaedic surgery and is associated with a substantial risk of complications. It can be difficult to achieve a stable, well-fixed

acetabular component in acetabular revisions with severe bone loss and/or pelvic discontinuity. Although each revision procedure must be individualized and no single method is appropriate for all patients, the focus of this chapter is to provide information for maximizing function and outcomes for acetabular reconstruction of segmental defects or pelvic discontinuity in revision THA. Impaction grafting, structural allografts, metal augments, hemispheric cups, antiprotrusio cages, and patient-specific triflanged components are discussed.

Classifying Bone Defects

Several classification systems have been developed to quantify the amount and location of acetabular bone loss in revision THA.[2-6] The American Academy of Orthopaedic Surgeons (AAOS) classification for acetabular defects is one such system.[2,3] This classification is di-

Table 1

AAOS Classification System for Acetabular Defects

Type	Description
I	Segmental defect
II	Cavitary defect
III	Combined segmental and cavitary defect
IV	Pelvic discontinuity
IVa	Discontinuity with mild segmental or cavitary bone loss
IVb	Discontinuity with moderate to severe segmental or cavitary bone loss
IVc	Discontinuity with prior pelvic irradiation
V	Hip arthrodesis

AAOS = American Academy of Orthopaedic Surgeons.

vided into five types and describes the pattern of acetabular bone loss (**Table 1**); however, it is not as descriptive as some other systems with regard to the location and the size of the defect and is less helpful in guiding treatment.

The Saleh and Gross classification system for acetabular defects also is divided into five types based on the amount of bone loss seen on preoperative AP and lateral radiographs.[4,5] It describes the defect as being contained or uncontained based on the ability of morcellized bone graft to fill the defect.

The Paprosky classification system for acetabular defects is divided into three types, with subdivisions based on four radiographic criteria from an AP pelvic radiograph: (1) superior migration of the hip center, (2) ischial osteolysis, (3) position of the implant relative to the Köhler line, and (4) acetabular teardrop osteolysis[6] (**Fig-ure 1**). Differences in the affected radiographic locations help to anatomically determine the area of acetabular deficiency and may predict the ability to obtain cementless fixation. Superior migration of the hip suggests bone loss of the acetabular dome involving the anterior and posterior columns. Superior and medial migration indicates greater involvement of the anterior column. Superior and lateral migration indicates involvement of the posterior column. Ischial osteolysis represents bone loss from the posterior column and wall. Teardrop osteolysis indicates bone loss from the medial and inferior acetabulum, including the inferior aspect of the anterior column, the lateral aspect of the pubis, and the medial wall. Migration of the prosthesis medial to the Köhler line represents medial acetabular bone loss and anterior column loss. The Köhler line is defined as a line connecting the pelvic brim and the most lateral aspect of the obturator foramen on an AP radiograph of the pelvis. The Paprosky classification is useful as a clinical predictor of acetabular bone loss and can guide treatment with regard to reconstructive options. (More information on classifications systems for acetabular defects is available in *Instructional Course Lectures, Volume 63*, chapter 19 [Advances in Acetabular Reconstruction in Revision Total Hip Arthroplasty: Maximizing Function and Outcomes After Treatment of Periacetabular Osteolysis Around the Well-Fixed Shell.]).

Bone Grafting

Bone grafting is common in acetabular revision surgery. The type of bone graft ranges from morcellized allograft or autograft used in impaction grafting to bulk allograft used in major column revision in the presence of larger acetabular defects.

Impaction Grafting

The technique of impaction grafting using allograft was first developed in the Netherlands and England and has been used as a biologic method of restoring bone stock in acetabular revision surgery. The technique involves the progressive compaction of allograft chips into the acetabular defect, followed by cementing of the prosthesis. This technique creates a three-layer matrix of graft, cement, and implant (**Figure 2**).

van Haaren et al[7] reported on the results of 71 acetabular revisions with impaction grafting, with an average

Dr. Maloney or an immediate family member has received royalties from Wright Medical Technology; serves as a paid consultant to or is an employee of Pipeline Orthopaedics; has stock or stock options held in Abbott, Gillead, ISTO Technologies, Johnson & Johnson, Merck, Moximed, Pfizer, Pipeline Orthopaedics, and TJO; and serves as a board member, owner, officer, or committee member of the American Joint Replacement Registry, The Knee Society, and the Western Orthopaedic Association. Dr. Paprosky or an immediate family member has received royalties from Wright Medical Technology and Zimmer; is a member of a speakers' bureau or has made paid presentations on behalf of Zimmer; serves as a paid consultant to or is an employee of Biomet and Zimmer; and serves as a board member, owner, officer, or committee member of The Hip Society. Dr. Ries or an immediate family member has received royalties from Smith & Nephew; serves as a paid consultant to or is an employee of Smith & Nephew and Stryker; has stock or stock options held in OrthAlign; and serves as a board member, owner, officer, or committee member of the Foundation for the Advancement of Research in Medicine. Dr. Saleh or an immediate family member has received royalties from Aesculap/B. Braun; is a member of a speakers' bureau or has made paid presentations on behalf of Carefusion; serves as a paid consultant to Aesculap/B. Braun, the Memorial Medical Center Co-Management Orthopaedic Board, and the Blue Cross Blue Shield Blue Ribbon Panel; has received research or institutional support from Smith & Nephew, the Orthopaedic Research and Education Foundation, and the National Institutes of Health/National Institute of Arthritis and Musculoskeletal Skin Diseases (R0-1); and serves as a board member, owner, officer, or committee member of the American Orthopaedic Association and the Orthopaedic Research and Education Foundation. None of the following authors or any immediate family member has received anything of value from or has stock or stock options held in a commercial company or institution related directly or indirectly to the subject of this chapter: Dr. Pope, Dr. Blankenship, Ms. Jones, and Ms. Robinson.

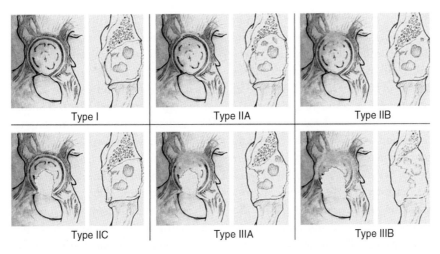

Figure 1 Illustrations of acetabular bone loss based on the Paprosky classification system. Type I acetabular bone loss has an intact rim with no distortion and intact columns. Type IIA has superomedial bone loss with intact columns and superior migration of less than 3 cm on radiographs. Type IIB has an uncontained superior rim defect of less than one third around the acetabulum but host bone contact of greater than 50%. Type IIC has a medial wall defect and a cup medial to the Köhler line. Type IIIA has superolateral cup migration and partial teardrop destruction on radiographic imaging, with an unsupportive dome intraoperatively. Type IIIB has severe ischial destruction, teardrop loss, and migration medial to the Köhler line on radiographic imaging, with pelvic discontinuity intraoperatively. (Reproduced with permission from Deirmengian GK, Zmistowski B, O'Neil JT, Hozack WJ: Management of acetabular bone loss in revision total hip arthroplasty. *J Bone Joint Surg Am* 2011;93(19):1842-1852.)

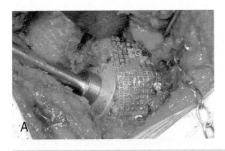 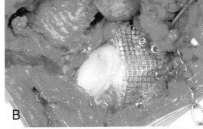

Figure 2 Intraoperative photographs showing (**A**) the last impactor, which is 4 mm larger than the definitive cup to allow for a circumferential 2-mm cement mantle, and (**B**) the definitive implanted cup. (Reproduced with permission from Buttaro MA, Comba F, Pusso R, Piccaluga F: Acetabular revision with metal mesh, impaction bone grafting, and a cemented cup. *Clin Orthop Relat Res* 2008;466(10):2482-2490.)

follow-up of 7.2 years. Twenty components required repeat revision for aseptic loosening, and component survival was 72% at the final follow-up. Seventy percent of the failed components had an AAOS type III or type IV defect.

Garcia-Cimbrelo et al[8] reported on a retrospective review of 165 patients (181 hips) treated with revision and

impaction grafting for major acetabular bone loss. Ninety-eight patients with type IIIA and 83 patients with type IIIB defects, according to the Paprosky system, were included. Minimal follow-up was 0.3 years, with an average follow-up of 7.5 years. The revision survival rate was 84% at 8 years for type IIIA defects and 82% for type IIIB defects. Twelve hips were rerevised for all causes, and 17 grafts showed bone resorption. Overall, the midterm results from this study showed promising results for impaction grafting in larger defects.

Graft Extenders

In addition to the use of morcellized allograft in impaction grafting, there has been interest in bone graft extenders, such as tricalcium phosphate and hydroxyapatite, to minimize the use of donor bone in revision surgery. These graft extenders may play a role in the treatment of pelvic discontinuity to stimulate union. Because of the risk of pathogen transmission and the cost and potential shortage of allografts, there is interest in allograft alternatives.[9-11] van Haaren et al[12] reported on the use of tricalcium phosphate and hydroxyapatite as bone graft extenders in impaction grafting in a human cadaver model. A tricalcium phosphate/hydroxyapatite allograft mix increased the risk of producing periprosthetic fractures in the femur during the impaction procedure but provided higher initial mechanical stability when compared with bone grafting alone.

Jacofsky et al[13] compared the biomechanical strength of calcium phosphate cement and reamed allograft in nine cadaver pelves. After a defect was created, it was filled with cement or allograft, reamed, and an uncemented component was placed. Biomechanical cycling was performed. Cemented defects lasted more cycles before failure and had greater stability and stiffness than the allograft-filled defects. These study results need verification from additional studies before reliable conclusions on their utility can be drawn.

Bulk Allograft

Bulk or structural allograft is also used in acetabular revisions. Structural allograft is most commonly used in Paprosky type IIIA defects because the severe bone loss necessitates additional structural support to obtain stability. Commonly, structural allograft is used in conjunction with a cementless acetabular implant, although this technique is also described with a cemented cup or cage. Because metal augments are becoming more popular, the use of structural allografts has declined.

The results of structural allograft in acetabular revision have been mixed. Lee et al[14] reported on a retrospective review of 74 patients (85 hips) treated with acetabular cup revision using minor column allografts. The allograft was used in uncontained acetabular defects involving 30% to 50% of the acetabulum. The minimum follow-up was 5 years (mean, 16 years). Twenty-three patients (27 hips) underwent a repeat revision for all causes. Cup survivorship was 61% and 55% at 15 and 20 years, respectively, with revision for any cause as the end point. Fifteen of the grafts failed, with an average time to failure of 6 years. With aseptic loosening as the end point, cup survivorship was 67% and 61% at 15 and 20 years, respectively.

Paprosky et al[15] treated 48 patients with type IIIA defects with a distal femoral allograft and a porous hemispheric shell. The initial survival rate of the shell was 94% at a mean follow-up of 6.1 years, with aseptic loosening as the end point. The results at an average 10-year follow-up for the same cohort found five components that re-

quired rerevision for aseptic loosening at an average of 5.3 years after the index procedure; however, the rerevisions did not require additional allograft. The allograft was believed to be effective in converting a type IIIA defect to a type II defect.[16] (More information on graft extenders and bone grafting in revision THA is available in *Instructional Course Lecture, Volume 63*, chapter 20 [Acetabular Reconstruction in Revision Total Hip Arthroplasty: Maximizing Function and Outcomes in Protrusio and Cavitary Defects.]).

Components
Hemispheric Cup

A cementless, hemispheric cup is the most common implant used in acetabular revision and is the first-line treatment for patients with type I, II, and IIIA defects, although type IIIA defects sometimes require augmentation as previously described.[17-19] Cemented implants have lost favor because of poor results compared with uncemented cups.[20-25] Tantalum implants boast a high volumetric porosity (ranging from 70% to 80%), a low modulus of elasticity, and a three-dimensional structure composed of a series of interconnected pores averaging 550 µm in diameter.[26] Tantalum has high frictional characteristics, with surface friction 40% to 75% higher than that of conventional porous coatings.[27] Encouraging short-term and midterm success has been reported in treating Paprosky type IIA to IIIB defects with these constructs.[18,28-33]

Jafari et al[34] retrospectively reviewed 283 patients treated with acetabular revision using either a hydroxyapatite-coated titanium cup or a porous tantalum cup. Although mechanical loosening was similar between the groups with minor acetabular deficiencies, a higher failure rate was reported in the group treated with the ti-

tanium cup (12% versus 24% with the tantalum cup) in patients with major acetabular bony deficiencies. In failed revisions, 80% of the tantalum cups failed before 6 months, whereas 80% of titanium cups failed after 6 months. The authors attributed this finding to a lack of bony ingrowth in the group with a titanium cup. Lachiewicz and Poon[35] reported on the use of an uncemented, titanium fiber, metal-coated hemispheric component with multiple screws in acetabular revisions in 56 patients, 21 of whom had AAOS type III defects. At an average follow-up of 5 years, they reported excellent implant survivorship with no radiographic evidence of loosening. Hydroxyapatite-coated shells should be used with caution in acetabular revisions because multiple studies have reported high failure rates.[36-38]

Jumbo Cups

If bone stock is limited (typically, Paprosky type IIIA or, potentially, Paprosky type IIIB defects), hemispheric cups with diameters greater than 66 mm for men and 62 mm for women can be used; these have been called jumbo cups.[39] By using a larger component, the contact area between the bone and the implant is maximized, the socket is filled, and the need for bone grafting is minimized. Hip biomechanics are also restored to a more anatomic position because the center of hip rotation is shifted both inferiorly and laterally. However, this concept has recently been challenged by Ries et al,[40] who used an in vitro computer and radiographic simulation to evaluate the position of the acetabular component. The authors found that as the reamer size increased, the hip center was shifted laterally, anteriorly, and superiorly. Radiographic analyses estimated that the hip joint center was elevated an average of 9.7 mm in males and 7.5 mm in females. Ries et al[40] recommended reaming inferiorly to the level of the obturator foramen to help maintain a more anatomic position of the acetabular component. Other drawbacks of a larger cup include permanent loss of bone stock and the inability of the component to fill oblong deficiencies in the superior-inferior plane without iatrogenic removal of remaining host bone.

Rees et al[41] reviewed 107 acetabular revisions using jumbo cups without bone grafting; 64 hips had moderate to severe bone loss based on the classification system developed by Saleh et al.[4] Of the 53 patients available for final follow-up at an average of 75.2 months, 3 patients had mechanical implant failure at an average of 13.3 months after revision; 1 of these patients had preoperative pelvic discontinuity and implant failure caused by acetabular migration into the pelvis. The other two patients with mechanical failures had type IV preoperative defects based on the system developed by Saleh et al;[4] implant failure was caused by loosening. Kaplan-Meier survivorship was 96.9% at 1 year and 95.2% at final follow-up.

Whaley et al[39] reported on acetabular revisions using jumbo cups in 89 hips at an average follow-up of 7.2 years. Most of the hips had combined segmental and cavitary acetabular bone loss prior to revision. Four patients required rerevisions, two for aseptic loosening. Two other patients had radiographic evidence of loosening, but rerevisions were not needed. Overall, the 8-year acetabular component survival rate was 93% with implant removal for any reason as the end point and 95% using radiographic evidence of loosening or revision for aseptic loosening as the end point.

Oblong Cups

With substantial superior migration of the acetabular component and the subsequent bone loss seen at the time of revision surgery, an oblong implant can return the hip center to a more anatomic position and fill the superior acetabular defect. Oblong components are expensive and technically more challenging to implant than standard hemispheric components. Because mixed results have been reported with failure rates ranging from none to 24% at midterm follow-up, these implants are rarely used in contemporary practice.[42-47]

Metal Augments

Uncemented, porous-coated acetabular components have greatly improved the survival rate of acetabular components in revision THAs. Using porous-coated metal augments in conjunction with these components has become popular in recent years. Metal augments fill cavitary defects, bring the hip center to a more anatomic position, allow biologic fixation, and are an attractive alternative to bulk allograft or oblong components.

Metal augments in conjunction with porous-coated acetabular components have shown promising results in treating large bony defects. Sporer and Paprosky[18] reported on 28 patients with Paprosky type IIIA defects (average follow-up of 3.1 years) who were treated with revision surgery using porous metal acetabular components and augments (**Figure 3**). One patient required revision for recurrent instability, and the other patients had stable implants. In another study, Weeden and Paprosky[19] reported on 43 patients after acetabular revision for Paprosky type IIIA or IIIB defects. Twenty-six patients received tantalum augments for bone loss. At a mean follow-up of 2.8 years, 1 component failed because of septic loosening, and 42 implants were stable (**Figure 4**).

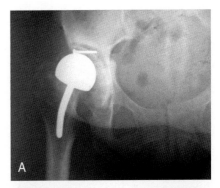
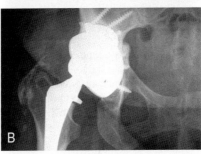

Figure 3 **A,** Preoperative radiograph of the hip of a 68-year-old woman with a type IIIA acetabular defect. **B,** Postoperative radiograph shows stable fixation achieved with a trabecular metal acetabular component and a superior augment. (Reproduced with permission from Sporer SM, Paprosky WG: The use of a trabecular metal acetabular component and trabecular metal augment for severe acetabular defects. *J Arthroplasty* 2006;21(6, suppl 2):83-86.)

Antiprotrusio Cages

For Paprosky type III defects in which stability is not possible with a porous-coated hemispheric component, an antiprotrusio cage, typically in conjunction with morcellized or structural bone graft or porous metal augments, can be used.[48] Antiprotrusio cages are typically available with varying combinations of ischial and iliac flanges, as well as an obturator hook. Historically, these cages were not porous coated, but porous-coated cages are now available that allow bony ingrowth. The cage is fixed to the pelvis with screws through the dome and the iliac flange. The ischial flange can either be fixed

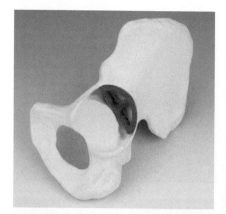

Figure 4 Photograph of an augment used to fill a cavitary defect and lower the hip center. (Reproduced with permission from Sporer SM: How to do a revision total hip arthroplasty: Revision of the acetabulum. *J Bone Joint Surg Am* 2011;93(14):1359-1366.)

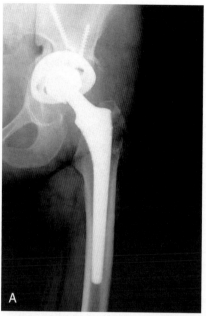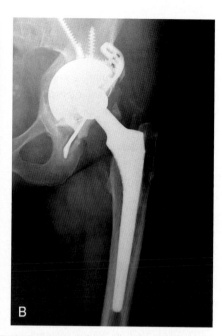

Figure 5 **A,** AP radiograph of the hip of a 65-year-old woman who presented with a loose uncemented cup and associated pelvic discontinuity. **B,** Postoperative radiograph taken 8 years after reconstruction with a cup-cage construct and morcellized bone grafting shows healing of the pelvic discontinuity. (Courtesy of Allan Gross, MD, Toronto, Ontario, Canada.)

with screws or press fit directly into the ischium.[49] A polyethylene cup can then be cemented into the cage at the appropriate abduction and anteversion. The cage can be cemented directly to the acetabulum to provide extra fixation.[50]

Regardless of the chosen fixation method, cages require an extensive approach for successful implantation. Advantages of the antiprotrusio cage include restoration of bone stock through bone grafting and return of the hip center to a nearly anatomic position. Even with these theoretic advantages, component survival rates at midterm follow-up have been lower than ideal, particularly in patients with large defects and pelvic discontinuity.[48,50,51]

Symeonides et al[52] reviewed 55 patients (57 hips) with acetabular deficiency treated with a Burch-Schneider antiprotrusio cage and bone grafting. At a mean follow-up of 11.5 years, the authors reported two hips with aseptic loosening and four hips with mechanical failure. Winter et al[53] also reported

no failures in 38 hips revised with a Burch-Schneider ring for AAOS type III and IV acetabular defects at an average follow-up of 7.3 years. Hansen et al[50] cemented the cage into the acetabulum in an attempt to decrease mechanical failure in 35 acetabular THA revisions with Paprosky type III defects or pelvic discontinuity. At an average follow-up of 59 months, 6 of 35 revisions required rerevision for loosening, and radiographic loosening was present in 2 other implants. Bostrom et al[54] evaluated 31 acetabular revisions in hips with Paprosky type IIB to type IIIB acetabular defects using the Contour cage (Smith & Nephew), which boasts a grit-blasted undersurface to theoretically allow more bony ingrowth. Two hips (7%) were revised for loosening, 16% showed radiographic signs of loosening, and only 45% had good or excellent clinical results at a mean follow-up of 30 months.[54] The success of hemi-

spheric cups in acetabular revision in patients with substantial bone loss, the advent of newer technologies that allow for bony ingrowth, and the success of custom triflange components have decreased the indications for antiprotrusio cages.[55]

Cup-Cage Constructs

Cup-cage combination constructs pair an antiprotrusio cage with a porous metal cup to encourage ingrowth and subsequent long-term stability (**Figure 5**). A porous metal cup is first placed into the acetabulum and followed by a cage, which is laid into the cup to increase the biomechanical strength of the construct until osteointegration of the porous metal cup occurs. Kosashvili et al[56] reviewed 26 hips treated with acetabular revision using a cup-cage construct with a mean follow-up of 44.6 months. Twenty-three of 26 hips showed no radiologic loosening at last follow-up.

Potential disadvantages of the cup-cage construct include unknown long-term durability and potential wear debris from the cage-cup interface.

Custom Triflanged Components

Custom triflanged components provide another good option for acetabular revision in patients with massive bone loss and/or pelvic discontinuity. These components are typically made of titanium, are porous- and/or hydroxyapatite-coated, and are reverse engineered via stereolithography from a model of the patient's hemipelvis based on preoperative three-dimensional CT reconstructions. The implant design typically consists of a dome centered in the acetabular defect, with three custom flanges augmented with 6.5-mm screws specifically designed to take advantage of the support provided by the remaining ilium, ischium, and pubis[57] (**Figure 6**).

Typically, a standard posterior surgical approach is used.[58,59] Placement of the component typically begins by flexing, abducting, and proximally shifting the hip to relax the abductor and facilitate placement of the iliac flange. Ischial and pubic flanges can then be rotated into place while extending the hip. Screw fixation begins in the ischium, which typically has the poorest quality bone. Augmentation may be considered if severe osteolysis is present both in the ischium and at the site of discontinuity.[59] The iliac flange can then be fixed with screws, which often reduces the discontinuity. The pubic flange does not usually support screw fixation, but porous metal on the backside of the flange supports ingrowth. Either a standard liner or, if stability is uncertain because of the integrity of the greater trochanter, a constrained liner can be locked into the flange. Postoperatively, patients should be kept at partial weight bearing for 6 to 8 weeks.[58,59]

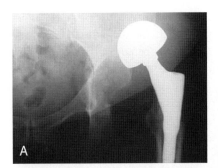
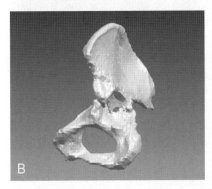
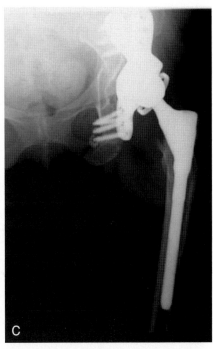

Figure 6 **A,** Preoperative AP radiograph of a failed acetabular component with pelvic discontinuity. **B,** Three-dimensional CT reconstruction of the acetabular defect. **C,** Postoperative radiograph of a triflanged component. (Reproduced with permission from Taunton MJ, Fehring TK, Edwards P, Bernasek T, Holt GE, Christie MJ: Pelvic discontinuity treated with custom triflanged component: A reliable option. *Clin Orthop Relat Res* 2012;470:428-434.)

The disadvantages of using custom triflanged components are that it takes approximately 4 to 8 weeks to make the implant, and the component cannot be modified intraoperatively if it does not fit appropriately. Another increasingly important concern is cost; however, Taunton et al[60] reported that the costs of custom triflanged components, cup-cage components, and cup-augment constructs were comparable.

Outcomes for custom triflanged components have been promising given the complex nature of the revision procedure. Taunton et al[60] retrospectively reviewed 57 patients with pelvic discontinuity treated with a custom triflange component. They reported that 54 of 57 patients had successful outcomes and were free of additional revision. Christie et al[58] retrospectively reviewed 76 patients (78 hips) treated with a custom trif-

langed component for severe bone loss or pelvic discontinuity. At an average follow-up of 53 months, 67 hips were available for review. The authors reported that no components had been removed, and Harris hip scores improved from 33.3 preoperatively to 82.1 postoperatively. Six patients had repeat revision surgery for recurrent dislocations.

DeBoer et al[59] reported on 20 hip revisions in 18 patients treated with a custom triflange component used for the treatment of a pelvic discontinuity (mean follow-up of 123 months). Mean Harris hip scores improved 39 points postoperatively, and no component needed rerevision. Holt and Dennis[57] retrospectively reviewed 26 patients who had massive periacetabular bone loss (Paprosky type IIIB) reconstructed with custom triflanged components and found that 23 of 26 hips were considered clinically successful at an average of 54 months. Three failures occurred because of the loss of ischial fixation. Joshi et al[61] reviewed 27 patients fitted with a custom triflanged acetabular component and reported 6 complications, including 2 wound infections (1 required implant removal and conversion to a Girdlestone pseudarthrosis), 2 partial sciatic nerve palsies, 1 complete sciatic nerve palsy, and 1 postoperative dislocation.

Plating

Plating of severe acetabular defects in conjunction with reconstruction cages or allografts is an alternative option in patients with pelvic discontinuity, although high complication and failure rates have been reported.[62,63] In a study by Stiehl et al,[62] 10 of 17 patients had pelvic discontinuity and were treated with structural allografts and plating. At 83 months, the implant survival rate was 50%, and the complication rate was 60%.

Pelvic Discontinuity

Pelvic discontinuity is defined as the separation of the cephalad aspect of the pelvis from the caudad aspect resulting from either traumatic injury or bone loss.[59] This challenging disorder is often encountered in revision THA in the setting of osteolysis, infection, or fracture. Diagnosing of pelvic discontinuity may be difficult because radiodense cement and implants can obscure the view of the underlying bone. The standard preoperative evaluation includes an AP pelvic radiograph and Judet oblique views to evaluate the anterior and posterior columns. Bone loss may involve both columns of the pelvis, or there may be a medial shift or rotation of the caudad hemipelvis in relationship to the cephalad hemipelvis. This results in disruption of the Köhler line and can cause asymmetry in the appearance of the obturator fo-

ramen on a standard AP pelvic radiograph.[64] If the diagnosis remains unclear, a preoperative CT scan may help determine the location and the amount of bone loss.[65] However, even with the available imaging techniques, some cases of severe bone loss may be diagnosed intraoperatively.

The treatment of pelvic discontinuity can be challenging and is dependent on the remaining host bone, the potential for healing of the discontinuity, and the potential for biologic ingrowth of acetabular components.[66] Because of the inherent lack of implant stability within the deficient acetabulum in patients with pelvic discontinuity, columnar fixation is often necessary to obtain adequate implant stability for ingrowth of the revision component and healing of the discontinuity to occur. Although anterior column fixation is not always feasible and the focus of most implant design has largely been posterior column fixation, bicolumnar fixation may be beneficial. Gililland et al[67] showed that bicolumnar fixation using a posterior column plate construct with an antegrade 4.5-mm anterior column screw provided a more stable construct when working with a composite hemipelvis compared with posterior column fixation alone.

Summary

Acetabular revision because of severe bone loss and pelvic discontinuity is likely to increase in frequency with the performance of more primary THAs. Although these revision surgeries will remain technically challenging, the development of porous metals, which encourage bony ingrowth into the prosthesis, has shown excellent results and will play a larger role in revision hip surgery. The hemispheric cup with some type of bone graft or metal augment will remain the workhorse in revision surgery, but custom triflanged

components appear to be an excellent option in patients who do not have sufficient bone stock to support a hemispheric component.

References

1. Kurtz S, Ong K, Lau E, Mowat F, Halpern M: Projections of primary and revision hip and knee arthroplasty in the United States from 2005 to 2030. *J Bone Joint Surg Am* 2007;89(4):780-785.

2. D'Antonio JA, Capello WN, Borden LS, et al: Classification and management of acetabular abnormalities in total hip arthroplasty. *Clin Orthop Relat Res* 1989;243: 126-137.

3. D'Antonio JA: Periprosthetic bone loss of the acetabulum: Classification and management. *Orthop Clin North Am* 1992;23(2): 279-290.

4. Saleh KJ, Holtzman J, Gafni A, Saleh L, et al: Development, test reliability and validation of a classification for revision hip arthroplasty. *J Orthop Res* 2001;19(1): 50-56.

5. Saleh KJ, Holtzman J, Gafni A, et al: Reliability and intraoperative validity of preoperative assessment of standardized plain radiographs in predicting bone loss at revision hip surgery. *J Bone Joint Surg Am* 2001;83(7):1040-1046.

6. Paprosky WG, Perona PG, Lawrence JM: Acetabular defect classification and surgical reconstruction in revision arthroplasty: A 6-year follow-up evaluation. *J Arthroplasty* 1994;9(1):33-44.

7. van Haaren EH, Heyligers IC, Alexander FG, Wuisman PI: High rate of failure of impaction grafting in large acetabular defects. *J Bone Joint Surg Br* 2007;89(3): 296-300.

8. Garcia-Cimbrelo E, Cruz-Pardos A, Garcia-Rey E, Ortega-Chamarro J: The survival and fate

of acetabular reconstruction with impaction grafting for large defects. *Clin Orthop Relat Res* 2010; 468(12):3304-3313.

9. Sugihara S, van Ginkel AD, Jiya TU, van Royen BJ, van Diest PJ, Wuisman PI: Histopathology of retrieved allografts of the femoral head. *J Bone Joint Surg Br* 1999; 81(2):336-341.

10. Cook SD, Salkeld SL, Prewett AB: Simian immunodeficiency virus (human HIV-II) transmission in allograft bone procedures. *Spine (Phila Pa 1976)* 1995; 20(12):1338-1342.

11. Conrad EU, Gretch DR, Obermeyer KR, et al: Transmission of the hepatitis-C virus by tissue transplantation. *J Bone Joint Surg Am* 1995;77(2):214-224.

12. van Haaren EH, Smit TH, Phipps K, Wuisman PI, Blunn G, Heyligers IC: Tricalcium-phosphate and hydroxyapatite bone-graft extender for use in impaction grafting revision surgery: An in vitro study on human femora. *J Bone Joint Surg Br* 2005; 87(2):267-271.

13. Jacofsky DJ, McCamley JD, Jaczynski AM, Shrader MW, Jacofsky MC: Improving initial acetabular component stability in revision total hip arthroplasty calcium phosphate cement vs reverse reamed cancellous allograft. *J Arthroplasty* 2012;27(2): 305-309.

14. Lee PT, Raz G, Safir OA, Backstein DJ, Gross AE: Long-term results for minor column allografts in revision hip arthroplasty. *Clin Orthop Relat Res* 2010; 468(12):3295-3303.

15. Paprosky WG, Bradford MS, Jablonsky WS: Acetabular reconstruction with massive acetabular allografts. *Instr Course Lect* 1996; 45:149-159.

16. Sporer SM, O'Rourke M, Chong P, Paprosky WG: The use of structural distal femoral allografts for acetabular reconstruction: Average ten-year follow-up. *J Bone Joint Surg Am* 2005;87(4): 760-765.

17. Sporer SM, Paprosky WG, O'Rourke MR: Managing bone loss in acetabular revision. *Instr Course Lect* 2006;55:287-297.

18. Sporer SM, Paprosky WG: The use of a trabecular metal acetabular component and trabecular metal augment for severe acetabular defects. *J Arthroplasty* 2006; 21(6):83-86.

19. Weeden SH, Paprosky WG: Porous-ingrowth revision acetabular implants secured with peripheral screws: A minimum twelve-year follow-up. *J Bone Joint Surg Am* 2006;88(6):1266-1271.

20. Pulido L, Rachala SR, Cabanela ME: Cementless acetabular revision: Past, present, and future. Revision total hip arthroplasty: the acetabular side using cementless implants. *Int Orthop* 2011; 35(2):289-298.

21. Kavanagh BF, Ilstrup DM, Fitzgerald RH Jr: Revision total hip arthroplasty. *J Bone Joint Surg Am* 1985;67(4):517-526.

22. Callaghan JJ, Salvati EA, Pellicci PM, Wilson PD Jr, Ranawat CS: Results of revision for mechanical failure after cemented total hip replacement, 1979 to 1982: A two to five-year follow-up. *J Bone Joint Surg Am* 1985;67(7):1074-1085.

23. Katz RP, Callaghan JJ, Sullivan PM, Johnston RC: Long-term results of revision total hip arthroplasty with improved cementing technique. *J Bone Joint Surg Br* 1997;79(2):322-326.

24. Lie SA, Havelin LI, Furnes ON, Engesaeter LB, Vollset SE: Failure rates for 4762 revision total hip arthroplasties in the Norwegian Arthroplasty Register. *J Bone Joint Surg Br* 2004;86(4):504-509.

25. Sternheim A, Abolghasemian M, Safir OA, Backstein D, Gross AE, Kuzyk PR: A long-term survivorship comparison between cemented and uncemented cups with shelf grafts in revision total hip arthroplasty after dysplasia. *J Arthroplasty* 2013;28(2): 303-308.

26. Levine B, Della Valle CJ, Jacobs JJ: Applications of porous tantalum in total hip arthroplasty. *J Am Acad Orthop Surg* 2006;14(12): 646-655.

27. Zhang Y, Ahn PB, Fitzpatrick DC: Interfacial frictional behavior: Cancellous bone, cortical bone, and a novel porous tantalum biomaterial. *J Musc Res* 1999; 81:907-914.

28. Sporer SM, Paprosky WG: Acetabular revision using a trabecular metal acetabular component for severe acetabular bone loss associated with a pelvic discontinuity. *J Arthroplasty* 2006;21(6): 87-90.

29. Van Kleunen JP, Lee GC, Lementowski PW, Nelson CL, Garino JP: Acetabular revisions using trabecular metal cups and augments. *J Arthroplasty* 2009;24(6): 64-68.

30. Davies JH, Laflamme GY, Delisle J, Fernandes J: Trabecular metal used for major bone loss in acetabular hip revision. *J Arthroplasty* 2011;26(8):1245-1250.

31. Weeden SH, Schmidt RH: The use of tantalum porous metal implants for Paprosky 3A and 3B defects. *J Arthroplasty* 2007;22(6): 151-155.

32. Flecher X, Sporer S, Paprosky W: Management of severe bone loss in acetabular revision using a trabecular metal shell. *J Arthroplasty* 2008;23(7):949-955.

33. Lachiewicz PF, Soileau ES: Tantalum components in difficult acetabular revisions. *Clin Orthop Relat Res* 2010;468(2):454-458.

34. Jafari SM, Bender B, Coyle C, Parvizi J, Sharkey PF, Hozack WJ: Do tantalum and titanium cups show similar results in revision hip

arthroplasty? *Clin Orthop Relat Res* 2010;468(2):459-465.

35. Lachiewicz PF, Poon ED: Revision of a total hip arthroplasty with a Harris-Galante porous-coated acetabular component inserted without cement: A follow-up note on the results at five to twelve years. *J Bone Joint Surg Am* 1998;80(7):980-984.

36. Manley MT, Capello WN, D'Antonio JA, Edidin AA, Geesink RG: Fixation of acetabular cups without cement in total hip arthroplasty: A comparison of three different implant surfaces at a minimum duration of follow-up of five years. *J Bone Joint Surg Am* 1998;80(8):1175-1185.

37. Lazarinis S, Kärrholm J, Hailer NP: Increased risk of revision of acetabular cups coated with hydroxyapatite. *Acta Orthop* 2010; 81(1):53-59.

38. Kim SY, Kim DH, Kim YG, Oh CW, Ihn JC: Early failure of hemispheric hydroxyapatite-coated acetabular cups. *Clin Orthop Relat Res* 2006;446:233-238.

39. Whaley AL, Berry DJ, Harmsen WS: Extra-large uncemented hemispherical acetabular components for revision total hip arthroplasty. *J Bone Joint Surg Am* 2001; 83(9):1352-1357.

40. Ries MD, Nwankwo CD, Dong NN, Heffernan CD: Scientific Exhibit No. SEO4: Do large (jumbo) cups cause hip center elevation in revision THA? *AAOS* 2013 *Annual Meeting Proceedings*. CD-ROM. Rosemont, IL, American Academy of Orthopaedic Surgeons, pp 478-479.

41. Rees HW, Fung DA, Cerynik DL, Amin NH, Johanson NA: Revision total hip arthroplasty without bone graft of high-grade acetabular defects. *J Arthroplasty* 2012;27(1):41-47.

42. Civinini R, Capone A, Carulli C, Villano M, Gusso MI: Acetabular revisions using a cementless ob-

long cup: Five to ten year results. *Int Orthop* 2008;32(2):189-193.

43. Herrera A, Martínez AA, Cuenca J, Canales V: Management of types III and IV acetabular deficiencies with the longitudinal oblong revision cup. *J Arthroplasty* 2006;21(6):857-864.

44. Köster G, Rading S: Revision of failed acetabular components utilizing a cementless oblong cup: An average 9-year follow-up study. *Arch Orthop Trauma Surg* 2009; 129(5):603-608.

45. Moskal JT, Shen FH: The use of bilobed porous-coated acetabular components without structural bone graft for type III acetabular defects in revision total hip arthroplasty: A prospective study with a minimum 2-year follow-up. *J Arthroplasty* 2004;19(7): 867-873.

46. Abeyta PN, Namba RS, Janku GV, Murray WR, Kim HT: Reconstruction of major segmental acetabular defects with an oblong-shaped cementless prosthesis: A long-term outcomes study. *J Arthroplasty* 2008;23(2): 247-253.

47. Chen WM, Engh CA Jr, Hopper RH Jr, McAuley JP, Engh CA: Acetabular revision with use of a bilobed component inserted without cement in patients who have acetabular bone-stock deficiency. *J Bone Joint Surg Am* 2000;82(2): 197-206.

48. Goodman S, Saastamoinen H, Shasha N, Gross A: Complications of ilioischial reconstruction rings in revision total hip arthroplasty. *J Arthroplasty* 2004;19(4): 436-446.

49. Regis D, Sandri A, Bonetti I, Bortolami O, Bartolozzi P: A minimum of 10-year follow-up of the Burch-Schneider cage and bulk allografts for the revision of pelvic discontinuity. *J Arthroplasty* 2012; 27(6):1057-1063, e1.

50. Hansen E, Shearer D, Ries MD: Does a cemented cage improve revision THA for severe acetabular defects? *Clin Orthop Relat Res* 2011;469(2):494-502.

51. Buttaro MA, de la Rosa DM, Comba F, Piccaluga F: High failure rate with the GAP II ring and impacted allograft bone in severe acetabular defects. *Clin Orthop Relat Res* 2012;470(11):3148-3155.

52. Symeonides PP, Petsatodes GE, Pournaras JD, Kapetanos GA, Christodoulou AG, Marougiannis DJ: The effectiveness of the Burch-Schneider antiprotrusio cage for acetabular bone deficiency: Five to twenty-one years' follow-up. *J Arthroplasty* 2009; 24(2):168-174.

53. Winter E, Piert M, Volkmann R, et al: Allogeneic cancellous bone graft and a Burch-Schneider ring for acetabular reconstruction in revision hip arthroplasty. *J Bone Joint Surg Am* 2001;83(6): 862-867.

54. Bostrom MP, Lehman AP, Buly RL, Lyman S, Nestor BJ: Acetabular revision with the Contour antiprotrusio cage: 2- to 5-year followup. *Clin Orthop Relat Res* 2006;453:188-194.

55. Hanssen AD, Lewallen DG: Acetabular cages: A ladder across a melting pond. *Orthopedics* 2004; 27(8):830-832, 832.

56. Kosashvili Y, Backstein D, Safir O, Lakstein D, Gross AE: Acetabular revision using an antiprotrusion (ilio-ischial) cage and trabecular metal acetabular component for severe acetabular bone loss associated with pelvic discontinuity. *J Bone Joint Surg Br* 2009; 91(7):870-876.

57. Holt GE, Dennis DA: Use of custom triflanged acetabular components in revision total hip arthroplasty. *Clin Orthop Relat Res* 2004; 429:209-214.

58. Christie MJ, Barrington SA, Brinson MF, Ruhling ME, DeBoer DK: Bridging massive acetabular defects with the triflange cup: 2- to 9-year results. *Clin Orthop Relat Res* 2001;393:216-227.

59. DeBoer DK, Christie MJ, Brinson MF, Morrison JC: Revision total hip arthroplasty for pelvic discontinuity. *J Bone Joint Surg Am* 2007;89(4):835-840.

60. Taunton MJ, Fehring TK, Edwards P, Bernasek T, Holt GE, Christie MJ: Pelvic discontinuity treated with custom triflange component: A reliable option. *Clin Orthop Relat Res* 2012; 470(2):428-434.

61. Joshi AB, Lee J, Christensen C: Results for a custom acetabular component for acetabular deficiency. *J Arthroplasty* 2002;17(5): 643-648.

62. Stiehl JB, Saluja R, Diener T: Reconstruction of major column defects and pelvic discontinuity in revision total hip arthroplasty. *J Arthroplasty* 2000;15(7): 849-857.

63. Springer BD, Berry DJ, Cabanela ME, Hanssen AD, Lewallen DG: Early postoperative transverse pelvic fracture: A new complication related to revision arthroplasty with an uncemented cup. *J Bone Joint Surg Am* 2005; 87(12):2626-2631.

64. Villanueva M, Rios-Luna A, Pereiro De Lamo J, Fahandez-Saddi H, Böstrom MP: A review of the treatment of pelvic discontinuity. *HSS J* 2008;4(2):128-137.

65. Noordin S, Duncan CP, Masri BA, Garbuz DS: Pelvic dissociation in revision total hip arthroplasty: Diagnosis and treatment. *Instr Course Lect* 2010;59:37-43.

66. Sporer SM, O'Rourke M, Paprosky WG: The treatment of pelvic discontinuity during acetabular revision. *J Arthroplasty* 2005;20(4):79-84.

67. Gililland JM, Anderson LA, Henninger HB, Kubiak EN, Peters CL: Biomechanical analysis of acetabular revision constructs: Is pelvic discontinuity best treated with bicolumnar or traditional unicolumnar fixation? *J Arthroplasty* 2013;28(1):178-186.

Acute Periprosthetic Fractures of the Acetabulum After Total Hip Arthroplasty

Anish G. Potty, MD
Jacqueline Corona, MD
Blaine T. Manning, BS
Amanda Le, BA
Khaled J. Saleh, BSc, MD, MSc, FRCS(C), MHCM

Abstract

Although periprosthetic fractures of the acetabulum are relatively uncommon after total hip arthroplasty, a variety of patient-, surgeon-, and implant-related risk factors can contribute to the occurrence of this serious complication. These risk factors, combined with the increased use of cementless acetabular cups, will likely result in an increased prevalence of these fractures in the future. By better understanding the risk factors, classification schemes, and treatment options for periprosthetic fractures of the acetabulum, orthopaedic surgeons can achieve better outcomes for their patients.

Instr Course Lect 2014;63:199-207.

By 2030, the number of total hip arthroplasties (THAs) is projected to nearly triple from current levels to almost 600,000 cases per year.[1] Although the procedure has proven to be successful in terms of functional outcomes and complication rates, the incidence of complications will likely increase with the growing number of THAs.[2] One major complication after THA is periprosthetic fracture of the acetabulum, which was first described by Miller[3] in 1972. Based on this study of nine women treated with THA, Miller postulated that several risk factors, including infection, obesity, and overreaming of the acetabulum, may lead to stress fractures. A later review by Peterson and Lewallen[4] reported 11 periprosthetic acetabular fractures in 23,850 THAs (0.07%) over a 20-year period. Given the increase in the use of cementless cups, the number of revision THAs, and the difficulty in managing these fractures, it is important for orthopaedic surgeons to understand acetabular THA fractures. This chapter reviews the epidemiology, risk factors (**Table 1**), classification, diagnosis, and treatment of intraoperative and postoperative periprosthetic acetabular fractures.

Risk Factors

Implant-Related Risk Factors

Of the nine acetabular fractures reported by Miller,[3] five fractures were associated with uncemented ring components. A 1974 study by McElfresh and Conventry[5] reported only 1 periprosthetic acetabular fracture in 5,400 THAs (< 0.02%) performed with cemented components. A subsequent study suggested a greater propensity for periprosthetic acetabular fractures when cementless cups are used.[6] In a review of 7,121 primary

Dr. Saleh or an immediate family member has received royalties from Aesculap/B. Braun; is a member of a speakers' bureau or has made paid presentations on behalf of Carefusion; serves as a paid consultant to Aesculap/B. Braun, the Memorial Medical Center Co-Management Orthopaedic Board, and the Blue Cross Blue Shield Blue Ribbon Panel; has received research or institutional support from Smith & Nephew, the Orthopaedic Research and Education Foundation, and the National Institutes of Health/National Institute of Arthritis and Musculoskeletal Skin Diseases (R0-1); and serves as a board member, owner, officer, or committee member of the American Orthopaedic Association and the Orthopaedic Research and Education Foundation. None of the following authors or any immediate family member has received anything of value from or has stock or stock options held in a commercial company or institution related directly or indirectly to the subject of this chapter: Dr. Potty, Dr. Corona, Mr. Manning, and Ms. Le.

Table 1

Risk Factors for Acetabular Periprosthetic Fracture

Surgeon-Related

Underreaming, forced cup fitting

Implant-Related

Monoblock elliptical cups, uncemented cups

Patient-Related

Age, female sex, traumatic injury, osteolysis, rheumatoid arthritis, peptic ulcer disease, heart disease, Paget disease

THAs, Haidukewych et al[6] reported 21 intraoperative acetabular fractures in the 5,329 patients treated with cementless components (0.4%). No fractures occurred in the 1,762 patients treated with cemented cups. Because of the increase in the use of cementless acetabular cups, the prevalence of acetabular intraoperative fractures is likely to increase.

Monoblock implant designs have been touted to reduce backside wear by providing uniform support and eliminating the migration of wear particles through screw holes. The lack of screw holes also maximizes the available surface area for osseous integration and solid fixation. Despite such advantages, monoblock elliptic components have been associated with an elevated risk of acetabular fracture in THA. Compared with a 0.3% fracture rate (7 fractures in 2,416 THAs) in procedures using elliptic modular acetabular shells, Haidukewych et al[6] reported an increased acetabular fracture rate of 3.5% (12 fractures in 339 THAs) when elliptic monoblock cups were used. Similar findings were reported when elliptic monoblock and hemispheric modular cups were compared. An acetabular fracture rate of 0.09% (2 fractures in 2,198 THAs) was reported in patients treated with hemispheric modular cups, whereas those receiving elliptic monoblock cups had an acetabular fracture rate of 3.5% (12 fractures in 339 THAs).[6]

Surgeon-Related Risk Factors

Surgical technique is also a potential cause of acetabular periprosthetic fractures because the underreaming required to press fit the acetabular cup without using screws often instigates the use of excessive impaction forces. A review of 13 patients with acetabular fractures who were treated with THA found that the acetabulum was underreamed from 1 to 3 mm in each patient, despite the use of various cementless components.[7] Impaction forces associated with a component oversized by 2 mm led to fractures in 4 of 15 acetabula; whereas 14 of 15 acetabula were fractured when components were oversized by 4 mm. The appropriate extent of underreaming depends on the size of the acetabulum; smaller and larger acetabula may require less or more underreaming, respectively. Although Schmalzried et al[8] suggested that oversizing the cup by up to 4 mm is feasible, a later study by Kim et al[9] recommended the currently accepted threshold of 2 mm for component oversizing.

Patient-Related Risk Factors

Acetabular fractures in association with THA may occur in the postoperative period because of trauma or osteolysis. Peterson and Lewallen[4] reported on 11 patients with postoperative fractures, 9 of whom received cemented components. Eight of the 11 fractures were attributable to trauma, 3 were spontaneous, and none was associated with component loosening or osteolysis. In a case series of three patients treated with THA, Sánchez-Sotelo et al[10] observed acetabular fractures in areas of the pelvis with severe osteolysis and subsequent structural failure. Of the 23,580 THAs in an institutional total joint registry, postop-erative acetabular fractures occurred in 13 patients (< 0.06%).[4] Another review of more than 3,500 revision THAs reported a 0.9% prevalence of acetabular fractures during the postoperative period.[11]

Certain demographic factors, such as age and female sex, also have been correlated with an increased risk of periprosthetic fractures in patients treated with THA.[12,13] Studies have reported that women have an increased risk of falling compared with men, thereby increasing their risk of traumatic injury.[14] Because many older women treated with THA have postmenopausal osteoporosis, the higher frequency of falls in this patient population may increase the prevalence of periprosthetic acetabular fractures.

Studies differ on the role of age as a risk factor.[12,13] A Scottish registry study reported that THA patients older than 70 years have an increased risk of periprosthetic fracture; however, Singh et al[12] associated older age with a decreased fracture risk, which was likely the result of the less demanding lifestyles of older patients compared with the more active lifestyles and participation in sports common in younger patients.[15] Rheumatoid arthritis, peptic ulcer disease, heart disease, and Paget disease are also known to elevate the risk for a periprosthetic THA fracture.[11,12,16]

Classification

There is no consensus on the best classification system for periprosthetic acetabular fractures. As the incidence of these fractures has increased, there has been an impetus to adopt a complete classification system that aids in guiding treatment. Classification systems have been based on a variety of factors.

In a 1996 retrospective analysis of the Total Joint Registry at the Mayo Clinic, Peterson and Lewallen[4] identified 11 periprosthetic acetabular fractures at a mean of 6.2 years after THA. The authors classified these fractures using a modified Letournel system that included a category for fractures of the medial wall of the acetabulum, and, perhaps more importantly, they classified fractures into two broad categories: type I (stable) and type II (unstable). Fractures were deemed to be type I (stable) if comparison of preoperative and postoperative fracture radiographs did not show any change in acetabular component positioning and little or no pain was elicited on passive range of motion of the hip; the opposite criteria were true for unstable type II fractures. The authors noted that the determination of fracture stability aided in choosing observation and activity modification versus surgical intervention as a treatment modality.

Similar to Peterson et al,[4] Callaghan et al[17] also described the stability of the prosthesis as a key classification component; however, based on prior in vitro work, the anatomic location of the fracture (for example, anterior wall, inferior wall, inferior lip, and transverse) was also judged to be important. The time at which the fracture was identified was also considered an important classification factor. Iatrogenic fractures can be found intraoperatively versus in the early postoperative period. Callaghan et al[17] described late postoperative fractures that present 6 to 12 months after surgery and postulated that these fractures occur secondary to increased activity after THA on bone with disuse osteopenia caused by years of painful osteoarthritis. Unlike iatrogenic fractures, late fractures are considered insufficiency fractures.

In 2003, Della Valle et al[18] presented a more comprehensive classification system that could be used to make specific recommendations. Fractures were organized according to five

Table 2

Classification of Periprosthetic Fractures of the Acetabulum Associated With THA

Type I	Intraoperative fractures secondary to acetabular component insertion IA: Fracture nondisplaced and component stable IB: Fracture displaced and acetabular component or column unstable IC: Fracture not recognized intraoperatively
Type II	Intraoperative fracture secondary to acetabular component removal IIA: Associated with loss < 50% of acetabular bone stock IIB: Associated with loss > 50% of acetabular bone stock
Type III	Traumatic fracture IIIA: Component stable IIIB: Component unstable
Type IV	Spontaneous fractures IVA: Associated with loss < 50% of acetabular bone stock IVB: Associated with loss > 50% of acetabular bone stock
Type V	Pelvic discontinuity VA: Associated with loss < 50% of acetabular bone stock VB: Associated with loss > 50% of acetabular bone stock VC: Associated with pelvic irradiation

(Reproduced from Della Valle CJ, Momberger NG, Paprosky WG: Periprosthetic fractures of the acetabulum associated with a total hip arthroplasty. *Instr Course Lect* 2003;52:281-290.)

main clinical presentations: intraoperative fracture secondary to acetabular component insertion, intraoperative fracture secondary to acetabular component removal, traumatic fracture, spontaneous fracture, and pelvic discontinuity. Fractures were further subdivided according to the stability of the prosthesis and the loss of acetabular bone stock (**Table 2**).

A 2008 review of periprosthetic THA fractures by Davidson et al[2] focused only on intraoperative fractures. The Davidson et al[2] classification was a modification of the Vancouver classification and focused on fracture stability, the presence of pelvic discontinuity, failure of the acetabular prosthesis, and the presence of osteolysis. Type I fractures are defined as undisplaced and stable. Type II fractures are undisplaced fractures that can compromise stability, such as transverse acetabular fractures with pelvic discontinuity and oblique fracture separating the anterior column, dome, and/or posterior column. Type III fractures are displaced fractures, assuming that the displacement causes instability of the acetabu-

lar component. Ideally, a classification system serves to guide treatment. In 2004, the treatment algorithm of Helfit and Ali[19] described a novel classification system (**Figure 1**).

Diagnosis

Periprosthetic acetabular fractures mainly occur intraoperatively or postoperatively in osteoporotic bone. Maintaining a high index of suspicion for intraoperative acetabular fractures is important because they are difficult to identify. When there is concern regarding a possible fracture, a full clinical and radiographic assessment of the affected hip is needed. Clinical symptoms of unresolved postoperative pain should be carefully assessed. Advanced metal suppression CT and MRI should be conducted to assess the periprosthetic bone stock. The stability of the acetabular cup is critical for implant survival and can be assessed intraoperatively when a fracture is suspected or postoperatively through clinical and radiologic testing. Intraoperative fracture assessment should include judicious examination of the

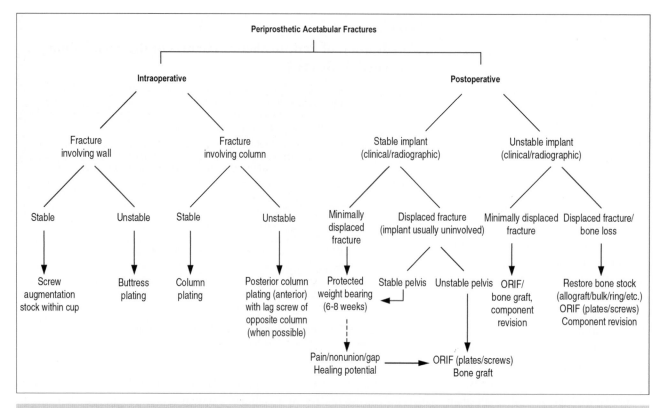

Figure 1   Treatment algorithm for periprosthetic fractures of the acetabulum. ORIF = open reduction and internal fixation. (Reproduced from Helfet DL, Ali A: Periprosthetic fractures of the acetabulum. *Instr Course Lect* 2004;53:93-98.)

columns and walls of the acetabulum. If the trial cup feels unstable during insertion, intraoperative radiographs should be obtained to assess for underlying fractures before further reaming is performed to insert a larger cup.

Treatment

General Principles

The decision for surgical management of a periprosthetic acetabular fracture can be based on information on the fracture's occurrence, stability, and location.[19] Generally, simple intraoperative fractures are treated with stable fixation of the implant and the fracture. Major intraoperative fractures require more aggressive reconstruction and plating of the columns.

Postoperative fractures associated with well-fixed implants are typically treated with open reduction and internal fixation. In a postoperative fracture

with an unstable implant, a systematic approach ranging from revision of the acetabular component to fracture stabilization and implant fixation may be required. In a study of 13 patients with periprosthetic acetabular fractures by Sharkey et al,[7] 6 patients were treated with additional acetabular screw fixation, 2 had stable implants and did not need additional fixation or a change in postoperative rehabilitation, and 1 patient did not require additional fixation but was treated with an 8-week postoperative non–weight-bearing regimen. Fracture union was observed in all nine patients. The four remaining postoperative fractures were associated with evidence of loosening on follow-up radiographs; two required cup revision. Failure often occurs if an unstable fracture is not stabilized, such as in instances of unrecognized fractures.

Intraoperative Acetabular Fractures

If the fracture is undisplaced and the component is stable, acetabular component screw fixation can be used intraoperatively to achieve stabilization. At least two to three acetabular screws, ideally at either end of the fracture line, are preferred over a single screw for greater stability and to prevent toggling. Eight to 12 weeks of light weight bearing should be instructed until healing occurs. For displaced fractures, the component is removed, and the fracture extent and location is precisely assessed. If the acetabular column is involved, buttress plating followed by gentle placement of a cementless acetabular component may be required. A careful reaming technique using gentle, high revolution spinning and low penetration should be used. Touchdown weight bearing is recommended for a minimum of 12 weeks until cup incorporation.

Della Valle et al[18] offered recommendations for treating intraoperative acetabular fractures. In patients with a nondisplaced fracture and a stable component, the prosthesis can remain in situ, and standard THA rehabilitation protocols can be applied. If the component is unstable, the structural integrity of the anterior and posterior columns must be assessed, and supplemental screw fixation can be used if necessary. A jumbo revision cup should be considered if there is marked instability and bone loss that necessitates a larger acetabular component. These fractures also should be treated with bone grafting. The patient should maintain protected weight bearing postoperatively until the fracture has healed. If there is substantial displacement at the fracture site, including the presence of pelvic dissociation, the posterior column should be treated with reduction and internal fixation. After the pelvis has been stabilized, the acetabulum can be reconstructed using standard THA techniques.

Acute Postoperative Acetabular Fractures

Postoperative acetabular fractures that are immediately diagnosed can be treated nonsurgically if the acetabular component is well fixed and the fracture pattern is stable. Nondisplaced fractures with radiographically stable components are treated with 12 weeks of touchdown weight bearing. Displaced fractures with component loosening require revision with wall or column fixation. Fixation with a reconstruction cage and subsequent bone grafting may be appropriate because the cage will bridge inferiorly to superiorly and allow temporary stabilization of the fracture during bone graft incorporation and fracture healing. If

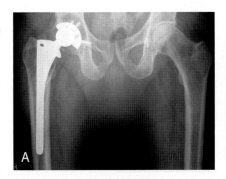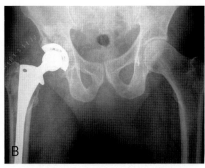

Figure 2 **A,** AP radiograph showing osteolysis of the acetabulum. **B,** Postoperative AP radiograph showing filling of the defect after an injection of calcium phosphate.

acetabular bone loss is so severe that a standard hemispheric cementless cup provides unreliable fixation and bone ingrowth, an alternate fixation method may be needed. In such instances, a porous metal cup may allow more rigid initial stability and more predictable ingrowth.[20]

Late Postoperative Acetabular Fractures

Late acetabular fractures are best treated based on clinical assessment, radiographic stability, and medical optimization of bone quality if nonsurgical medical treatment is required. In instances of minor symptomatic osteolysis with evidence of loosening in two or more Charley zones, either injection of bone substitutes (**Figure 2**) or component revision may be needed. With clear radiographic evidence of acetabular loosening and an unstable acetabular cup, component revision is required. If fractures extend to the anterior or posterior columns, plated column fixation is combined with revision. In patients with extensive fractures with large acetabular bone defects or severe osteolysis (**Figure 3, A**), it may be necessary to use cage fixation (**Figure 3, B** and **C**), tantalum, or allograft augments with plate augmentation to secure hemipelvic continuity. If the bone stock cannot be reconstructed because of severe pelvic dis-

continuity, the use of a custom-made implant may be warranted (**Figure 4**).

Periprosthetic Fractures in Revision THA

Periprosthetic fractures in revision THAs usually occur during implant removal. The choice of fixation can depend on the extent of the fracture. Most often, these are undisplaced fractures and can be treated with additional screws for stability. With two-column fractures, additional fixation based on the general principles previously described is recommended. In 2005, Springer et al[20] reported on seven women who had a delayed transverse fracture of the acetabulum after revision THA with a porous metal cup. The authors believed that these fractures were not caused intraoperatively but were related to the patients' osteoporotic weak bone stock. They noted that the cups failed after resuming activity. The cause of the fractures and their displacement over time suggested that the cup that bridges from superiorly to inferiorly has a higher capacity for bone ingrowth.

Boscainos et al[21] reported good early results in 14 patients treated with a cup-cage construct; however, a high rate of recurrent dislocations was reported, with 2 of the 14 patients requiring revision to a constrained acetabular liner. Both Springer et al[20]

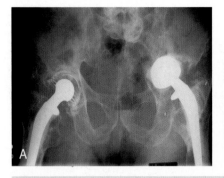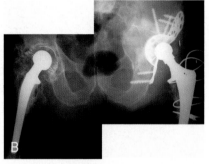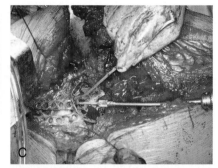

Figure 3 **A,** Left AP hip radiograph showing pelvic discontinuity and severe osteolysis. **B,** Left postoperative AP hip radiograph after reconstruction with a cage. **C,** Intraoperative photograph showing placement of the cage screws during acetabular reconstruction.

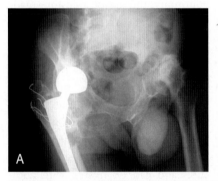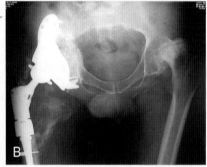

Figure 4 **A,** AP radiograph showing pelvic discontinuity with osteolysis. **B,** Postoperative AP radiograph after reconstruction with a custom-made implant.

and Boscainos et al[21] described the use of this technique in revision THA. The use of this technique for intraoperative acetabular fractures has not been reported.

Prevention and Medical Management

The prevention of periprosthetic fractures requires preoperative planning to assess the risk factors associated with their occurrence. A detailed patient history and surgical plan are needed. Full-length, adequate, preoperative radiographs (including Judet views) should be obtained to fully appreciate any deformity or areas of bone loss that may increase the risk of fracture. All potential reconstructive options should be carefully planned, with templating of preoperative radiographs to

anticipate the likely sizes of the components. It should be emphasized that, if the implant chosen on the basis of the templating is not stable, the surgeon should carefully inspect the femur to make sure a fracture is not creating instability and fixation failure.

During surgery, careful attention must be given to the parts of the procedure that are associated with the highest risk of fracture, such as hip dislocation, cement removal (in revision cases), canal preparation, and component insertion. Adequate soft-tissue releases are necessary to minimize the force required to obtain sufficient exposure. If necessary, adjunctive surgical strategies, such as an extended trochanteric osteotomy, should be considered. This is particularly relevant for removing well-fixed cement-

less and precoated cemented stems. The use of cerclage wires at the distal extent of a trochanteric osteotomy or a periprosthetic fracture should be considered to prevent fracture propagation. Appropriate, thin hemispheric osteotomes can be used for acetabular component extraction. In the setting of a complex revision procedure, intraoperative radiographs can be obtained to ensure proper implant positioning by optimizing reaming. Immediate postoperative radiographs should be made to assess potential fractures that were not appreciated intraoperatively.

Pharmacologic management includes maintenance of appropriate calcium intake (≥ 1,000 mg per day) and vitamin D levels (≥ 20 ng per mL serum) because their importance in bone maintenance and fracture healing is well known.[22-24] Parathyroid hormone also has gained attention as a bone-forming agent.[25] Numerous animal studies have documented the effectiveness of parathyroid hormone in complex bone healing scenarios, such as critical bone-size defects, host-allograft integration, distraction osteogenesis, and corticosteroid use.[26-29] In an animal study, Reynolds et al[27] tried to reduce complications that shortened the functional life of large bone allografts. It was found that daily injections of teriparatide into mice treated with femoral defect reconstruction aided in graft-host integration. In a recent study of 65 postmenopausal women, Peichl et al[30] reported that parathyroid hormone 1-84 accelerated healing and improved functional outcomes in patients with pelvic fracture. In addition to anabolic agents, bisphosphonates also have been successful in treating osteoporosis, which has led to animal studies and randomized controlled trials in humans on their effectiveness in preventing periprosthetic osteolysis.[31-36] One study found that treatment with intramuscular clodronate for 1 year after THA resulted in a substantial reduction in bone loss.[31] Although the results have been encouraging, there is controversy regarding reports that suggest that bisphosphonates can delay fracture healing.[37,38] Gong et al[39] recently reported that bisphosphonate treatment had no effect on fracture healing in patients with an osteoporotic distal radial fracture. Further investigations are needed to determine the efficacy of bisphosphonate therapy on periprosthetic fractures.

Sclerostin antibodies are among the newest therapeutic innovations for preventing implant loosening and periprosthetic osteolysis caused by polyethylene particles.[40,41] In animal models, the infusion of polyethylene particles caused pathologic changes in tissues bordering areas of osteolysis.[42] Sclerostin antibodies act by blocking the damaging effect of polyethylene particles and have been shown to increase the rate of bone formation while decreasing bone resorption in rat models.[40,43]

Summary

Periprosthetic fracture of the acetabulum in primary and revision THAs will continue to affect patient outcomes. The limited visualization associated with minimally invasive techniques and press-fit components requires meticulous attention to prevent and, if necessary, appropriately address intraoperative fractures. The increasing prevalence of THAs combined with the influence of osteolysis and osteoporosis suggest a rise in the future prevalence of late postoperative periprosthetic fractures. A thorough awareness of the risk factors, the classification schemes, and the treatment options for periprosthetic acetabular fractures will allow the orthopaedic surgeon to effectively manage this adverse event before it develops into a more complex and serious complication.

References

1. Kurtz S, Ong K, Lau E, Mowat F, Halpern M: Projections of primary and revision hip and knee arthroplasty in the United States from 2005 to 2030. *J Bone Joint Surg Am* 2007;89(4):780-785.

2. Davidson D, Pike J, Garbuz D, Duncan CP, Masri BA: Intraoperative periprosthetic fractures during total hip arthroplasty: Evaluation and management. *J Bone Joint Surg Am* 2008;90(9): 2000-2012.

3. Miller AJ: Late fracture of the acetabulum after total hip replacement. *J Bone Joint Surg Br* 1972; 54(4):600-606.

4. Peterson CA, Lewallen DG: Periprosthetic fracture of the acetabulum after total hip arthroplasty. *J Bone Joint Surg Am* 1996; 78(8):1206-1213.

5. McElfresh EC, Coventry MB: Femoral and pelvic fractures after total hip arthroplasty. *J Bone Joint Surg Am* 1974;56(3):483-492.

6. Haidukewych GJ, Jacofsky DJ, Hanssen AD, Lewallen DG: Intraoperative fractures of the acetabulum during primary total hip arthroplasty. *J Bone Joint Surg Am* 2006;88(9):1952-1956.

7. Sharkey PF, Hozack WJ, Callaghan JJ, et al: A report of 13 cases. *J Arthroplasty* 1999; 14(4):426-431.

8. Schmalzried TP, Wessinger SJ, Hill GE, Harris WH: The Harris-Galante porous acetabular component press-fit without screw fixation: Five-year radiographic analysis of primary cases. *J Arthroplasty* 1994;9(3):235-242.

9. Kim YS, Callaghan JJ, Ahn PB, Brown TD: Fracture of the acetabulum during insertion of an oversized hemispherical component. *J Bone Joint Surg Am* 1995; 77(1):111-117.

10. Sánchez-Sotelo J, McGrory BJ, Berry DJ: Acute periprosthetic fracture of the acetabulum associated with osteolytic pelvic lesions: A report of 3 cases. *J Arthroplasty* 2000;15(1):126-130.

11. Berry DJ, Lewallen DG, Hanssen AD, Cabanela ME: Pelvic discontinuity in revision total hip arthroplasty. *J Bone Joint Surg Am* 1999;81(12):1692-1702.

12. Singh JA, Jensen MR, Lewallen DG: Patient factors predict periprosthetic fractures after revision total hip arthroplasty. *J Arthroplasty* 2012;27(8):1507-1512.

13. Meek RM, Norwood T, Smith R, Brenkel IJ, Howie CR: The risk of peri-prosthetic fracture after primary and revision total hip and knee replacement. *J Bone Joint Surg Br* 2011;93(1):96-101.

14. Sattin RW: Falls among older persons: A public health perspective. *Annu Rev Public Health* 1992;13:489-508.

15. Huch K, Müller KA, Stürmer T, Brenner H, Puhl W, Günther KP: Sports activities 5 years after total knee or hip arthroplasty: The Ulm Osteoarthritis Study. *Ann Rheum Dis* 2005;64(12):1715-1720.

16. Mitchell PA, Greidanus NV, Masri BA, Garbuz DS, Duncan CP: The prevention of periprosthetic fractures of the femur during and after total hip arthroplasty. *Instr Course Lect* 2003;52: 301-308.

17. Callaghan JJ, Kim YS, Pederson DR, Brown TD: Periprosthetic fractures of the acetabulum. *Orthop Clin North Am* 1999;30(2): 221-234.

18. Della Valle CJ, Momberger NG, Paprosky WG: Periprosthetic fractures of the acetabulum associated with a total hip arthroplasty. *Instr Course Lect* 2003;52:281-290.

19. Helfet DL, Ali A: Periprosthetic fractures of the acetabulum. *Instr Course Lect* 2004;53:93-98.

20. Springer BD, Berry DJ, Cabanela ME, Hanssen AD, Lewallen DG: Early postoperative transverse pelvic fracture: A new complication related to revision arthroplasty with an uncemented cup. *J Bone Joint Surg Am* 2005; 87(12):2626-2631.

21. Boscainos PJ, Kellett CF, Maury AC, Backstein D, Gross AE: Management of periacetabular bone loss in revision hip arthroplasty. *Clin Orthop Relat Res* 2007;465: 159-165.

22. Rebolledo BJ, Unnanuntana A, Lane JM: A comprehensive approach to fragility fractures. *J Orthop Trauma* 2011;25(9): 566-573.

23. Nawabi DH, Chin KF, Keen RW, Haddad FS: Vitamin D deficiency in patients with osteoarthritis undergoing total hip replacement: A cause for concern? *J Bone Joint Surg Br* 2010;92(4):496-499.

24. McCabe MP, Smyth MP, Richardson DR: Current concept review: Vitamin D and stress fractures. *Foot Ankle Int* 2012;33(6): 526-533.

25. Barnes GL, Kakar S, Vora S, Morgan EF, Gerstenfeld LC, Einhorn TA: Stimulation of fracture-healing with systemic intermittent parathyroid hormone treatment. *J Bone Joint Surg Am* 2008; 90(suppl 1):120-127.

26. Komatsu DE, Brune KA, Liu H, et al: Longitudinal in vivo analysis of the region-specific efficacy of parathyroid hormone in a rat cortical defect model. *Endocrinology* 2009;150(4):1570-1579.

27. Reynolds DG, Takahata M, Lerner AL, O'Keefe RJ, Schwarz EM, Awad HA: Teriparatide therapy enhances devitalized femoral allograft osseointegration and biomechanics in a murine model. *Bone* 2011;48(3):562-570.

28. Seebach C, Skripitz R, Andreassen TT, Aspenberg P: Intermittent parathyroid hormone (1-34) enhances mechanical strength and density of new bone after distraction osteogenesis in rats. *J Orthop Res* 2004;22(3):472-478.

29. Bostrom MP, Gamradt SC, Asnis P, et al: Parathyroid hormone-related protein analog RS-66271 is an effective therapy for impaired bone healing in rabbits on corticosteroid therapy. *Bone* 2000;26(5):437-442.

30. Peichl P, Holzer LA, Maier R, Holzer G: Parathyroid hormone 1-84 accelerates fracture-healing in pubic bones of elderly osteoporotic women. *J Bone Joint Surg Am* 2011;93(17):1583-1587.

31. Trevisan C, Ortolani S, Romano P, et al: A 1-year randomized controlled study. *Calcif Tissue Int* 2010;86(6):436-446.

32. Arabmotlagh M, Pilz M, Warzecha J, Rauschmann M: Changes of femoral periprosthetic bone mineral density 6 years after treatment with alendronate following total hip arthroplasty. *J Orthop Res* 2009;27(2):183-188.

33. Shetty N, Hamer AJ, Stockley I, Eastell R, Willkinson JM: Clinical and radiological outcome of total hip replacement five years after pamidronate therapy: A trial extension. *J Bone Joint Surg Br* 2006;88(10):1309-1315.

34. Wang CJ, Wang JW, Ko JY, Weng LH, Huang CC: Three-year changes in bone mineral density around the knee after a six-month course of oral alendronate following total knee arthroplasty: A prospective, randomized study. *J Bone Joint Surg Am* 2006;88(2): 267-272.

35. Wilkinson JM, Eagleton AC, Stockley I, Peel NF, Hamer AJ, Eastell R: Effect of pamidronate on bone turnover and implant migration after total hip arthroplasty: A randomized trial. *J Orthop Res* 2005;23(1):1-8.

36. Yamaguchi K, Masuhara K, Yamasaki S, Nakai T, Fuji T: Cyclic therapy with etidronate has a therapeutic effect against local osteoporosis after cementless total hip arthroplasty. *Bone* 2003;33(1): 144-149.

37. Jørgensen NR, Schwarz P: Effects of anti-osteoporosis medications on fracture healing. *Curr Osteoporos Rep* 2011;9(3):149-155.

38. Mehsen N, Paccou J, Confavreux CB, David C, Leboime A, Laroche M: Management of patients with incident fractures during osteoporosis treatment. *Joint Bone Spine* 2010;77(suppl 2):S133-S138.

39. Gong HS, Song CH, Lee YH, Rhee SH, Lee HJ, Baek GH: Early initiation of bisphosphonate does not affect healing and outcomes of volar plate fixation of osteoporotic distal radial fractures. *J Bone Joint Surg Am* 2012; 94(19):1729-1736.

40. Atkins GJ, Haynes DR, Howie DW, Findlay DM: Role of polyethylene particles in periprosthetic osteolysis: A review. *World J Orthop* 2011;2(10): 93-101.

41. Virdi AS, Liu M, Sena K, et al: Sclerostin antibody increases bone volume and enhances implant fixation in a rat model. *J Bone Joint Surg Am* 2012;94(18):1670-1680.

42. Ma T, Huang Z, Ren PG, et al: An in vivo murine model of continuous intramedullary infusion of polyethylene particles. *Biomaterials* 2008;29(27):3738-3742.

43. Tian X, Jee WS, Li X, Paszty C, Ke HZ: Sclerostin antibody increases bone mass by stimulating bone formation and inhibiting bone resorption in a hindlimb-immobilization rat model. *Bone* 2011;48(2):197-201.

19

Advances in Acetabular Reconstruction in Revision Total Hip Arthroplasty: Maximizing Function and Outcomes After Treatment of Periacetabular Osteolysis Around the Well-Fixed Shell

Adam Hall, MD
Mark Eilers, MD
Rachel Hansen, BS
Brooke S. Robinson, MPH
William J. Maloney, MD
Wayne G. Paprosky, MD
Michael D. Ries, MD
Khaled J. Saleh, BSc, MD, MSc, FRCS(C), MHCM

Abstract

As the incidence of primary and revision hip arthroplasty increases, the need for a comprehensive approach to acetabular revision cannot be overstated. In the presence of osteolysis, there is a substantial population of patients with a well-fixed acetabular shell. It will be helpful to orthopaedic surgeons to review the classification of acetabular defects, techniques for exposing an acetabular component when the femoral component will be retained, methods of facilitating access to osteolytic lesions, the priciples of bone grafting, options for liner fixation, and when removal of a well-fixed shell is necessary.

Instr Course Lect 2014;63:209-218.

As the numbers of primary and revision hip arthroplasties increase, a comprehensive approach to acetabular revision is needed. A substantial number of patients with radiographic osteolysis in the hip after a total hip arthroplasty (THA) have a well-fixed acetabular shell. This chapter describes the classification and treatment of these patients, including the exposure of the

acetabular component with a retained, well-functioning femoral component; access to osteolytic lesions; bone grafting; liner fixation; and when to make the decision to remove the well-fixed acetabular shell.

THA is the definitive treatment for adult end-stage diseases of the hip. Few other treatment modalities have similar clinical success as THA, which has led

to an increased demand for the procedure. It is projected that by 2030, there will be more than 572,000 primary THAs and 97,000 revision THAs performed in the United States alone.[1]

With the advent of enhanced bearing surfaces and materials, total hip replacements are lasting longer than their predecessors. However, even with this improved durability, failure secondary to aseptic loosening, instability, malpositioning, infection, and polyethylene wear remain problematic. Aseptic loosening secondary to periprosthetic osteolysis is one of the leading causes of revision hip arthroplasty.[2,3]

With osteolysis and polyethylene wear in association with an osseointegrated acetabular shell, the surgeon must decide whether to exchange the polyethylene liner alone or undertake

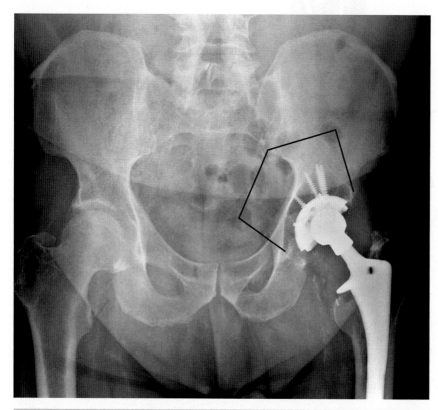

Figure 1 AP pelvic radiograph showing osteolysis (expansile type) around an uncemented acetabular component as indicated by the black outline.

path is at the cement-bone interface. This results in a linear pattern of osteolysis, manifested as a progressive radiolucent line at the cement-bone interface. These radiolucent regions occur predominantly in zone III, according to the classification system of DeLee and Charnley,[10] but may also occur in zone I.[6,11-13] Linear or focal osteolysis in two or three DeLee and Charnley acetabular zones has been associated with a prevalence of cemented socket loosening of 71% and 94%, respectively.[7,8,14] According to some authors, the socket is considered loose if the radiolucency encompasses the entire circumference of the cement-bone interface, irrespective of thickness.[15] However, other authors have reported that a circumferential radiolucency with a thickness of 2 mm or greater is required to consider the socket to be loose.[11-13]

In contrast, cementless porous-coated acetabular components have bone ingrowth into the porous coating by way of pseudopods of bone, with these areas being resistant to fluid and particles.[8,12,15] Areas without ingrowth then become the path of least resistance and provide access channels for fluid developing in the supra-acetabular space, forming expansile lesions[6,7,11-14] (**Figure 1**). These lesions occur predominantly in DeLee and Charnley zones II and III but may occur in any of the zones.[6,12] Expansile lesions around uncemented acetabular components can occur without affect-

the more difficult task of revising the acetabular cup.

The decision-making process is complex, and the goal of this chapter's authors is to review treatment options in revision arthroplasty in the face of a well-fixed acetabular component.

Preoperative Planning

The importance of preoperative planning cannot be overstated. Preoperative planning involves the patient history, the physical examination, the

diagnostic workup to rule out infection, and a thorough review of radiographs to determine the type of acetabular osseous defect.

It is important to note the pattern of osteolysis, which differs between cemented and uncemented components, and the implications for radiographic loosening, which differ between the two. Particle-laden joint fluid typically follows the path of least resistance within the effective joint space.[4-9] In the case of cemented components, that

Dr. Maloney or an immediate family member has received royalties from Wright Medical Technology; serves as a paid consultant to or is an employee of Pipeline Orthopaedics; has stock or stock options held in Abbott, Gillead, ISTO Technologies, Johnson & Johnson, Merck, Moximed, Pfizer, Pipeline Orthopaedics, and Total Joint Orthopedics; and serves as a board member, owner, officer, or committee member of the American Joint Replacement Registry, The Knee Society, and the Western Orthopaedic Association. Dr. Paprosky or an immediate family member has received royalties from Wright Medical Technology and Zimmer; is a member of a speakers' bureau or has made paid presentations on behalf of Zimmer; serves as a paid consultant to or is an employee of Biomet and Zimmer; and serves as a board member, owner, officer, or committee member of The Hip Society. Dr. Ries or an immediate family member has received royalties from Smith & Nephew; serves as a paid consultant to or is an employee of Smith & Nephew and Stryker; has stock or stock options held in OrthAlign; and serves as a board member, owner, officer, or committee member of the Foundation for the Advancement of Research in Medicine. Dr. Saleh or an immediate family member has received royalties from Aesculap/B. Braun; is a member of a speakers' bureau or has made paid presentations on behalf of Carefusion; serves as a paid consultant to or is an employee of Aesculap/B. Braun, the Memorial Medical Center Co-Management Orthopaedic Board and the Blue Cross Blue Shield Blue Ribbon Panel; has received research or institutional support from Smith & Nephew, the Orthopaedic Research and Education Foundation, and National Institutes of Health/National Institute of Arthritis and Musculoskeletal Skin Diseases (RO-I); and serves as a board member, owner, officer, or committee member of the American Orthopaedic Association and the Orthopaedic Research and Education Foundation. None of the following authors or any immediate family member has received anything of value from or has stock or stock options held in a commercial company or institution related directly or indirectly to the subject of this chapter: Dr. Hall, Dr. Eilers, Ms. Hansen, and Ms. Robinson.

ing implant stability, with one study citing a 48% rate of silent osteolysis identifiable CT.[16]

Cemented components generally do not remain well fixed because of the linear pattern of osteolysis noted at the cement-bone interface. However, cementless components may remain well fixed despite expansile osteolytic lesions.

Currently, radiography is the standard for both detecting and monitoring osteolytic defects. However, radiographs typically underestimate the size of the osteolytic lesions and are unable to detect smaller lesions altogether. Using both radiography and spiral CT, Puri et al[17] evaluated 50 hips that had been treated with primary cementless THA. Osteolysis was identified on the radiographs of 16 hips and on the CT scans of 26 hips. Furthermore, radiographs underestimated the extent of osteolysis in 13 hips (**Figure 2**). In another study, Leung et al[18] found that only 39% of lesions were detected on AP pelvic radiographs. Adding an iliac oblique radiograph increased detection to 52%, and CT scans identified 87% of the defects.

When reviewing radiographs, the accurate classification of acetabular defects is necessary. Classification systems are an important tool in evaluating acetabular defects and allow for a systematic approach to managing these defects. There are a number of good classification systems. This chapter's authors use the Saleh and Gross classification because this system has been validated and previously shown to have interobserver reliability.[19,20] This classification system also lends itself to a logical reconstruction paradigm.

The Saleh and Gross classification system distinguishes between segmental and cavitary defects and is based on the anticipated remaining bone stock after removal of the failed implant.[19,20] Five types of defects are de-

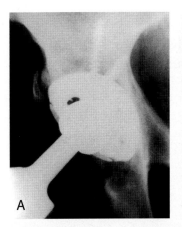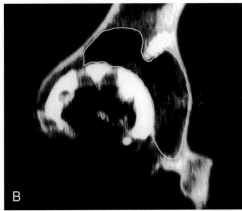

Figure 2   Imaging studies of a hip with osteolysis in an asymptomatic 70-year-old man who had undergone THA. **A,** AP radiograph made approximately 7 years postoperatively shows minimal evidence of osteolysis. **B,** Sagittal CT reconstruction made 7 years postoperatively shows the portion of the osteolytic lesion behind the acetabular cup that is not apparent on the standard AP radiograph. (Reproduced with permission from Puri L, Wixson RL, Stern SH, Kohli J, Hendrix RW, Stulberg SD: Use of helical CT for the assessment of acetabular osteolysis after total hip arthroplasty. *J Bone Joint Surg Am* 2002;84(4):609-614.)

Table 1

Saleh and Gross Classification System for Acetabular Bone Loss

Type	Description
I	No notable loss of bone stock. The amount of bone loss is less than that which would require a revision component. There has been no migration of the primary component into the ilium, and both columns are largely intact.
II	Contained loss of bone stock. There is cavitary or volumetric enlargement of the acetabulum. If the cup extends beyond the ilioischial line (protrusio), the defect can still be considered type II, provided the columns are intact.
III	Uncontained (segmental) loss of bone stock involving less than 50% of the acetabulum, primarily affecting either the anterior or the posterior column. Bone loss is considered uncontained if it is not amenable to treatment with morcellized bone graft. The sum of all segments of bone loss in either the anterior or the posterior column allows 50% or more of cup coverage by host bone (as assessed preoperatively with templates).
IV	Uncontained (segmental) loss of bone stock of more than 50% of the acetabulum affecting both the anterior and the posterior column. Type IV is identical to type III, except that the sum of the segmental bone loss in the columns exceeds 50%. There is no pelvic discontinuity.
V	Acetabular defect with contained loss of bone stock in association with pelvic discontinuity. Any pelvic discontinuity is considered a type V defect regardless of the amount of bone loss.

scribed in the classification system (**Table 1**). Type I has no notable loss of bone stock (a well-fixed cup with osteolysis). Type II has contained (cavitary) loss of bone stock. Type III has uncontained (segmental) loss of bone stock involving less than 50% of the acetabulum affecting one column. Type IV has uncontained (segmental) loss of bone stock of more than 50% of the acetabulum affecting both columns, and type V has an acetabular

Table 2

Treatment Algorithm for Pelvic Osteolysis Around Uncemented Cups as Proposed by Rubash et al[21-22] and Maloney et al[23]

Type I[a]: Radiographically stable cup

  Retain shell

  Exchange liner

  Graft may or may not be used

Type II[b]: Radiographically stable cup

  Revise component

  Graft may or may not be used

Type III: Radiographically unstable cup

  Revise component

  Graft may or may not be used

---

[a]For type I cups, six criteria must be met to perform a liner exchange. See text for a list of the criteria.
[b]Type II cups do not meet at least one of the type I criteria, but the cup is radiographically stable.

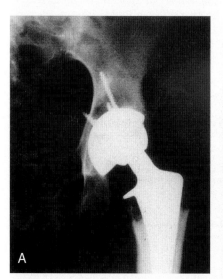 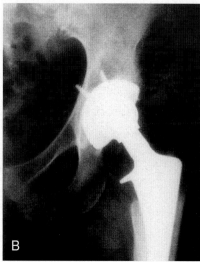

Figure 3 Radiographs of a hip with a type I cup. **A,** Preoperative radiograph showing that the polyethylene liner is worn, and there is radiographic evidence of osteolysis of the pelvis. The metal shell is well fixed. **B,** A radiograph, made 2 years after liner exchange and downsizing of the femoral head from a 32-mm head to a 28-mm femoral head, shows that the osteolytic lesion appears to have partially healed. The femoral head remains centered in the shell, and the socket remains radiographically stable. (Reproduced with permission from Maloney WJ, Paprosky W, Engh CA, Rubash H: Surgical treatment of pelvic osteolysis. *Clin Orthop Relat Res* 2001;393:78-84.)

metal augment. Type IV requires major structural grafts and/or large metallic augments. Type V defects require restoration of bone stock with structural grafts and a fixation device that bridges the defect.[19,20]

The Saleh and Gross classification system is useful when revision or reconstruction of the acetabular shell is planned. What about the well-fixed shell? The system described by Rubash et al[21,22] and Maloney et al[23] has been devised to guide treatment with regard to retention of stable acetabular shells and exchangeability of the polyethylene liner in cementless components. This classification system divides uncemented cups into three types on the basis of radiographic stability of the porous-coated shell and the possibility of exchanging the polyethylene liner while retaining the shell[21-23] (**Table 2**). In type I, the osteolysis is focal, and the cup is radiographically stable; however, the polyethylene liner is worn, with an eccentric position of the femoral head within the cup noted on radiographs. Hips with true type I cups are treated with polyethylene liner exchange, débridement of granulomatous material, and filling of accessible osteolytic lesions with graft material, if needed[21-23] (**Figure 3**). According to this classification system, six criteria must be met to perform a liner exchange: (1) the cup must not be malpositioned, (2) the locking mechanism for the modular acetabular component must be intact, (3) the metal shell must not be damaged secondary to head penetration, (4) the polyethylene liner replacement must be of adequate thickness, (5) the implant should be one with an acceptable track record, and (6) the implant should be a modular implant.

If any of the aforementioned criteria are not met, but the shell is radiographically stable, then it is classified as type II. In these cases, the surgeon

defect with contained loss of bone stock in association with pelvic discontinuity. Type I defects can be managed either with a conventional cemented or cementless acetabular component, or with retention and bone grafting if the cup is well fixed and functioning. Type II defects are cavitary lesions that can be managed with a large cementless cup, by creating a high hip center, and by morcellized cancellous graft impaction. Segmental defects are managed in accordance with the loss of bone stock. Type III can be managed with a cementless acetabular component and/or minor column graft or must be prepared to remove an ingrown metal shell. A high-speed metal cutting burr should be available to remove the socket piecemeal, if necessary. In addition, further instrumentation, including the explant system, curved gouges, osteotomes, and antiprotrusio cages, and bone graft material should be available.[21-23]

Type III cups have radiographic evidence of migration or complete implant-bone radiolucency and are thus considered unstable. Type III cups require acetabular shell revision.[21-23]

Using this classification system, Maloney et al[23] evaluated 124 failed cementless sockets preoperatively and found 40 that met type I criteria and 28 that met type II criteria. In the patients with type I cups, the polyethylene liner was exchanged, and the osteolytic lesions were débrided but not grafted in 11 patients, whereas allograft bone chips were packed into the defect in the remaining 29 patients. At a mean follow-up of 3.5 years, all of the acetabular components were radiographically stable, and no new osteolytic lesions were identified. Approximately one third of the lesions had resolved completely regardless of whether they were grafted. The remaining two thirds of the lesions had decreased in size. The patients with type II cups underwent socket revision, and all were radiographically stable at the final follow-up.[23]

It is important to remember that intraoperative assessment is the definitive method to assess loosening of the components. This chapter's authors recommend intraoperative testing of the shell by applying manual force to the nonarticulating surface (the superolateral aspect of the exposed shell) and looking for movement or seepage of blood between the bone-metal interface.

Preoperative planning can be imprecise in that a shell or femoral com-

ponent that appears well fixed radiographically may be determined to be loose intraoperatively. Thus, even when planning for an isolated polyethylene liner exchange, the surgeon should always be prepared to revise the shell. The necessary equipment, including revision components, graft, porous-coated and cemented components, and reconstruction rings, should be available.

The following sections describe the approach to managing periacetabular osteolysis around the well-fixed uncemented acetabular component. Cemented fixation of the acetabular component has largely fallen out of favor in primary arthroplasty, but cemented shells are still encountered for revision. When treating a patient with a cemented acetabular component, the surgeon may attempt to follow this approach but should expect to revise the cemented acetabular component.

Exposure With a Retained Femoral Component

Adequate exposure is the cornerstone of success in revision THA. This may require extensile methods not commonly used in primary arthroplasty. The exposure technique is influenced by the number of components to be revised (for example, liner, shell, femoral head, and/or femoral stem), the previous fixation technique (for example, cemented or uncemented), the degree of bone loss and/or the need for reconstruction, the component modularity, and the previous surgical approach.

When both the femoral and the acetabular components need to be revised, particularly with a nonmodular femoral component, the use of a trochanteric osteotomy or extended trochanteric osteotomy may be necessary.[24-33] This technique is not without risk, because poor bone quality secondary to stress shielding as well

as osteolysis may lead to trochanteric nonunion and subsequently to instability.[34] This has led to alternative exposure techniques when both components are revised.[34,35]

In a hip with a well-fixed femoral stem with a modular head-neck junction, it is desirable to revise the acetabular component while retaining the femoral stem. This avoids the potential morbidity of femoral stem removal, including intraoperative fracture, prolonged surgical time, and increased blood loss. Moskal et al[36] reviewed the cases of 32 patients treated with isolated revision acetabuloplasty without removal of a well-fixed femoral component. At an average follow-up of 8.1 years (range, 6.4 to 12.5 years) after the revision surgery (an average of 17 years after the primary surgical procedure), 97% of the primary femoral components were stable and well fixed. They observed no dislocations, nerve palsies, or intraoperative fractures in their series using a modified direct lateral surgical approach.[36,37] Neil and Solomon[38] described a posterior surgical approach in which a pocket is created by reflecting the capsule from the anterior aspect of the acetabulum where the femoral neck (or femoral head with a nonmodular prosthesis) of the femoral prosthesis can be displaced and held with a Hohmann retractor. In addition to providing exposure, this technique also protects the trunion from inadvertent injury.

Access to Acetabular Osteolytic Lesions

For acetabular shell revision, access to osteolytic lesions is facilitated by the exposure of the shell and its subsequent removal. In hips in which the shell is retained, alternative routes must be found. In this regard, Sablan and Lieberman[8] suggested three ways to access these lesions. The first option is to locate an egress hole at the periphery of the shell and, if necessary, widen the hole to allow access for débridement and grafting. If the retained shell has existing screw or dome holes, these may also be used, and they may be adequate when osteolysis is limited to the region of these holes. Alternatively, a trapdoor may be created superior or posterior to the rim of the component.[8] This chapter's authors prefer to make a rectangular window approximately 2 cm superior to the retained component. This creates access to débride and graft lesions both anterior and posterior to the shell. After bone grafting the lesions, the rectangular cortical segment can then be placed into the window and rotated 90° to help contain the graft material.

Principles of Bone Grafting

The use of bone graft in the treatment of osteolysis can serve osteoconductive, osteoinductive, osteogenic, and mechanical functions. The need for each function varies on the basis of the size and the type of defect. With a well-fixed shell, the osteolytic lesions are often cavitary and do not require the level of mechanical support that would be desirable with pelvic discontinuity.

In a review of the basic science and clinical applications of bone grafts in revision hip arthroplasty, Goldberg[39] explained that autogenous bone is superior to allogeneic graft in restoring bone loss. Autogenous bone is limited by supply and donor-site morbidity; thus, allograft is often used in place of or in conjunction with autogenous graft. Local autogenous donor sites include the greater trochanter and the anterior and posterior iliac crest.

In the treatment of cavitary defects around a well-fixed shell, access for grafting is often limited; thus, many authors have described the use of particulate or morcellized graft products. This form of graft material is often limited in its mechanical support but

can be superior in osteoinductive and osteogenic potential. Autograft remains the gold standard and is known to produce new bone within 4 to 8 weeks.[39-41] Further, cancellous bone has greater potential for promoting bone formation because of its larger surface area relative to cortical bone.[39]

Allograft is useful as a primary and adjunct source of graft in treating osteolysis. It avoids the potential drawbacks of autograft, including donor-site morbidity, and it should not be limited by supply if arrangements are made for its availability. It does, however, have its own set of risks. Allogeneic bone is well known to create an immune response in the recipient.[42,43] In addition, there is a risk of disease transmission (hepatitis B, hepatitis C, or HIV) when any transplanted tissue is used, although this risk can be reduced when grafts are obtained from sources that follow the standards of the American Association of Tissue Banks.[39,44] The risk of HIV transmission from allograft sources is estimated to be approximately 1 in 1.6 million.[44,45] These risks are minimized when bone tissues are processed to eliminate cells and tissue factors, although this eliminates their osteoinductive and osteogenic potential. Demineralized bone matrix retains osteoinductive properties while maintaining the potential risks of allograft. Demineralized bone matrix products lack osteoconductive and mechanical supportive properties but have the advantage of faster incorporation by host bone.[39]

Another potential option lies in the use of bioresorbable cement. The use of calcium phosphate-based cements has been suggested as a stand-alone agent and as a graft extender by mixing with bone allograft in revision hip arthroplasty, but the in vitro and in vivo data to support its use are very limited in the arthroplasty literature.[46-48] These preliminary studies suggest that

it may enhance the mechanical properties of particulate graft materials.

Each of the graft options has distinct advantages and disadvantages. Autograft has the best all-around graft properties while minimizing rejection and disease transmission risks. Although limited in its local supply, its role remains vital and can often be incorporated with the use of the other sources as graft extenders.

Liner Fixation

To retain a well-fixed acetabular shell, adequate liner fixation is essential. In the simplest scenario, an intact locking mechanism in an undamaged shell can be used to secure a liner of adequate thickness. Alternatively, either complete shell revision or securing the liner by cementing it into the metal shell can be done (**Figure 4**).

The technique of cementing the liner into a well-fixed shell has been previously described in conjunction with both modular and nonmodular shell designs.[49-52] To apply this technique, the well-fixed shell should not be malpositioned and should be able to accept a liner of adequate diameter and thickness. Biomechanical studies support its use and suggest that it does not affect polyethylene wear rates.[53] Clinical studies have shown promising outcomes, but caution is advised when considering the technique in patients with hip instability.[54-56]

When cementing a liner into a well-fixed shell, this chapter's authors prefer to texture the outer surface of the liner and the inner surface of the shell with a metal cutting burr to facilitate stability of the interface. Texturing of polyethylene liners in this technique improves torsional and lever-out strength.[57] If an oversized liner is used, a circumferential pattern (rather than cruciform) can improve the biomechanical strength of the interface.[58]

When To "Call It" and Remove the Shell

In the setting of a well-fixed shell, the choice of liner exchange or revision of the acetabular shell is challenging. Given the complexity of making this decision and the risk of complications, some advocate removal and revision of the well-fixed shell in the presence of osteolysis.[59-61] This chapter's authors recommend a systematic consideration of criteria previously described by one of the senior authors (WJM) for liner exchange as discussed in the preoperative planning section. If these criteria are met, but the center of rotation and/or mechanical stability cannot be restored, then revision of both the acetabular and the femoral components must be considered.

First, attention should be paid to the clinical track record of the implant and, in particular, the intraoperative assessment of the locking mechanism. If the implant is known to have a high failure rate with polyethylene breakage or fixation failure, such as has occurred with the Acetabular Cup System (DePuy), then removal of the shell with revision should be strongly considered.[62,63]

Some components, such as the Harris-Galante porous-coated acetabular component (Zimmer), have shown good results in primary and revision arthroplasty.[64-67] However, this component also has had several reports of dislodgment of the polyethylene liner from the metal shell.[68-70] Most recently, Talmo et al[71] reported on 128 revision THAs involving well-fixed Harris-Galante acetabular components. Of those treated with isolated liner exchange, 25% of the patients required rerevision at a minimum follow-up of 2 years. More than 50% of these revisions were related to liner dislodgment despite intraoperative assessment of the locking mechanism. The authors concluded that complete

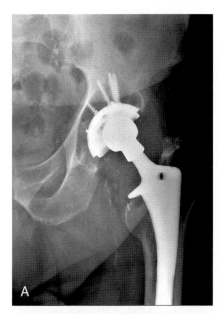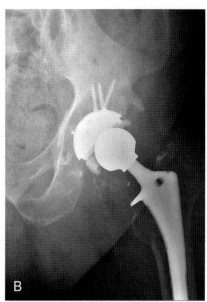

Figure 4   Radiographs of the hip of a patient who had osteolysis around an acetabular shell that was well fixed at the time of surgery. **A,** Preoperative radiograph. **B,** Radiograph made 6 months after the patient was treated with grafting through the acetabular holes and a trapdoor in the ilium. A new liner was then cemented into the existing shell.

revision is a more reliable option with a well-fixed Harris-Galante shell.[71] Alternatively, this chapter's authors routinely cement highly cross-linked polyethylene liners into well-fixed Harris-Galante shells when they are well positioned and the center of rotation can be restored.

Postoperative Care

Postoperative care should begin with physical therapy, routine postoperative wound care, and appropriate venous thromboembolism and infection prophylaxis during the hospital stay. The degree of bone loss, condition of host bone, mechanical strength of the graft, and stability of the implants will influence weight-bearing status. Many authors advocate limited weight bearing during the initial postoperative period. However, some evidence has suggested that early, full weight bearing does not have detrimental effects and may, in fact, have beneficial remodeling effects

when morcellized impacted grafts are used.[72,73] Abduction bracing may be considered in patients having revision THA in an attempt to minimize early dislocation and allow for soft-tissue healing; however, data to support this as a routine practice are limited, and its use has been challenged by more recent studies.[74-78]

Summary

As the numbers of primary and revision THAs increase, there is a need for a comprehensive approach to acetabular revision. A substantial number of patients with radiographic osteolysis have a well-fixed acetabular shell. The classification and treatment of these patients has been described, including exposure of the acetabular component with a retained femoral component, access to osteolytic lesions, bone grafting, liner fixation, and when to make the decision to remove the well-fixed acetabular shell.

References

1. Kurtz S, Ong K, Lau E, Mowat F, Halpern M: Projections of primary and revision hip and knee arthroplasty in the United States from 2005 to 2030. *J Bone Joint Surg Am* 2007;89(4):780-785.

2. Harris WH: The problem is osteolysis. *Clin Orthop Relat Res* 1995;311:46-53.

3. Desai MA, Bancroft LW: The case: Diagnosis. Periprosthetic osteolysis. *Orthopedics* 2008; 31(6):518, 615-618.

4. Archibeck MJ, Jacobs JJ, Roebuck KA, Glant TT: The basic science of periprosthetic osteolysis. *Instr Course Lect* 2001;50:185-195.

5. Beck RT, Illingworth KD, Saleh KJ: Review of periprosthetic osteolysis in total joint arthroplasty: An emphasis on host factors and future directions. *J Orthop Res* 2012;30(4):541-546.

6. Chiang PP, Burke DW, Freiberg AA, Rubash HE: Osteolysis of the pelvis: Evaluation and treatment. *Clin Orthop Relat Res* 2003;417: 164-174.

7. Saleh KJ, Thongtrangan I, Schwarz EM: Osteolysis: Medical and surgical approaches. *Clin Orthop Relat Res* 2004;427:138-147.

8. Sablan NK, Lieberman JR: *Arthritis and Arthroplasty: The Hip*. Philadelphia, PA, Saunders; 2009, pp 387-397.

9. Schmalzried TP, Jasty M, Harris WH: Periprosthetic bone loss in total hip arthroplasty: Polyethylene wear debris and the concept of the effective joint space. *J Bone Joint Surg Am* 1992;74(6): 849-863.

10. DeLee JG, Charnley J: Radiological demarcation of cemented sockets in total hip replacement. *Clin Orthop Relat Res* 1976;121: 20-32.

11. Harris WH: Wear and periprosthetic osteolysis: The problem.

Clin Orthop Relat Res 2001;393: 66-70.

12. Sinha RK, Shanbhag AS, Maloney WJ, Hasselman CT, Rubash HE: Osteolysis: Cause and effect. *Instr Course Lect* 1998;47:307-320.

13. Zicat B, Engh CA, Gokcen E: Patterns of osteolysis around total hip components inserted with and without cement. *J Bone Joint Surg Am* 1995;77(3):432-439.

14. Hodgkinson JP, Shelley P, Wroblewski BM: The correlation between the roentgenographic appearance and operative findings at the bone-cement junction of the socket in Charnley low friction arthroplasties. *Clin Orthop Relat Res* 1988;228:105-109.

15. Maloney WJ, Herzwurm P, Paprosky W, Rubash HE, Engh CA: Treatment of pelvic osteolysis associated with a stable acetabular component inserted without cement as part of a total hip replacement. *J Bone Joint Surg Am* 1997; 79(11):1628-1634.

16. Stulberg SD, Wixson RL, Adams AD, Hendrix RW, Bernfield JB: Monitoring pelvic osteolysis following total hip replacement surgery: An algorithm for surveillance. *J Bone Joint Surg Am* 2002; 84(suppl 2):116-122.

17. Puri L, Wixson RL, Stern SH, Kohli J, Hendrix RW, Stulberg SD: Use of helical computed tomography for the assessment of acetabular osteolysis after total hip arthroplasty. *J Bone Joint Surg Am* 2002;84(4):609-614.

18. Leung S, Naudie D, Kitamura N, Walde T, Engh CA: Computed tomography in the assessment of periacetabular osteolysis. *J Bone Joint Surg Am* 2005;87(3): 592-597.

19. Johanson NA, Driftmier KR, Cerynik DL, Stehman CC: Grading acetabular defects: The need for a universal and valid system. *J Arthroplasty* 2010;25(3): 425-431.

20. Saleh KJ, Holtzman J, Gafni A, et al: Reliability and intraoperative validity of preoperative assessment of standardized plain radiographs in predicting bone loss at revision hip surgery. *J Bone Joint Surg Am* 2001;83(7):1040-1046.

21. Rubash HE, Sinha RK, Paprosky W, Engh CA, Maloney WJ: A new classification system for the management of acetabular osteolysis after total hip arthroplasty. *Instr Course Lect* 1999;48:37-42.

22. Rubash HE, Sinha RK, Maloney WJ, Paprosky WG: Osteolysis: Surgical treatment. *Instr Course Lect* 1998;47:321-329.

23. Maloney WJ, Paprosky W, Engh CA, Rubash H: Surgical treatment of pelvic osteolysis. *Clin Orthop Relat Res* 2001;393:78-84.

24. Charnley J, Ferreiraade S: Transplantation of the greater trochanter in arthroplasty of the hip. *J Bone Joint Surg Br* 1964;46: 191-197.

25. Dall D: Exposure of the hip by anterior osteotomy of the greater trochanter: A modified anterolateral approach. *J Bone Joint Surg Br* 1986;68(3):382-386.

26. Glassman AH, Engh CA, Bobyn JD: A technique of extensile exposure for total hip arthroplasty. *J Arthroplasty* 1987;2(1): 11-21.

27. Aribindi R, Paprosky W, Nourbash P, Kronick J, Barba M: Extended proximal femoral osteotomy. *Instr Course Lect* 1999; 48:19-26.

28. Chen WM, McAuley JP, Engh CA Jr, Hopper RH Jr, Engh CA: Extended slide trochanteric osteotomy for revision total hip arthroplasty. *J Bone Joint Surg Am* 2000;82(9):1215-1219.

29. McGrory BJ, Bal BS, Harris WH: Trochanteric osteotomy for total hip arthroplasty: Six variations and indications for their use. *J Am Acad Orthop Surg* 1996;4(5): 258-267.

30. Meek RM, Greidanus NV, Garbuz DS, Masri BA, Duncan CP: Extended trochanteric osteotomy: Planning, surgical technique, and pitfalls. *Instr Course Lect* 2004;53:119-130.

31. Miner TM, Momberger NG, Chong D, Paprosky WL: The extended trochanteric osteotomy in revision hip arthroplasty: A critical review of 166 cases at mean 3-year, 9-month follow-up. *J Arthroplasty* 2001;16(8):188-194.

32. Peters PC Jr, Head WC, Emerson RH Jr: An extended trochanteric osteotomy for revision total hip replacement. *J Bone Joint Surg Br* 1993;75(1):158-159.

33. Younger TI, Bradford MS, Magnus RE, Paprosky WG: Extended proximal femoral osteotomy: A new technique for femoral revision arthroplasty. *J Arthroplasty* 1995;10(3):329-338.

34. Head WC, Mallory TH, Berklacich FM, Dennis DA, Emerson RH Jr, Wapner KL: Extensile exposure of the hip for revision arthroplasty. *J Arthroplasty* 1987;2(4):265-273.

35. McMinn DJ, Roberts P, Forward GR: A new approach to the hip for revision surgery. *J Bone Joint Surg Br* 1991;73(6):899-901.

36. Moskal JT, Shen FH, Brown TE: The fate of stable femoral components retained during isolated acetabular revision: A six-to-twelve-year follow-up study. *J Bone Joint Surg Am* 2002;84(2):250-255.

37. Moskal JT, Mann JW III: A modified direct lateral approach for primary and revision total hip arthroplasty: A prospective analysis of 453 cases. *J Arthroplasty* 1996;11(3):255-266.

38. Neil MJ, Solomon MI: A technique of revision of failed acetabular components leaving the femoral component in situ.

J Arthroplasty 1996;11(4):482-483.

39. Goldberg VM: Selection of bone grafts for revision total hip arthroplasty. *Clin Orthop Relat Res* 2000;381:68-76.

40. Burwell RG: Osteogenesis in cancellous bone grafts: Considered in terms of cellular changes, basic mechanisms and the perspective of growth-control and its possible aberrations. *Clin Orthop Relat Res* 1965;40:35-47.

41. Gray JC, Elves MW: Early osteogenesis in compact bone isografts: A quantitative study of contributions of the different graft cells. *Calcif Tissue Int* 1979;29(3):225-237.

42. Stevenson S, Li XQ, Davy DT, Klein L, Goldberg VM: Critical biological determinants of incorporation of non-vascularized cortical bone grafts: Quantification of a complex process and structure. *J Bone Joint Surg Am* 1997;79(1):1-16.

43. Stevenson S, Horowitz M: The response to bone allografts. *J Bone Joint Surg Am* 1992;74(6):939-950.

44. Mroz TE, Joyce MJ, Steinmetz MP, Lieberman IH, Wang JC: Musculoskeletal allograft risks and recalls in the United States. *J Am Acad Orthop Surg* 2008;16(10):559-565.

45. Boyce T, Edwards J, Scarborough N: Allograft bone: The influence of processing on safety and performance. *Orthop Clin North Am* 1999;30(4):571-581.

46. Jacofsky DJ, McCamley JD, Jaczynski AM, Shrader MW, Jacofsky MC: Improving initial acetabular component stability in revision total hip arthroplasty calcium phosphate cement vs reverse reamed cancellous allograft. *J Arthroplasty* 2012;27(2):305-309.

47. Nich C, Sedel L: Bone substitution in revision hip replacement. *Int Orthop* 2006;30(6):525-531.

48. Speirs AD, Oxland TR, Masri BA, Poursartip A, Duncan CP: Calcium phosphate cement composites in revision hip arthroplasty. *Biomaterials* 2005;26(35):7310-7318.

49. Heck DA, Murray DG: In vivo construction of a metal-backed, high-molecular-weight polyethylene cup during McKee-Farrar revision total joint arthroplasty: A case report. *J Arthroplasty* 1986;1(3):203-206.

50. Jiranek WA: Acetabular liner fixation by cement. *Clin Orthop Relat Res* 2003;417:217-223.

51. LaPorte DM, Mont MA, Pierre-Jacques H, Peyton RS, Hungerford DS: Technique for acetabular liner revision in a nonmodular metal-backed component. *J Arthroplasty* 1998;13(3):348-350.

52. Springer BD, Hanssen AD, Lewallen DG: Cementation of an acetabular liner into a well-fixed acetabular shell during revision total hip arthroplasty. *J Arthroplasty* 2003;18(7):126-130.

53. Delanois RE, Seyler TM, Essner A, Schmidig G, Mont MA: Cementation of a polyethylene liner into a metal shell. *J Arthroplasty* 2007;22(5):732-737.

54. Beaulé PE, Ebramzadeh E, Le Duff M, Prasad R, Amstutz HC: Cementing a liner into a stable cementless acetabular shell: The double-socket technique. *J Bone Joint Surg Am* 2004;86(5):929-934.

55. Callaghan JJ, Hennessy DW, Liu SS, Goetz KE, Heiner AD: Cementing acetabular liners into secure cementless shells for polyethylene wear provides durable mid-term fixation. *Clin Orthop Relat Res* 2012;470(11):3142-3147.

56. Yoon TR, Seon JK, Song EK, Chung JY, Seo HY, Park YB: Cementation of a metal-inlay polyethylene liner into a stable metal shell in revision total hip arthroplasty. *J Arthroplasty* 2005;20(5): 652-657.

57. Haft GF, Heiner AD, Callaghan JJ, et al: Polyethylene liner cementation into fixed acetabular shells. *J Arthroplasty* 2002;17(4): 167-170.

58. Bonner KF, Delanois RE, Harbach G, Bushelow M, Mont MA: Cementation of a polyethylene liner into a metal shell: Factors related to mechanical stability. *J Bone Joint Surg Am* 2002;84(9): 1587-1593.

59. Hozack WJ, Mesa JJ, Carey C, Rothman RH: Relationship between polyethylene wear, pelvic osteolysis, and clinical symptomatology in patients with cementless acetabular components: A framework for decision making. *J Arthroplasty* 1996;11(7):769-772.

60. Kavanagh BF, Callaghan JJ, Leggon R, Heekin RD, Wold L: Pelvic osteolysis associated with an uncemented acetabular component in total hip arthroplasty. *Orthopedics* 1996;19(2):159-163.

61. Mallory TH, Lombardi AV Jr, Fada RA, Adams JB, Kefauver CA, Eberle RW: Noncemented acetabular component removal in the presence of osteolysis: The affirmative. *Clin Orthop Relat Res* 2000;381:120-128.

62. Bono JV, Sanford L, Toussaint JT: Severe polyethylene wear in total hip arthroplasty: Observations from retrieved AML PLUS hip implants with an ACS polyethylene liner. *J Arthroplasty* 1994; 9(2):119-125.

63. Manley MT, Capello WN, D'Antonio JA, Edidin AA, Geesink RG: Fixation of acetabular cups without cement in total hip arthroplasty: A comparison of three different implant surfaces at a minimum duration of follow-up of five years. *J Bone Joint Surg Am* 1998;80(8):1175-1185.

64. Clohisy JC, Harris WH: The Harris-Galante porous-coated acetabular component with screw fixation: An average ten-year follow-up study. *J Bone Joint Surg Am* 1999;81(1):66-73.

65. Hallstrom BR, Golladay GJ, Vittetoe DA, Harris WH: Cementless acetabular revision with the Harris-Galante porous prosthesis: Results after a minimum of ten years of follow-up. *J Bone Joint Surg Am* 2004;86(5):1007-1011.

66. Jamali AA, Dungy DS, Mark A, Schule S, Harris WH: Isolated acetabular revision with use of the Harris-Galante Cementless Component: Study with intermediate-term follow-up. *J Bone Joint Surg Am* 2004;86(8):1690-1697.

67. Petersen MB, Poulsen IH, Thomsen J, Solgaard S: The hemispherical Harris-Galante acetabular cup, inserted without cement: The results of an eight to eleven-year follow-up of one hundred and sixty-eight hips. *J Bone Joint Surg Am* 1999;81(2):219-224.

68. González della Valle A, Ruzo PS, Li S, Pellicci P, Sculco TP, Salvati EA: Dislodgment of polyethylene liners in first and second-generation Harris-Galante acetabular components: A report of eighteen cases. *J Bone Joint Surg Am* 2001;83(4):553-559.

69. Mihalko WM, Papademetriou T: Polyethylene liner dissociation with the Harris-Galante II acetabular component. *Clin Orthop Relat Res* 2001;386:166-172.

70. Min BW, Song KS, Kang CH, Won YY, Koo KH: Polyethylene liner failure in second-generation Harris-Galante acetabular components. *J Arthroplasty* 2005;20(6): 717-722.

71. Talmo CT, Kwon YM, Freiberg AA, Rubash HE, Malchau H: Management of polyethylene wear associated with a well-fixed modular cementless shell during revision total hip arthroplasty. *J Arthroplasty* 2011;26(4):576-581.

72. Ornstein E, Franzén H, Johnsson R, Stefánsdóttir A, Sundberg M, Tägil M: Hip revision with impacted morselized allografts: Unrestricted weight-bearing and restricted weight-bearing have similar effect on migration. A radiostereometry analysis. *Arch Orthop Trauma Surg* 2003; 123(6):261-267.

73. Wang JS, Tägil M, Aspenberg P: Load-bearing increases new bone formation in impacted and morselized allografts. *Clin Orthop Relat Res* 2000;378:274-281.

74. Dorr LD, Wolf AW, Chandler R, Conaty JP: Classification and treatment of dislocations of total hip arthroplasty. *Clin Orthop Relat Res* 1983;173:151-158.

75. Ritter MA: Dislocation and subluxation of the total hip replacement. *Clin Orthop Relat Res* 1976; 121:92-94.

76. Dewal H, Maurer SL, Tsai P, Su E, Hiebert R, Di Cesare PE: Efficacy of abduction bracing in the management of total hip arthroplasty dislocation. *J Arthroplasty* 2004;19(6):733-738.

77. Murray TG, Wetters NG, Moric M, Sporer SM, Paprosky WG, Della Valle CJ: The use of abduction bracing for the prevention of early postoperative dislocation after revision total hip arthroplasty. *J Arthroplasty* 2012;27(8): 126-129.

78. Patel PD, Potts A, Froimson MI: The dislocating hip arthroplasty: Prevention and treatment. *J Arthroplasty* 2007;22(4):86-90.

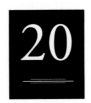

Acetabular Reconstruction in Revision Total Hip Arthroplasty: Maximizing Function and Outcomes in Protrusio and Cavitary Defects

Brian Dahl, MD
Christian McNeely, BS
Brooke S. Robinson, MPH
William J. Maloney, MD
Wayne G. Paprosky, MD
Michael D. Ries, MD
Khaled J. Saleh, BSc, MD, MSc, FRCS(C), MHCM

Abstract

Osteolysis in the periacetabular region is a common long-term complication of total hip arthroplasty that can lead to bone loss, implant loosening, and protrusio. Several systems have been developed for classifying osteolysis and guiding treatment. Options such as bone grafting or augmentation, with exchange of the bearing surface and, in some cases, revision of the acetabular component, can be used for treatment. Most cavitary and protrusio defects can be treated with a cementless revision cup using screw fixation and grafting with morcellized bone. However, structural augmentation, custom components, or cage reconstruction may occasionally be necessary for managing larger defects with severe loss of acetabular bone stock.

Instr Course Lect 2014;63:219-225.

The number of total hip arthroplasties (THAs) being performed in the United States is increasing each year.[1] Late complications, such as polyethylene wear and subsequent osteolysis, are becoming increasingly common. Fortunately, orthopaedic surgeons have many options for managing osteolysis-associated bone loss during revision surgery.

Osteolysis after THA is primarily caused by a macrophage-mediated inflammatory reaction in response to wear-related polyethylene debris. (More information on osteolysis after

Dr. Maloney or an immediate family member has received royalties from Wright Medical Technology; serves as a paid consultant to or is an employee of Pipeline Orthopaedics; has stock or stock options held in Abbott, Gillead, ISTO Technologies, Johnson & Johnson, Merck, Moximed, Pfizer, Pipeline Orthopaedics, and TJO; and serves as a board member, owner, officer, or committee member of the American Joint Replacement Registry, The Knee Society, and the Western Orthopaedic Association. Dr. Paprosky or an immediate family member has received royalties from Wright Medical Technology and Zimmer; is a member of a speakers' bureau or has made paid presentations on behalf of Zimmer; serves as a paid consultant to or is an employee of Biomet and Zimmer; and serves as a board member, owner, officer, or committee member of The Hip Society. Dr. Ries or an immediate family member has received royalties from Smith & Nephew; serves as a paid consultant to or is an employee of Smith & Nephew and Stryker; has stock or stock options held in OrthAlign; and serves as a board member, owner, officer, or committee member of the Foundation for the Advancement of Research in Medicine. Dr. Saleh or an immediate family member has received royalties from Aesculap/B. Braun; is a member of a speakers' bureau or has made paid presentations on behalf of Carefusion; serves as a paid consultant to Aesculap/B. Braun, the Memorial Medical Center Co-Management Orthopaedic Board, and the Blue Cross Blue Shield Blue Ribbon Panel; has received research or institutional support from Smith & Nephew, the Orthopaedic Research and Education Foundation, and National Institutes of Health/National Institute of Arthritis and Musculoskeletal Skin Diseases (RO-I) and serves as a board member, owner, officer, or committee member of the American Orthopaedic Association and the Orthopaedic Research and Education Foundation. None of the following authors or any immediate family member has received anything of value from or has stock or stock options held in a commercial company or institution related directly or indirectly to the subject of this chapter: Dr. Dahl, Mr. McNeely, and Ms. Robinson.

THA is available in *Instructional Course Lecture, Volume 63*, chapter 16, Advances in Acetabular Osteolysis: Biomarkers, Imaging, and Pharmacologic Management. It may take several years for bony defects to be visualized with radiography, and some defects may be seen only on oblique radiographs.[2] CT has a much higher sensitivity than standard radiography for detecting osteolysis.[3] Patterns of osteolysis can differ based on implant fixation. Cemented cups exhibit a more linear pattern of osteolysis that is commonly associated with acetabular loosening, whereas uncemented components are more likely to be associated with larger defects that are localized and expansile but are less often associated with component loosening.[4] However, with time, such components are at risk for late cup loosening, which is often associated with severe bone loss that can greatly complicate the revision procedure.[5]

Bone Defect Assessment

Accurate bone defect assessment and classification is an important facet of acetabular reconstruction in revision THA because it helps guide treatment decisions and can predict results. Failure to accurately identify and classify defects preoperatively and appropriately plan for them can lead to recurrent failure.

Three standard radiographic views are recommended, especially in posterior cavitary defects in which the acetabular implant obscures all or part of the lytic lesion, making it difficult to fully visualize on an AP view. Using the 45° iliac-oblique and 60° obturator-oblique views allows for better detection of osteolysis versus the AP view alone[2] (**Figure 1**). CT is substantially more sensitive than standard radiography for detecting osteolysis, especially in the acetabular rim and ischium, and has a much higher corre-

lation with intraoperative findings. CT images can be distorted by metal artifact, particularly from cobalt-chromium implants. Metal artifact reduction protocols, which improve the quality of images in proximity to metal implants, are now available.[6] Because of the high radiation associated with CT, it should be reserved for use in preoperative planning or when there is clinical suspicion of osteolytic lesions that cannot be seen with routine radiography.[3]

Several classification schemes have been published for grading acetabular bony defects in revision THA.[7-12] The main functions of these classification systems are to provide an organizational structure that can be used for research purposes and help guide treatment decisions. Although the most commonly used systems have several similarities, they all have unique grading scales for defect progression from mild to severe bone loss. The classification scheme proposed by the American Academy of Orthopaedic Surgeons divides defects by anatomic location and type but does not address treatment.[10] The Saleh and Gross classification system is based on the estimated bone stock available after implant removal, is predictive of intraoperative findings, and has a high level of interobserver reliability.[12,13] The Paprosky classification system is based on the presence or absence of supporting structures and the degree of prosthetic migration.[8]

Protrusio is a cavitary deformity in which the femoral head has migrated medial to the Köhler line (the line on an AP radiograph that extends from the lateral border of the sciatic notch to the medial border of the obturator foramen), indicating anterior column bone loss[14,15] (**Figure 2**). Protrusio defects are typically categorized as a type II defect in the Saleh and Gross classification system or as type IIc defects in the Paprosky system. Clini-

cally, the divisions between classes within a given grading system are important because they can help dictate optimal treatment decisions. The Paprosky and Saleh and Gross classification systems detail treatment options for each class.[9-16] For example, Paprosky type IIc is a protrusion defect that can usually be treated with a cementless cup with adjunctive screw fixation alone, whereas more severely graded deformities, such as Paprosky type III, may require augmentation because of the loss of the acetabular rim or supporting columns.[17] (More information about these classification systems and deformities requiring structural augmentation is available in *Instructional Course Lectures, Volume 63*, chapter 17 [Maximizing Function and Outcomes in Acetabular Reconstruction: Segmental Bony Defects and Pelvic Continuity] and chapter 19 [Advances in Acetabular Reconstruction in Revision Total Hip Arthroplasty: Maximizing Function and Outcomes After Treatment of Periacetabular Osteolysis Around the Well-Fixed Shell]).

Surgical Treatment

Approaches

The posterior approach has been the workhorse for revision THA, although anterior and anterolateral approaches also can be used. The posterior approach provides excellent exposure of the acetabulum and proximal femur, and it can be extended with a trochanteric osteotomy, and, if needed, the release of the gluteus maximus tendon. However, this approach is associated with a higher risk of posterior dislocation. The anterior approach yields excellent exposure with less risk of dislocation; however, the approach is not as extensible.

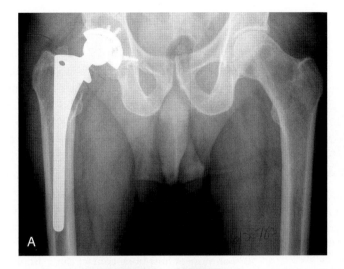

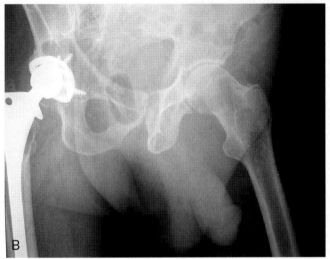

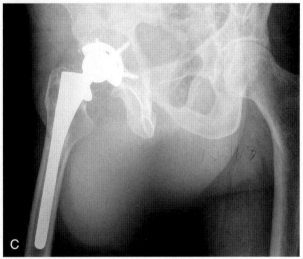

Figure 1   AP (**A**), 45° obturator-oblique (**B**), and 45° iliac-oblique (**C**) radiographic views of a right acetabular cup with evidence of a large osteolytic lesion. The full extent of the lesion cannot be appreciated on the AP pelvic view alone.

Liner Exchange and Bone Grafting

Patients with cavitary lesions with well-fixed and well-oriented acetabular components can be treated with an isolated liner exchange. Bone grafting the defect through the screw holes is technically easy to perform and may help replenish bone stock over time; however, some authors have suggested that bone grafting these defects has no value. After removing the polyethylene liner, bone stock can be assessed with a small curet or depth gauge passed through the screw holes in the acetab-

ular component. All loose screws should be removed, leaving well-fixed screws in place. Although 6.5-mm hex screwdrivers fit most acetabular components, other variations exist; therefore, preoperative identification of the implanted component is critical to ensure that the correct screwdrivers are available at the time of the revision procedure. Lesions behind a well-fixed cup are usually filled with granulomatous tissue that lightly adheres to the bony wall; these lesions should be curettaged and grafted with morcellized bone. After grafting, the appropriate

cross-linked polyethylene liner is inserted using the existing locking mechanism. Knowledge of the size and the name of the manufacturer of the current implant is critical to ensure the availability of replacement implants or trials. If the locking mechanism is destroyed or the correct polyethylene liner is unavailable, an appropriately sized polyethylene liner can be cemented into the cup after roughening the interior of the shell and backside of the liner with a burr to facilitate fixation.[18] Because dislocation is the most common complication in a revised

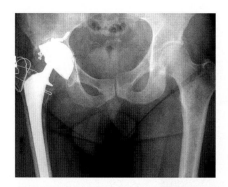

Figure 2 AP radiograph showing a protrusio deformity. The medial border of the acetabular component is medial to the Köhler line from the lateral border of the sciatic notch to the medial border of the obturator foramen.

THA, the largest head size that will fit in a well-fixed cup is typically used. Trialing the femoral head size and neck length before final implantation is recommended to ensure final stability.

Shell Revision

Loose or malpositioned acetabular components should be revised. The polyethylene should be removed without damaging the locking mechanism if possible in the event a liner exchange alone is warranted. Retroverted cups and vertical cup positions of more than 50° should be revised because they can lead to instability and abnormally increased wear that propagates osteolysis.[19]

To remove cementless components, the Explant system (Zimmer) or an equivalent device can be used to minimize bone loss. The Explant system consists of curved cutting blades that are specifically sized to the outer diameter of the cup and pass around it directly adjacent to the porous coating to free the area of bony ingrowth.[20] If a cemented component is being removed, this chapter's authors prefer to use curved osteotomes to divide the cement-component interface to loosen

and remove the implant. The cement is then removed with handheld cement removal instruments or a burr.[16]

In acetabular protrusio, there is medial migration of the cup, which generally leaves an intact peripheral rim. Because the rim is left intact, most cavitary and protrusio defects encountered during revision THA can be treated with a morcellized graft and a cementless hemispheric component. The amount of host bone that contacts and supports the cup helps dictate the management of these defects. When 50% or more of host bone contact can be obtained with the implant, an uncemented cup has been shown to be a reliable option.[16] With the advent of osteophilic porous metal coated implants, it may be possible to achieve stable fixation with even less host bone contact. A cementless component may be supplemented with additional screw fixation for added stability.[21] Large defects that are not contained may require porous metal augments to provide structural support for the revision acetabular component. Several choices of porous metal augments are available that allow the surgeon to size and orient the pieces to match the acetabular deficiency. These augments can be used alone or in combination with allograft to further individualize the graft to fit the defect.[20]

The preferred technique of this chapter's authors is to ream the bony rim to the smallest possible diameter necessary for circumferential fit. The component size is chosen to be approximately 1 to 2 mm larger in diameter than this reamer size, including the porous coating on the shell. The contained defect can be filled with morcellized bone graft and packed by reverse reaming 2 mm smaller than the last reamer. Next, the first reamer is also used on reverse to further pack the bone graft. The cup is then inserted and malleted into place in the appro-

priate position, avoiding retroversion or vertical cup positioning while maintaining 50% coverage for a press fit.

For extensive but contained defects without appropriate rim fit for stable osseointegration, large sized acetabular components can be used. These jumbo cups (62 mm or larger mm in women and 66 mm or larger in men) increase the host bone contact area and allow more stable fixation.[22] Some anterior wall can be sacrificed when reaming to preserve the posterior column and achieve 50% rim fit; however, if the implant protrudes anteriorly into the soft tissues, it can cause iliopsoas tendinitis. These components will alter the center of rotation, so limb length and stability must be considered before reaming for large diameter cups.

In certain revision procedures, superior migration of the implant can create an oblong defect. In these situations, reconstruction options include superior structural augmentation or high placement of a cementless cup with screw fixation.[20,22,23] When the defect is not contained, allografts are often used to create a suitable base for the component. Allografts can include femoral head, distal femoral, and partial or total acetabular transplants. For larger defects, and in cases of column loss and pelvic discontinuity, reconstruction cages may be necessary for definitive fixation. (More information on the role of allografts and structural implants in THA revisions is available in *Instructional Course Lectures, Volume 63*, chapter 17 [Maximizing Function and Outcomes in Acetabular Reconstruction: Segmental Bony Defects and Pelvic Continuity]).

Graft Preparation

Autograft has superior incorporation compared with allograft; however, this approach is limited because there is often too little autograft available to repair defects other than small cavitary lesions, and host morbidity is associated with the procedure.

Allogeneic graft is the most common source of material for bone grafting. This type of graft, which is typically obtained from the cancellous bone of the femoral head, has been shown to have long-term durability.[24] Cortical bone is a more recently used alternative to cancellous allografts. One study comparing the effect of cortical versus cancellous bone found that cortical bone had better radiologic and clinical outcomes after 5 years. Further studies are needed to determine the effect of the bone source on long-term graft durability.[25]

The optimal preparation of allograft is important to achieve the highest stability and strength. The distribution of particle sizes is one contributing factor. To maximize the interlocking of particles, a broad range of particle sizes (a well-graded mixture) allows for the production of a more compact graft compared with a graft composed of uniform particles. Biomechanically, a well-graded mixture can withstand substantially more shear stress than a more homogeneous mixture.[26] Particle size is another factor that has been shown to affect the structural integrity of the graft. Mixtures with large particle sizes (8 to 10 mm) confer greater stability to the acetabular component than a graft made predominantly of smaller chips. The best mixture appears to be one that contains large bone chips and a well-graded mixture of smaller particles.[27]

Washing the bone mixture before impaction increases the shear strength of the graft. Using 0.9% saline solution to remove the fat and marrow fluid results in a substantial increase in shear strength compared with an unwashed bone mixture. Without washing, marrow fluid and fat remain in the graft. These substances are believed to reduce bone compaction and also function as a sort of lubricant.[26] Anti-

genic factors may also be removed in the washing process, resulting in better graft incorporation because of a reduction in the host immune response.[28]

Graft Extenders

Bone graft substitutes have been increasingly explored in recent years because of the limited supply of grafts, possible transmission of viruses, poor integration with host bone, and rejection caused by the host's immune response. Bone graft substitutes are also cost-efficient, with costs as little as 10% of the price of allografts. Several products are available that can be used as either 1:1 mixtures with morcellized graft or as a pure bone graft substitute for acetabular revisions with impaction grafting.

Hydroxyapatite granules in a 1:1 mixture have similar long-term clinical outcomes to pure allograft in terms of revision occurrence and function for acetabular reconstruction. Good clinical outcomes have been reported with exclusive hydroxyapatite grafts.[27,29,30] Calcium phosphate ceramics and sulfate are other options that have demonstrated favorable results in 1:1 mixtures and as pure bone graft substitutes.[31-34] Two studies have evaluated glass ceramics for acetabular reconstruction. One study yielded encouraging long-term clinical results and the other reported high rates of early loosening.[35,36]

Despite the literature supporting bone graft substitutes as potential comparable alternatives in acetabular reconstruction in THA revision surgery, there is a lack of randomized controlled trials comparing allografts and substitutes. Until more high-quality data are available, it is advisable to choose bone replacement products with published data supporting their safety and long-term clinical results.[37] (More information on graft extenders in revision THA is available in *Instruc-

tional Course Lecture, Volume 63*, chapter 17 [Maximizing Function and Outcomes in Acetabular Reconstruction: Segmental Bony Defects and Pelvic Continuity.])

Principles of Screw Fixation

In revision THA, the success of implants depends on adequate bone ingrowth, which, in turn, depends on the mechanical stability of the component and the acetabulum. Minimal micromotion (< 50 μm) promotes osseointegration of the implant, whereas excessive motion (> 150 μm) leads to bone resorption and fibrosis and ultimately results in fixation failure.[38] Although screw fixation is often not required for stability in primary THA, the use of screws is often necessary for optimal initial fixation strength in the revision setting. Many studies have reported successful long-term outcomes with multiple screws for cementless acetabular reconstruction.[39-41]

For screw insertion, the main consideration is to avoid neurovascular structures while drilling into the best available bone stock. A map of four clinically useful quadrants is used to define some of the anatomic structures at risk in each area. These quadrants are formed by drawing a line from the anterior superior iliac spine through the center of the acetabulum and a perpendicular line through the center of the acetabulum, thus making four quadrants.[42] Drilling superiorly into the posterior column toward the sciatic notch, which lies in the posterior superior quadrant, poses the least neurovascular risk and provides the best bone stock for screw fixation. The bone depth in this column allows the use of up to 50-mm screw lengths. The posterior inferior quadrant is also relatively safe; however, there is generally less bone stock in this quadrant, so screws less than 25 mm in length should be used.[42] Additional screw fixation into the ischium should be performed if possible because this enhances the mechanical stability of the component.[43] The anterior quadrants should be avoided because these areas have less available bone stock and pose the greatest risk of injury to the external iliac and obturator structures.

Summary

Bony defects of the acetabulum without segmental loss or pelvic discontinuity can usually be managed effectively with morcellized bone grafting. Although a modular exchange of the femoral head and liner can be used for well-fixed and appropriately positioned cups associated with wear and/or osteolysis, shell revision should be undertaken for components that are loose or malpositioned. Protrusio deformity can develop in association with loose acetabular components and can generally be reconstructed with a cementless acetabular component that is lateralized by reaming just the acetabular rim and bone grafting medially with morcellized cancellous bone and multiple screws for adjunctive fixation. In more complex defects, porous metal augments, structural grafts, or reconstruction cages can be used to achieve adequate fixation to host bone.

References

1. Kurtz S, Ong K, Lau E, Mowat F, Halpern M: Projections of primary and revision hip and knee arthroplasty in the United States from 2005 to 2030. *J Bone Joint Surg Am* 2007;89(4):780-785.

2. Southwell DG, Bechtold JE, Lew WD, Schmidt AH: Improving the detection of acetabular osteolysis using oblique radiographs. *J Bone Joint Surg Br* 1999;81(2):289-295.

3. Garcia-Cimbrelo E, Tapia M, Martin-Hervas C: Multislice computed tomography for evaluating acetabular defects in revision THA. *Clin Orthop Relat Res* 2007;463:138-143.

4. Zicat B, Engh CA, Gokcen E: Patterns of osteolysis around total hip components inserted with and without cement. *J Bone Joint Surg Am* 1995;77(3):432-439.

5. Urban RM, Hall DJ, Della Valle C, Wimmer MA, Jacobs JJ, Galante JO: Successful long-term fixation and progression of osteolysis associated with first-generation cementless acetabular components retrieved post mortem. *J Bone Joint Surg Am* 2012;94(20):1877-1885.

6. Ries MD, Link TM: Monitoring and risk of progression of osteolysis after total hip arthroplasty. *J Bone Joint Surg Am* 2012;94(22):2097-2105.

7. Gustilo RB, Pasternak HS: Revision total hip arthroplasty with titanium ingrowth prosthesis and bone grafting for failed cemented femoral component loosening. *Clin Orthop Relat Res* 1988;235:111-119.

8. Engh CA, Glassman AH: Cementless revision of failed total hip replacement: An update. *Instr Course Lect* 1991;40:189-197.

9. Paprosky WG, Perona PG, Lawrence JM: Acetabular defect classification and surgical reconstruction in revision arthroplasty: A 6-year follow-up evaluation. *J Arthroplasty* 1994;9(1):33-44.

10. D'Antonio JA: Periprosthetic bone loss of the acetabulum: Classification and management. *Orthop Clin North Am* 1992;23(2):279-290.

11. Gross AE, Allan DG, Catre M, Garbuz DS, Stockley I: Bone grafts in hip replacement surgery: The pelvic side. *Orthop Clin North Am* 1993;24(4):679-695.

12. Saleh KJ, Holtzman J, Gafni A, Saleh L, et al: Development, test reliability and validation of a classification for revision hip arthroplasty. *J Orthop Res* 2001;19(1):50-56.

13. Johanson NA, Driftmier KR, Cerynik DL, Stehman CC: Grading acetabular defects: The need for a universal and valid system. *J Arthroplasty* 2010;25(3):425-431.

14. Gates HS III, Callaghan JJ, McCollum DE: Radiographic measurements in protrusio acetabuli. *J Arthroplasty* 1989;4(4):347-351.

15. Ries MD: Total hip arthroplasty in acetabular protrusio. *Orthopedics* 2009;32(9):666-668.

16. Burstein G, Yoon P, Saleh KJ: Component removal in revision total hip arthroplasty. *Clin Orthop Relat Res* 2004;420:48-54.

17. Hansen E, Ries MD: Revision total hip arthroplasty for large medial (protrusio) defects with a rim-fit cementless acetabular component. *J Arthroplasty* 2006;21(1):72-79.

18. Callaghan JJ, Parvizi J, Novak CC, et al: A constrained liner cemented into a secure cementless acetabular shell. *J Bone Joint Surg Am* 2004;86(10):2206-2211.

19. Masri BA, Mitchell PA, Duncan CP: Removal of solidly fixed implants during revision hip and knee arthroplasty. *J Am Acad Orthop Surg* 2005;13(1):18-27.

20. Mitchell PA, Masri BA, Garbuz DS, Greidanus NV, Wilson D, Duncan CP: Removal of well-fixed, cementless, acetabular components in revision hip arthroplasty. *J Bone Joint Surg Br* 2003;85(7):949-952.

21. Deirmengian GK, Zmistowski B, O'Neil JT, Hozack WJ: Management of acetabular bone loss in revision total hip arthroplasty. *J Bone Joint Surg Am* 2011;93(19):1842-1852.

22. Wedemeyer C, Neuerburg C, Heep H, et al: A retrospective review of a case series. *Arch Orthop Trauma Surg* 2008;128(6):545-550.

23. Civinini R, Capone A, Carulli C, Villano M, Gusso MI: Acetabular revisions using a cementless oblong cup: Five to ten year results. *Int Orthop* 2008;32(2):189-193.

24. Oakes DA, Cabanela ME: Impaction bone grafting for revision hip arthroplasty: Biology and clinical applications. *J Am Acad Orthop Surg* 2006;14(11):620-628.

25. Kligman M, Padgett DE, Vered R, Roffman M: Cortical and cancellous morselized allograft in acetabular revision total hip replacement: Minimum 5-year follow-up. *J Arthroplasty* 2003;18(7): 907-913.

26. Dunlop DG, Brewster NT, Madabhushi SP, Usmani AS, Pankaj P, Howie CR: Techniques to improve the shear strength of impacted bone graft: The effect of particle size and washing of the graft. *J Bone Joint Surg Am* 2003; 85(4):639-646.

27. McNamara IR: Impaction bone grafting in revision hip surgery: Past, present and future. *Cell Tissue Bank* 2010;11(1):57-73.

28. van der Donk S, Weernink T, Buma P, Aspenberg P, Slooff TJ, Schreurs BW: Rinsing morselized allografts improves bone and tissue ingrowth. *Clin Orthop Relat Res* 2003;408:302-310.

29. Aulakh TS, Jayasekera N, Kuiper JH, Richardson JB: Long-term clinical outcomes following the use of synthetic hydroxyapatite and bone graft in impaction in revision hip arthroplasty. *Biomaterials* 2009;30(9):1732-1738.

30. Oonishi H, Iwaki Y, Kin N, et al: Hydroxyapatite in revision of total hip replacements with massive acetabular defects: 4- to 10-year clinical results. *J Bone Joint Surg Br* 1997;79(1):87-92.

31. Müller M, Stangl R: [Norian SRS augmentation in revision of acetabular cup of total hip arthroplasty: A follow up of six patients]. *Unfallchirurg* 2006; 109(4):335-338.

32. Blom AW, Wylde V, Livesey C, et al: Impaction bone grafting of the acetabulum at hip revision using a mix of bone chips and a biphasic porous ceramic bone graft substitute. *Acta Orthop* 2009;80(2):150-154.

33. Schwartz C, Bordei R: Biphasic phospho-calcium ceramics used as bone substitutes are efficient in the management of severe acetabular bone loss in revision total hip arthroplasties. *Eur J Orthop Surg Traumatol* 2005;15:191-196.

34. Egawa H, Ho H, Huynh C, Hopper RH Jr, Engh CA: A three-dimensional method for evaluating changes in acetabular osteolytic lesions in response to treatment. *Clin Orthop Relat Res* 2010;468(2):480-490.

35. Kawanabe K, Iida H, Matsusue Y, Nishimatsu H, Kasai R, Nakamura T: A-W glass ceramic as a bone substitute in cemented hip arthroplasty: 15 hips followed 2-10 years. *Acta Orthop Scand* 1998;69(3):237-242.

36. Engelbrecht E, von Foerster G, Delling G: Ionogran in revision arthroplasty. *J Bone Joint Surg Br* 2000;82(2):192-199.

37. Beswick A, Blom AW: Bone graft substitutes in hip revision surgery: A comprehensive overview. *Injury* 2011;42(suppl 2):S40-S46.

38. Cook SD, Barrack RL, Thomas KA, Haddad RJ Jr: Quantitative analysis of tissue growth into human porous total hip components. *J Arthroplasty* 1988;3(3): 249-262.

39. Jones CP, Lachiewicz PF: Factors influencing the longer-term survival of uncemented acetabular components used in total hip revisions. *J Bone Joint Surg Am* 2004; 86(2):342-347.

40. Templeton JE, Callaghan JJ, Goetz DD, Sullivan PM, Johnston RC: Revision of a cemented acetabular component to a cementless acetabular component: A ten to fourteen-year follow-up study. *J Bone Joint Surg Am* 2001; 83(11):1706-1711.

41. Clohisy JC, Harris WH: The Harris-Galante porous-coated acetabular component with screw fixation: An average ten-year follow-up study. *J Bone Joint Surg Am* 1999;81(1):66-73.

42. Wasielewski RC, Cooperstein LA, Kruger MP, Rubash HE: Acetabular anatomy and the transacetabular fixation of screws in total hip arthroplasty. *J Bone Joint Surg Am* 1990;72(4):501-508.

43. Meneghini RM, Stultz AD, Watson JS, Ziemba-Davis M, Buckley CA: Does ischial screw fixation improve mechanical stability in revision total hip arthroplasty? *J Arthroplasty* 2010;25(7):1157-1161.

Video Reference

Francisco C, Villanueva M, Rojo-Manaute JM, Pérez-Diaz M, Fernández-Mariño J, Vaquero-Martin J: *Stoppa Approach for Removal of the Intrapelvic Cup for Acetabular Revision* [video]. Rosemont, IL, American Academy of Orthopaedic Surgeons, 2013. *Orthopaedic Video Theater 3.* http://orthoportal.aaos.org/emedia/singleVideoPlayer.aspx?resource=EMEDIA_OSVL_13 _03. Accessed November 20, 2013.

21

Direct Anterior Total Hip Arthroplasty

Anthony S. Unger, MD
Benjamin M. Stronach, MS, MD
Patrick F. Bergin, MD
Michael Nogler, MD, MA, MAS, MsC

Abstract

The direct anterior approach to hip arthroplasty has become a popular technique. This technique, which was described almost 70 years ago, allows the surgeon to approach the hip through an internervous and intermuscular plane. Preliminary studies show that direct anterior hip arthroplasty may allow patients to recover faster with a lower dislocation rate. It is helpful to understand the history, scientific basis, and surgical technique of direct anterior hip arthroplasty.

Instr Course Lect 2014;63:227-238.

Total hip arthroplasty (THA) is one of the most successful orthopaedic surgical procedures because it has the ability to provide excellent pain relief, restore function, increase mobility, and correct deformity in patients with debilitating disease. THA is used to treat many different types of hip pathology, including osteoarthritis, posttraumatic arthritis, inflammatory arthritis, postseptic arthritis, osteonecrosis, and hip dysplasia. Approximately 250,000 primary THAs were performed in the United States in 2010, and it is expected that 500,000 THAs will be performed annually by 2030.[1]

Surgical techniques for THA continue to evolve as orthopaedic surgeons attempt to meet the increasingly high expectations of their patients. Current joint replacement patients are younger, more active, and demand higher function than the initial population the procedure was designed to treat. Patients, surgeons, and hospitals want to minimize the recovery period and complications associated with THA surgery. These efforts may hasten the patient's return to activities and employment, improve the use of hospital resources, and allow surgeons to treat more patients to meet the growing demand for this procedure. These goals can be accomplished by providing rapid functional recovery with a safe, reproducible surgical procedure that minimizes pain and soft-tissue injury.

Multiple approaches to the hip joint have been described, including medial, anterior, anterolateral, lateral and posterior approaches, with the latter four approaches used for THA. Each approach provides distinct advantages and potential risks for complications. Extensive modifications and variations to each THA approach have been made, with the goals of decreasing soft-tissue damage, allowing adequate exposure, and decreasing surgical risks.

The direct anterior approach to the hip is unique because it provides the only intermuscular and internervous exposure of the joint. This approach was first described for hip replacement in 1949 by Smith-Petersen[2] and has recently gained increased popularity because of the possibility for rapid patient recovery, decreased concern for dislocation, more accurate component positioning, and reliable restoration of limb length.[3-8]

Dr. Unger or an immediate family member has received royalties from Biomet and Innomed; is a member of a speakers' bureau or has made paid presentations on behalf of Biomet and Stryker; serves as a paid consultant to Biomet, Stryker, and Corin USA; and has received research or institutional support from Zimmer. Dr. Nogler or an immediate family member is a member of a speakers' bureau or has made paid presentations on behalf of Stryker and DJO; serves as a paid consultant to Stryker and DJO; and has received research or institutional support from Stryker and Heraeus Intrinsic Bone Glass. Neither of the following authors nor any immediate family member has received anything of value from or owns stock in a commercial company or institution related directly or indirectly to the subject of this chapter: Dr. Stronach and Dr. Bergin.

History

In 2009, Rachbauer et al[9] published a comprehensive history of the anterior approach to the hip. The first description of the anterior approach to the hip is credited to Hueter in 1881, who used it to resect the femoral head.[8] Smith-Petersen[10] subsequently used and further developed the approach, which provided a wide exposure to the anterior portion of the pelvis. The anterior approach to the hip is commonly referred to as the Smith-Petersen approach because of his interest in and use of the exposure. Smith-Petersen is also credited with performing the first joint replacement procedure through an anterior exposure.[2] In its early stages in the 1970s, the anterior approach was preferred by Wagner[11] for hip resurfacing procedures because it allowed preservation of the blood supply to the femoral head and intermuscular dissection. In the 1980s in France, Judet and Judet[12] used the anterior approach with a specialized fracture table to help position the leg. They preferred the anterior approach because it decreased damage to muscles and bone compared with other available techniques. Their technique was an extensile approach compared with modern standards; the tensor fascia lata was removed from the iliac crest with release of the reflected head of the rectus femoris.

Kennon et al[5] reported on 2,132 patients treated with the anterior THA approach. The authors describe a technique that does not require a specialized operating table and frequently uses multiple incisions to complete the procedure. Berger[13] and Berger and Duwelius[14] subsequently developed a minimally invasive two-incision technique that used an anterior approach with a small incision for cup preparation and placement and a small posterolateral incision for femoral preparation and component placement. The two-incision technique uses the Smith-Petersen interval for acetabular placement. The femur is placed through a separate gluteal stab wound. The technique is tedious and requires the extensive use of radiographic monitoring. Most advocates of the technique use a full beaded distal fixation stem, which may not be the stem of choice of some surgeons. Multiple studies have reported that the two-incision technique offers no benefits and concerns have been expressed about increased muscle damage and delayed recovery.[15-18] Many surgeons who reported on the two-incision technique subsequently abandoned it for other techniques. Despite the fact that this approach has lost popularity, a specialized retractor system and some instruments developed for the two-incision approach have been adopted for use in direct anterior THA.[14]

Encouraging outcomes reported in two large studies resulted in renewed interest in direct anterior THA using a specialized fracture table.[6,19] In a study of 1,037 patients, Siguier et al[19] reported a low dislocation rate of 0.96% with adequate component positioning. Matta et al[6] reported similar findings in a study of 437 patients. Over the past century, the direct anterior approach has been gradually modified and improved to provide an exposure that may reduce soft-tissue trauma and allow surgeons to accurately and reproducibly place arthroplasty components.

Anatomy and Approach

The classically described Smith-Petersen approach is an extensile approach to the hip that uses the anterior superior iliac spine (ASIS) as an anatomic landmark, with the incision extending superiorly and inferiorly.[2,10] The superior limb provides access to the iliac wing and supra-acetabular pelvis, with the inferior limb providing access to the hip joint. The current method of direct anterior hip arthroplasty uses the inferior limb of this classic incision (**Figure 1**).

This approach is the most direct approach to the hip with the least overlying fat, even in morbidly obese patients. The palpable osseous landmarks are the ASIS and greater trochanter (**Figure 2**). One technique used to plan the skin incision involves drawing a line between the osseous landmarks of the ASIS and greater trochanter, starting the superior incision at the halfway point of this line, and aiming it slightly posteriorly.[20] Another option is to measure 2 cm laterally and distally to the ASIS and extend the incision distally from this point, aiming it slightly posteriorly.[6] The lateral femoral cutaneous nerve (LFCN) is at risk during this approach. This structure exits medially to the ASIS and is protected by basing the incision slightly laterally (**Figure 3**).

The direct anterior approach is an intermuscular and internervous approach, with the superficial dissection carried out between the tensor fascia lata muscle (superior gluteal nerve) laterally and the sartorius muscle (femoral nerve) medially. The tensor fascia lata must be accurately identified. It has a deep blue coloration in relation to the white gluteal fascia and is located just posterior to it. The tensor fascia lata also can be identified by the posterior penetrating vessels. Proper identification is critical because confusing the sartorius muscle for the tensor fascia lata will bring the surgeon in close proximity to the femoral bundle, with the associated dangers of dissection in this area. After the tensor fascia lata is identified, its fascia is incised midline, and finger dissection is carried out deep and medially along the muscle belly to reach the deep intermuscular interval that lies between the gluteus medius muscle (superior gluteal nerve)

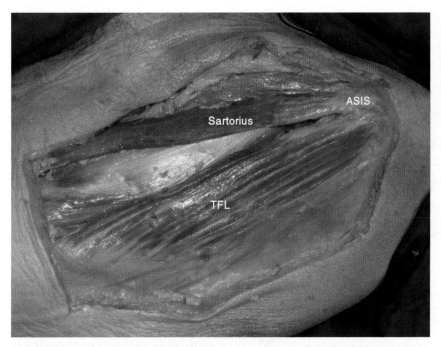

Figure 1 Photograph of the superficial hip anatomy important in making the incision using the direct anterior approach. TFL = tensor fascia lata muscle.

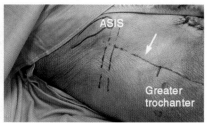

Figure 2 The location of the initial incision (arrow) is shown with the palpable osseous landmarks. The most proximal parallel line represents the anatomic landmark of the superior extent of the initial incision. The second parallel line is the preferred starting point for the incision when using the direct anterior approach.

An easily identified fat layer defines the deep interval and the ascending branch of the lateral femoral circumflex vascular bundle, which crosses the interval in this plane (**Figure 5**). The number and diameter of the vessels in the bundle are variable and must be ligated, stapled, or cauterized. Ligation is the most reliable option to prevent intraoperative bleeding and postoperative hematoma. A sharp Hohmann retractor is placed deep to the hip abductors on the outer portion of the hip capsule between the greater trochanter and superior femoral neck. The hip is then flexed 30° to relax the hip capsule and allow placement of a blunt Hohmann retractor under the medial femoral neck. The reflected head of the rectus femoris attaches to the anterior hip capsule and acetabular rim and is elevated off of the capsule with a Cobb elevator or electrocautery to expose the capsule. This retraction and dissection provides excellent exposure of the anterior hip capsule; capsulotomy and intra-articular exposure are then performed (**Figure 6**).

Surgical Technique Using a Specialized Table

Many instruments are available for direct anterior hip arthroplasty, includ-

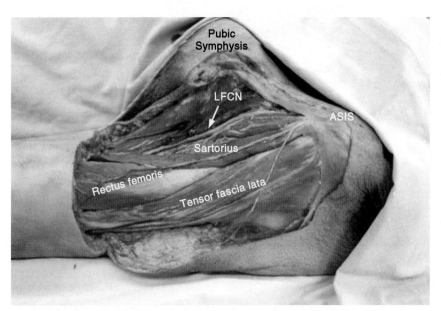

Figure 3 Cadaver dissection showing position of the LFCN (arrow) on top of the sartorius.

laterally and the rectus femoris muscle (femoral nerve) medially (**Figure 4**). The classic Smith-Petersen approach developed the interval between the sartorius and tensor fascia lata muscles, which placed branches of the LFCN at risk during dissection and retraction. This modification through the tensor fascia lata better protects the LFCN for the remainder of the procedure.

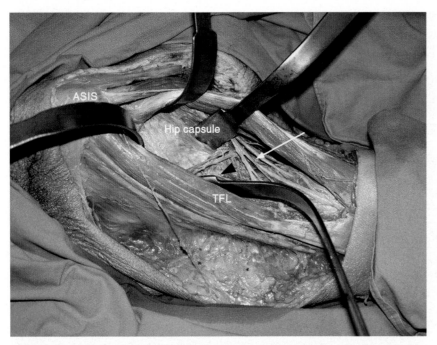

Figure 4 Cadaver photograph of the deep dissection anatomy. Arrowhead points to the rectus femoris. Arrow points to the deep branch of the femoral nerve to the rectus femoris. TFL = tensor fascia lata muscle.

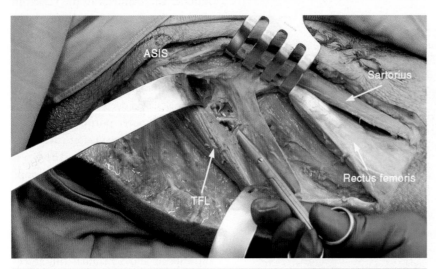

Figure 5 Cadaver photograph showing ligation of the lateral circumflex vessels. TFL = tensor fascia lata muscle.

ing specialized retractor sets, implant positioning guidance systems (computer navigation and fluoroscopic grid), and specialized orthopaedic tables to facilitate patient positioning. Many techniques also are available to perform the procedure based on the surgeon's preference and available resources. The specialized orthopaedic table is not required for direct anterior hip arthroplasty, but it is preferred by many surgeons (**Figure 7**).

The use of a specialized orthopaedic table allows for control of rotation, abduction, flexion, and traction of the surgical extremity and has a wide range of potential positions. Fluoroscopy also can be use to aid in intraoperative component positioning and limb-length determination. When using this specialized table, however, the leg cannot be freely tested for stability in the traditional manner, and the table is a mechanical device that can cause injury if not used with care. The cost and availability of the table are also potential drawbacks.

The patient is positioned supine on the table with a perineal post, and both legs are placed in the provided boots to secure the limbs. The nonsurgical hip is placed in a neutral position in all planes; this can be verified with fluoroscopy. Fluoroscopy also may be used during the procedure for assistance with limb-length and offset determinations. Gentle traction with fluoroscopy can be used to level the pelvis at this point in the procedure. Sequential compression devices are placed on both extremities, and the operative leg is draped in a sterile fashion.

After exposing the anterior hip capsule, a capsulotomy is performed, and an anterior capsulectomy also may be performed or the capsule can be tagged and preserved for repair at closure. The Hohmann retractors placed outside the capsule can now be placed within the capsule on the superior and inferior femoral neck. Several options are available for the femoral neck osteotomy. Matta et al[6] describe a technique to dislocate the hip prior to the osteotomy. The authors prefer to cut the neck in situ and subsequently remove the femoral head because of concerns about the increased torque placed on the operative leg with the dislocation technique. The in situ resection is performed using a long, narrow oscillating saw blade and can include one osteotomy or two parallel resections in a napkin-ring fashion to provide more space for removing the femoral head (**Figure 8**). Preoperative templating is referenced to determine this resection level. Gentle traction on the operative leg can assist in removing the femoral head; a Steinmann pin or power corkscrew device is placed into the head for removal.

The acetabulum is now prepared with component placement. Using gentle traction, the leg is positioned in 45° of external rotation. This facilitates exposure of the acetabulum and moves the greater trochanter posteriorly. A blunt Hohmann retractor is retained in the same position around the medial femoral neck. An acetabular retractor is placed directly inferior to the fovea against the transverse acetabular ligament. The anterior retractor is placed at the 9-o' clock position, and the anterior musculature is mobilized (**Figure 9**). Several stab incisions can be made into the posterior capsule to increase mobility if it is under tension, and a posterior retractor can be placed within the capsule around the posterior acetabular rim if needed for further exposure. Next, the foveal tissue and labrum are removed under direct visualization. The acetabulum is reamed in 10° to 15° of anteversion, with 40° to 45° of anteversion (**Figure 10**). Reaming is directly visualized, and fluoroscopy is then used for the final reaming to set the component size and depth. The selected implant is sized and impacted into position under fluoroscopic guidance, with screw insertion if needed. A curved acetabular inserter can be used to facilitate adequate soft-tissue clearance (**Figure 11**). The final liner is inserted, appropriate seating is verified, and any exposed osteophytes are removed from the acetabular rim (**Figure 12**).

The proximal femur is then exposed in preparation for insertion of the femoral stem. Traction is released on the leg, and it is returned to a position of neutral rotation. A femoral hook, which attaches to a connector

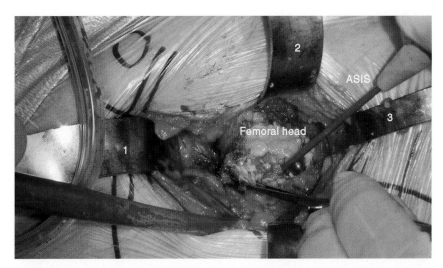

Figure 6   The capsule is resected. (1) Medial neck retractor. (2) Anterior retractor. (3) Superior neck retractor.

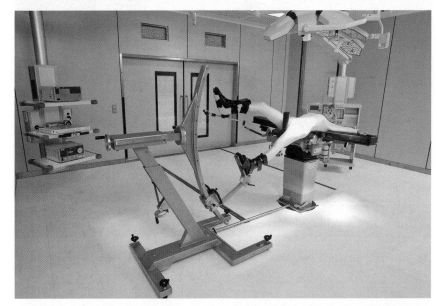

Figure 7   Photograph of the specialized orthopaedic table.

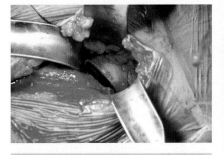

Figure 8   Intraoperative photograph of osteotomy of the femoral head before removal.

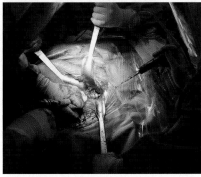

Figure 9   Position of the acetabular retractors.

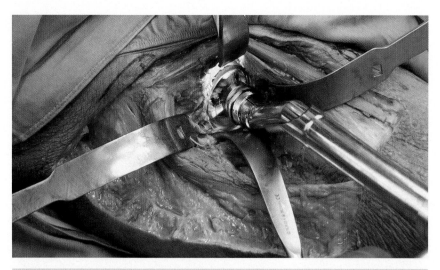

Figure 10   The acetabulum is reamed.

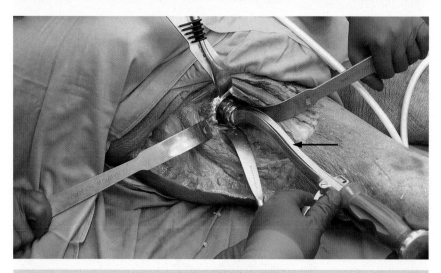

Figure 11   Placement of the cup. A curved acetabular inserter (arrow) facilitates insertion.

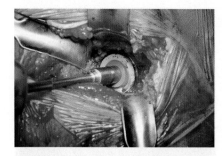

Figure 12   The final liner is inserted.

arm on the surgical table, aids in exposing the proximal femur. The connector arm can then be elevated to deliver the femur anteriorly, providing clearance for broach and stem insertion. Prior to the placement of this device, the superior and the medial capsules are removed. A bone hook is used to place anterior tension on the proximal femur to assess mobility; further releases of the piriformis, obturator internus, and gemelli can be performed in a sequential fashion. The posterior capsule, obturator externus, and quadratus femoris are always preserved. After adequate mobility is obtained, the S-hook is placed below the vastus lateralis ridge on the posterior

femur, and the leg is externally rotated 90°, adducted, and extended. The hook is attached to the connection bracket on the table and the hook is elevated. Undue tension should not be placed on the hook because of the risk of a proximal femoral fracture. Adequate releases (as described) must be performed to prevent complications and allow for adequate exposure.

The femur is prepared by removing any remaining lateral femoral neck; this is followed by broaching the femoral canal. This chapter's authors prefer to use an offset broach handle, which greatly facilitates access to the femoral canal by providing adequate soft-tissue clearance. There is a risk of femoral canal perforation laterally if the broach handle cannot be brought down to the appropriate position because of soft-tissue impingement. A short, taper-fit stem is routinely used because it allows for ease of insertion and preparation. Preoperative templating is helpful in determining the stem size. The broach also is assessed intraoperatively for adequate stability and canal fill. Proximal or distal mismatch as seen in a Dorr type A femoral bone can be addressed using flexible reamers distally. Stem designs that require femoral reaming are technically more challenging to use in direct anterior hip arthroplasty because of the difficulty with reaming and the increased concern for femoral fracture with stem insertion.

The final broach is impacted into position with the placement of a trial head and neck. The hip is reduced by removing the hook, the leg is internally rotated to neutral with release of traction, and the femoral head is guided into the acetabulum.

Limb length and femoral offset are evaluated with fluoroscopy. A typical surgical fluoroscope can only image one hip at a time; however, new, large-diameter fluoroscopes can display an entire pelvic image. Several methods have been described for evaluating the position of the implant. With standard fluoroscopy, the image of the contralateral hip can be obtained and printed, and the same process can be performed on the operative extremity. The two printed images are then laid over one another, with proper limb length and offset determined by direct comparison with the contralateral extremity.[6] Another option with a standard or large-diameter machine is the use of a fluoroscopic grid. The grid is placed on the surgical table prior to the procedure and provides visible reference lines for determining offset and limb length on fluoroscopic images. This method has been shown to increase the percentage of acetabular components placed in the so-called safe zone and allows improved restoration of limb length and offset in comparison with fluoroscopy alone.[21] If desired, the leg can be removed from the traction spar to allow for stability testing. The leg must be appropriately draped to prevent contamination of the sterile field. The hip is dislocated by replacing the hook and applying traction and external rotation. Trial components can be removed with impaction of the femoral prosthesis, placement of the femoral head, and reduction of the hip.

The wound is irrigated, and anterior capsular closure is performed if a capsulectomy was not performed. The fascia lata interval is closed in a running fashion and is followed by subcutaneous and skin closure with the surgeon's preferred method. The patient is allowed to immediately bear weight as tolerated. Hip precautions are not required.[22]

Surgical Technique Using a Standard Table

The use of a standard table for direct anterior THA has several advantages over a specialized table. There is no in-

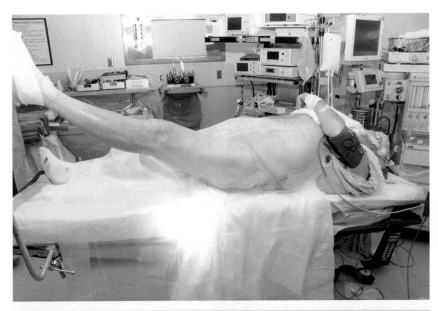

Figure 13   Photograph of a patient on a standard operating room table. The table is turned around to allow extension of the hip for femur insertion.

creased cost associated with the purchase of a specialized table, the operative extremity is not attached to the table and can be examined with ease, and there is no need for a nonsterile staff member to control the leg. The table must be radiolucent if fluoroscopy is used during the procedure or the advantage of fluoroscopy is lost.

With a standard operating table, direct anterior THA is performed in a similar manner as the procedure using a specialized table, but a slightly different setup is required (**Figure 13**). The patient is positioned supine with the hip joint at the level of the table break. This position allows the hips to be hyperextended during femoral preparation. A perineal post can be used if preferred. The post secures the patient on the table during the procedure but makes adduction of the leg more difficult. An arm board is attached to the contralateral side of the bed to support the nonoperative leg in an abducted position and allows for adduction of the operative extremity during femoral preparation. The surgeon has the option of draping only the operative ex-

tremity or both extremities into the sterile field. Inclusion of both legs allows the operative leg to be crossed under the nonoperative leg and facilitates femoral exposure. It also allows for quick limb-length measurement by palpation of the bilateral malleoli. This chapter's authors routinely drape only the operative leg and place compression stockings with a sequential compression device on the nonoperative leg.

The exposure and acetabular preparation with cup insertion is carried out as previously described. The leg is then placed in a figure-of-4 position and the medial capsule is released until the lesser trochanter is completely seen. The leg is then returned to a neutral position, and a bone hook is used to verify adequate mobilization of the proximal femur to provide clearance of the acetabulum. This requires release of the superior capsule and frequently the piriformis. The distal portion of the surgical table is then dropped 40°, allowing for hyperextension of the hip with the addition of the Trendelenburg position to keep the foot of the bed

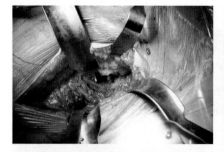

Figure 14 Position of the retractors for femoral preparation.

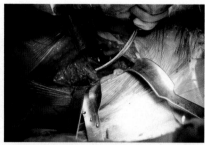

Figure 15 A curved canal finder is used to open the femur prior to broaching.

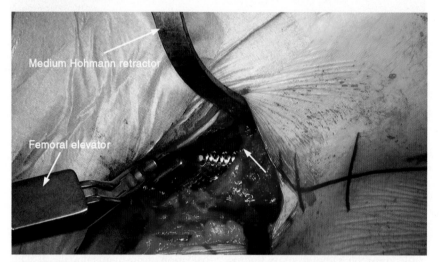

Figure 16 Double-offset broaching is preferred for femoral preparation because it allows adequate soft-tissue clearance, provides a better angle for alignment with the femoral canal, and minimizes the need for femoral elevation. The arrow points to the medial aspect of the femoral neck.

from dropping too close to the floor. The contralateral limb is abducted onto the arm board and the operative limb is adducted and externally rotated with the knee kept in extension. Further adduction can be obtained if both legs are draped into the field by allowing the operative limb to cross under the contralateral limb. A bone hook is used to pull the proximal femur anteriorly and laterally to clear the acetabulum; a specialized femoral retractor is then placed behind the greater trochanter to assist with soft-tissue retraction and hold the femur in position (**Figure 14**). Care must be taken with this retractor because it is not meant to elevate the femur but to retract soft tis-

sue; excessive force on the retractor can damage the tensor fascia lata. A second retractor is placed proximal to the lesser trochanter in the calcar region to retract the medial soft tissues; a retractor can be placed laterally if necessary. A retraction system has been described for the proximal femur that attaches to the surgical bed and provides an elevation arm similar to the S-hook used with the specialized table.[23]

A box osteotome is used to remove any remaining lateral femoral neck, and the femoral canal is identified using an angled curette (**Figure 15**). A curved rasp or opening broach is then used to remove lateral bone in the region of the greater trochanter. Double-

offset broach handles are preferred for femoral preparation because they allow adequate clearance of soft tissues, provide a better angle for alignment with the femoral canal, and minimize the need for femoral elevation[24] (**Figure 16**). Broaching is completed, and a trial head and neck are placed. The foot of the bed is leveled, and the Trendelenburg position is then removed from the table. The hip is reduced with gentle traction and internal rotation by the assistant, with the surgeon directly guiding the femoral head into the acetabulum. Limb length can be assessed by bringing the ankles together and palpating the malleoli. Fluoroscopy can be used to assess implant alignment, offset, and limb length. Hip stability and range of motion are also assessed at this time.

The hip is then dislocated with gentle traction on the leg and a bone hook around the femoral neck pulling anteriorly, laterally, and distally. Retractors are again placed, the trial head and neck are removed, and a bone hook is used to elevate the proximal femur. The table is then positioned to allow extension of the leg. The final implants are inserted with reduction of the hip joint. The hip can then be assessed clinically and fluoroscopically if desired. Closure is carried out as previously described (**Figure 17**).

Results

There has recently been renewed interest in direct anterior hip arthroplasty because of the potential for rapid recovery with less soft-tissue damage. A study comparing gait analysis in patients treated with the anterolateral approach and the direct anterior approach found that patients treated with the direct anterior approach had an earlier return to a normal gait pattern and substantially improved gait parameters.[25] Patients treated with the direct anterior approach have less pain, substantially more improvement in functional outcome scores, and quicker recovery in comparison with those treated with the lateral approach.[3,26] In a clinical comparative study of 182 consecutive patients (195 hips), Nakata et al[8] reported a faster functional recovery, with limp resolution and independent ambulation, along with increased accuracy of component placement in the direct anterior approach group (99 hips) compared with those treated with the posterior approach (96 hips).

The improved recovery seen in direct anterior THA is attributed to the use of an intermuscular and internervous interval, with no muscle splitting as required in other approaches. A cadaver study by Meneghini et al[27] compared muscle damage between the posterior and anterior approaches and found increased muscle damage to the gluteus minimus in the posterior group, increased tensor fascia lata and rectus femoris damage in the anterior group, and similar damage to the gluteus medius in both groups. A 2011 study quantitatively compared the presence of inflammatory markers and markers of muscle damage in patients treated with direct anterior and posterior hip arthroplasty and found the group treated with the posterior approach had significantly increased levels of creatine kinase ($P < .01$), which was consistent with increased muscle damage, although the clinical importance of this is unclear.[4] This finding supports the hypothesis that direct anterior hip arthroplasty has the potential for less muscle damage than other hip approaches.

The risk of dislocation after arthroplasty exists in all approaches. Special hip precautions have been routinely advocated for 6 to 12 weeks to prevent dislocation after THA. There is a higher risk of dislocation in the first 3 months after surgery as the capsule

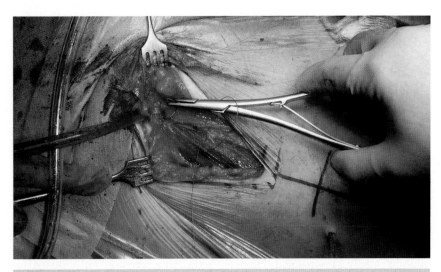

Figure 17 Closure of the tensor fascia lata with running suture.

and supportive soft tissues of the hip joint heal.[28,29] Hip precautions result in increased costs because of the need for specialized assistive devices and aids and limit the patient's range of activities during the first months of recovery. Several large series have reported dislocation rates of 0.6% to 1.3% for direct anterior THA[5,6,19,30]; these rates are generally lower in comparison with those reported for other approaches.[28,29] Because hip precautions are not necessary to prevent dislocation with the anterior approach, the patient can return to his or her normal activities without concerns about dislocation, no dislocation precaution education is needed, and costs are decreased because no special equipment is required.[22]

There is a learning curve associated with the direct anterior approach for THA. Seng et al[26] reported on the learning curve in a high-volume arthroplasty practice. They found a substantial decrease in surgical time after treatment of the first 37 patients over a 6-month period. The initial patient selection was highly selective, with the procedure performed only on thin women with a high femoral neck offset; difficult cases, such as those involving muscular men or obese pa-

tients, were avoided. Masonis et al[31] examined a single surgeon's initial consecutive series of 300 THAs using the direct anterior approach and found substantial improvement in surgical and fluoroscopy times and minimization of limb-length discrepancy after treatment of the first 100 patients. A similar investigation, which evaluated 81 patients treated with direct anterior THA, reported improving surgeon proficiency over time, with a substantial decrease in surgical and fluoroscopy times and estimated blood loss.[32] A large, multicenter study of 1,152 patients reported a substantial decline in the complication rate after a surgeon performed 100 THAs using a single-incision anterior approach.[30] There is a well-defined learning curve associated with a surgeon performing 40 to 100 THAs with the direct anterior approach. Most of the studies were conducted in high-volume centers in which hip arthroplasty was routinely performed.

Specific complications are associated with each THA approach; the specific risks of the direct anterior approach have been well characterized. The most frequent intraoperative concerns are LFCN injury, lower extremity fracture, and implant malalignment.

The LFCN is at risk of injury during exposure and during retraction. This risk has been minimized by modification of the exposure with dissection through the fascia of the tensor fascia lata instead of between the tensor fascia lata and sartorius muscles. Most studies have reported rates of LCFN neurapraxia at or below 1%.[26,30,32,33] In a study of patients treated with the anterior approach, Goulding et al[34] reported LFCN neurapraxia in 53 of 60 patients (88%) at the first follow-up, with complete resolution after 12 months in only a few patients. Despite the high rate of neurapraxia, no functional limitations were identified in these patients.

Fracture of the operative extremity can occur during the femoral portion of the procedure and with manipulation of the leg on the specialized table. Femoral perforation can occur during preparation or implant insertion because of inadequate exposure and the inability to obtain in-line access to the femur.[26,30] The greater trochanter can be fractured by excessive traction on the elevation hook or manipulation. The femoral calcar also can be fractured during implant preparation and insertion. Ankle fracture has been caused by excessive torsion on the extremity with the use of a specialized table.[6] This chapter's authors recommend the use of specialized broaches and instrumentation for direct anterior THA to minimize the risk of femoral perforation and prefer an implant that is conducive to this approach (reduced distal geometry and lateral shoulder).

The primary postoperative concerns are hip dislocation and hematoma formation. Because the dislocation rate is low, this chapter's authors do not recommend the routine use of hip precautions with the direct anterior approach. Hematoma risk can be minimized by proper ligation of the lateral femoral circumflex vascular bundle and obtaining intraoperative hemostasis. Barton and Kim[35] provide a thorough description the complications of the direct anterior approach to hip arthroplasty and recommendations to minimize their occurrence.

The concept of direct anterior hip arthroplasty is not novel, and there are several centers that have been performing arthroplasty through this approach for decades with excellent outcomes.[5,6,36] The indications for the direct anterior approach extend beyond THA and can be used for trauma, head resurfacing, revision arthroplasty, infection, and impingement.[37,38]

Summary

The direct anterior approach to THA is attracting renewed interest because of the desire for faster recovery in high-demand patients, the ability to avoid hip precautions, and the surgeon's ability to reproducibly restore limb length and offset with accurate component placement. It is a technically demanding procedure with a well-defined learning curve.

This chapter's authors recommend advanced preparation such as cadaver dissection, attendance at a course on direct anterior THA, or consultation with a surgeon who is experienced with the approach. When initially performing the procedure, patients should be carefully selected. The ideal patient is a thin woman with high femoral offset, which minimizes the soft-tissue envelope and provides adequate clearance of the femur and acetabulum. More technically difficult cases, including the treatment of muscular men, obese patients, and those with posttraumatic arthritis or atypical anatomy, should be avoided until the surgeon gains experience in the direct anterior approach. There has been some evidence of improvement in short-term outcomes associated with direct anterior THA, and it may provide quicker functional recovery with less soft-tissue damage, although further randomized controlled trials are needed.

References

1. Kurtz S, Ong K, Lau E, Mowat F, Halpern M: Projections of primary and revision hip and knee arthroplasty in the United States from 2005 to 2030. *J Bone Joint Surg Am* 2007;89(4):780-785.

2. Smith-Petersen MN: Approach to and exposure of the hip joint for mold arthroplasty. *J Bone Joint Surg Am* 1949;31A(1):40-46.

3. Alecci V, Valente M, Crucil M, Minerva M, Pellegrino CM, Sabbadini DD: Comparison of primary total hip replacements performed with a direct anterior approach versus the standard lateral approach: Perioperative findings. *J Orthop Traumatol* 2011;12(3):123-129.

4. Bergin PF, Doppelt JD, Kephart CJ, et al: Comparison of minimally invasive direct anterior versus posterior total hip arthroplasty based on inflammation and muscle damage markers. *J Bone Joint Surg Am* 2011;93(15):1392-1398.

5. Kennon RE, Keggi JM, Wetmore RS, Zatorski LE, Huo MH, Keggi KJ: Total hip arthroplasty through a minimally invasive anterior surgical approach. *J Bone Joint Surg Am* 2003;85(suppl 4):39-48.

6. Matta JM, Shahrdar C, Ferguson T: Single-incision anterior approach for total hip arthroplasty on an orthopaedic table. *Clin Orthop Relat Res* 2005;441:115-124.

7. Moskal JT, Capps SG: Minimally invasive anterior approach with a fracture table for total hip arthroplasty: Letter to the editor. *J Arthroplasty* 2010;25(7):1171-1172, author reply 1172-1173.

8. Nakata K, Nishikawa M, Yamamoto K, Hirota S, Yoshikawa H: A clinical comparative study of

the direct anterior with mini-posterior approach: Two consecutive series. *J Arthroplasty* 2009; 24(5):698-704.

9. Rachbauer F, Kain MS, Leunig M: The history of the anterior approach to the hip. *Orthop Clin North Am* 2009;40(3):311-320.

10. Smith-Petersen MN: A new supra-articular subperiosteal approach to the hip joint. *J Bone Joint Surg Am* 1917;15(8):592-595.

11. Wagner H: Surface replacement arthroplasty of the hip. *Clin Orthop Relat Res* 1978;134:102-130.

12. Judet J, Judet R: The use of an artificial femoral head for arthroplasty of the hip joint. *J Bone Joint Surg Br* 1950;32(2):166-173.

13. Berger RA: Total hip arthroplasty using the minimally invasive two-incision approach. *Clin Orthop Relat Res* 2003;417:232-241.

14. Berger RA, Duwelius PJ: The two-incision minimally invasive total hip arthroplasty: Technique and results. *Orthop Clin North Am* 2004;35(2):163-172.

15. Krych AJ, Pagnano MW, Wood KC, Meneghini RM, Kaufmann K: No benefit of the two-incision THA over mini-posterior THA: A pilot study of strength and gait. *Clin Orthop Relat Res* 2010; 468(2):565-570.

16. Mardones R, Pagnano MW, Nemanich JP, Trousdale RT: Muscle damage after total hip arthroplasty done with the two-incision and mini-posterior techniques. *Clin Orthop Relat Res* 2005;441:63-67.

17. Pagnano MW, Trousdale RT, Meneghini RM, Hanssen AD: Slower recovery after two-incision than mini-posterior-incision total hip arthroplasty: A randomized clinical trial. *J Bone Joint Surg Am* 2008;90(5):1000-1006.

18. Van Oldenrijk J, Hoogervorst P, Schaap GR, van Dijk CN, Schafroth MU: Two-incision minimally invasive total hip arthro-plasty: Results and complications. *Hip Int* 2011;21(1):81-86.

19. Siguier T, Siguier M, Brumpt B: Mini-incision anterior approach does not increase dislocation rate: A study of 1037 total hip replacements. *Clin Orthop Relat Res* 2004;426:164-173.

20. Bender B, Nogler M, Hozack WJ: Direct anterior approach for total hip arthroplasty. *Orthop Clin North Am* 2009;40(3):321-328.

21. Gilliland JM, Anderson LA, Boffeli SL, Pelt CE, Peters CL, Kubiak EN: A fluoroscopic grid in supine total hip arthroplasty: Improving cup position, limb length, and hip offset. *J Arthroplasty* 2012;27(8)111-116.

22. Restrepo C, Mortazavi SM, Brothers J, Parvizi J, Rothman RH: Hip dislocation: Are hip precautions necessary in anterior approaches? *Clin Orthop Relat Res* 2011;469(2):417-422.

23. Berend KR, Lombardi AV Jr, Seng BE, Adams JB: Enhanced early outcomes with the anterior supine intermuscular approach in primary total hip arthroplasty. *J Bone Joint Surg Am* 2009; 91(suppl 6):107-120.

24. Nogler M, Krismer M, Hozack WJ, Merritt P, Rachbauer F, Mayr E: A double offset broach handle for preparation of the femoral cavity in minimally invasive direct anterior total hip arthroplasty. *J Arthroplasty* 2006;21(8): 1206-1208.

25. Mayr E, Nogler M, Benedetti MG, et al: A prospective randomized assessment of earlier functional recovery in THA patients treated by minimally invasive direct anterior approach: A gait analysis study. *Clin Biomech (Bristol, Avon)* 2009;24(10):812-818.

26. Seng BE, Berend KR, Ajluni AF, Lombardi AV Jr : Anterior-supine minimally invasive total hip arthroplasty: Defining the learning curve. *Orthop Clin North Am* 2009;40(3):343-350.

27. Meneghini RM, Pagnano MW, Trousdale RT, Hozack WJ: Muscle damage during MIS total hip arthroplasty: Smith-Petersen versus posterior approach. *Clin Orthop Relat Res* 2006;453:293-298.

28. Khatod M, Barber T, Paxton E, Namba R, Fithian D: An analysis of the risk of hip dislocation with a contemporary total joint registry. *Clin Orthop Relat Res* 2006; 447:19-23.

29. Phillips CB, Barrett JA, Losina E, et al: Incidence rates of dislocation, pulmonary embolism, and deep infection during the first six months after elective total hip replacement. *J Bone Joint Surg Am* 2003;85(1):20-26.

30. Bhandari M, Matta JM, Dodgin D, et al: Outcomes following the single-incision anterior approach to total hip arthroplasty: A multicenter observational study. *Orthop Clin North Am* 2009;40(3):329-342.

31. Masonis J, Thompson C, Odum S: Safe and accurate: Learning the direct anterior total hip arthroplasty. *Orthopedics* 2008;31(12).

32. Goytia RN, Jones LC, Hungerford MW: Learning curve for the anterior approach total hip arthroplasty. *J Surg Orthop Adv* 2012; 21(2):78-83.

33. Sendtner E, Borowiak K, Schuster T, Woerner M, Grifka J, Renkawitz T: Tackling the learning curve: Comparison between the anterior, minimally invasive (Micro-hip®) and the lateral, transgluteal (Bauer) approach for primary total hip replacement. *Arch Orthop Trauma Surg* 2011; 131(5):597-602.

34. Goulding K, Beaulé PE, Kim PR, Fazekas A: Incidence of lateral femoral cutaneous nerve neuropraxia after anterior approach hip arthroplasty. *Clin Orthop Relat Res* 2010;468(9):2397-2404.

35. Barton C, Kim PR: Complications of the direct anterior ap-

proach for total hip arthroplasty. *Orthop Clin North Am* 2009; 40(3):371-375.

36. Light TR, Keggi KJ: Anterior approach to hip arthroplasty. *Clin Orthop Relat Res* 1980;152: 255-260.

37. Kreuzer S, Leffers K, Kumar S: Direct anterior approach for hip resurfacing: Surgical technique and complications. *Clin Orthop Relat Res* 2011;469(6):1574-1581.

38. Kennon R, Keggi J, Zatorski LE, Keggi KJ: Anterior approach for total hip arthroplasty: Beyond the minimally invasive technique. *J Bone Joint Surg Am* 2004; 86(suppl 2):91-97.

Video Reference

Unger AS: Video.
Direct Anterior Hip Arthroplasty.
Washington, DC, 2013.

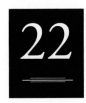

Let's Do a Revision Total Knee Arthroplasty

Edward M. Vasarhelyi, MD, MSc, FRCSC
Steven J. MacDonald, MD, FRCSC
Craig J. Della Valle, MD
Thomas Parker Vail, MD

Abstract

Numerous steps are required to successfully complete a revision total knee arthroplasty. A review of the technical details of each step will be helpful to arthroplasty surgeons, along with a discussion of reoperative planning, complex surgical exposure techniques, component removal, and the choice of prosthetic components. A review of common difficult issues, including bone loss, ligamentous instability, and management of the extensor mechanism, will also aid in achieving a successful revision total knee arthroplasty.

Instr Course Lect 2014;63:239-251.

The incidence of primary total knee arthroplasty (TKA) has been increasing in the United States over the past several years. It is now estimated that more than 4% of the population older than 50 years is living with a TKA.[1] As a result of the increasing number of TKAs being performed, it is anticipated that the revision burden will continue to increase.

With an expected increased volume, it is important that arthroplasty surgeons have a thorough understanding of the steps to follow in revision TKA. It can be a technically challenging procedure, even for experienced surgeons. This chapter discusses the importance of thorough preoperative planning and key factors that should be identified prior to surgery. The

steps to a successful exposure and component removal are included, along with a review of the types of revision components and their indications and the management of extensor mechanism disruption.

Preoperative Planning

Revision TKA can be a technically demanding procedure, even for experienced arthroplasty surgeons. Thorough preoperative planning is essential to improve the quality and efficiency of surgery and reduce the rate of complications associated with revision surgery.

Preoperative planning is necessary to accomplish several goals. It helps to ensure that the correct tools are available for component removal and the correct implant trials and grafts are available for placement. Detailed preoperative planning also provides the opportunity for a mental rehearsal of the surgical procedure and allows a review of the decision-making process for the surgery, including all fallback options and alternative plans.

Planning Checklist

Prior to beginning a revision TKA, a preoperative checklist should be fol-

Dr. Vasarhelyi or an immediate family member has received research or institutional support from DePuy, Smith & Nephew, and Stryker. Dr. MacDonald or an immediate family member has received royalties from DePuy; serves as a paid consultant to or is an employee of DePuy; has received research or institutional support from DePuy, Smith & Nephew, and Stryker; and serves as a board member, owner, officer, or committee member of the Knee Society. Dr. Della Valle or an immediate family member serves as a paid consultant to or is an employee of Biomet, Convatec, and Smith & Nephew; has stock or stock options held in CD Diagnostics; has received research or institutional support from Smith & Nephew and Stryker; and serves as a board member, owner, officer, or committee member of the American Association of Hip and Knee Surgeons, the Arthritis Foundation, and the Knee Society. Dr. Vail or an immediate family member has received royalties from DePuy; serves as a paid consultant to or is an employee of DePuy; has stock or stock options held in Pivot Medical and Biomimedica; and serves as a board member, owner, officer, or committee member of the American Board of Orthopaedic Surgery, the American Association of Hip and Knee Surgeons, and the Knee Society.

lowed. The first step is to ensure that the patient does not have an infection. Laboratory analyses should include an erythrocyte sedimentation rate and C-reactive protein level, followed by knee aspiration if the result of either analysis is elevated or if the clinical suspicion of infection is high.

Identifying the original implants aids in component removal and is especially important if some of the components will be retained. Ideally, this information should be retrieved from implant stickers because dictation or transcription errors in medical records are common. Obtaining past surgical reports can yield useful information pertaining to the past exposure, important intraoperative findings, and the concerns of the operating surgeon.

Preoperative radiography is another component of the preoperative plan. Radiographs should include dedicated views of the knee to evaluate the implant interfaces and bony structure. Long, standing leg radiographs should be used to evaluate the limb for alignment and deformities; they also allow evaluation of the hip and identification of pertinent factors, such as the presence of an ipsilateral total hip arthroplasty.

Before a revision TKA, it is important to identify and understand the mechanism of failure so the surgeon can develop a plan to fix the problem. Caution should be exercised in performing a revision TKA if the cause of the patient's pain is unclear. A review of preoperative radiographs can be helpful because a patient who had minimal degenerative joint disease before the initial arthroplasty procedure is unlikely to be satisfied after further revision surgery.

Templating allows the surgeon to preoperatively plan for the implant size and positioning and determine if augments and/or stems are necessary. The goals for implant sizing are to cap the tibia without an overhang. On the femoral side, the sizing is typically the same as used for the tibia or slightly larger. In the revision setting, there is often a large flexion gap, which can be reduced by upsizing the femur. In implant positioning, the goal is to establish neutral tibial alignment that is perpendicular to the long axis of the tibia. The femoral component should be placed in 5° to 7° of valgus. Excessive anterior placement of the femoral component should be avoided to prevent overstuffing the anterior compartment and reduce the flexion space to maintain matching flexion and extension spaces. It may be necessary to use an offset stem to achieve these objectives on either the tibial or the femoral component. In addition to the goal of achieving neutral alignment, preserving as much bone stock as possible is typically preferred. The use of metal augments or bone grafts helps prevent overresectioning of bone and fills segmental defects. Augments on the femoral side are used distally to fill the extension gap and posteriorly to fill the flexion gap.

Preoperative planning for implants involves decision making regarding the use of stems and sleeves and the fixation method (press-fit with metaphyseal cement only or fully cemented). Each implant type has merits; the choice will be dictated by a combination of surgeon preference and host factors.

Steps in the Surgical Procedure

When planning a revision TKA, it is important to be aware of the series of steps applicable to all cases. After exposure is achieved and the old implants are removed, the sequence of steps is as follows: reestablish a tibial platform, measure the flexion and extension spaces, and then reconstruct the femur to equally fill those spaces.

Surgical Exposures in Revision TKA

Obtaining an adequate surgical exposure is among the first and most important steps in performing a revision TKA. Goals of this part of the procedure include protecting the extensor mechanism, safely removing the implanted components without damaging host bone, and obtaining adequate visualization to prepare the bony surfaces for the revision components. Challenges to these goals include prior skin incisions, dense scarring, and, in some patients, the presence of patella baja, which can greatly complicate attempts at safely exposing the revision TKA.

The Skin Incision

The first step in obtaining exposure is selecting a skin incision. The blood supply to the skin over the anterior aspect of the knee is predominantly derived medially; therefore, if multiple skin incisions are present, the most lateral one that can reasonably be used to perform the procedure is selected.[2] Because the blood supply to the skin of the anterior knee runs just above the deep fascia, any skin flaps that are raised must be full thickness to avoid damage to the dermal blood supply.[3] If skin bridges are required, they should be wide (greater than 6 cm between parallel incisions); if prior incisions are crossed, acute angles of less than 60° should be avoided to decrease the risk of dermal necrosis. If transverse incisions are present (which were often used in the past to perform high tibial osteotomies or patellectomies), these incisions can be crossed perpendicularly. When incising the skin incision and performing subcutaneous dissection, many surgeons find it helpful to extend the incision into normal tissues proximally and distally to assist in finding the extensor mechanism.

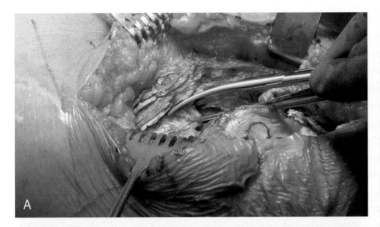

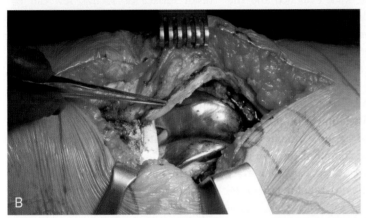

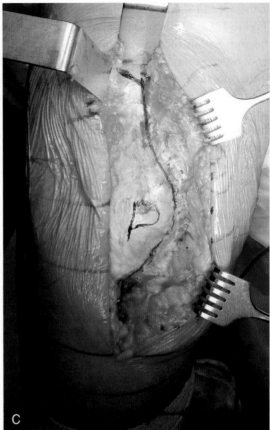

Figure 1   **A,** Intraoperative photograph of the excision of scar tissue deep to the extensor mechanism to facilitate mobilization of the proximal extensor mechanism. **B,** Excision of the scar tissue between the patellar tendon and proximal tibia facilitates exposure and mobilization of the patella. Care must be taken not to avulse the patellar tendon insertion on the tibia. **C,** The quadriceps snip maneuver is an oblique apical extension of the medial parapatellar arthrotomy within the substance of the quadriceps tendon. A side-to-side repair can be made when closing.

Medial Parapatellar Approach

The medial parapatellar approach is the workhorse exposure of revision TKA. This approach is familiar to most orthopaedic surgeons and is easily converted to a more extensile approach if needed. When performed in conjunction with a thorough intra-articular synovectomy, the medial parapatellar approach provides adequate exposure for most revision TKAs encountered in practice.[4,5]

The arthrotomy itself is generally performed in the revision setting from the apex of the quadriceps tendon proximally to the medial aspect of the tibial tubercle distally. A medial flap is then raised around the posteromedial aspect of the tibia. A thorough and generous medial release will facilitate external rotation of the tibia, which decreases stresses on the extensor mechanism. Next, the medial and lateral gutters are reestablished by excising scar tissue from underneath the extensor mechanism (**Figure 1, A**). A plane is usually easy to identify, and complete excision of the scar tissue will greatly enhance mobilization of the extensor mechanism proximally. A similar plane is developed between the patellar tendon and the proximal aspect of the anterolateral tibia by resecting scar tissue in this interval. This technique will greatly enhance exposure; however, care must be taken to avoid injury to the patellar tendon or its insertion to the proximal tibia (**Figure 1, B**). At this point, the modular polyethylene liner is removed, and an attempt is made to subluxate (preferred) or evert the patella. If the exposure is suboptimal or if the patella cannot be mobilized, the surgeon can attempt to peel soft tissue from the lateral edge of the patella to increase its mobility or, if required, can perform a formal lateral release.

Quadriceps Snip

If at this point in the procedure the exposure is inadequate, the quadriceps snip is the most straightforward technique to improve the exposure.[6] The quadriceps snip is an oblique, apical extension of the arthrotomy across the proximal aspect of the patellar tendon at the apex of the medial arthrotomy (**Figure 1, C**). It is important to make the snip within the substance of the tendon (as opposed to more cephalad in the substance of the rectus femoris muscle) because this facilitates a secure side-to-side repair. The advantages of this approach include its technical simplicity, the maintenance of an unaltered postoperative physical therapy regimen, and clinical outcomes that appear to be the same as those achieved using a medial parapatellar approach alone.[7,8]

V-Y Quadricepsplasty

The V-Y quadricepsplasty is a proximal release of the extensor mechanism that connects a medial parapatellar arthrotomy with a lateral release that extends proximally across the quadriceps tendon.[9] Although excellent exposure can be obtained, this procedure is rarely used in current clinical practice because extensor lag and weakness can occur, as well as necrosis of the extensor mechanism if the blood supply is completely disrupted.[8,10] The primary indication for this procedure is severe stiffness, which is believed to be secondary to contracture of the extensor mechanism proximally.

Tibial Tubercle Osteotomy

The tibial tubercle osteotomy allows for distal release of the extensor mechanism. In contemporary practice, it is most commonly used to assist with the removal of intramedullary stems and/or cement. Although excellent exposure can be obtained and good results have been reported, complications (including painful hardware and tibial shaft fracture) can occur.[11-14] The postoperative regimen may need to be altered if this exposure is used.

The osteotomy is usually made with a saw and performed medially to laterally, which creates a cut that is typically 5 to 8 cm in length. Ideally, a bone bridge of 1 cm or more is maintained proximally to help prevent proximal migration. The osteotomy is generally tapered proximally. It is important to hinge the osteotomy open and maintain soft-tissue attachments laterally to facilitate healing via maintenance of the blood supply. After the osteotomy is hinged open, the knee is flexed, and (typically) the patella is easily everted.

At the conclusion of the procedure, the osteotomy is rotated back into its bed, with the knee extended and the tibial tubercle osteotomy repaired with wires that are looped around the fragment but not around the tibia itself because of the high risk of neurovascular injury. If the surgeon prefers screw fixation, care must be taken to avoid fracturing the osteotomy; an appropriate trajectory to avoid intramedullary stems that are commonly used in revision procedures is necessary. One strategy to decrease the risk of fracture is to predrill the screw holes before performing the osteotomy.

Component Removal Techniques

The primary goal of implant removal in a revision TKA is to preserve the host bone stock. This goal must be accomplished while avoiding pitfalls, such as damage to the extensor mechanism, collateral ligament or vascular injury, and iatrogenic fracture of the femoral condyles or tibial plateau.

Femoral Component Removal

The method and tools used for removing the femoral component are dependent on the type of component. Before removal, full exposure should be obtained, with the implant-cement and implant-bone interfaces visualized both medially and laterally. Removal is performed at the implant-cement interface if the component is cemented or the implant-bone interface in a cementless implant. The preferred method of this chapter's authors is to use an oscillating saw with a large blade to cut along the anterior surface and a small blade to cut along the chamfer and distal surfaces. A curved 0.25-inch osteotome is used at the posterior condylar surfaces. If a cruciate-retaining implant is being removed, a 0.25-inch straight osteotome can be used through the notch. If additional freeing of the interface is required, stacked osteotomes can be used at the distal surface or a Gigli saw can be used at the anterior surface and anterior chamfer, although care must be taken to avoid excessive bone resection if this technique is used. The component can then be impacted gently with a punch and a mallet.[15]

The same initial steps as previously described are followed when removing a revision femoral component with a press-fit stem. Caution must be exercised in metaphyseal offset stems with cement fixation. In this scenario, a small anterior cortical window can be a useful adjunct to facilitate component removal. With a fully cemented stem, the same steps should initially be followed. The removal technique will depend on whether the component fixation is well fixed or loose. If the component is loose, extraction can be relatively straightforward. If the cement is still well fixed to the stem (but the stem itself has loosened from the surrounding bone), caution must be taken to ensure that the mass of cement does not cause a distal femoral fracture during extraction. In this case, the cement mantle should be fractured before extraction, or the implant-cement interface should be exploited to remove the component. In the event that the implant is well fixed, an anterior cortical trough can be created to facilitate cement debonding. When implanting the revision stem, it is important that this trough is bypassed with a longer stem, with or without a cortical strut graft. At this point in the procedure, it is advisable to leave any remaining cement on the femur because it can assist with retraction by reinforcing the osteopenic/osteolytic bone during tibial exposure. If the femoral bone is very osteopenic, the surgeon should consider placing the removed femoral component loosely back onto the femur to protect it.

Tibial Component Removal

The type of primary tibial component that was implanted will dictate the removal method. A primary all-polyethylene tibial component is the simplest to remove. An oscillating saw with a large blade is used at the cement-polyethylene interface. The saw is used to cut through the keel, which is then removed with osteotomes.

Most commonly, a primary modular component will be encountered. An oscillating saw with a small blade is used to separate the implant, either at the implant-cement interface or the bone-implant interface if the component is cementless. The geometry of the keel or lug will dictate the direction of the saw. Most commonly, the saw is blocked when attempting to saw in an anterior to posterior direction. As a result, the small blade should be passed in a medial to lateral direction, taking care to ensure that the blade does not advance beyond the posterior tibial cortical margin. Before disimpacting the tray, the surgeon should ensure that the posteromedial and posterolateral corners are released to minimize the risk of a tibial fracture. Care must be taken to avoid collapsing the often soft metaphyseal bone when using osteotomes to remove the tibial tray. Using stacked osteotomes to separate the tray is an effective technique. The widest osteotome should remain on the bone interface to distribute the load as broadly as possible across the proximal tibia. Gentle impaction with a punch and mallet is usually able to remove the tibial component; however, specialized extraction tools may be needed.

When revising stemmed components, the same concepts apply as previously outlined in this chapter regarding femoral stem removal. Caution should be taken when removing offset stems. The tibia is more conical in shape than the femur, making it less susceptible to fracture when removing a cemented stem with a solid cement-implant bond. This is not the case when cement has extruded from the tibia, which most commonly occurs secondary to posterior cortical perforation from a posterior tibial retractor during implantation of the previous component.

Removal of the Femoral and the Tibial Cement

This chapter's authors prefer to begin with cement removal from the femur because cement debris falls onto the tibia. This is accomplished with a combination of osteotomes, cement splitters, crochet hooks, and a high-speed burr. It is important to recognize that in aseptic cases, cement that is well fixed to the underlying bone can be retained if preferred.

Patellar Component Removal

The method of fixation of the implant to the patella dictates the removal technique. The removal of a cemented polyethylene button is best accomplished with an oscillating saw through the polyethylene-cement interface, with sawing directly through the pegs. The pegs then can be removed with a high-speed burr. Cementless patellar components can be very challenging to remove while preserving remaining patellar bone. There is often underlying osteolysis, which predisposes the patella to fracture. An oscillating saw with a small blade should be used circumferentially around the button but will be blocked by the lugs. At this point, the implant can be checked to see whether it can be removed; however, prying between the implant and bone should not be attempted. A metal cutting wheel or a burr then can be used to cut the remaining pegs.

Dealing With Bone Loss

General Considerations

Preoperative planning can help the surgeon prepare for the lack of bony support by making available techniques and devices that are proven to be successful. In general, there are a few key points that should be considered when planning a revision TKA involving bone loss. The overall health of the patient needs to be evaluated because medical conditions such as rheumatoid arthritis, renal disease, and other chronic medical conditions can lead to substantial osteoporosis as well as a predisposition to segmental bone loss associated with deformity. The health, age, and activity level of the patient may help determine if a bone graft (younger patient) or segmental metallic replacement (older and less active patient) is chosen to manage the bone loss.

A physical examination of the extremity is necessary to document the neurovascular status, the quality of the skin, and the presence of ligamentous insufficiency. Significant instability associated with bone loss that creates either an unrecoverable flexion-extension gap mismatch or the loss of bone that extends to the attachment of supporting ligamentous structures may require a constrained implant. Standard radiographs may not completely show the amount of bone loss present, and, in some cases, a CT scan may be helpful for preoperative planning and assessment.

Classification of Bone Loss

The Anderson Orthopaedic Research Institute established one of several useful bone defect classification systems for revision TKA to guide treatment decisions and research.[16] In a type 1 defect, there is a full metaphyseal segment without substantial damage. Often, good bone is available, and the revision can be accomplished with primary components. If the bone is excessively osteopenic and cannot support the primary prosthesis, the addition of a short, fully cemented stem will add stability. Further damage to the metaphyseal bone leads to type 2 bone loss. If the defects are less than 10 mm, then treatment is with polymethyl methacrylate (PMMA) augmentation. In type 3 bone loss, the metaphysis can be completely deficient.

Management of Smaller Contained and Peripheral Bone Defects

Small defects (range, 5 to 10 mm) on both the femoral and tibial sides of the joint can be managed using allograft, autograft, metallic augments, or PMMA cement. Filling a peripheral defect becomes more difficult if it is uncontained; however, successful results have been reported with screw reinforcement of the cement mantle on the tibial side.[17] To effectively decrease the size of the defect, the tibial implant can be translated away (to some extent) from the deficient area onto the available bone. There are limits to this strategy because the tibial component must be compatible with the femoral component and, in some systems, the tibial and femoral implants must be within one or two sizes of one another. Translation of a component to the point that it creates an overhang (especially medially on the tibia and laterally on the femur) can be associated with pain or can adversely affect collateral ligament tension and patellar tracking.

Bone Loss Greater Than 10 mm

When bone defects exceed 10 mm, PMMA cement may be inadequate to fill the void. In such situations, prosthetic augments have been used successfully.[18] The use of wedges or block augments may require further resection of bone to create a match between the bone defect and the predetermined off-the-shelf augment size. The prime benefits of an augment are that modular augments fill defects and assist with maintaining the joint line and proper ligament tensioning. Medial tibial uncontained defects have been successfully treated using wedges, with 96% good to excellent results at 5-year follow-up.[19] The disadvantage of wedge and cemented augments is that they rely on cement for fixation in bone that is often sclerotic and not ideal for cement penetration. Cementless, porous metallic augments may offer the option of both defect filling and enhanced fixation to remaining bone.

Massive Bone Loss

Managing more substantial bone loss in the revision setting can be more complex and may require specialized reconstructive techniques.[20,21] Structural grafts, although attractive in younger patients in whom bone stock restoration is desired, present the risks of malunion, nonunion, and late collapse. In these scenarios, long-stem components are required to support the reconstruction and protect the allograft.

Union rates of 82% with uncontained medial tibial autografts have been reported.[22] In a study of 30 patients treated with TKA by Engh et al,[23] 35 structural allografts were used, including 29 femoral head allografts, 5 distal femoral allografts, and 1 proximal tibial allograft. Eighty-seven percent of the patients had a good or excellent clinical result. There were no cases of graft collapse.

Clatworthy et al[24] studied 52 revision TKAs treated with structural allografts for defects and reported a 75% success rate at 10 years, similar to the results reported in a 2009 study by Bauman et al.[25] The authors reported that five knees had graft resorption and two knees had a nonunion between the graft and the host bone. The remainder of the failures in the study by Bauman et al[25] resulted from infection (four patients) and the lack of a 20-point improvement in the knee score. In patients with severe defects, a rotating hinge knee replacement can be used to manage massive bone loss and instability. Early experience with a hinge prosthesis demonstrated loosening and failure, resulting from stresses transferred to the interface of the implant. Short-term studies on a rotating hinge design suggest more encouraging results, with no evidence of loosening at 2-year follow-up.[26]

The limitations of allografts have led to the development of porous metal augments and metaphyseal cones that function as void fillers and serve to enhance fixation through biologic incorporation of bone into the porous metal substrate.[27-29] The use of cones is a departure from the use of augments that are direct extensions of the implant because the augments can be positioned independently of the prosthesis. Recent studies on the use of modular cones and augments on both sides of the joint have reported excellent early outcomes in terms of fixation and function.[30]

Patellar Component Revision

In most instances, revision of the patellar component is not required at the time of revision TKA. Even if the implanted component is not from the same manufacturer or is not the same design, retention in the face of revision of the tibiofemoral articulation during revision TKA is associated with a low rate of failure.[31,32] Revision of a well-fixed patellar component is often difficult because even small amounts of bone loss associated with the removal of a well-fixed component can result in a thin patellar remnant that can be challenging to reconstruct. Indications for revision or removal of the patella component include chronic deep periprosthetic joint infection; the presence of an older generation metal-backed patella, which has a high risk of damaging the femoral component; or an overly thick patella that is grossly malpositioned or malsized. Barrack et al[32] recommended caution if the patellar component was sterilized with gamma radiation in air.

If the patellar component requires revision and the remaining bone is greater than 12 mm in thickness, the surgeon can use the standard reconstruction techniques used for primary procedures. If the patellar remnant is thinner, more specialized techniques may be required. If the loss of bone stock is severe but relatively contained (with an intact cortical rim), a straightforward alternative is using a biconvex all-polyethylene patellar component.[33,34] Erak et al[34] reported on the use of an inset, single peg, biconvex patellar component for remnants with a mean thickness of 8 mm and a component that was either 13 or 17 mm in thickness. The overall results were encouraging, with 97% implant survivorship at 10 years; failures were associated with remnants of less than 6 mm in thickness.

Another option is using a porous, tantalum-backed patellar component.[35] The surgical technique includes reaming the remnant with a convex reamer to create a concave bed into which the component is secured

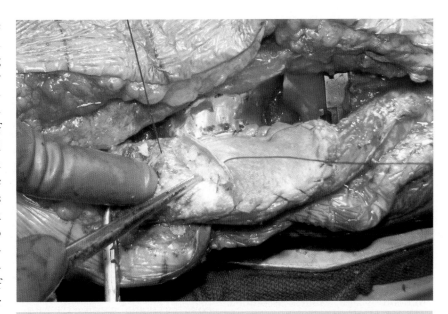

Figure 2   Bone graft is packed into a sutured soft-tissue pocket to reconstitute a bone-deficient patella.

with suture. Lessons learned from published studies include the importance of using this component in situations in which a bony shell is present (as opposed to securing it into only soft tissue).[36,37]

Impaction grafting is another potential solution for treating a patella with bony deficiency. As described in the original technique, a soft-tissue flap is raised from native tissues lateral to the patella that is used to contain the graft.[36] Suture is used to secure the soft-tissue flap around the periphery, and a bone graft is then packed into the pocket that is created (**Figure 2**). An alternative to using native tissues is soft-tissue graft substitutes, such as those used to augment rotator cuff or hernia repairs. These grafts can make the reconstruction technically easier, but the cost of the soft-tissue graft substitutes must be considered.

If none of the aforementioned techniques is believed to be technically feasible, resection arthroplasty of the patella should be avoided because it is associated with less than optimal results.[38,39] In these scenarios, a final option is the use of a so-called gull-wing

osteotomy. In this technique, the patella is split longitudinally to create a convex surface. Two small series showed that this technique appears to be successful at containing the patellar remnant to avoid lateral tracking and dislocation, which can occur if the patellar remnant is left untreated.[40,41]

Managing Ligamentous Instability

General Considerations

Instability is the third most common cause of failure in TKA, after infection and aseptic loosening.[42,43] Subtle instability after knee replacement is not only an important cause of revision but also an underreported factor in patient dissatisfaction after TKA. Although joint stability is critically dependent on implant sizing, ligament integrity, and implant alignment, it is important to understand the role of implant positioning on joint stability after knee replacement. When examining a patient, determining the presence or absence of collateral ligaments will be important in surgical decision making. When a collateral ligament is absent, increased prosthetic constraint is indicated. In contrast, when a collateral ligament is present (end point detectable with a stress examination), but the knee is not stable, balancing the knee without adding additional constraint is possible. Instability can be clinically relevant and should be separately assessed in the coronal plane (varus/valgus laxity) throughout the range of motion, the sagittal plans (anteroposterior laxity), and in combination (global laxity).

The clinical presentation of an unstable knee often reflects the pattern of instability, but the presentation can be nonspecific or even associated with arthrofibrosis and stiffness as chronic manifestations of a mechanically unbalanced knee. Persistent effusion can be a manifestation of a chronically unstable knee. A patient will commonly report a lack of confidence in his or her knee. Posterior cruciate insufficiency or excessive anteroposterior laxity can cause patellofemoral pain, limited flexion (resulting from posterior impingement of the tibial plateau), problems initiating gait, and limited extension (resulting from a mechanical disadvantage of the quadriceps mechanism). Coronal imbalance is most often related to unequal flexion and extension gaps or a trapezoidal (rather than rectangular) gap in flexion or extension. The most common clinical pattern in the presence of unbalanced flexion and extension gaps is a tight extension gap (leading to extensor lag) combined with a larger flexion gap, which causes instability with stair descent or incline walking. In the absence of a true ligamentous deficiency, most of the common patterns of instability can be managed by correcting the flexion and extension gap balance along with component rotation.[44]

Recognizing and Managing the Common Causes of Early-Onset Knee Instability

Instability in the first 12 to 24 months after TKA, which is not associated with gross ligament rupture or damage, is most often related to component alignment and sizing or flexion-extension imbalance.[45] Although any combination of flexion and extension gap mismatch is theoretically possible, the most common pattern is a flexion gap that is substantially larger than the extension gap. The situation can be remedied by increasing the extension gap through additional distal femoral bone resection to equalize the gaps. It must be considered that proximal movement of the joint line has an effect on collateral ligament function and patellar contact stress. The distal femoral bone cannot be resected to the point that it compromises ligament attachments or creates a patella infera, with resultant patellar component impingement on the tibial tray in flexion.

Another common cause of instability in flexion is the inadequate release of the posterior capsule in a patient with a flexion contracture. This leads to a tight extension gap as the posterior capsule comes into tension, masking the unbalanced collateral ligaments. As the knee is flexed and the posterior capsule is no longer tight, the collateral ligaments will again control the varus/valgus stability of the knee.

Component alignment is the second crucial requirement for a balanced knee. Component alignment can be divided into coronal and axial alignment. The coronal alignment of the tibial and femoral components correlates with overall limb alignment and collateral ligament stability in extension. Excessive valgus in the coronal plane can cause lateral patellar instability, thigh chafing during gait, and diminished quadriceps power. Axial alignment of the tibial and femoral components is critical for proper patellar tracking and maintaining the appropriate step angle during gait. Internal rotation of the components can lead to lateral patellar tracking and external rotation of the limb.

The size and rotation of the femoral component is critical to the stability of the knee in flexion. An undersized or anteriorly translated femoral component also can lead to flexion instability. An internally rotated femoral component will create a trapezoidal flexion gap, lateral laxity, and instability in knee flexion. The goal of revision surgery is to create rotational alignment in flexion of a properly sized femoral component that results in a rectangular flexion gap when the tibia is cut perpendicular to the mechanical axis.

Common Causes and Treatments of Late Knee Instability and Ligamentous Insufficiency

Common causes of total knee instability include polyethylene wear, ligament injury or attrition (posterior collateral ligament or collateral ligament), ligament insufficiency related to bone loss, and extensor mechanism problems. When the knee is unstable in both flexion and extension but the gaps are equally lax, the instability pattern is balanced. A balanced pattern of instability is the least common scenario, but it is the easiest scenario to manage. For example, when polyethylene wear creates a globally unstable knee, but the knee has balanced instability in both flexion and extension, polyethylene liner exchange is an appropriate treatment. Another pattern of instability that is relatively easy to manage is late posterior cruciate ligament insufficiency. This pattern of instability can be managed by revising a cruciate-sparing knee implant to a cruciate-substituting implant. Cruciate substitution alone will not be sufficient in the presence of collateral ligament insufficiency.

When a collateral ligament is truly compromised as the result of attrition, rupture, or bone loss, the only solution is to increase the varus-valgus constraint at the articulation commensurate with the degree of instability. In the most severe cases of ligament incompetence or gap mismatch, a hinged component is required.[46]

Recurvatum patterns resulting from extensor mechanism or posterior capsular insufficiency will most likely require additional articular constraint or a hinge in the most severe cases. A weak extensor mechanism leads to a recurvatum gait pattern that forces the center of gravity behind the midcoronal axis to prevent collapse of the knee in extension. The result of this abnormal mechanical loading of the posterior capsule is posterior capsular laxity.

An Algorithm for Treating Instability in Revision TKA

Simplifying the management of knee instability in revision TKAs involves creating a simple algorithm of treatment. In one simple work flow, the tibia is cut first. After the tibial platform is established, the gaps can be balanced, and the femoral component rotation can be determined using the tibia as a point of reference. Other general guidelines are to match the degree of constraint with the degree of instability after obtaining the best possible ligament and gap balance, component alignment, and component sizing. Ligament reconstruction can be considered for isolated ligament injuries with optimal component alignment and balance.

Stems: When and Which Type?

Stems are generally used during revision TKA; however, the optimal fixation method for stems in revision TKA is unclear. The role of a stem is to transfer loads to the diaphysis, which has a protective role in preventing failure of the metaphyseal interfaces.[47] No single type of stem is appropriate for all patients. Because uncemented and cemented stems have advantages and disadvantages, each fixation method should be in the armamentarium of the arthroplasty surgeon.

Uncemented stems have several advantages over cemented stems. They are expeditious to use, and, for most systems, stem preparation is compatible with intramedullary-based instrumentation. Given the diaphyseal-filling objective of these stems, they can more reliably ensure limb alignment.[48] If component removal is required, uncemented stems are generally easier to remove than fully cemented stems.

The disadvantages of uncemented stems include an indeterminate degree of long-term fixation, even though the stems can offload metaphyseal stresses.[49] Analogous to total hip arthroplasty, there is the potential for pain at the end of the stem, with reported incidences of approximately 20% in solid stems and 8% in slotted stems.[50] The potential for canal deformities and improper orientation make it difficult to achieve a proper diaphyseal fit and can introduce component malalignment. Although uncemented stems are widely used, several variables, including optimal length, surface finish, and preparation technique, have not been fully studied to establish the most effective application.

When using uncemented stems, preoperative templating is useful in planning the revision surgery. Offset stems on the femoral side and offset trays on the tibial side are often needed to prevent the stem from forcing the implant into a suboptimal position. Using longer stems help ensure dia-

physeal engagement. Short stems that do not engage the diaphysis are of questionable benefit.

A fully cemented stem is much less commonly used in the practices of this chapter's authors. Its use can be advantageous in the setting of abnormal canal geometry because the smaller stem allows more latitude in adjusting component placement. The lack of canal-filling ability introduces a greater potential for component malalignment, so care must be taken when definitively inserting the revision components. A fully cemented stem provides excellent initial stability in metaphyseal and diaphyseal bone; however, component removal may be difficult. Some evidence in the literature suggests that short, cemented stems (particularly on the tibial side) can lead to aseptic loosening in the long-term, secondary to a reduction in the load distribution to metaphyseal bone.[51]

Fully cemented stems are indicated in revision TKAs in patients with very osteoporotic bone and capacious canals. This type of bone makes achieving diaphyseal fit difficult, and iatrogenic fracture is possible. If the canal geometry will not permit the placement of an uncemented stem, cemented stems provide additional options. Cemented stems also are preferred in patients with sclerotic or damaged metaphyseal bone if there will be an inadequate interface with the component after reconstruction unless cementation is extended into the canal. When cementing stems, the surgeon should use cement restrictors and a cement gun for appropriate pressurization; antibiotic cement is recommended.

The literature is inclusive on guiding the choice of which type of technique should be used in revision TKA. There is evidence that both hybrid and cemented revision techniques provide equal stability and implant survivorship and have a similar risk of aseptic loosening.[52] However, these studies have many shortcomings, including the broad range of implants used and the unique characteristics of each patient that make it difficult to generalize results. Many of the reports present only midterm results, and there have been no randomized controlled trials comparing techniques. After reviewing the relative advantages and disadvantages of each option, the arthroplasty surgeon should consider patient factors and bony anatomy, along with his or her comfort level, before deciding on a system and a technique for revision TKA.

Managing the Extensor Mechanism

Managing the extensor mechanism may be a secondary concern for the surgeon performing revision TKAs because the extensor mechanism may not be the primary reason for revision surgery. However, many of the integral steps in revision TKA concern protecting the extensor mechanism from injury and optimizing its function after the tibiofemoral articulation has been reconstructed. A thorough understanding of the basic principles of managing the extensor mechanism is critical to a surgeon who performs revision TKA as part of his or her practice.

As with any complication, prevention is preferable to treatment. The extensor mechanism is the main impediment to exposure during revision TKA and must be protected throughout the procedure. Patients with patella baja, those undergoing revision for knee stiffness, or patients in whom the exposure is difficult for some other reason (such as obesity) are at highest risk for intraoperative disruption of the extensor mechanism.

Intraoperative and Acute Extensor Mechanism Disruption

Acute extensor mechanism disruption most commonly occurs at the insertion of the patellar tendon into the tibial tubercle. If encountered, an attempt should be made at primary repair back to the tibial tubercle using either suture anchors or bone tunnels, with the use of a running locking stitch and heavy nonabsorbable suture for fixation into the tendon itself. Although few studies are available on the management of this complication, augmentation of the repair with autogenous semitendinosus graft, allograft, or polypropylene mesh is recommended.[53-56] If a semitendinosus graft is used, the technique includes proximal harvest while maintaining the tibial insertion intact, followed by looping the tendinous portion either around or through the patella, and then a distal side-to-side repair.[56] Rigid immobilization is recommended for 6 weeks and is followed by gradual mobilization in a hinged knee brace because stiffness is generally easier to manage than incompetence of the extensor mechanism.

In the early postoperative period, patellar tendon disruptions can occur secondary to fractures of the inferior pole of the patella; a small portion of the inferior pole of the patella is oftentimes present but is too small to allow for internal fixation. Surgical treatment includes a soft-tissue repair, with the placement of two running locking sutures into the patellar tendon proximally to distally and then proximally again to create four strands that are placed through drill holes in the patella. This repair can be augmented with autograft or allograft tissue and is followed by rigid immobilization for 6 weeks, after which gradual range of motion in a hinged knee brace is recommended.

Acute tears of the quadriceps tendon after TKA seem to be less common, but equally poor results have been reported.[57] The recommended technique includes the use of running locking sutures placed into the tendon and then tied through drill holes as previously described, typically with autograft, allograft, or polypropylene mesh augmentation. The previously described postoperative protocol is recommended.

Managing Chronic Extensor Mechanism Disruption

If the initial attempt at primary extensor mechanism repair fails, repeated attempts at repair are not recommended because of the high risk of infection and the low likelihood that repeated attempts will restore extensor mechanism function. In these situations, a complete extensor mechanism allograft can be used or, in patients with a chronic patellar tendon rupture, an Achilles tendon allograft with a calcaneal bone block can be used.[55,58-60] The principal advantage of the Achilles tendon allograft is that the patella is retained. The complete extensor allograft, however, allows for more robust fixation proximally and for coverage of the entire allograft with host tissue, whereas the Achilles tendon allograft lies superficial to the remaining extensor mechanism underneath the skin.

The basic principles of reconstruction using a complete extensor mechanism allograft include using appropriately sided (right as opposed to left) allografts that are fresh frozen and nonirradiated. Concomitant component revisions are common to optimize knee stability and component rotation. The surgeon should be prepared to exchange the modular polyethylene liner and revise the components, if necessary. A midline approach down the center of the quadriceps tendon,

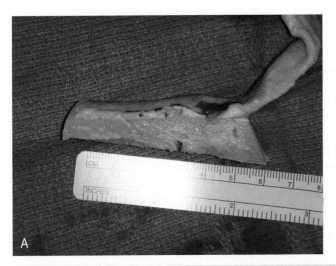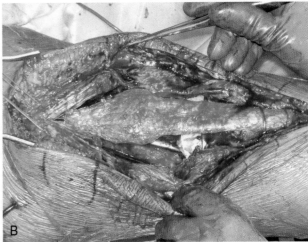

Figure 3 **A,** A bone block of approximately 5 cm in length to allow for a press-fit into a corresponding tibial trough and adjunctive fixation is crafted from the allograft extensor mechanism. **B,** The allograft should be covered as completely as possible with native tissue and tensioned while in extension.

the patella, and the tibial tubercle is used expose and retain all of the remaining host tissue, which is used to cover the allograft at the conclusion of the procedure. A bone block of approximately 5 cm in length is crafted from the allograft that includes the tibial tubercle, with a bevel cut proximally to augment stability (**Figure 3, A**); a matching trough is made in the host proximal tibia. The bone block is then press-fit into the trough with wires or a screw used for adjunctive fixation. The optimal length of the allograft quadriceps tendon is approximately 5 cm. Using two nonabsorbable heavy sutures, four strands are created by running the suture up and down the tendon in a running locking fashion. The allograft tissue is then tightly tensioned in full extension and covered as completely as possible with native tissue using additional sutures that run through both the native and the allograft tissues (**Figure 3, B**). The allograft patella is not resurfaced, and, after tensioning, the repair is not trialed. Rigid immobilization for 6 weeks is recommended, followed by gradual range of motion in a hinged knee brace. Outcomes with a full extensor mechanism allograft show a high rate of restoration of active knee extension, with stiffness rarely reported as a complication.[55,58,59]

Summary

Revision TKA can be a technically demanding procedure. Successful surgery is predicated on comprehensive preoperative planning and knowledge of common challenges and strategies to address those challenges. Preoperative planning is integral to establishing the mechanism of failure so that it can be addressed in the revision procedure. In the planning phase, it is important to identify potential challenges and bony and soft-tissue deficiencies that are likely to be encountered. Intraoperatively, care must be taken to ensure the exposure is carried out in a systematic fashion, using extensile exposures when necessary. Component removal can proceed after adequate exposure has been obtained. Care must be taken to preserve as much bone stock as possible, with attention to preserving soft-tissue attachments. When choosing revision components, the quality of the patient's bone stock and soft-tissue adequacy will determine the types of components used. Careful surgical technique during the revision procedure is important to avoid extensor mechanism disruption, which is a potentially devastating complication.

References

1. Weinstein AM, Rome BN, Reichmann WM, et al: Estimating the burden of total knee replacement in the United States. *J Bone Joint Surg Am* 2013;95(5):385-392.

2. Colombel M, Mariz Y, Dahhan P, Kénési C: Arterial and lymphatic supply of the knee integuments. *Surg Radiol Anat* 1998;20(1):35-40.

3. Haertsch PA: The blood supply to the skin of the leg: A post-mortem investigation. *Br J Plast Surg* 1981;34(4):470-477.

4. Della Valle CJ, Berger RA, Rosenberg AG: Surgical exposures in revision total knee arthroplasty. *Clin Orthop Relat Res* 2006;446:59-68.

5. Sharkey PF, Homesley HD, Shastri S, Jacoby SM, Hozack WJ, Rothman RH: Results of revision total knee arthroplasty after exposure of the knee with extensor

mechanism tenolysis. *J Arthroplasty* 2004;19(6):751-756.

6. Garvin KL, Scuderi G, Insall JN: Evolution of the quadriceps snip. *Clin Orthop Relat Res* 1995;321: 131-137.

7. Meek RM, Greidanus NV, McGraw RW, Masri BA: The extensile rectus snip exposure in revision of total knee arthroplasty. *J Bone Joint Surg Br* 2003;85(8): 1120-1122.

8. Barrack RL, Smith P, Munn B, Engh G, Rorabeck C: Comparison of surgical approaches in total knee arthroplasty. *Clin Orthop Relat Res* 1998;356:16-21.

9. Aglietti P, Buzzi R, D'Andria S, Scrobe F: Quadricepsplasty with the V-Y incision in total knee arthroplasty. *Ital J Orthop Traumatol* 1991;17(1):23-29.

10. Trousdale RT, Hanssen AD, Rand JA, Cahalan TD: V-Y quadricepsplasty in total knee arthroplasty. *Clin Orthop Relat Res* 1993;286: 48-55.

11. Mendes MW, Caldwell P, Jiranek WA: The results of tibial tubercle osteotomy for revision total knee arthroplasty. *J Arthroplasty* 2004; 19(2):167-174.

12. Ries MD, Richman JA: Extended tibial tubercle osteotomy in total knee arthroplasty. *J Arthroplasty* 1996;11(8):964-967.

13. Whiteside LA: Exposure in difficult total knee arthroplasty using tibial tubercle osteotomy. *Clin Orthop Relat Res* 1995;321:32-35.

14. Young CF, Bourne RB, Rorabeck CH: Tibial tubercle osteotomy in total knee arthroplasty surgery. *J Arthroplasty* 2008;23(3): 371-375.

15. Laskin RS: Ten steps to an easier revision total knee arthroplasty. *J Arthroplasty* 2002;17(4):78-82.

16. Engh GA, Ammeen DJ: Bone loss with revision total knee arthroplasty: Defect classification and alternatives for reconstruction.

Instr Course Lect 1999;48: 167-175.

17. Ritter MA, Keating EM, Faris PM: Screw and cement fixation of large defects in total knee arthroplasty: A sequel. *J Arthroplasty* 1993;8(1):63-65.

18. Rand JA: Modular augments in revision total knee arthroplasty. *Orthop Clin North Am* 1998; 29(2):347-353.

19. Pagnano MW, Trousdale RT, Rand JA: Tibial wedge augmentation for bone deficiency in total knee arthroplasty: A followup study. *Clin Orthop Relat Res* 1995; 321:151-155.

20. Ghazavi MT, Stockley I, Yee G, Davis A, Gross AE: Reconstruction of massive bone defects with allograft in revision total knee arthroplasty. *J Bone Joint Surg Am* 1997;79(1):17-25.

21. Rorabeck CH, Smith PN: Results of revision total knee arthroplasty in the face of significant bone deficiency. *Orthop Clin North Am* 1998;29(2):361-371.

22. Aglietti P, Buzzi R, Scrobe F: Autologous bone grafting for medial tibial defects in total knee arthroplasty. *J Arthroplasty* 1991;6(4): 287-294.

23. Engh GA, Herzwurm PJ, Parks NL: Treatment of major defects of bone with bulk allografts and stemmed components during total knee arthroplasty. *J Bone Joint Surg Am* 1997;79(7):1030-1039.

24. Clatworthy MG, Ballance J, Brick GW, Chandler HP, Gross AE: The use of structural allograft for uncontained defects in revision total knee arthroplasty: A minimum five-year review. *J Bone Joint Surg Am* 2001;83(3):404-411.

25. Bauman RD, Lewallen DG, Hanssen AD: Limitations of structural allograft in revision total knee arthroplasty. *Clin Orthop Relat Res* 2009;467(3):818-824.

26. Jones RE, Skedros JG, Chan AJ, Beauchamp DH, Harkins PC:

Total knee arthroplasty using the S-ROM mobile-bearing hinge prosthesis. *J Arthroplasty* 2001; 16(3):279-287.

27. Cohen R: A porous tantalum trabecular metal: Basic science. *Am J Orthop (Belle Mead NJ)* 2002; 31(4):216-217.

28. Lewallen DG, Fehring TK, Dennis DA, Scuderi GR: Revision total knee arthroplasty: Surgical techniques. *J Bone Joint Surg Am* 2009;91(suppl 5):69-71.

29. Meneghini RM, Lewallen DG, Hanssen AD: Use of porous tantalum metaphyseal cones for severe tibial bone loss during revision total knee replacement: Surgical technique. *J Bone Joint Surg Am* 2009;91(suppl 2, pt 1):131-138.

30. Lachiewicz PF, Bolognesi MP, Henderson RA, Soileau ES, Vail TP: Can tantalum cones provide fixation in complex revision knee arthroplasty? *Clin Orthop Relat Res* 2012;470(1):199-204.

31. Lonner JH, Mont MA, Sharkey PF, Siliski JM, Rajadhyaksha AD, Lotke PA: Fate of the unrevised all-polyethylene patellar component in revision total knee arthroplasty. *J Bone Joint Surg Am* 2003; 85(1):56-59.

32. Barrack RL, Rorabeck C, Partington P, Sawhney J, Engh G: The results of retaining a well-fixed patellar component in revision total knee arthroplasty. *J Arthroplasty* 2000;15(4):413-417.

33. Maheshwer CB, Mitchell E, Kraay M, Goldberg VM: Revision of the patella with deficient bone using a biconvex component. *Clin Orthop Relat Res* 2005;440:126-130.

34. Erak S, Bourne RB, MacDonald SJ, McCalden RW, Rorabeck CH: The cemented inset biconvex patella in revision knee arthroplasty. *Knee* 2009;16(3):211-215.

35. Nelson CL, Lonner JH, Lahiji A, Kim J, Lotke PA: Use of a trabecular metal patella for marked pa-

tella bone loss during revision total knee arthroplasty. *J Arthroplasty* 2003;18(7):37-41.

36. Hanssen AD: Bone-grafting for severe patellar bone loss during revision knee arthroplasty. *J Bone Joint Surg Am* 2001;83(2): 171-176.

37. Ries MD, Cabalo A, Bozic KJ, Anderson M: Porous tantalum patellar augmentation: The importance of residual bone stock. *Clin Orthop Relat Res* 2006;452: 166-170.

38. Barrack RL, Matzkin E, Ingraham R, Engh G, Rorabeck C: Revision knee arthroplasty with patella replacement versus bony shell. *Clin Orthop Relat Res* 1998;356: 139-143.

39. Garcia RM, Kraay MJ, Conroy-Smith PA, Goldberg VM: Management of the deficient patella in revision total knee arthroplasty. *Clin Orthop Relat Res* 2008; 466(11):2790-2797.

40. Vince KR, Blackburn D: Gull-wing sagittal patellar osteotomy in total knee arthroplasty. *Tech Knee Surg* 2002;1:106-112.

41. Klein GR, Levine HB, Ambrose JF, Lamothe HC, Hartzband MA: Gull-wing osteotomy for the treatment of the deficient patella in revision total knee arthroplasty. *J Arthroplasty* 2010;25(2): 249-253.

42. Fehring TK, Odum S, Griffin WL, Mason JB, Nadaud M: Early failures in total knee arthroplasty. *Clin Orthop Relat Res* 2001;392: 315-318.

43. Sharkey PF, Hozack WJ, Rothman RH, Shastri S, Jacoby SM: Why are total knee arthroplasties failing today? *Clin Orthop Relat Res* 2002;404:7-13.

44. McAuley JP, Engh GA, Ammeen DJ: Treatment of the unstable total knee arthroplasty. *Instr Course Lect* 2004;53:237-241.

45. Fehring TK, Valadie AL: Knee instability after total knee arthroplasty. *Clin Orthop Relat Res* 1994; 299:157-162.

46. Naudie DD, Rorabeck CH: Managing instability in total knee arthroplasty with constrained and linked implants. *Instr Course Lect* 2004;53:207-215.

47. Murray PB, Rand JA, Hanssen AD: Cemented long-stem revision total knee arthroplasty. *Clin Orthop Relat Res* 1994;309:116-123.

48. Parsley BS, Sugano N, Bertolusso R, Conditt MA: Mechanical alignment of tibial stems in revision total knee arthroplasty. *J Arthroplasty* 2003;18(7):33-36.

49. Beckmann J, Lüring C, Springorum R, Köck FX, Grifka J, Tingart M: Fixation of revision TKA: A review of the literature. *Knee Surg Sports Traumatol Arthrosc* 2011;19(6):872-879.

50. Barrack RL, Stanley T, Burt M, Hopkins S: The effect of stem design on end-of-stem pain in revision total knee arthroplasty. *J Arthroplasty* 2004;19(7): 119-124.

51. Nakama GY, Peccin MS, Almeida GJ, Lira Neto OdeA, Queiroz AA, Navarro RD: Cemented, cementless or hybrid fixation options in total knee arthroplasty for osteoarthritis and other non-traumatic diseases. *Cochrane Database Syst Rev* 2012;10:CD006193.

52. Sah AP, Shukla S, Della Valle CJ, Rosenberg AG, Paprosky WG: Modified hybrid stem fixation in revision TKA is durable at 2 to 10 years. *Clin Orthop Relat Res* 2011; 469(3):839-846.

53. Parker DA, Dunbar MJ, Rorabeck CH: Extensor mechanism failure associated with total knee arthroplasty: Prevention and management. *J Am Acad Orthop Surg* 2003;11(4):238-247.

54. Schoderbek RJ Jr, Brown TE, Mulhall KJ, et al: Extensor mechanism disruption after total knee arthroplasty. *Clin Orthop Relat Res* 2006;446:176-185.

55. Burnett RS, Berger RA, Paprosky WG, Della Valle CJ, Jacobs JJ, Rosenberg AG: Extensor mechanism allograft reconstruction after total knee arthroplasty: A comparison of two techniques. *J Bone Joint Surg Am* 2004;86(12):2694-2699.

56. Cadambi A, Engh GA: Use of a semitendinosus tendon autogenous graft for rupture of the patellar ligament after total knee arthroplasty: A report of seven cases. *J Bone Joint Surg Am* 1992; 74(7):974-979.

57. Dobbs RE, Hanssen AD, Lewallen DG, Pagnano MW: Quadriceps tendon rupture after total knee arthroplasty: Prevalence, complications, and outcomes. *J Bone Joint Surg Am* 2005;87(1): 37-45.

58. Nazarian DG, Booth RE Jr: Extensor mechanism allografts in total knee arthroplasty. *Clin Orthop Relat Res* 1999;367:123-129.

59. Emerson RH Jr, Head WC, Malinin TI: Extensor mechanism reconstruction with an allograft after total knee arthroplasty. *Clin Orthop Relat Res* 1994;303:79-85.

60. Crossett LS, Sinha RK, Sechriest VF, Rubash HE: Reconstruction of a ruptured patellar tendon with Achilles tendon allograft following total knee arthroplasty. *J Bone Joint Surg Am* 2002;84(8):1354-1361.

Video Reference

Karim A, Incavo SJ, Dominues B: *Surgical Techniques for the Removal of the Infected Primary TKA and 2nd Stage Revision.* [video]. Rosemont, IL, American Academy of Orthopaedic Surgeons, 2013. *Orthopaedic Video Theater 17.* http://orthoportal.aaos.org/emedia/singleVideoPlayer.aspx?resource=EMEDIA_OSVL_13_17. Accessed 11/20/13.

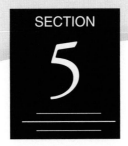
Spine

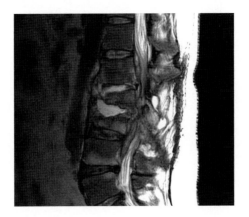

Spine

23

Current Concepts in Cervical Spine Trauma

Louis F. Amorosa, MD
Alexander R. Vaccaro, MD, PhD

Abstract

Much has been written about cervical spine trauma. Although occipitocervical dislocations result in high mortality rates at the scene of the injury, more patients are surviving this injury as a result of safety improvements. Injuries to this region of the spine are often undiagnosed, even by experienced spine surgeons and radiologists. Substantial controversy and debate remain surrounding cervical spinal clearance, spinal cord injury, odontoid fractures, traumatic spondylolisthesis of C2 on C3, and subaxial cervical spine facet subluxations and dislocations. Although debate regarding appropriate treatment algorithms for these injuries still exists, management recommendations based on the available evidence will be helpful to the treating surgeon.

Instr Course Lect 2014;63:255-262.

Several recently published studies can guide spine surgeons in the best evidence-based practices for treating cervical spine injuries. This chapter will review the most commonly encountered and challenging clinical scenarios and the evidence-based guidelines for treatment. Although a comprehensive review of all aspects of cervical spine trauma is beyond the scope of this chapter, the most controversial areas of this subject will be discussed, and proper treatment recommendations will be provided.

Evaluating the Cervical Spine

Cervical spine injuries occur in 1% to 3% of all patients with blunt trauma.[1] Historically, as part of the Advanced Trauma Life Support protocol, a lateral radiograph of the cervical spine was obtained to diagnose fractures, malalignment, and soft-tissue swelling suggestive of ligamentous injury. At most trauma centers, the lateral radiograph is now bypassed, and a CT scan, often of the entire body, is the first test obtained. Although this "pan scan" is appropriate in severely injured patients to quickly diagnose all injuries, in less severely injured or awake patients, a CT scan, particularly of the neck and thyroid gland, has the potential to increase radiation and cancer risks.[2,3] In the era of medical cost containment and evidence-based medicine, less expensive tests should be used if appropriate.[4,5]

In awake patients with blunt trauma who are not obtunded and have no distracting injuries, a physical examination is adequate to safely evaluate the cervical spine. A recent metaanalysis of 14 prospective studies with 61,989 patients included various evaluation protocols, including the National Emergency X-Radiography Utilization Study and the Canadian C-Spine Rule, in its analysis. It was concluded that an awake and alert patient without distracting injuries and no neurologic deficit had a negative predictive value for cervical spine injury of 99.8%; therefore, no radio-

Dr. Vaccaro or an immediate family member has received royalties from Aesculap/B. Braun, DePuy, Globus Medical, Medtronic Sofamor Danek, Stout Medical, Progressive Spinal Technology, and Applied Spinal Intellectual Properties; has stock or stock options held in Globus Medical, Progressive Spinal Technologies, Advanced Spinal Intellectual Properties, Computational Biodynamics, Stout Medical, Paradigm Spine, K2M, Replication Medica, Spinology, Spine Medica, Orthovita, Vertiflex, Small Bone Technologies, NeuCore, Crosscurrent, Syndicom, In Vivo, Flagship Surgical, Location Based Intelligence, Gamma Spine, and Spinicity; has received research or institutional support from AO North America and Cerapeutics; has received nonincome support (such as equipment or services), commercially derived honoraria, or other non–research-related funding (such as paid travel) from Nuvasive; and serves as a board member, owner, officer, or committee member of the Cervical Spine Research Society and AO North America. Neither Dr. Amorosa nor any immediate family member has received anything of value from or has stock or stock options held in a commercial company or institution related directly or indirectly to the subject of this chapter.

graphic evaluation was necessary.[1] Both geriatric and pediatric patients were assessed.

A more challenging clinical scenario is evaluating the cervical spine with a negative CT scan, in a patient who is obtunded and with blunt trauma, a patient with a distracting injury, or a patient with persistent neck pain after trauma. Options include obtaining an acute MRI versus delayed dynamic flexion and extension lateral cervical spine radiographs when the patient is more awake and paraspinal spasm has subsided. Waiting has obvious disadvantages, including a longer immobilization time for the patient, which can be especially detrimental in the setting of an intensive care unit. However, MRI also has disadvantages, including cost, the practical problem of obtaining MRI for a polytraumatized patient, and the lack of availability of MRI at some institutions.

Recent studies have attempted to determine if CT alone is an adequate study to evaluate the cervical spine.[6,7] A recent retrospective study reviewed 389 patients with blunt trauma and persistent neck pain or obtundation who were observed to be moving all four extremities.[6] Of the 389 patients, 199 had abnormal cervical spinal CT findings. In the remaining 190 patients with normal CT scans, 12% of those with persistent neck pain had ligamentous edema or injuries not seen with CT but identified with MRI. Twenty percent of the obtunded patients with no abnormal CT findings had ligamentous edema or injury found on MRI. However, none of the injuries missed with CT and later found with MRI required surgical intervention. The authors recommended that a cervical collar can be safely removed after a negative CT scan in patients with persistent neck pain or obtundation if they can move all extremities.

In a recent meta-analysis of 17 studies with 14,327 patients, modern CT had a greater than 99.9% sensitivity and specificity for detecting cervical spinal injuries requiring surgery.[7] Although this is a controversial topic, if a modern CT scan is negative for a cervical spinal injury in a patient with blunt trauma who is obtunded but moving all extremities or who has persistent neck pain but no focal neurologic deficit, MRI may be bypassed and the cervical spine safely evaluated.

Spinal Cord Injury

The timing of spinal cord decompression in a patient with an acute spinal cord injury is controversial. The Surgical Timing in Acute Spinal Cord Injury Study prospectively followed 313 patients from six spinal cord injury centers across the United States and Canada.[8] The study reported a significant difference in the American Spinal Injury Association grade of improvement between patients treated with early decompression (mean, 14.2 hours after injury) compared with patients treated with later spinal decompression (mean, 48.3 hours after injury). There was no difference in the complication rates between the two groups. Based on the results of this study, early surgical decompression of the compressed spinal cord can be considered, followed by stabilization when the patient is medically stable and qualified personnel are available.

Steroids are often given acutely in the presence of spinal cord injury based on the results of the second and third National Acute Spinal Cord Injury Studies (NASCISs).[9,10] Some authors have questioned the methodology and the conclusions of the NASCISs.[11,12] However, many institutions continue to follow the NASCIS protocol, in part because of the fear of litigation if steroids are not administered.[13] Some investigators believe that high-dose steroids do not improve outcomes and may increase complications such as wound infection, gastrointestinal ulcers, and steroid-induced myopathy.[11,14] A recent Cochrane review by the lead author of NASCIS examined seven randomized controlled studies, including the three NASCIS trials, comparing high-dose methylprednisolone with placebo, and found that patients given steroids in the acute period were more likely to recover pinprick sensation and some degree of motor recovery below the level of injury.[15] Based on the Cochrane review, it was recommended that if injury occurred within 3 hours, 30 mg/kg of methylprednisolone loading dose over 15 minutes followed 45 minutes later by 5.4 mg/kg for the ensuing 24 hours should be administered. If the injury occurred from 3 to 8 hours prior, the steroids should be continued for a total of 48 hours. Although many institutions follow this protocol, the argument for administering steroids remains controversial, and more research is needed.

Therapeutic hypothermia for the treatment of spinal cord injuries recently gained widespread attention in the lay press after a high cervical spine fracture-dislocation and complete spinal cord injury occurred in an American professional football player. The patient was treated acutely with intravenous cooled fluids and early spinal cord decompression. Excellent motor function in the lower extremities was subsequently recovered. Although the patient's neurologic recovery may have resulted, in part, from the early therapeutic hypothermia, it is also possible it resulted from timely transport and imaging, intravenous steroid administration, and early spinal cord decompression.[16]

The excellent clinical evidence that early therapeutic hypothermia prevents brain ischemia in cardiac arrest

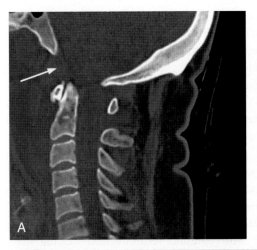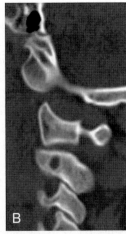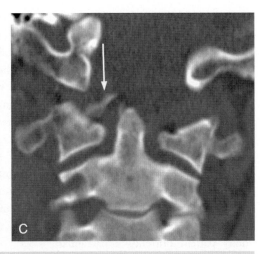

Figure 1 Subtle CT findings typical of occipitocervical instability include an increased basion-dens interval (arrow) (**A**), occipitoatlantal subluxation (**B**), and increased height of the lateral atlantoaxial joint (**C**). Note the associated bony avulsion of the transverse alar ligament (arrow). (Reproduced with permission from Radcliff K, Kepler C, Reitman C, Harrop J, and Vaccaro A: CT and MRI-based diagnosis of craniocervical dislocations: The role of the occipitoatlantal ligament. *Clin Orthop Relat Res* 2012;470(6):1602-1613.)

patients who are successfully resuscitated has made such therapy the standard of care for those patients. Although several animal models have shown promising results, there is sparse clinical evidence for using therapeutic hypothermia in patients with spinal cord injuries.[17] More research is needed before therapeutic hypothermia can be considered a routine treatment for patients with a cervical spinal cord injury.

Occipitocervical Junction and Upper Cervical Spine Injuries

Occipitocervical dislocations are associated with a high mortality rate at the scene of the injury. However, with better safety mechanisms, patients with unstable injuries to the occipitocervical junction are more frequently surviving the scene of injury. A recent study retrospectively reviewed 69 patients diagnosed with occipitocervical dissociation at a level I trauma center.[18] Forty-seven of these patients were diagnosed only at postmortem; of the remaining 22 patients, only 7 patients survived their injury to discharge

from the hospital. A higher score on the Glasgow Coma Scale and a lower basion-dens interval were associated with survival. A similar review of a trauma database found that nonsurvivability was associated with complete spinal cord injury and a high Injury Severity Score.[19]

Often, because of distracting serious injuries and the subtlety of radiographic findings, injuries to the occipitocervical complex and occipitocervical instability can be easily missed, even with CT (**Figure 1**). A delay in diagnosing and stabilizing these injuries puts patients at risk for sudden paralysis, respiratory arrest, and death with mobilization. A recent retrospective review of cervical CT scans from a large database of polytraumatized patients reported that five patients had an occipitocervical injury based on the amount of displacement on CT or MRI scans.[20] The injury had been initially missed in three of the five patients despite review of imaging studies by a trained neuroradiologist.

A prospectively collected spinal cord injury database identified 18 patients with disruptions of the cranio-

cervical ligaments diagnosed on MRI.[21] Two types of associated injury patterns were found. Patients with type I injuries had atlantoaxial injuries alone, and those with type II injuries had combined occipitoatlantal-atlantoaxial injuries. A complete spinal cord injury was more likely in patients with type II injuries. Type I injuries were treated with C1-C2 fusion, whereas type II injuries were treated with fusion of the occiput to C2. A high index of suspicion must be maintained for occipitocervical spinal injuries in high-energy injuries, and MRI should be obtained if CT suggests ligamentous instability to the occipitocervical complex.

Occipital condyle fractures are rarely associated with occipitocervical instability. A recent retrospective review of 24,745 trauma patients at a level I trauma center over a 6-year period identified 100 patients (0.4%) with 106 occipital condyle fractures.[22] Two of these patients showed evidence of concurrent occipitocervical instability or malalignment and were treated with occipitocervical fusion without complication. The remaining patients were successfully treated with either a hard cervical collar or counseling. A prospective study of 31 occipital condyle fractures also found that these fractures can be successfully treated nonsurgically if they are not associated with occipitocervical instability.[23]

Odontoid Fractures

Odontoid fractures are increasing in prevalence as the population ages.[24] An odontoid fracture with an associated neurologic deficit in an elderly patient portends a particularly poor prognosis. A recent study of geriatric patients identified 20 patients with an odontoid fracture and associated neurologic deficit. Nine of the 20 patients died in the hospital; patients with an odontoid fracture and complete spinal cord injury were 9.33 times more likely to die.[25]

Type I avulsion fractures of the odontoid not associated with occipitoatlantal or atlantoaxial instability and type III odontoid fractures with little displacement have presumed high union rates with nonsurgical treatment in a hard cervical orthosis. The treatment of type II odontoid fractures is more controversial and is associated with increased mortality in the geriatric population. A recent retrospective study of 156 patients 65 years and older with a type II odontoid fracture reported a 39% mortality rate at 3 years postoperatively regardless of the intervention, including collar or halo immobilization, or surgery.[26]

Type II odontoid fractures occur at the base of the dens, a watershed vascular zone, and are at increased risk for nonunion. Although painless nonunion is not clinically important in the absence of myelopathy, instability or callous hypertrophy can in some cases lead to neurologic compromise. Elderly patients with type II odontoid fractures who are treated with halo vests have been shown to have poor

outcomes and high mortality rates.[27] However, surgical and nonsurgical mortality rates vary among studies, and high-level evidence regarding surgical versus nonsurgical treatment are lacking in the literature.[28]

Previously accepted indications for surgery in patients with type II odontoid fractures have included polytrauma, neurologic deficit, associated cervical spine injuries, and painful nonunion.[29] However, the results of a large, multicenter, prospective study of 159 patients 65 years or older with type II odontoid fractures who were either treated surgically or nonsurgically were recently presented.[30] The patients treated surgically had significantly better functional outcomes as measured by the Medical Outcomes Short Form 36-Item bodily pain score (P = 0.0014) and the Neck Disability Index (P = 0.0071) and showed a trend in lower mortality rates at 1 year after injury, although this did not rise to statistical significance (P = 0.059).

The type of surgical fixation for odontoid fractures is also controversial. Reducible, type II odontoid fractures with an oblique fracture pattern extending from anterior cephalad to posterior caudad may be amenable to osteosynthesis using one or two odontoid screws from an anterior approach.[31] The benefit of direct osteosynthesis is the preservation of atlantoaxial rotation, which contributes to approximately 50% of the overall rotation of the cervical spine.[32] Although this is usually not as clinically important in elderly patients, in younger patients, motion should be preserved, and anterior fixation chosen for an amenable fracture pattern. In elderly patients, anterior screw fixation should be used with caution because of issues concerning bone density.[33,34]

A recent retrospective study of 33 patients older than 65 years treated with anterior odontoid screw fixation

had a failure rate of 36.4%.[33] Failure of anterior odontoid screw fixation was associated with atlanto-odontoid arthritis, osteoporosis, poor reduction, poor screw placement, inadequate compression, and a comminuted fracture pattern. In a prospective study of 69 patients with odontoid fractures, 68 were followed to successful healing.[34] Thirty-one patients were treated with cervical orthosis, 25 with posterior transarticular fixation, and 13 with anterior screw fixation. The authors recommended treating stable fractures with a cervical orthosis, treating type II or III fractures in patients younger than 75 years with anterior screw fixation, and treating patients older than 75 years with C1-C2 transarticular fixation.

Because closed reduction of posteriorly displaced odontoid fractures has been associated with acute respiratory distress caused by retropharyngeal swelling, prophylactic nasotracheal intubation should be considered before reduction.[35] Heavy sedation should be avoided because it is necessary to assess the patient's neurologic status during and after closed reduction. Odontoid fractures, especially type II odontoid fractures in elderly patients, remain a challenging and controversial injury, and more research is necessary to reach more definitive treatment guidelines.

Traumatic Spondylolisthesis of the Axis

Traumatic spondylolisthesis of C2 on C3, otherwise known as a hangman's fracture, most commonly occurs from a high-energy mechanism. The injury is a fracture of the C2 pars interarticularis and causes a variable degree of displacement of C2 on C3. The Levine-Edwards modification of the Effendi classification system is most commonly used to describe these injuries.[36,37] Type I injuries have less than 3 mm of displacement and no angulation and can be treated with a cervical orthosis. Type II injuries are displaced more than 3 mm and can be managed with closed reduction and traction followed by a halo vest. Many clinicians treat this subtype with a collar or halo vest alone without reduction. Type IIa injuries have no listhesis but are substantially angulated; reduction with traction should be avoided to help prevent overdistraction. Type III injuries are both displaced and angulated and include C2-3 facet fracture or dislocation. Although management is controversial and multiple studies have reported on surgical and nonsurgical treatments, surgery is generally reserved for type IIa and type III injuries, nonunions, or the presence of neurologic deficit.[38]

The optimal approach and the form of fixation for hangman's fractures are also controversial. Evidence for one form of surgical treatment over another is based only on retrospective reviews. Anterior cervical diskectomy and fusion of C2 and C3 has been reported in retrospective series to improve neck pain and function and has high fusion rates and low complication rates.[39,40] Posterior cervical fusion of C2 and C3 offers the advantages of direct visualization of the facets and ease of reduction and also has been shown to have good results, improved function, and low complication rates.[41] A small case series reported good short-term results and one vertebral artery injury with direct repair of the pars with reduction and pedicle screw fixation of C2.[42] This technique offers the theoretic advantage of motion preservation; however, because the C2-C3 disk complex is usually injured, Xie et al[43] reported on combined fusion of the C2-C3 disk space in conjunction with direct osteosynthesis of the pars fracture to prevent instability.

Table 1
The Subaxial Injury Classification System[a]

Morphology	Points
No abnormality	0
Compression	1
Burst	+ 1 = 2
Distraction (for example, facet perch, hyperextension)	3
Rotation/translation (for example, facet dislocation, unstable teardrop or advanced-stage flexion compression injury)	4
Diskoligamentous complex	
Intact	0
Indeterminant (for example, isolated interspinous widening, MRI signal change only)	1
Disrupted (for example, widening of disk space, facet perch, or dislocation)	2
Neurologic status	
Intact	0
Root injury	1
Complete cord injury	2
Incomplete cord injury	3
Continuous cord compression in setting of neurodeficit (neuromodifier)	+ 1

[a]This scoring system entails three primary categories related to injury morphology, the status of the diskoligamentous complex, and neurologic status. The scores are totaled, and the total score may help guide subsequent treatment. Low scores (less than 4) indicate nonsurgical treatment; higher scores (greater than 4) indicate a need for surgical stabilization and possible decompression. (Reproduced with permission from Vaccaro AR, Hulbert RJ, Patel AA, et al; Spine Trauma Study Group: The subaxial cervical spine injury classification system: A novel approach to recognize the importance of morphology, neurology, and integrity of the disco-ligamentous complex. *Spine* 2007; 32:2365-2374.)

Subaxial Cervical Spine Trauma

Cervical facet dislocations are commonly caused by high-energy flexion-distraction mechanisms and result in varying degrees of neurologic injury, which may be the result of the injury mechanism, the amount of displacement, and whether the injury is unilateral or bilateral.[44,45] A recent prospective cohort study from several North American spinal cord injury centers examined whether patients with facet dislocations and associated spinal cord injuries had worse motor recovery at 1 year after injury compared with those patients with cervical spinal cord injury without associated facet dislocation. At 1-year follow-up, the 135 patients with facet dislocations were less

likely to have achieved motor recovery compared with the 286 patients without facet dislocation.[45]

The Spine Trauma Study Group introduced the Subaxial Injury Classification in 2007 as a scoring system to better classify and predict the best form of treatment for patients with cervical spinal injuries.[46] The Subaxial Injury Classification is based on three parameters: the injury mechanism, the integrity of the diskoligamentous complex, and the neurologic status of the patient (**Table 1**). Intraobserver and interobserver reliability of this classification system was shown to be comparable with conventional subaxial spinal trauma injury classifications. This classification has been used as a tool for evidence-based research on cervical spine trauma, although it has not been widely adopted for clinical use.

One controversial issue is the algorithm for treating cervical facet subluxations and dislocations. Surveys of members of the Spine Trauma Study Group have shown that there is poor interobserver and intraobserver agreement among spine trauma experts on the proper algorithm of diagnosis and treatment—whether to obtain an MRI before treatment, perform a closed reduction before MRI, or proceed directly to surgery.[47,48] The best consensus concerns the treatment of patients with complete spinal cord injuries. It is generally agreed that a closed reduction should be obtained as soon as possible, before MRI is performed, because there is minimal risk and greater potential benefit in relieving spinal cord pressure as early as possible after the injury. In an awake patient who is neurologically intact, one argument for an initial closed reduction with traction before obtaining an MRI is that there has never been a reported case of permanent neurologic decline after closed traction reduction of a cervical facet dislocation in an awake patient.[49] If neurologic decline occurs during the reduction, traction can be stopped or easily reversed. The logic for this argument is that in most institutions, MRI is time consuming, especially during nighttime hours. Generally, if closed reduction can be successfully obtained preoperatively in an awake, neurologically intact patient, only one procedure is usually necessary: either a posterior fusion or an anterior decompression and fusion. A combined approach is performed if more stability is believed to be necessary. In patients with cervical facet subluxation or dislocation who are obtunded or have an incomplete neurologic deficit, the most agreed-on algorithm is to obtain an MRI before attempted reduction.

Summary

The diagnosis and treatment of cervical spine trauma has evolved rapidly over the past decade. Spinal cord trauma, however, remains a challenging problem with a poor long-term prognosis for both patients and society because most spinal cord injuries occur in young people in the prime of life. Continued high-level research is necessary to address this problem and improve the lives of patients. Controversy still exists in the proper treatment of both upper and lower cervical spine injuries. More research and better reporting of outcomes is needed to work toward more standardized treatments.

References

1. Anderson PA, Muchow RD, Munoz A, Tontz WL, Resnick DK: Clearance of the asymptomatic cervical spine: A meta-analysis. *J Orthop Trauma* 2010;24(2): 100-106.

2. Richards PJ, Summerfield R, George J, Hamid A, Oakley P: Major trauma and cervical clearance radiation doses and cancer induction. *Injury* 2008;39(3): 347-356.

3. Biswas D, Bible JE, Bohan M, Simpson AK, Whang PG, Grauer JN: Radiation exposure from musculoskeletal computerized tomographic scans. *J Bone Joint Surg Am* 2009;91(8):1882-1889.

4. Andrawis JP, Chenok KE, Bozik KJ: Health policy implications of outcome measurements in orthopaedics. *Clin Orthop Relat Res* 2013;471(11):3475-3481.

5. Mahoney E, Agarwal S, Li B, et al: Evidence-based guidelines are equivalent to a liberal CT scan protocol for initial patient evaluation but are associated with decreased computed tomography scan use, cost, and radiation exposure. *J Trauma Acute Care Surg* 2012;73(3):573-578.

6. Soult MC, Weireter LJ, Britt RC, et al: A utility analysis. *Am Surg* 2012;78(7):741-744.

7. Panczykowski DM, Tomycz ND, Okonkwo DO: Comparative effectiveness of using computed tomography alone to exclude cervical spine injuries in obtunded or intubated patients: Meta-analysis of 14,327 patients with blunt trauma. *J Neurosurg* 2011;115(3): 541-549.

8. Fehlings MG, Vaccaro A, Wilson JR, et al: Results of the Surgical Timing in Acute Spinal Cord Injury Study (STASCIS). *PLoS One* 2012;7(2):e32037.

9. Bracken MB, Shepard MJ, Collins WF, et al: A randomized, controlled trial of methylprednisolone or naloxone in the treatment of acute spinal-cord injury: Results of the Second National Acute Spinal Cord Injury Study. *N Engl J Med* 1990;322(20):1405-1411.

10. Bracken MB, Shepard MJ, Holford TR, et al: Administration of methylprednisolone for 24 or 48 hours or tirilazad mesylate for 48 hours in the treatment of acute spinal cord injury: Results of the Third National Acute Spinal Cord Injury Randomized Controlled Trial. National Acute Spinal Cord Injury Study. *JAMA* 1997; 277(20):1597-1604.

11. Coleman WP, Benzel D, Cahill DW, et al: A critical appraisal of the reporting of the National Acute Spinal Cord Injury Studies (II and III) of methylprednisolone in acute spinal cord injury. *J Spinal Disord* 2000;13(3): 185-199.

12. Sayer FT, Kronvall E, Nilsson OG: Methylprednisolone treatment in acute spinal cord injury: The myth challenged through a structured analysis of published literature. *Spine J* 2006;6(3): 335-343.

13. Hurlbert RJ, Hamilton MG: Methylprednisolone for acute spinal cord injury: 5-year practice

reversal. *Can J Neurol Sci* 2008;
35(1):41-45.

14. Qian T, Guo X, Levi AD, Vanni
    S, Shebert RT, Sipski ML: High-
    dose methylprednisolone may
    cause myopathy in acute spinal
    cord injury patients. *Spinal Cord*
    2005;43(4):199-203.

15. Bracken MB: Steroids for acute
    spinal cord injury. *Cochrane Data-
    base Syst Rev* 2012;1:CD001046.

16. Cappuccino A, Bisson LJ, Car-
    penter B, Marzo J, Dietrich WD
    III, Cappuccino H: The use of
    systemic hypothermia for the
    treatment of an acute cervical
    spinal cord injury in a professional
    football player. *Spine (Phila Pa
    1976)* 2010;35(2):E57-E62.

17. Dietrich WD, Levi AD, Wang M,
    Green BA: Hypothermic treat-
    ment for acute spinal cord injury.
    Neurotherapeutics 2011;8(2):
    229-239.

18. Cooper Z, Gross JA, Lacey JM,
    Traven N, Mirza SK, Arbabi S:
    Identifying survivors with trau-
    matic craniocervical dissociation:
    A retrospective study. *J Surg Res*
    2010;160(1):3-8.

19. Chaput CD, Torres E, Davis M,
    Song J, Rahm M: Survival of
    atlanto-occipital dissociation cor-
    relates with atlanto-occipital dis-
    traction, Injury Severity Score,
    and neurologic status. *J Trauma*
    2011;71(2):393-395.

20. Chaput CD, Walgama J, Torres E,
    et al: Defining and detecting
    missed ligamentous injuries of the
    occipitocervical complex. *Spine
    (Phila Pa 1976)* 2011;36(9):
    709-714.

21. Radcliff K, Kepler C, Reitman C,
    Harrop J, Vaccaro A: CT and
    MRI-based diagnosis of craniocer-
    vical dislocations: The role of the
    occipitoatlantal ligament. *Clin
    Orthop Relat Res* 2012;470(6):
    1602-1613.

22. Maserati MB, Stephens B,
    Zohny Z, et al: Clinical decision
    rule and surgical management.

J Neurosurg Spine 2009;11(4):
388-395.

23. Mueller FJ, Fuechtmeier B, Kin-
    ner B, et al: Prospective follow-up
    of 31 cases within 5 years at a
    level 1 trauma centre. *Eur Spine J*
    2012;21(2):289-294.

24. Smith HE, Kerr SM, Fehlings
    MG, et al: 20-year experience at a
    model system spine injury tertiary
    referral center. *J Spinal Disord
    Tech* 2010;23(8):501-505.

25. Patel A, Smith HE, Radcliff K,
    Yadlapalli N, Vaccaro AR: Odon-
    toid fractures with neurologic
    deficit have higher mortality and
    morbidity. *Clin Orthop Relat Res*
    2012;470(6):1614-1620.

26. Schoenfeld AJ, Bono CM, Reich-
    mann WM, et al: Do treatment
    type and medical comorbidities
    affect mortality in elderly patients?
    Spine (Phila Pa 1976) 2011;
    36(11):879-885.

27. Tashjian RZ, Majercik S, Biffl
    WL, Palumbo MA, Cioffi WG:
    Halo-vest immobilization in-
    creases early morbidity and mor-
    tality in elderly odontoid frac-
    tures. *J Trauma* 2006;60(1):
    199-203.

28. Pal D, Sell P, Grevitt M: Type II
    odontoid fractures in the elderly:
    An evidence-based narrative re-
    view of management. *Eur Spine J*
    2011;20(2):195-204.

29. Elgafy H, Dvorak MF, Vaccaro
    AR, Ebraheim N: Treatment of
    displaced type II odontoid frac-
    tures in elderly patients. *Am J
    Orthop (Belle Mead NJ)* 2009;
    38(8):410-416.

30. Vaccaro AR, Kopjar B, Chap-
    man J, et al: Function and
    quality-of-life outcomes in geriat-
    ric patients with type-II dens frac-
    ture. *J Bone Joint Surg Am* 2013;
    95(3):729-735.

31. Grauer JN, Shafi B, Hilibrand AS,
    et al: Proposal of a modified,
    treatment-oriented classification
    of odontoid fractures. *Spine J*
    2005;5(2):123-129.

32. White AA III, Panjabi MM: *Clin-
    ical Biomechanics of the Spine*,
    ed 2. Philadelphia, PA, Lippincott
    Williams & Wilkins, 1990.

33. Osti M, Philipp H, Meusburger
    B, Benedetto KP: Analysis of fail-
    ure following anterior screw fixa-
    tion of type II odontoid fractures
    in geriatric patients. *Eur Spine J*
    2011;20(11):1915-1920.

34. Konieczny MR, Gstrein A, Müller
    EJ: Treatment algorithm for dens
    fractures: Non-halo immobiliza-
    tion, anterior screw fixation, or
    posterior transarticular C1-C2
    fixation. *J Bone Joint Surg Am*
    2012;94(19):e144(1-6).

35. Harrop JS, Vaccaro A, Przybylski
    GJ: Acute respiratory compromise
    associated with flexed cervical
    traction after C2 fractures. *Spine
    (Phila Pa 1976)* 2001;26(4):
    E50-E54.

36. Effendi B, Roy D, Cornish B,
    Dussault RG, Laurin CA: Frac-
    tures of the ring of the axis: A
    classification based on the analysis
    of 131 cases. *J Bone Joint Surg Br*
    1981;63-B(3):319-327.

37. Levine AM, Edwards CC: The
    management of traumatic spon-
    dylolisthesis of the axis. *J Bone
    Joint Surg Am* 1985;67(2):
    217-226.

38. Li XF, Dai LY, Lu H, Chen XD:
    A systematic review of the
    management of hangman's frac-
    tures. *Eur Spine J* 2006;15(3):
    257-269.

39. Ying Z, Wen Y, Xinwei W, et al:
    Anterior cervical discectomy and
    fusion for unstable traumatic
    spondylolisthesis of the axis. *Spine
    (Phila Pa 1976)* 2008;33(3):
    255-258.

40. Xu H, Zhao J, Yuan J, Wang C:
    Anterior discectomy and fusion
    with internal fixation for unstable
    hangman's fracture. *Int Orthop*
    2010;34(1):85-88.

41. Ma W, Xu R, Liu J, et al: Poste-
    rior short-segment fixation and
    fusion in unstable Hangman's

fractures. *Spine (Phila Pa 1976)* 2011;36(7):529-533.

42. ElMiligui Y, Koptan W, Emran I: Transpedicular screw fixation for type II Hangman's fracture: A motion preserving procedure. *Eur Spine J* 2010;19(8):1299-1305.

43. Xie N, Khoo LT, Yuan W, et al: Combined anterior C2-C3 fusion and C2 pedicle screw fixation for the treatment of unstable hangman's fracture: A contrast to anterior approach only. [Published online ahead of print Feb 10] *Spine (Phila Pa 1976)* 2010.

44. Andreshak JL, Dekutoski MB: Management of unilateral facet dislocations: A review of the literature. *Orthopedics* 1997;20(10): 917-926.

45. Wilson JR, Vaccaro A, Harrop JS, et al: The impact of facet dislocation on clinical outcomes after cervical spinal cord injury: Results of a multicenter North American prospective cohort study. *Spine (Phila Pa 1976)* 2013;38(2): 97-103.

46. Vaccaro AR, Hulbert RJ, Patel AA, et al: The subaxial cervical spine injury classification system: A novel approach to recognize the importance of morphology, neurology, and integrity of the disco-ligamentous complex. *Spine (Phila Pa 1976)* 2007;32(21): 2365-2374.

47. Grauer JN, Vaccaro AR, Lee JY, et al: The timing and influence of MRI on the management of patients with cervical facet dislocations remains highly variable: A survey of members of the Spine Trauma Study Group. *J Spinal Disord Tech* 2009;22(2):96-99.

48. Nassr A, Lee JY, Dvorak MF, et al: Variations in surgical treatment of cervical facet dislocations. *Spine (Phila Pa 1976)* 2008;33(7): E188-E193.

49. Wimberley DW, Vaccaro AR, Goyal N, et al: Acute quadriplegia following closed traction reduction of a cervical facet dislocation in the setting of ossification of the posterior longitudinal ligament: Case report. *Spine (Phila Pa 1976)* 2005;30(15):E433-E438.

Video Reference

Valencia M, De La Fuente P, Abara S, Novoa F, Leiva A, Olid A: *Fixation of Odontoid Fractures With an Anterior Screw: Surgical Technique* [video]. Rosemont, IL, American Academy of Orthopaedic Surgeons, 2014. *Orthopaedic Video Theater 40.* http://orthoportal.aaos.org/emedia/singleVideoPlayer.aspx?resource=EMEDIA_OSVL_14_40. Accessed January 8, 2014.

Recent Advances in the Prevention and Management of Complications Associated With Routine Lumbar Spine Surgery

Louis G. Jenis, MD
Wellington K. Hsu, MD
Joseph R. O'Brien, MD, MPH
Peter G. Whang, MD, FACS

Abstract

Lumbar spine surgery is often associated with complications in the perioperative and postoperative periods. Evidence-based literature in the prevention and management of adverse events, including surgical site infection, venous thromboembolism, and positioning-related complications, has advanced the understanding of the etiology of these complications and preventive measures. Cost-effective measures to reduce intraoperative bleeding can lead to a lower incidence of infection, disease transmission, and morbidity in the postoperative period. As the healthcare system receives additional scrutiny with value-based assessments, surgeons, hospitals, and administrators will need to make critical decisions to prevent and manage the complications of lumbar spine surgery.

Instr Course Lect 2014;63:263-270.

In 2009, more than 448,000 patients were treated with spinal arthrodesis in the United States.[1] Complications have been reported to range from 4% to 19%, depending on the nature of the spinal surgery.[2] Some of the most commonly encountered yet highly preventable complications are surgical site infection and hemorrhagic and/or thromboembolic complications. With this in mind, prevention of infection should be a paramount concern for all spine surgeons. Recent areas of focus have been on eradication of normal bacterial skin flora before surgery via skin antisepsis and nasal decolonization, the application of topical antibiotics, and perioperative glycemic management, as well as insights into sterile processing.

This chapter focuses on recent evidence surrounding the identification and the prevention of these common occurrences and complications.

Postoperative Surgical Site Infection

It is estimated that surgical site infections make up nearly 22% of all health-care associated infections. With up to 27 million surgical procedures performed each year in the United States, it is estimated that there are 300,000 to 500,000 annual postopera-

Dr. Jenis or an immediate family member has received royalties from Stryker; is a member of a speakers' bureau or has made paid presentations on behalf of Nuvasive; and serves as a paid consultant to or is an employee of Nuvasive and Stryker. Dr. Hsu or an immediate family member serves as a paid consultant to or is an employee of AO North America, Lifenet, Medtronic, Pioneer Surgical, Stryker, Terumo, and Zimmer; has received research or institutional support from Baxter; and serves as a board member, owner, officer, or committee member of the American Academy of Orthopaedic Surgeons, the Lumbar Spine Research Society, and the North American Spine Society. Dr. O'Brien or an immediate family member has received royalties from Nuvasive and Globus; serves as a paid consultant to or is an employee of Stryker, Nuvasive, Globus, and Relievant; has stock or stock options held in Doctors Research Group; and has received research or institutional support from Bioset, Nuvasive, and Globus. Dr. Whang or an immediate family member is a member of a speakers' bureau or has made paid presentations on behalf of Medtronic and Stryker; serves as a paid consultant to or is an employee of Cerapedics, Medtronic, the Musculoskeletal Transplant Foundation, Paradigm Spine, ProFibrix, Relievant, Stryker, Trans1, and Vertiflex; serves as an unpaid consultant to DiFusion; and has stock or stock options held in DiFusion.

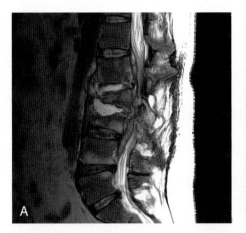
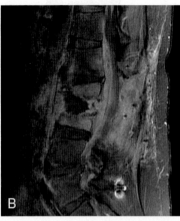

Figure 1 **A,** T2-weighted sagittal MRI scan of the lumbar spine, confirming the presence of increased signal intensity within the L1-L2 and L2-L3 disk space as well as vertebral body erosion consistent with diskitis. **B,** T1-weighted sagittal MRI scan with gadolinium enhancement, depicting the presence of increased signal within the vertebral bodies as well as enhancement within the spinal canal consistent with osteomyelitis and epidural abscess formation.

tive surgical site infections. Although patient comorbidities affect infection rates, many preoperative, intraoperative, and postoperative factors can affect risk as well.[3-9] Postoperative surgical site infection is a costly complication, leading to both direct and indirect expenditures affecting hospital and physician practices.

The recognition of specific features of postoperative surgical site infection is critical for establishing a treatment plan. However, there are no specific pathognomonic features that are reliable for the clinician based on the varied surgical techniques, approaches, associated use of spinal implants, and patient characteristics and their risks for infection. The diagnosis of surgical site infection can be challenging, and a high index of suspicion is necessary. The diagnosis is established by a combination of clinical, radiographic, and laboratory investigations. The most common clinical presentation is increased pain after surgery that develops following a brief period of relief of normal postoperative pain, sometimes up to 2 to 3 weeks after the index surgery. The discomfort may range from inci-

sional discomfort to a deep, aching pain that may be associated with systemic symptoms of fever and chills, although the patient may also feel remarkably well. Pain out of proportion to the expected course of recovery should be considered a red flag for potential surgical site infection. New-onset neurologic signs in association with any of these symptoms should serve as a clue to surgical site infection. Examination of the surgical wound may reveal inflammatory changes along the incisional margin, swelling, or tenderness accompanied by serous or purulent drainage. However, it is also important to consider that a relatively benign appearance of a surgical wound does not preclude the presence of a deep infection.

Measuring inflammatory serum mediators is a more reliable method of confirming the presence of postoperative surgical site infection. After surgery, an elevation of the neutrophil count and a decrease in the lymphocyte percentage are proportionate to the extent of the surgical intervention, and these laboratory studies normally return to presurgical levels within 4 to

21 days. Takahashi et al[10] showed that persistent lymphopenia was evident in patients who had lumbar arthrodesis with instrumentation that was complicated by surgical site infection. Acute phase reactants, including the erythrocyte sedimentation rate and the C-reactive protein level, reflect the degree of inflammatory and surgical damage.[11] The C-reactive protein level is more reliable and predictable with half-life kinetics of 2.6 days.[12] Therefore, within 1 to 2 weeks after surgery, it is reasonable to expect C-reactive protein levels to have normalized, whereas the erythrocyte sedimentation rate may remain variably elevated for weeks. A persistently elevated C-reactive protein level should alert the clinician to a surgical site infection, even in the absence of important clinical features or limited symptoms.

Radiographic imaging studies often lag behind the clinical and laboratory changes after surgical site infection. Radiographs may reveal early loss of fixation of instrumentation within the pedicle, end-plate dissolution, or rapid disk space collapse. Although MRI shows greater soft-tissue and osseous detail, the results must be interpreted cautiously. Pathologic changes on MRI are similar to normal postoperative inflammatory responses, even in the presence of gadolinium-enhanced images. Signs of surgical site infection on MRI include rim enhancement of fluid collections, vertebral body marrow changes, epidural abscess formation, and disk space enhancement (**Figure 1**). Alternative imaging studies that may be used for additional information include CT and positron emission tomography (PET) scans, although these studies are limited by expense and patient radiation risk.[13] The radiation risk for PET is similar to that for CT, given that a radionuclide is used for PET followed by a CT scan.

Nasal and Skin Decolonization

Nasal colonization of methicillin-sensitive *Staphylococcus aureus* or methicillin-resistant *S aureus* is very common throughout the community, as well as in the hospital setting, where more than one third of orthopaedic surgeons are carriers of methicillin-sensitive *S aureus*.[14] The ability to detect bacterial colonization in patients being admitted to hospitals has paralleled the development of screening techniques, including the use of rapid polymerase chain reaction detection techniques. These tools allow for determination of the presence of bacteria within minutes of a nasal swab. Treatment with 2% intranasal mupirocin (Bactroban; GlaxoSmithKline) as a topical antimicrobial for two to three times each day up to 5 days is successful in eradicating these nasal bacteria.[15] Eradication of microbial flora may also decrease the risk of postoperative surgical site infection. In a recent single-center study of patients having arthroplasty and spine surgery, identification of nasal colonization of methicillin-resistant *S aureus* that was treated with Bactroban resulted in a significant reduction of postoperative surgical site infection.[16]

In addition to nasal decolonization with very specific focus on *S aureus* species, attempts at eradication of nonspecific skin flora from the surgical site have become the standard of care in preoperative preparation for surgery. Common bacterial floras overlying the area of the lumbar spine are ubiquitous. Routine scrub-paint solutions of povidone-iodine have been used for some time as broad spectrum topical antiseptic agents with variable efficacy, whereas the use of combined solutions, such as 2% chlorhexidine and 70% isopropyl alcohol (ChloraPrep; Carefusion) or 0.7% iodine and 74% isopropyl alcohol (DuraPrep; 3M Corpo-

ration), eradicate skin flora and possibly have an effect on postoperative surgical site infection.[17] The preoperative use of these agents, as well as skin preparation in the operating room before incision, has become standard technique to diminish the risk of surgical site infection.

The application of adhesive drapes after skin preparation has also become a routine aspect of care, but extensive reviews have not shown any significant effect on the rate of infection with the use of iodine-impregnated or clear plastic adhesive drapes or the use of drapes at all.[18]

Topical Antibiotic Therapy

Another means of preventing surgical site infection in addition to perioperative systemic intravenous antibiotic therapy is to administer topical antibiotics directly onto the wound. Numerous studies have now focused on the application of 1 to 2 g of vancomycin powder placed directly into the wound at the completion of surgery before closure. Given the slow resorption of topical vancomycin, the systemic effect is exceptionally low, and no evidence of local toxicity, such as wound complications, has been reported based on the knowledge of this chapter's authors.[19] Recent studies have suggested that this adjunct of local application may substantially decrease postoperative surgical site infection in procedures using posterior spinal instrumentation.[19,20]

Perioperative Glycemic Management

Serum glucose levels undergo fluctuations after a stress response from surgery or injury. Unrecognized diabetes or poorly controlled hyperglycemia leads to a higher perioperative risk of complications, including infection. Improving blood glucose control in the perioperative period may limit the

detrimental consequences of hyperglycemia, and this has become a recent focus of awareness for the clinician and hospital team. Careful preoperative evaluation is critical in patients with diabetes, and a multidisciplinary approach is recommended to follow these patients. Prior to a planned surgical procedure, the blood glucose level in the patient should be maintained within a target range (90 to 130 mg/dL preprandially) as should the hemoglobin A1C level (< 7.0%).[21,22] It may be advisable to delay elective surgery until satisfactory glucose control has been obtained. Recent studies have suggested that higher preoperative, early (within 24 hours), as well as postoperative day-5 glucose levels have been related to surgical site infection, and aggressive management to control glucose levels is imperative.[23]

Sterile Processing

Surgeon and infection-control group involvement in hospital processes can lead to decreased postoperative infection rates.[9] The preparation of spinal implants and instruments merits special mention. Spine surgery deals with durable tissues, including bone, anulus fibrosus, and ligaments. These materials are not as easily removed from instruments, especially once they have dried after a surgical case. Often, spinal instruments and implants are shipped from hospital to hospital and undergo cleansing 1 to 2 days before surgery. However, there is no standardized routine for the cleansing of instruments and implants. Loaner sets arriving at the hospital have been found to have bone or biologic material on or in them.[24] Hospital policy should include mechanical preparation of all sets coming into the facility, with a 48-hour requirement for elective cases, so that they can be adequately evaluated and prepared in time for surgery. Also, efficient and effective removal of bone from instruments can be difficult, and mechanical washing by operating-room assistants during and after surgery is vital. It is necessary to have a rigorous education program with sterile-processing staff regarding adequate cleaning of instruments.[24] Flash sterilization of instruments and/or implants is not an acceptable practice.[25]

Additionally, surgeons should give special attention to having consigned surgical sets to ensure quality control with regard to sets residing in the hospital. Recently, the use of prepackaged sterile implants has gained attention. The benefits of this practice are the standardization of sterilization methods as well as the elimination of the need for repetitive cycles for sterilization.

In addition to the preparation of instruments and implants, maintenance of implant sterility is vital. Spine surgery instruments and implant sets can often be heavy and may weigh more than 15 lb (6.8 kg). Transport or movement of sets can lead to inadvertent tears in the packaging and compromise sterility. Corner protectors for sets heavier than 8 lb (3.6 kg) as well as the use of metal pans should be considered to maintain sterility of the spinal surgery set.

Intraoperative Bleeding

Surgery of the lumbar spine has the potential for substantial blood loss, which may lead to increased morbidity and mortality in the immediate postoperative period. Not surprisingly, the prevalence of uncontrolled hemorrhage is likely to be greater for patients with a preexisting coagulopathy or other bleeding diathesis as well as for cases of greater complexity, such as multilevel arthrodesis and deformity correction. In these situations, allogeneic blood transfusions may be required to maintain an appropriate he-

matocrit, but transfusions expose patients to the risks of immunologic reactions and infectious disease transmission. The cost-effectiveness of routine autologous blood donation has been questioned because it is expensive and frequently results in wasted resources.[26]

In an attempt to mitigate the adverse effects of prolonged hypovolemia, several strategies have been adopted by spinal surgeons to minimize intraoperative bleeding. In addition to ensuring that the abdomen is positioned free of any undue pressure to decrease venous oozing into the epidural space, electrocautery (monopolar versus bipolar) and topical hemostatic agents, such as thrombin-soaked gelatin sponges or fibrin-based matrices, are routinely used to inhibit active bleeding.[27] Hypotensive and hemodilution anesthetic techniques are advocated as adjunctive methods for reducing blood loss during lumbar spine procedures.[28-30]

One method for bolstering blood-cell counts before surgery involves the injection of recombinant human erythropoietin (epoetin alfa), which stimulates erythrocyte production within the bone marrow. The administration of this synthetic protein raises preoperative hematocrit levels and decreases both the rate of transfusion and the length of hospital stay of both pediatric and adult patients undergoing surgical correction of spinal deformities.[31,32] However, this technique may not be practical for every patient because it typically involves a regimen of multiple injections, which must be done over the course of several weeks, and the cost of this medication may be prohibitively high.[33] Although red blood-cell augmentation does not increase the prevalence of thrombovascular events after other orthopaedic procedures, concerns have been raised regarding its safety for spinal surgery.[34]

For example, in a recent prospective, randomized, multicenter study, deep vein thromboses (DVTs) were more prevalent among a cohort of patients receiving epoetin alfa before major elective spinal surgery compared with the corresponding control group (4.7% versus 2.1%, respectively).[35]

Antifibrinolytic agents, including aminocaproic acid, tranexamic acid, and aprotinin, represent another pharmacologic method for addressing intraoperative bleeding. This class of drugs functions to slow plasmin-mediated fibrin clot dissolution and has been widely used for a wide range of cardiac, trauma, and orthopaedic interventions. Multiple investigations have reported that the intraoperative infusion of these drugs may reduce blood loss and transfusion requirements associated with instrumented thoracolumbar arthrodesis with no significant increase in bleeding complications.[36-39] In general, caution must be exercised with aprotinin because data suggest that this naturally occurring compound may exhibit greater renal toxicity than tranexamic acid and other synthetic lysine analogues.[37] As a result of these concerns, aprotinin has been taken off the market and is no longer available for routine clinical use in the United States.

Intraoperative blood salvage is another option that is commonly used for clinical scenarios in which considerable blood loss is anticipated (for example, complex spinal reconstructions). The amount of blood that must be retrieved to allow reinfusion is dependent on several factors, including the patient's hematocrit level and the dimensions of the fluid reservoir specific to each system. Although these systems may decrease the need for allogeneic transfusions, in many instances, the volume collected may be insufficient for processing so that any autologous blood products recovered during the case cannot be reclaimed.[40-42] Given that this technique entails specialized equipment and dedicated operating-room personnel, the cost-benefit ratio of so-called cell-saver devices remains a matter of some debate.[40,41] At this time, there continues to be a paucity of level I evidence justifying the widespread adoption of this and most other strategies for mitigating blood loss during routine lumbar spinal procedures.[43] This chapter's authors believe that the specific hemostatic regimen should largely be based on several factors, including the comorbidities of the patient, the preference and experience of the surgeon, and the type of surgical procedure and its potential for excessive bleeding.

Venous Thromboembolism

As with other orthopaedic procedures, lumbar spine surgery predisposes patients to DVT and thromboembolic events. Although the true prevalence of these events has been less well defined for this population, systematic reviews of the literature have estimated the rate of DVT and pulmonary embolism after elective spine surgery to be approximately 1% to 2% and 0.06% to 0.3%, respectively.[44,45] Various patient-related and procedural factors associated with clot formation in the lower extremities, including a history of a thromboembolic event, pre-existing hypercoagulable state, diagnosis of traumatic injury or spinal deformity, lumbar procedures, and either an anterior or circumferential surgical approach, have been identified.[46-49]

To prevent the formation of DVT after lumbar spine procedures, surgeons often implement one or several different prophylactic measures, ranging from mechanical compression stockings or pneumatic sleeves to pharmacologic anticoagulation with aspirin, warfarin, or either unfraction-

ated or a low-molecular-weight heparin.[44,50] The benefits of any of these strategies must be weighed against the potential for wound hemorrhage or epidural hematoma. Even though multiple studies have determined that the prevalence of clinically important bleeding with chemical prophylaxis is relatively low, permanent neurologic deficits arising from compression of the neural elements as a consequence of these drugs have been reported.[45,51] For patients who are at high risk for venous thromboembolism but are not candidates for anticoagulation, the placement of inferior vena cava filters is safe and effective for preventing pulmonary embolism. These devices may be removed when they are no longer needed.[52,53] Nevertheless, there is still no level I evidence establishing the superiority of one particular treatment nor is there a universally accepted protocol defining the indications, timing, or duration of treatment.[44,46,47,50] Similarly, there are also no standardized guidelines available to direct the perioperative management of chronic anticoagulation medications before and after spinal procedures.[54] The specific type of prophylaxis initiated should continue to be left to the discretion of the surgeon according to the level of concern for venous thromboembolism with each patient.

Positioning-Related Complications

Because of the expected surgical time, estimated blood loss, and complexity of spine surgery, careful positioning of a patient in the operating room is critical to reduce the prevalence of potentially catastrophic complications. Intraoperative injuries to skin, eyes, nerve structures, and underlying soft tissues can occur if proper technique is not used.

In the prone position, patients often require multiple safety straps,

bumps, and taping for security during surgery. Patients at a higher risk for complications related to improper pressure relief include those with diabetes mellitus, vascular disease, and obesity and elderly patients.

Similarly, peripheral nerve injury can occur either from direct compression or traction during positioning. Nerve palsies are associated with longer operating room times and obesity.[55] The upper extremities can either be tucked close to the body with a sheet or secured to arm boards at the level of the head. When the arms are kept away from the body, proper technique ensures that the shoulder and elbow joint are placed at a 90° angle to avoid peripheral nerve root or brachial plexus compression. Neurapraxia from brachial plexus and ulnar nerve traction is the most common symptom in the upper extremity after spine procedures, presenting as paresthesia and/or pain in the affected distribution. Excessive traction force with shoulder tape during tucking of the arms can lead to a stretch injury, manifesting in pain, weakness, and numbness in the dermatomes of the brachial plexus postoperatively. In the lower extremity, placement of pads to limit compression of the lateral femoral cutaneous nerve can help avoid meralgia paresthetica postoperatively. Positioning of the knees and ankles in flexion (30° and 60°, respectively) will help limit traction on the femoral and peroneal nerves.

Although rare, positioning-related compartment syndrome can lead to a catastrophic complication.[56] In a study involving eight healthy volunteers, anterior compartment intramuscular pressures were elevated in the so-called 90/90 kneeling position (with both hips and knees at 90° of flexion) compared with a so-called 45/45 suspended position.[57] Because elevated pressure correlated with volunteer weight in this study, the authors concluded that the 45/45 suspended position should be considered during decompressive procedures in patients with risk factors to minimize the risk of compartment syndrome.

Perioperative blindness is also a rare but devastating complication after spine surgery. The overall prevalence has been reported to range from 0.028% to 0.094%, with a higher rate in scoliosis correction and posterior lumbar arthrodesis.[58,59] Risk factors include external compression of the orbit from a frame, estimated blood loss of more than 1,000 mL, prolonged anesthesia times of more than 6 hours, intraoperative hypotension, and associated comorbidities, such as peripheral vascular disease, smoking, and diabetes mellitus.[58,60] Clinical presentation manifests as a painless visual field deficit that may be either unilateral or bilateral. Ischemic optic neuropathy is the most common etiology, with a central retinal artery occlusion as the second most common cause. Alterations in local blood flow explain the acute pathophysiology behind blindness, either from decreased perfusion or increased intraocular pressure. Treatment measures include correction of associated anemia, increased mean arterial pressure of more than 85 mm Hg, and urgent ophthalmologic consultation; however, the prognosis for improvement of perioperative blindness is poor.[61] Prevention of such events is critical by aggressive management of perioperative hypotension, avoiding direct eye pressure (possibly with use of a Mayfield pin holder), and the staging of expected long procedures.

Summary

Although the complete eradication of complications in lumbar spine surgery is unlikely, in this era of cost-effectiveness and patient safety, it is more critical to identify the causes of these adverse events and manage them as they develop. In addition, financial incentives, including enhanced payment for optimum performance and reduction of the prevalence of complications, as well as diminished reimbursement because of the occurrence of these adverse events, will likely continue to be developed.

References

1. HCUP: Statistics on Hospital-Based Care in the United States, 2009. Healthcare cost and utilization project (HCUP) agency for healthcare research and quality. http://www.hcup-us.ahrq.gov/reports/factsandfigures/2009/pdfs/FF_report_2009.pdf. Accessed February 8, 2012.

2. Dekutoski MB, Norvell DC, Dettori JR, Fehlings MG, Chapman JR: Surgeon perceptions and reported complications in spine surgery. *Spine (Phila Pa 1976)* 2010;35(9):S9-S21.

3. Yokoe DS, Mermel LA, Anderson DJ, et al: A compendium of strategies to prevent healthcare-associated infections in acute care hospitals. *Infect Control Hosp Epidemiol* 2008;29(suppl 1):S12-S21.

4. Chen KW, Yang HL, Lu J, et al: Risk factors for postoperative wound infections of sacral chordoma after surgical excision. *J Spinal Disord Tech* 2011;24(4):230-234.

5. Fang A, Hu SS, Endres N, Bradford DS: Risk factors for infection after spinal surgery. *Spine (Phila Pa 1976)* 2005;30(12):1460-1465.

6. Friedman ND, Sexton DJ, Connelly SM, Kaye KS: Risk factors for surgical site infection complicating laminectomy. *Infect Control Hosp Epidemiol* 2007;28(9):1060-1065.

7. Apisarnthanarak A, Jones M, Waterman BM, Carroll CM, Bernardi R, Fraser VJ: Risk factors for spinal surgical-site infections in a community hospital: A case-control study. *Infect Control Hosp Epidemiol* 2003;24(1):31-36.

8. Banco SP, Vaccaro AR, Blam O, et al: Variations in incidence during the academic year. *Spine (Phila Pa 1976)* 2002;27(9):962-965.

9. Boston KM, Baraniuk S, O'Heron S, Murray KO: Risk factors for spinal surgical site infection, Houston, Texas. *Infect Control Hosp Epidemiol* 2009;30(9):884-889.

10. Takahashi J, Shono Y, Hirabayashi H, et al: Usefulness of white blood cell differential for early diagnosis of surgical wound infection following spinal instrumentation surgery. *Spine (Phila Pa 1976)* 2006;31(9):1020-1025.

11. Takahashi J, Ebara S, Kamimura M, et al: Early-phase enhanced inflammatory reaction after spinal instrumentation surgery. *Spine (Phila Pa 1976)* 2001;26(15):1698-1704.

12. Mok JM, Pekmezci M, Piper SL, et al: Comparison with erythrocyte sedimentation rate as predictor of early postoperative infectious complications. *Spine (Phila Pa 1976)* 2008;33(4):415-421.

13. De Winter F, Gemmel F, Van De Wiele C, Poffijn B, Uyttendaele D, Dierckx R: 18-Fluorine fluorodeoxyglucose positron emission tomography for the diagnosis of infection in the postoperative spine. *Spine (Phila Pa 1976)* 2003;28(12):1314-1319.

14. Schwarzkopf R, Takemoto RC, Immerman I, Slover JD, Bosco JA: Prevalence of Staphylococcus aureus colonization in orthopaedic surgeons and their patients: A prospective cohort controlled study. *J Bone Joint Surg Am* 2010;92(9):1815-1819.

15. Bode LG, Kluytmans JA, Wertheim HF, et al: Preventing surgical-site infections in nasal carriers of Staphylococcus aureus. *N Engl J Med* 2010;362(1):9-17.

16. Kim DH, Spencer M, Davidson SM, et al: Institutional prescreening for detection and eradication of methicillin-resistant Staphylococcus aureus in patients undergoing elective orthopaedic surgery. *J Bone Joint Surg Am* 2010;92(9): 1820-1826.

17. Darouiche RO, Wall MJ Jr, et al: Chlorhexidine-alcohol versus povidone-iodine for surgical-site antisepsis. *N Engl J Med* 2010; 362(1):18-26.

18. Webster J, Alghamdi AA: Use of plastic adhesive drapes during surgery for preventing surgical site infection. *Cochrane Database Syst Rev* 2007;17(4):CD006353.

19. Sweet FA, Roh M, Sliva C: Intra-wound application of vancomycin for prophylaxis in instrumented thoracolumbar fusions: Efficacy, drug levels, and patient outcomes. *Spine (Phila Pa 1976)* 2011; 36(24):2084-2088.

20. O'Neill KR, Smith JG, Abtahi AM, et al: Reduced surgical site infections in patients undergoing posterior spinal stabilization of traumatic injuries using vancomycin powder. *Spine J* 2011;11(7): 641-646.

21. Richards JE, Kauffmann RM, Zuckerman SL, Obremskey WT, May AK: Relationship of hyperglycemia and surgical-site infection in orthopaedic surgery. *J Bone Joint Surg Am* 2012;94(13):1181-1186.

22. Godoy DA, Di Napoli M, Biestro A, Lenhardt R: Perioperative glucose control in neurosurgical patients. *Anesthesiol Res Pract* 2012; 2012:690362.

23. Olsen MA, Nepple JJ, Riew KD, et al: Risk factors for surgical site infection following orthopaedic spinal operations. *J Bone Joint Surg Am* 2008;90(1):62-69.

24. Tosh PK, Disbot M, Duffy JM, et al: Outbreak of Pseudomonas aeruginosa surgical site infections after arthroscopic procedures: Texas, 2009. *Infect Control Hosp Epidemiol* 2011;32(12):1179-1186.

25. Lopansri B, Taylor C, Anderson V, Pombo D, Burke J: Abstract: Protracted outbreak of post-arthroscopy infections associated with flash sterilization of instruments. Decennial International Conference on Healthcare-Associated Infections, March 18-22, 2010. https://shea.confex.com/shea/2010/webprogram/Paper2792.html. Accessed June 11, 2013.

26. Bess RS, Lenke LG, Bridwell KH, Steger-May K, Hensley M: Wasting of preoperatively donated autologous blood in the surgical treatment of adolescent idiopathic scoliosis. *Spine (Phila Pa 1976)* 2006;31(20):2375-2380.

27. Lee TC, Yang LC, Chen HJ: Effect of patient position and hypotensive anesthesia on inferior vena caval pressure. *Spine (Phila Pa 1976)* 1998;23(8):941-947, discussion 947-948.

28. Joseph SA Jr, Mariller MM, et al: A retrospective review of patients refusing blood transfusion. *Spine (Phila Pa 1976)* 2008;33(21): 2310-2315.

29. Copley LA, Richards BS, Safavi FZ, Newton PO: Hemodilution as a method to reduce transfusion requirements in adolescent spine fusion surgery. *Spine (Phila Pa 1976)* 1999;24(3):219-222, discussion 223-224.

30. Hur SR, Huizenga BA, Major M: Acute normovolemic hemodilution combined with hypotensive anesthesia and other techniques to avoid homologous transfusion in spinal fusion surgery. *Spine (Phila Pa 1976)* 1992;17(8):867-873.

31. Vitale MG, Stazzone EJ, Gelijns AC, Moskowitz AJ, Roye DP Jr: The effectiveness of preoperative erythropoietin in averting allogenic blood transfusion among children undergoing scoliosis surgery. *J Pediatr Orthop B* 1998; 7(3):203-209.

32. Shapiro GS, Boachie-Adjei O, Dhawlikar SH, Maier LS: The use of Epoetin alfa in complex spine deformity surgery. *Spine (Phila Pa 1976)* 2002;27(18):2067-2071.

33. Keating EM, Meding JB: Perioperative blood management practices in elective orthopaedic surgery. *J Am Acad Orthop Surg* 2002;10(6):393-400.

34. Parr AM, Wang MY: Preoperative erythropoietin prior to spinal surgery increases DVT risk. *Neurosurgery* 2010;66(2):N16.

35. Stowell CP, Jones SC, Enny C, Langholff W, Leitz G: An open-label, randomized, parallel-group study of perioperative epoetin alfa versus standard of care for blood conservation in major elective spinal surgery: Safety analysis. *Spine (Phila Pa 1976)* 2009; 34(23):2479-2485.

36. Urban MK, Beckman J, Gordon M, Urquhart B, Boachie-Adjei O: The efficacy of antifibrinolytics in the reduction of blood loss during complex adult reconstructive spine surgery. *Spine (Phila Pa 1976)* 2001;26(10):1152-1156.

37. Okubadejo GO, Bridwell KH, Lenke LG, et al: Aprotinin may decrease blood loss in complex adult spinal deformity surgery, but it may also increase the risk of acute renal failure. *Spine (Phila Pa 1976)* 2007;32(20):2265-2271.

38. Wong J, El Beheiry H, Rampersaud YR, et al: Tranexamic acid reduces perioperative blood loss in adult patients having spinal fusion surgery. *Anesth Analg* 2008; 107(5):1479-1486.

39. Baldus CR, Bridwell KH, Lenke LG, Okubadejo GO: Can we safely reduce blood loss during lumbar pedicle subtraction osteotomy procedures using tranexamic acid or aprotinin? A comparative study with controls. *Spine (Phila Pa 1976)* 2010;35(2): 235-239.

40. Behrman MJ, Keim HA: Perioperative red blood cell salvage in spine surgery: A prospective analysis. *Clin Orthop Relat Res* 1992; 278:51-57.

41. Reitman CA, Watters WC III, Sassard WR: The Cell Saver in adult lumbar fusion surgery: A cost-benefit outcomes study. *Spine (Phila Pa 1976)* 2004;29(14): 1580-1583, discussion 1584.

42. Siller TA, Dickson JH, Erwin WD: Efficacy and cost considerations of intraoperative autologous transfusion in spinal fusion for idiopathic scoliosis with predeposited blood. *Spine (Phila Pa 1976)* 1996;21(7):848-852.

43. Elgafy H, Bransford RJ, McGuire RA, Dettori JR, Fischer D: Blood loss in major spine surgery: Are there effective measures to decrease massive hemorrhage in major spine fusion surgery? *Spine (Phila Pa 1976)* 2010;35(9): S47-S56.

44. Glotzbecker MP, Bono CM, Wood KB, Harris MB: Thromboembolic disease in spinal surgery: A systematic review. *Spine (Phila Pa 1976)* 2009;34(3):291-303.

45. Sansone JM, del Rio AM, Anderson PA: The prevalence of and specific risk factors for venous thromboembolic disease following elective spine surgery. *J Bone Joint Surg Am* 2010;92(2):304-313.

46. Geerts WH, Bergqvist D, Pineo GF, et al: Prevention of venous thromboembolism: American College of Chest Physicians Evidence-Based Clinical Practice Guidelines (8th Edition). *Chest* 2008;133(6):381S-453S.

47. Cheng JS, Arnold PM, Anderson PA, Fischer D, Dettori JR: Anticoagulation risk in spine surgery. *Spine (Phila Pa 1976)* 2010;35(9): S117-S124.

48. Oda TFuji T, Kato Y, Fujita S, Kanemitsu N: Deep venous thrombosis after posterior spinal surgery. *Spine (Phila Pa 1976)* 2000;25(22):2962-2967.

49. Dearborn JT, Hu SS, Tribus CB, Bradford DS: Thromboembolic complications after major thoracolumbar spine surgery. *Spine (Phila Pa 1976)* 1999;24(14): 1471-1476.

50. Glotzbecker MP, Bono CM, Harris MB, Brick G, Heary RF, Wood KB: Surgeon practices regarding postoperative thromboembolic prophylaxis after high-risk spinal surgery. *Spine (Phila Pa 1976)* 2008;33(26):2915-2921.

51. Glotzbecker MP, Bono CM, Wood KB, Harris MB: Postoperative spinal epidural hematoma: A systematic review. *Spine (Phila Pa 1976)* 2010;35(10):E413-E420.

52. Ozturk C, Ganiyusufoglu K, Alanay A, Aydogan M, Onat L, Hamzaoglu A: Efficacy of prophylactic placement of inferior vena cava filter in patients undergoing spinal surgery. *Spine (Phila Pa 1976)* 2010;35(20):1893-1896.

53. Dazley JM, Wain R, Vellinga RM, Cohen B, Agulnick MA: Prophylactic inferior vena cava filters prevent pulmonary embolisms in high-risk patients undergoing major spinal surgery. *J Spinal Disord Tech* 2012;25(4):190-195.

54. Thakur NA, Czerwein JK, Butera JN, Palumbo MA: Perioperative management of chronic anticoagulation in orthopaedic surgery.

J Am Acad Orthop Surg 2010; 18(12):729-738.

55. Patel N, Bagan B, Vadera S, et al: Relation to perioperative complications. *J Neurosurg Spine* 2007; 6(4):291-297.

56. Geisler FH, Laich DT, Goldflies M, Shepard A: Anterior tibial compartment syndrome as a positioning complication of the prone-sitting position for lumbar surgery. *Neurosurgery* 1993;33(6): 1117.

57. Leek BT, Meyer RS, Wiemann JM, Cutuk A, Macias BR, Hargens AR: The effect of kneeling during spine surgery on leg intramuscular pressure. *J Bone Joint Surg Am* 2007;89(9):1941-1947.

58. Patil CG, Lad EM, Lad SP, Ho C, Boakye M: Visual loss after spine surgery: A population-based study. *Spine (Phila Pa 1976)* 2008;33(13):1491-1496.

59. Chang SH, Miller NR: The incidence of vision loss due to perioperative ischemic optic neuropathy associated with spine surgery: The Johns Hopkins Hospital Experience. *Spine (Phila Pa 1976)* 2005; 30(11):1299-1302.

60. Myers MA, Hamilton SR, Bogosian AJ, Smith CH, Wagner TA: Visual loss as a complication of spine surgery: A review of 37 cases. *Spine (Phila Pa 1976)* 1997;22(12):1325-1329.

61. Stambough JL, Dolan D, Werner R, Godfrey E: Ophthalmologic complications associated with prone positioning in spine surgery. *J Am Acad Orthop Surg* 2007;15(3):156-165.

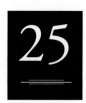

Developing a Toolkit for Comparing Safety in Spine Surgery

Sohail K. Mirza, MD, MPH
Brook I. Martin, PhD, MPH
Robert Goodkin, MD
Robert A. Hart, MD
Paul A. Anderson, MD

Abstract

Safety information in spine surgery is important for informed patient choice and performance-based payment incentives, but measurement methods for surgical safety assessment are not standardized. Published reports of complication rates for common spinal procedures show wide variation. Factors influencing variation may include differences in safety ascertainment methods and procedure types. In a prospective cohort study, adverse events were observed in all patients undergoing spine surgery at two hospitals during a 2-year period. Multiple processes for adverse occurrence surveillance were implemented, and the associations between surveillance methods, surgery invasiveness, and observed frequencies of adverse events were examined.

The study enrolled 1,723 patients. Adverse events were noted in 48.3% of the patients. Reviewers classified 25% as minor events and 23% as major events. Of the major events, the daily rounding team reported 38.4% of the events using a voluntary reporting system, surgeons reported 13.4%, and 9.1% were identified during clinical conferences. A review of medical records identified 86.7% of the major adverse events. The adverse events occurred during the inpatient hospitalization for 78.1% of the events, within 30 days for an additional 12.5%, and within the first year for the remaining 9.4%. A unit increase in the invasiveness index was associated with an 8.2% increased risk of a major adverse event. A Current Procedural Terminology–based algorithm for quantifying invasiveness correlated well with medical records–based assessment.

Increased procedure invasiveness is associated with an increased risk of adverse events. The observed frequency of adverse events is influenced by the ascertainment modality. Voluntary reports by surgeons and other team members missed more than 50% of the events identified through a medical records review. Increased surgery invasiveness, measured from medical records or billing codes, is quantitatively associated with an increased risk of adverse events.

Instr Course Lect 2014;63:271-286.

Patients routinely weigh the anticipated benefits and risks when considering surgical options; however, information concerning individualized patient features and local practice settings is frequently lacking. Published reports do not consistently provide information about complications and often show wide ranges for common adverse events.[1-4]

Comparing safety for spine surgery is problematic for several reasons. Spinal procedures can be performed at multiple vertebral levels, and multilevel procedures generally carry a greater risk of complications.[5] Each spine surgery can involve varying types of surgical elements, such as neurologic decompression, vertebral fusion, and spinal instrumentation. The risk of complications is greater with more extensive surgeries, such as decompression combined with instrumented fusion.[6,7] Spine surgery can be performed through anterior, posterior, or combined anterior-posterior surgical approaches; there is greater safety risk in the combined anterior-posterior procedures.[8] Patients with degenerative lumbar disease may be offered different types of surgery for the same presenting symptoms, imaging findings, and spinal diagnosis.[9] The strongest predictor for the type of surgery offered is based on surgeon preference, not patient factors.[10] Even for homogeneous patient populations, varying combinations of vertebral levels, procedure types, and surgical approaches make aggregate safety comparisons difficult in spine surgery.

Spine surgery procedures are common, expensive, and high-risk interventions.[11,12] Furthermore, adverse events may be underreported in the literature because of conflicts of interest.[1] The rates of adverse events also vary by surgeon and hospital.[13,14] The efficacy of common procedures, such as fusion for back pain, remains uncertain.[15] Despite this uncertainty, the national rates of spinal surgery show rapid growth.[16] When selecting surgery, a surgeon, and a hospital, patients need specific comparative safety information.[11] Such quality-related performance information is not readily available for most spine surgical procedures and settings.

To address this deficiency locally, the quality improvement department at the University of Washington partnered with a National Institutes of Health research team and designed a program to provide site-specific information on the risks of spine surgery.[17]

The program sought to create a system and culture of routinely and rigorously monitoring adverse events in all patients undergoing spine surgery at two hospitals within a single healthcare system. This chapter's authors attempted to integrate the data collection methods developed for this study with quality improvement surveillance of routine clinical care (**Figure 1**).

Materials and Methods
Study Design
This chapter reports on data collected in a prospective observational cohort study of patients undergoing spine surgery during the 2-year study period from 2003 through 2004.[17-23] The study was performed at two hospitals (Harborview Medical Center and the University of Washington Medical Center) within a single, regional academic institution, the University of Washington. The detailed study protocol has been previously reported.[17] The institutional review board at the University of Washington approved the study.

Patient Enrollment
All patients undergoing spine surgery during calendar years 2003 and 2004 were eligible for this study. Patients scheduled for spine surgery were offered enrollment in the Spine End Results Registry during outpatient visits. Operating room logs were reviewed to identify patients admitted through the

emergency department and those missed by the outpatient study coordinators. Registry enrollment required completion of health status surveys and follow-up interviews. If a patient declined enrollment, only his or her medical records were reviewed to identify adverse events.[17]

Selection of Data Elements
The study was designed to develop predictive models for adverse events, including reoperations, readmissions, infections, and life-threatening complications.[17] Patient characteristics, comorbidity measures, spinal disease classification, and treatment invasiveness were selected as major domains for adverse occurrence prediction models.[17,18] Data elements were identified through a literature review and a consensus process and were guided by a clinical research methodology team.[17] Reviewer agreement and reproducibility for adverse event categorization scales were also tested.[17]

Creation of Safety Surveillance Infrastructure
For this study, this chapter's authors developed the processes and the training methods and recruited the staff for measuring and reporting adverse events associated with spine surgery. Multimodal surveillance was implemented for 176 prospectively defined adverse events.[17] Surgeons and other

Dr. Mirza or an immediate family member serves as a board member, owner, officer, or committee member of the North American Spine Society. Dr. Hart or an immediate family member has received royalties from DePuy and SeaSpine; is a member of a speakers' bureau or has made paid presentations on behalf of DePuy, Kyphon, Medtronic, and Synthes; serves as a paid consultant to or is an employee of DePuy, Eli Lilly, and Medtronic; has stock or stock options held in Spine Connect; has received research or institutional support from DePuy, Medtronic, Synthes, and the Orthopaedic Research and Education Foundation; and serves as a board member, owner, officer, or committee member of the American Academy of Orthopaedic Surgeons, the American Orthopaedic Association, the Cervical Spine Research Society, the Lumbar Spine Research Society, the North American Spine Society, the Oregon Association of Orthopaedics, the Orthopaedic Research and Education Foundation, and the Scoliosis Research Society. Dr. Anderson or an immediate family member has received royalties from Pioneer and Stryker; serves as a paid consultant to or is an employee of Aesculap and Pioneer Surgical; serves as an unpaid consultant to Expanding Orthopedics, SI Bone, Spartec, and Titan Surgical; has stock or stock options held in Expanding Orthopedics, Pioneer Surgical, SI Bone, Spartec, and Titan Surgical; and serves as a board member, owner, officer, or committee member of the American Academy of Orthopaedic Surgeons, the ASTM, the Lumbar Research Society, the North American Spine Society, the Spine Arthroplasty Society, and the Spine section of the American Association of Neurological Surgeons/Congress of Neurological Surgeons. Neither of the following authors nor any immediate family member has received anything of value from or has stock or stock options held in a commercial company or institution related directly or indirectly to the subject of this chapter: Dr. Martin and Dr. Goodkin (deceased).

Source of Funding
This work was supported by grants from the National Institutes of Health/National Institute of Arthritis, Musculoskeletal, and Skin Disorders 5K23AR48979 and 5P60-AR48093. It was also supported in part by the quality improvement departments of Harborview Medical Center and the University of Washington Medical Center and by the Spine End Results Research Fund at the University of Washington through gifts from Surgical Dynamics (since acquired by other companies) and Synthes Spine (Paoli, PA).

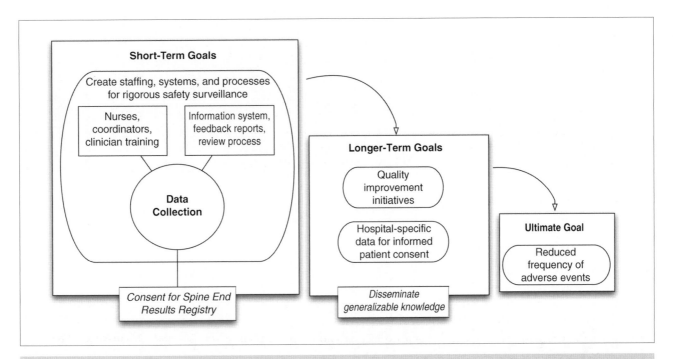

Figure 1   Illustration showing the conceptual framework for program goals and the integration of rigorous safety surveillance in routine clinical practice with observational research and the generation of generalizable knowledge. This report involved a subset of the clinical patient population enrolled in the prospective patient outcomes registry (those enrolled in the Spine End Results Registry). This report focused on the success rate of data collection methods and the observed frequency of adverse events.

team members were trained to voluntarily report adverse events by phone, e-mail, or written forms. Research nurses were trained to identify adverse events during clinical conferences and daily inpatient rounds. Research nurses also performed a daily review of medical record notes to identify documented events.

Pilot Program to Integrate Research and Quality Improvement Goals

The research team worked with surgeons to reengineer safety surveillance methods in spine surgery to meet the University of Washington's intermediate- and long-term quality improvement goals. The new system leveraged statutory protections afforded to potentially highly sensitive adverse event information. Although the long-term goal for this pilot program was the prevention of adverse

events, the immediate goal was to successfully implement a surveillance system, and the intermediate-term goal was to enhance the University of Washington's local quality improvement process (**Figure 1**). Clinical teams, supported by departmental and hospital funding, gathered, categorized, and classified primary data on adverse events. This methodology allowed the research staff access to only de-identified information, which is consistent with the requirements of the institutional review board and the Health Insurance Portability and Accountability Act.[24]

The medical documentation was redesigned to provide more consistent information on each patient's spinal diagnosis, neurologic status, and spinal surgery. Specific documents were developed to detail (1) the diagnosis by International Classification of Diseases (ICD) Version 9 codes,[25] with an

additional neurologic status designation; (2) treatment by Current Procedural Terminology (CPT) codes;[26] (3) details of the surgical spinal levels, implants, grafts, neurologic status, and intraoperative fluids;[17,18] (4) adverse events during hospitalization, discharge disposition, discharge neurologic status, and at follow-up; and (5) patient health status, neurologic status, and late adverse events. Medical records committees of both participating institutions approved the forms for placement in the patient's chart as part of the permanent medical record.

The hospital computer systems were supplemented with software that generated reports to provide feedback in real time to participating surgeons. A Microsoft Access (Microsoft Corporation) database was developed that contained the collected patient information. This program was placed on a secure network file server in the

Table 1
Adverse Events: Description of Codes

Description	Code	Description	Code	Description	Code	Description	Code	Description	Code
No adverse or unexpected occurrence	aa01	Difficult intubation	ma07	CVA/TIA	mn01	Patient to OR without surgical H&P	pp11	Muscle, compartmental syndrome	ti11
Death	aa02	Endobronchial intubation	ma08	Cerebral perfusion	mn02	Patient to OR without test results	pp12	Neural, erectile dysfunction	ti12
Cardiopulmonary resuscitation	aa03	Esophageal intubation	ma09	Delirium	mn03	Other process occurrence	pp00, ppzz	Neural, intraoperative root injury	ti13
Identification of patient or incision site	aa04	Inability/difficult to ventilate	ma10	Diabetes insipidus	mn04	Anesthetic equipment failure	td01	Neural, laryngeal nerve injury/hoarseness	ti14
Surgery aborted after incision	aa05	Inadequate ventilation/oxygenation in OR	ma11	Electrolyte change	mn05	Cervical traction–related occurrence	td02	Neural, new cord/cauda equina injury	ti15
Reoperation, unexpected	aa06	Laryngospasm	ma12	Meningitis	mn06	Contamination of surgical field	td03	Neural, new radiculopathy	ti16
ICU transfer, unexpected	aa07	Premature extubation	ma13	SAH	mn07	Count difficulty, spinal level	td04	Neural pressure palsy	ti17
Ventilator, unexpected	aa08	Other airway occurrence	ma00, mazz	Seizure	mn08	Count discrepancy, instrument/sponge/needle	td05	Neural, retrograde ejaculation	ti18
Code blue/199 activation for any reason	aao09	Air embolism	mc01	Withdrawal, alcohol	mn09	Count discrepancy, spinal level	td06	Neural, worsening of cord injury	ti19
Delay, disposition, or placement for hospital discharge	dl01	Arrest	mc02	Withdrawal, narcotic	mn10	Failure to achieve reduction	td07	Neural, worsening of radiculopathy	ti20
Delay, patient condition (number of days)	dl02	Arrhythmia	mc03	Other neurologic occurrence	mn00, mnzz	Failure of closed treatment	td08	Pressure sore, brace or cast	ti21
Delay, imaging availability (number of days)	dl03	CHF	mc04	Acute respiratory distress syndrome	mr01	Fracture at/above/below implant	td09	Pressure sore, face/head/pressure alopecia	ti22
Delay, SEP availability (number of days)	dl04	Hypertension	mc05	Empyema	mr02	Graft settling/displacement/dislodgement	td10	Pressure sore, sacral	ti23
Delay, OR turnover (number of hours)	dl05	Hypotension	mc06	Hemothorax	mr03	Halo ring– or frame-related occurrence	td11	Pressure sore, other body area	ti24
Delay, implant availability (number of hours)	dl06	Infarction	mc07	Pleural effusion	mr04	Implant breakage	td12	Swallowing difficulty	ti25
Delay, surgeon availability (number of hours)	dl07	Inappropriate or inadequate fluid therapy	mc08	Postoperative hypoxia	mr04p	Implant choice suboptimal	td13	Ureteral injury	ti26
Other delay	dl00, dlzz	Ischemia	mc09	Pneumonia	mr05	Implant migration or loosening	td14	Vessel injury, artery	ti27
Delayed recognition of adverse occurrence	dxo1	Thermoregulation	mc10	Pneumothorax	mr06	Implant placement suboptimal	td15	Vessel injury, vein	ti28
Suboptimal preoperative evaluation resulting in adverse occurrence	dx02	Other cardiac occurrence	mc00, mczz	Pulmonary embolus	mr07	Line failure, arterial	td16	Pseudomeningocele	ti29
Delayed diagnosis of neural deficit	dx03	Drug/allergic reaction	md01	Respiratory arrest	mr08	Line failure, central	td17	Unintended dural opening	ti30

Table 1 (Continued)
Adverse Events: Description of Codes

Description	Code	Description	Code	Description	Code	Description	Code	Description	Code
Missed diagnosis of neural deficit	dx04	Drug choice	md02	Other respiratory	mr09, mr00, mrzz	Line failure, infiltration	td18	Unintended pleural/peritoneal opening	ti31
Delayed diagnosis of vertebral injury	dx05	Drug dosage	md03	Foley catheter trauma	mu01	Line failure, intravenous disconnect	td19	Other technical occurrence	ti00, tizz
Missed diagnosis of vertebral injury	dx06	Drug interaction	md04	Renal insufficiency	mu02	Line placement, arterial	td20	Abscess, epidural	wh01
Other diagnosis occurrence	dx00, dxzz	Drug neuromuscular block management	md05	Urinary retention	mu03	Line placement, central	td21	Abscess, paraspinal	wh02
Change in anesthetic plan	ec01	Other drug occurrence	md00, mdzz	Urinary tract infection	mu04	Loss of spinal alignment	td22	Bacteremia	wh03 b
Change in surgical plan	ec02	Ascites	mg01	Other urologic event	mu00, muzz	Retained foreign body	td23	Cerebral spinal fluid leak	wh03 c
Delay in extubation in OR	ec03	Colitis	mg02	Blindness (PION)	mv01	Surgical positioning occurrence	td24	Drainage, prolonged	wh04
Delay in extubation in PACU	ec04	GI bleeding	mg03	Corneal abrasion	mv02	Other technical occurrence	td00, tdzz	Dehiscence	wh05
Extra drugs required during surgery	ec05	Ileus	mg04	Other visual event	mv00, mvzz	Awareness or recall	ti01	Fever, unknown etiology	wh06
Extra tests required during surgery	ec06	Obstruction	mg05	Anesthesia team not called	pp01	Bladder injury	ti02	Hematoma, wound/epidural (required OR)	wh07
Prolonged stay in PACU	ec07	Pancreatitis	mg06	Surgical team not called	pp02	Bowel injury	ti03	Sepsis	wh08
Reintubation	ec08	Perforation	mg07	Cancellation of procedure before incision	pp03	Burn (thermal) injury	ti04	Wound infection, deep	wh09
Other escalation of care	ec00, eczz	Peritonitis	mg08	Implant or instrumentation defective	pp04	Dental or denture injury	ti05	Wound infect, superficial	wh10, wh00, whzz
Airway edema	ma01	Other GI occurrence	mgzz	Implant or instrumentation set incomplete	pp05	Employee exposure, body fluid	ti06	Late deformity	zh01
Airway trauma	ma02	Coagulopathy	mh01	Implant or instrumentation unavailable	pp06	Employee exposure, sharp	ti07	Late instability	zh02
Airway obstruction	ma03	DVT (confirmed by imaging)	mh02	Implant or instrumentation unfamiliar	pp07	Esophageal injury	ti08	Late junctional arthrosis	zh03
Aspiration	ma04	OR hemorrhage > 3,000 cc	mh03	Implant, wasted/wrong one opened	pp08	Monitoring, EMG neurotonic activity	ti09	Late nonunion	zh04
Bronchospasm (wheezing/nebulizer/steroid)	ma05	Transfusion occurrence	mh04	Patient to OR needing more tests	pp09	Monitoring, SSEP decrease > 50%	ti10	Other late occurrence	zh00, zhzz
Accidental extubation	ma06	Other hematologic occurrence	mh00, mhzz	Patient to OR without adequate consent	pp10				

CHF = congestive heart failure, CVA/TIA = cerebrovascular accident/transient ischemic accident, DVT = deep vein thrombosis, EMG = electromyography, GI = gastrointestinal, H&P = history and physical, ICU = intensive care unit, OR = operating room, PACU = postanesthesia care unit, PION = posterior ischemic optic neuropathy, SAH = subarachnoid hemorrhage, SEP = sensory evoked potential, SSEP = somatosensory evoked potential.

Treatment Levels							
Disease	Posterior			Anterior			
Levels	Dec	Fus	Ins	Dec	Fus	Ins	VP
	None	None	None	None	None	None	None
C0	[ ]	[ ]	[ ]	[ ]	[ ]	[ ]	[ ]
C1	[ ]	[ ]	[ ]	[ ]	[ ]	[ ]	[ ]
C2	[ ]	[ ]	[ ]	[ ]	[ ]	[ ]	[ ]
C3	[ ]	[ ]	[ ]	[ ]	[ ]	[ ]	[ ]
C4	[ ]	[ ]	[ ]	[ ]	[ ]	[ ]	[ ]
C5	[ ]	[ ]	[ ]	[ ]	[ ]	[ ]	[ ]
C6	[ ]	[ ]	[ ]	[ ]	[ ]	[ ]	[ ]
C7	[ ]	[ ]	[ ]	[ ]	[ ]	[ ]	[ ]
T1	[ ]	[ ]	[ ]	[ ]	[ ]	[ ]	[ ]
T2	[ ]	[ ]	[ ]	[ ]	[ ]	[ ]	[ ]
T3	[ ]	[ ]	[ ]	[ ]	[ ]	[ ]	[ ]
T4	[ ]	[ ]	[ ]	[ ]	[ ]	[ ]	[ ]
T5	[ ]	[ ]	[ ]	[ ]	[ ]	[ ]	[ ]
T6	[ ]	[ ]	[ ]	[ ]	[ ]	[ ]	[ ]
T7	[ ]	[ ]	[ ]	[ ]	[ ]	[ ]	[ ]
T8	[ ]	[ ]	[ ]	[ ]	[ ]	[ ]	[ ]
T9	[ ]	[ ]	[ ]	[ ]	[ ]	[ ]	[ ]
T10	[ ]	[ ]	[ ]	[ ]	[ ]	[ ]	[ ]
T11	[ ]	[ ]	[ ]	[ ]	[ ]	[ ]	[ ]
T12	[ ]	[ ]	[ ]	[ ]	[ ]	[ ]	[ ]
L1	[ ]	[ ]	[ ]	[ ]	[ ]	[ ]	[ ]
L2	[ ]	[ ]	[ ]	[ ]	[ ]	[ ]	[ ]
L3	[ ]	[ ]	[ ]	[ ]	[ ]	[ ]	[ ]
L4	[ ]	[ ]	[ ]	[ ]	[ ]	[ ]	[ ]
L5	[ ]	[ ]	[ ]	[ ]	[ ]	[ ]	[ ]
S1	[ ]	[ ]	[ ]	[ ]	[ ]	[ ]	[ ]
S2	[ ]	[ ]	[ ]	[ ]	[ ]	[ ]	[ ]
S3	[ ]	[ ]	[ ]	[ ]	[ ]	[ ]	[ ]
S4	[ ]	[ ]	[ ]	[ ]	[ ]	[ ]	[ ]
CC	[ ]	[ ]	[ ]	[ ]	[ ]	[ ]	[ ]
IL	[ ]	[ ]	[ ]	[ ]	[ ]	[ ]	[ ]

Figure 2 The complexity of surgery was measured quantitatively using the spine surgery invasiveness index. The anterior and posterior interventions performed on individual vertebrae were marked on the grid. The invasiveness index is the sum of the total vertebral procedures performed on a patient. The following five scenarios provide calculation examples of the invasiveness index. (1) An L5-S1 posterior diskectomy = 1. (2) An L4-S1 laminectomy = 3. (3) An L4-S1 posterior fusion with pedicle screws = 6. (4) An L4-L5 posterior interbody fusion, with an L4 and L5 laminectomy and L4-5 interbody fusion with cages = 10. (5) A T1 ilium posterior fusion, with pedicle screws placed bilaterally at T1, T4, T8, L1, L2, L4, L5, S1, and the ilium; a laminectomy L1 to S1; and interbody fusion with cages at L1-2, L2-3, and L4-5 = 47. Dec = decompression, Fus = fusion, Ins = instrumentation, VP = vertebroplasty.

hospital's computing network. Surgeons, clinicians, and study team members could access the program from any workstation in the inpatient and outpatient areas. The program supplied reports summarizing surgical details, discharge information, and adverse events during hospitalization. The research team members could also generate de-identified reports for each adverse occurrence.

Four spine surgery teams were trained in the infrastructure of the redesigned safety surveillance system. Pocketbooks, which contained phone numbers, adverse event definitions and codes, and instruction on the use of new safety surveillance software implemented through the hospital informatics system, were provided to the spine surgery teams. A list of the adverse event codes and descriptions are shown in **Table 1**. As a further aid, the phone number of a voicemail box dedicated to spine surgery surveillance was supplied. Surgery and adverse event data were collated into reports that provided clinicians with feedback on their surgical activity and safety performance. Surgeons had the opportunity to review reports and provide corrections and additional information.

Study Interventions

A research team member who was not involved in patient care used the surveillance documentation, electronic records, and meeting discussions to determine the source of an adverse event report. There were four sources for adverse events: a surgeon, a clinical team, a meeting discussion, and a record review. The surgeon could report the adverse event on the back of the operating room note (operating room summary) or the outpatient visit note. The clinical team could report the adverse event in the study database or to a study team member by phone, e-mail, or in person. It could be discussed at each hospital's monthly morbidity and mortality conference. The adverse event also could be noted in the medical record. Multiple sources could exist for the report of a particular event. The credit for reporting the adverse event was assigned to the first source that reported the event. For example, a nerve root injury during surgery could be reported by the surgeon and clinical team, could be discussed at a monthly morbidity and mortality conference, and could appear in the medical record. If the surgeon reported the nerve root injury on the operating room form the surgeon would be credited as the source. If the surgeon did not report the injury on the operating room form, but discussed it in the dictated surgical note, then record review would be credited as the source.

The study team collected the surveillance documentation and entered it into the study database. The anesthesia record for each surgery was reviewed for surgical information and adverse events. A research team member, who was not involved in patient care, reviewed each dictated surgical report for operated levels, implants, grafts, the estimated blood loss, and the duration of surgery from incision to wound closure. Neurologic status based on the American Spinal Injury Association[27] impairment scale, motor score, and neurologic level at admission was recorded on specially designed medical record templates to be used at admission, surgery, and discharge.

Rationale for the Invasiveness Index

A trained research coordinator reviewed standardized, brief surgical note forms and full, dictated surgical reports to calculate an invasiveness score for each surgical procedure[17,18] (**Figure 2**). The invasiveness index was designed to quantitatively account for the surgical approach and the number of vertebral levels decompressed, fused, and instrumented. The index assigns a unit value for each vertebral level included in decompression, fusion, and instrumentation from the posterior approach and a unit value for the anterior approach. The index was coded using the format shown in **Figure 2**. The invasiveness score for a particular spinal procedure can range from 0, for procedures such as débridement for infection or removal of spinal fixation, to more than 40, for procedures that involve multiple-level anterior and posterior thoracic and lumbar fusion with instrumentation.

The invasiveness score showed high reproducibility across observers (intraclass correlation coefficient = 0.99).[17] The construct validity of this index was demonstrated by a strong correlation between an invasiveness score and both intraoperative blood loss and the duration of a surgical procedure.[18] In a multivariate regression model, which included patient characteristics, disease attributes, and treatment factors, the index value explained 44% of the variation in blood loss and 52% of the variation in the length of surgery.[18] The index accounted for more variation compared with any other factor in the model. By comparison, the number of vertebral levels involved in the surgery explained 32% of the variation in blood loss and 38% of the variation in duration of the surgery; the surgical approach explained 20% of the variation in the blood loss and 32% of the variation in surgery; and the type of surgical procedure (decompression or fusion) explained only 10% of the variation in blood loss and 20% of the variation in surgery. Each unit value of the invasiveness index was associated with an 11.5% increase in blood loss and an increment of 12.8 minutes in the duration of surgery.[18] Modifications of the index based on relative weights for anterior and posterior decompression in fusion and instrumentation did not further increase the amount of variation explained by the

multivariate model.

The invasiveness index also correlated with the risk of surgical site infection.[19] In that analysis, the quantitative association of the invasiveness index with the overall risk of adverse events was examined. This chapter's authors examined the association between the invasiveness index and the occurrence of adverse events after surgery using a logistic regression model that incorporated the invasiveness score and controlled for other factors.

CPT-Based Invasiveness Index

Nearly all elements of the medical record required for scoring the invasiveness index can be obtained from the CPT codes for spinal procedures.[26] CPT codes specify the number of vertebral levels operated, the surgical approach, the use of instrumentation, and varying combinations of these procedure elements. The precision of CPT codes is somewhat limited by ranges for certain procedures specified in the codes, such as instrumentation codes that use ranges of two to three levels, four to seven vertebral levels, and more than seven vertebral levels. This chapter's authors developed CPT code invasiveness values based on clinical judgment (**Table 2**). CPT codes for spine procedures that did not involve decompression, fusion, or fixation of vertebrae were assigned an invasiveness score of zero and are not shown in **Table 2**. For a subset of the study population (n = 564) for whom billing records were available, an invasiveness score was calculated from the billing CPT codes and compared with the invasiveness score derived from the medical records.

Data Analyses

Counts and percentages for adverse events were reported, and separate logistic regressions were performed to assess the association of 15 adverse event

categories with the invasiveness index, with adjustments for age, sex, body mass index, smoking history, the Charlson comorbidity score, spinal diagnosis, preoperative neurologic status, spinal level, and revision surgery.[17,28] The correlation coefficient and the intraclass correlation coefficient between CPT-derived and medical record–derived invasiveness scores were calculated. De-identified datasets were assembled using SAS/STAT software (SAS Institute), and analyses were performed using STATA 10 (StataCorp).

Results

Patient Sample

During the 2-year study interval, 1,745 patients had spine surgery at the participating institution; of these, 1,723 patients were enrolled in the prospective observational study (**Figures 3** and **4**). Twenty-two patients were excluded because of a missing surgical report or an anesthetic record.

The mean age of the patients was 49 years (SD, 16 years), and 43% of the patients were female (**Table 3**). The most common diagnoses were degenerative disease (57%) and trauma (26%). Cervical spine surgery was performed in 34% of the patients, and thoracic-lumbar surgery was performed in 66%. The surgeries involved both decompression and fusion in 53% of the patients. Combined anterior-posterior surgery through a single posterior approach was performed in 20% of the patients and consisted primarily of costotransversectomy for thoracic procedures and interbody fusion for lumbar procedures. All of the fusion procedures included instrumentation. All of the patients had a 2-year medical record review after surgery, and 46% of the participants enrolled in the Spine End Results Registry for pain and functional status surveys.

Table 2
Invasiveness (Inv) Scores Assigned to CPT Codes[a]

Inv Score	CPT Code	Inv Score	CPT Code	Inv Score	CPT Code	Inv Score	CPT Code	Inv Score	CPT Code	Inv Score	CPT Code
16	22804	16	22844	10	22802	10	22812	10	22843	10	22847
5	22810	5	22842	5	22846	4	22630	4	22632	4	22650
4	22800	4	49215	4	63015	4	63016	4	63017	3	22590
3	22808	3	22848	3	22849	2	22210	2	22212	2	22214
2	22216	2	22220	2	22222	2	22224	2	22226	2	22318
2	22319	2	22325	2	22326	2	22327	2	22328	2	22523
2	22524	2	22525	2	22532	2	22533	2	22534	2	22548
2	22554	2	22556	2	22558	2	22585	2	22595	2	22600
2	22610	2	22612	2	22614	2	22840	2	22841	2	22845
2	22851	2	63001	2	63003	2	63005	2	63055	2	63056
2	63057	2	63064	2	63081	2	63082	2	63085	2	63087
2	63088	2	63090	1	22100	1	22101	1	22102	1	22103
1	22110	1	22112	1	22114	1	22116	1	22520	1	22521
1	22522	1	63012	1	63020	1	63030	1	63035	1	63040
1	63042	1	63043	1	63044	1	63045	1	63046	1	63047
1	63048	1	63075	1	63076	1	63077	1	63300	1	63301
1	63302	1	63303	1	63304	1	63305	1	63306	1	63307
1	63709										

[a]Data from Abraham M, Glenn RL, O'Heron MR, eds: *CPT 2013 Professional Edition*. Chicago, IL, American Medical Association, 2012, pp 104-114, 331-340.

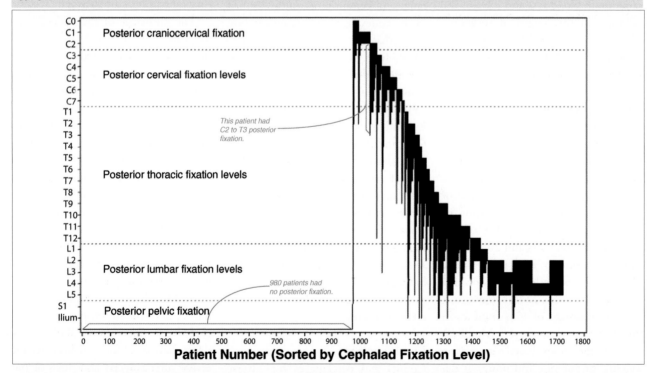

Figure 3 Graph showing the levels of posterior fixation for each of the 1,743 patients in the study sample. Patients were sorted by the cranial-most level of posterior fixation, and a vertical line was drawn from the cephalad to the caudad level of posterior fixation in each patient.

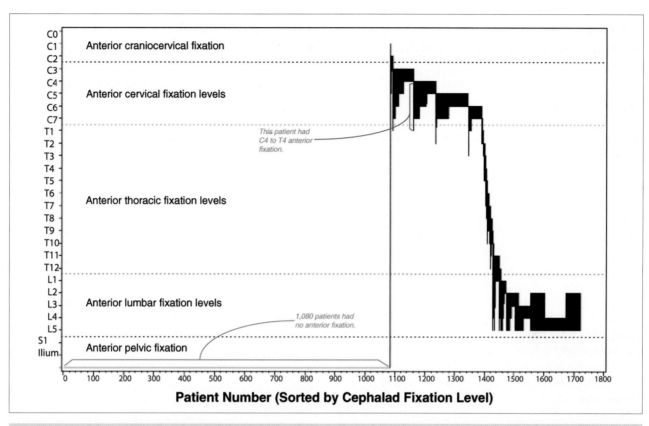

Figure 4 Graph showing the levels of anterior fixation for each of the 1,743 patients in the study sample. Patients were sorted by the cranial-most level of anterior fixation, and a vertical line was drawn from the cephalad to the caudad level of anterior fixation in each patient.

Source, Accuracy, and Timing of Adverse Events

Clinicians did not use standardized medical record templates for documenting brief surgical notes, discharge summaries, or outpatient visits. Compared with the full surgical report, surgeons reported information on the surgical time, the amount of blood loss, and the spinal level of the procedure on standard forms in fewer than 30% of the patients. Documentation of neurologic status at admission and discharge peaked at the end of the first study year, reaching more than 90% of the patients in only one of four teams; performance deteriorated in the second study year.

No adverse events were identified in 891 of the 1,723 patients (51.7%), and major adverse events occurred in 401 of 1,723 patients (23.3%) (**Table 4**). The pilot surveillance system iden-

tified only a minority of adverse events (**Tables 4** and **5**). A review of medical records identified most of the adverse events (82%, range 22% to 99%) but missed events related to the process of care, such as delays and equipment or staffing issues. Surgeons reported only 13% of the major adverse events (**Table 5**), although they did report more than 50% of the delays, the unavailability of equipment or staff, and other process of care events (**Table 4**). Most adverse events (78.1%) occurred during inpatient hospitalization. An additional 12.5% of adverse events occurred within 30 days of surgery, and 9.4% occurred more than 30 days after surgery (**Table 6**).

Association of the Invasiveness Index With Adverse Events

A unit increase in the invasiveness

score was associated with an odds ratio of 1.07 (95% confidence interval [CI]: 1.06 to 1.09), which indicated a 7% increased risk of adverse events with a unit value increase in the invasiveness index (**Table 7**). When minor complications (those judged by clinicians not to affect the length of hospitalization) and major complications (those judged by clinicians as likely to prolong hospitalization) were examined separately, the invasiveness index was not associated with the occurrence of minor complications. In contrast, the association between the invasiveness index and major complications was stronger, with an adjusted odds ratio of 1.08 (95% CI: 1.06 to 1.10). The invasiveness score was also associated with an increased risk of cardiac events, hematologic events, neurologic events, respiratory problems, technical

Table 3
Characteristics of the Study Population

	Number of Patients	%
Age (decade of life)		
0	6	0.3
10th	72	4.2
20th	179	10.4
30th	243	14.1
40th	411	23.9
50th	369	21.4
60th	224	13.0
70th	172	10.0
80th	44	2.6
90th	3	0.2
Sex		
Male	989	57.4
Female	734	42.6
Body mass index (BMI)		
Underweight (BMI < 18.5)	59	3.4
Normal (BMI ≥ 18.5 and < 25)	561	32.6
Overweight (BMI ≥ 25 and < 30)	532	30.9
Obese (BMI ≥ 30)	455	26.4
Unknown	116	6.7
Diagnosis group		
Degeneration	978	56.8
Trauma	441	25.6
Neoplasm	128	7.4
Infection	71	4.1
Other diagnosis	65	3.8
Unknown	40	2.3
Spinal region		
Thoracic, lumbar, or sacral spine	1,131	65.6
Cervical spine	592	34.4
Neurologic status		
Normal	711	41.3
Sensory deficit	398	23.1
Motor deficit	361	21.0
Cord deficit	253	14.7

Table 3 (Continued)
Characteristics of the Study Population

	Number of Patients	%
Revision surgery		
Primary surgery	1,371	79.6
Revision surgery	312	18.1
Unknown	40	2.3
Charlson comorbidity score		
0	280	16.3
> 2	848	49.2
1 or 2	595	34.5
Smoking history		
No	1,063	61.7
Yes	480	27.9
Unknown	180	10.4
Type of surgery		
Both decompression and fusion	911	52.9
Decompression only	521	30.2
Fusion only	154	8.9
Neither fusion nor decompression	137	8.0
Approach category		
Any posterior approach	959	55.7
Combined anterior and posterior approaches	341	19.8
Any anterior approach	333	19.3
Other approach	90	5.2
Number of vertebrae		
0	90	5.2
1	202	11.7
2	530	30.8
3	353	20.5
4	174	10.1
5	136	7.9
6 or more	238	13.8
All operations	**1,723**	**100**

occurrences, iatrogenic injury, and wound problems (**Table 7**).

Correlation of Medical Record– and CPT-Based Invasiveness Scores

The association between an invasiveness score derived from CPT codes in billing records using three different methods was examined. A CPT index was initially calculated based on each occurrence of a given CPT code. This methodology created erroneous values of invasiveness (greater than 100) in situations in which repeated CPT codes occurred in a patient's administrative billing data. A CPT-based index in which each CPT code could be included only once from the billing records was then calculated, with the exception that codes that defined additional vertebral levels would be included as often as they occurred in the billing records. This method of calculating a CPT index also tended to overestimate the invasiveness score, but it had a moderate correlation with the medical records–based index (correlation coefficient 0.71, $P < 0.001$). The CPT-based invasiveness index was

Table 4

Frequency of Adverse Occurrences

Adverse Event Category	Number of Patients	%	Identified By				Adverse Event Codes
			Surgeon[a] (%)	Team[b] (%)	Conference[c] (%)	Records[d] (%)	
No adverse occurrence	891	51.7					aa01
Wound healing problem	101	5.9	21.2	46.2	9.2	83.7	wh00, 01, 03 b, 03 c, 04, 05, 06, 07, 08, 10
Infection requiring surgery	59	3.4	31.1	42.5	7.5	81.1	wh02, wh09
Spinal fluid leak/dural laceration	148	8.6	59.8	23.7	8.9	79.5	ti30
New neurologic deficit	68	3.9	14.7	35.3	10.8	85.3	ti12 to ti20
Repeat surgery	140	8.1	12.3	26.9	26.9	99.0	aa06
Death[f]	32	1.9	0.7	83.7	15.0	78.2	aa02
CPR/ICU/mechanical ventilation	55	3.2	10.3	53.3	13.1	74.8	aa03, aa05, aa07, aa08, aa09
Iatrogenic injury[e]	147	8.5	30.0	26.5	5.1	80.5	ti00 to ti11, ti21 to ti29, ti31, tizz
Surgical/technical event	166	9.6	40.0	39.3	6.7	74.0	td01 to td24, tdzz
Anesthetic event	88	5.1	29.0	26.0	6.0	74.0	ec00 to ec08,eczz, ma00 to ma13, mazz
Medical events	465	27.0	7.9	32.1	4.7	89.5	any m*** code
Cardiac	103	6.0	16.6	29.0	4.7	88.8	mc00 to mc10, mczz
Respiratory	134	7.8	2.9	30.1	5.9	89.7	mr00 to mr09
Genitourinary	131	7.6	3.3	20.2	16.4	95.1	mu000 to mu04,muzz
Gastrointestinal	54	3.1	1.2	43.0	5.8	83.7	mg00 to mg08, mgzz
Neurologic[f]	101	5.9	4.3	44.3	7.1	88.6	mn00 to mn10, mnzz
Hematologic	121	7.0	18.3	33.0	4.7	88.5	mh00 to mh04, mhzz
Pharmacologic	40	2.3	6.8	35.6	0.0	86.4	md00 to md05, mdzz
Visual	15	0.9	0.0	45.0	10.0	90.0	md00 to md05, mdzz
Delays	52	30.0	50.6	43.0	6.3	20.3	dl00 to dl07, dlzz
Process-related events	37	2.1	50.9	29.1	3.6	45.4	pp00 to pp12, ppzz

[a]Reported in the surveillance system directly by the attending surgeon through forms, phone, e-mail, or verbal reports to clinical team or research staff.

[b]Reported in the surveillance system directly by the resident, nurse, physician assistant, or spine fellow rounding daily with the team, through forms, phone, e-mail, or verbally.

[c]Adverse events identified by trained research staff through clinical conferences, such as weekly surgical indications conference or the monthly morbidity and mortality conference.

[d]Identified by trained research staff through prospective, daily review of progress notes, imaging reports, or other reports in each patient's medical records.

[e]Excluding dural laceration and new spinal cord or nerve root deficit.

[f]Excluding spinal cord or nerve root deficit.

then further modified by assigning only a single score for each unique CPT code. This method tended to underestimate the invasiveness score slightly, but it had the best correlation with the medical records–based index (correlation coeffi-

cient, 0.87; intraclass correlation coefficient, 0.97; $P < 0.001$).

Discussion

This study shows a failure of a voluntary surveillance system for monitor-

ing adverse events in spine surgery. Medical records review was able to identify approximately 90% of the observed adverse events. The team of physicians and nurses conducting inpatient rounds identified fewer than

Table 5
Frequency of Major Adverse Occurrences

Adverse Event Category	Number of Patients	%	Identified By				Adverse Events Codes
			Surgeon[a] (%)	Team[b] (%)	Conference[c] (%)	Records[d] (%)	
Major adverse	401	23.3	13.4	38.4	9.1	86.7	aa02, 03, 06, 09, ec08, ma04, 06, 11, 12, 13, mc01, 02, 03, 04, 06, 07, 09, mg02, 07, mh01, 03, mn01, 02, 03, 06, 07, 08, mr01, 04, 05, 07, 09, mn02, mv01, td09, 10, ti02, 03, 08, 13, 14, 15, 16, 19, 26, 27, 28, wh01, 02, 07, 08, 09
Minor adverse events	431	25.0	27.6	33.6	6.3	77.3	All codes not included in major category
Death	32	1.9	0.7	83.7	15.0	78.2	aa02
Life-threatening event	56	3.3	10.6	52.9	13.5	75.0	aa03, 04, 05, 07, 09
Major wound problem	99	5.7	27.1	40.7	8.5	84.2	wh01, 02, 03 b, 03 c, 07, 08, 09
Major iatrogenic injury[e]	70	4.1	24.7	29.3	10.7	82.7	ti02, 03, 08, 13-16, 19, 20, 26-28
Major technical event	25	1.5	26.3	42.1	5.3	89.5	td09, 10
Major medical events							
Cardiac	90	5.2	16.9	28.4	5.4	87.8	mc01-04, 06, 07, 09
Respiratory	104	6.0	2.1	27.8	5.7	89.9	mr01, 04, 05, 07, 09
Genitourinary	14	0.8	0.0	28.6	0.0	85.7	mu02
Gastrointestinal	2	0.1	0.0	25.0	25.0	100	mg02, 007
Neurologic[f]	73	4.2	3.0	43.4	7.1	89.9	mn01-03, 06, 07, 09, mv01
Hematologic	50	2.9	43.6	17.9	9.0	84.6	mh01, 03

[a]Reported in the surveillance system directly by the attending surgeon through forms, phone, e-mail, or verbal reports to clinical team or research staff.

[b]Reported in the surveillance system directly by the resident, nurse, physician assistant, or spine fellow rounding daily with the team, through forms, phone, e-mail, or verbally.

[c]Adverse events identified by trained research staff through clinical conferences, such as the weekly surgical indications conference or the monthly morbidity and mortality conference.

[d]Identified by trained research staff through prospective daily review of progress notes, imaging reports, or other reports in each patient's medical records.

[e]Excluding dural laceration and new spinal cord or nerve root deficit.

[f]Excluding spinal cord or nerve root deficit.

50% of the events, and surgeons identified fewer than 15%. Efforts to improve safety can be prioritized to focus on less expensive surveillance methods, such as medical records review or an analysis of administrative claims.

Focusing surveillance on the periods of acute hospitalization and the subsequent 30 days will capture more than 90% of adverse events in patients undergoing spine surgery. Longer periods of surveillance of medical records and in-person clinic visits add costs without achieving a significant yield of clinically recognized events. Directing longer surveillance to patient-reported outcome and safety measures, as opposed to adverse event racking, will be a more efficient strategy for longer surveillance.

The assignment of an invasiveness score to a CPT code based on clinical judgment correlated well with medical records–based invasiveness scores (**Figure 5**). The calculation of the invasiveness score from billing records may be further refined based on the sensitivity analysis examining the outlying variables and determining specific weights for CPT codes. Empiric methods of assigning weights to unique CPT codes may also be feasible.

The observed rates of adverse events are determined by the modes of ascer-

Table 6

Timing of Major Adverse Events

Adverse Event Category	Operating Room (%)	Inpatient (%)	30 Days (%)	1 Year (%)	2 Years (%)	Adverse Event Codes
Death	0.0	78.1	12.5	9.4	0.0	aa02
Life-threatening event	25.5	74.5	0.0	0.0	0.0	aa03, 04, 05, 07, 09
Major wound problem	15.2	42.4	27.2	14.1	1.1	wh01, 02, 03 b, 03 c, 07, 08, 09
Major iatrogenic injury[a]	52.3	40.0	3.1	3.1	1.5	ti02, 03, 08, 13-16, 19, 20, 26-28
Major technical event	13.0	8.7	17.4	60.9	0.0	td09, 10
Major medical events						
Cardiac	48.2	50.6	0	1.2	0.0	mc01-04, 06, 07, 09
Respiratory	10.6	78.7	9.6	1.1	0.0	mr01, 04, 05, 07, 09
Genitourinary	25.0	66.7	8.3	0.0	0.0	mu02
Gastrointestinal	0.0	100.0	0.0	0.0	0.0	mg02, 007
Neurologic[b]	26.1	71.0	2.9	0.0	0.0	mn01-03, 06, 07, 09, mv01
Hematologic	85.1	14.9	0.0	0.0	0.0	mh01, 03

[a]Excluding dural laceration and new spinal cord or nerve root deficit.
[b]Excluding spinal cord or nerve root deficit.

tainment. Multimodal methods capture the most events, followed in progressively decreasing yield order by medical record reviews, team conferences, voluntary team reports, and reports by the surgeon. Data provided directly by surgeons are often inaccurate and incomplete. Surgeons tended to underestimate adverse events, except for intraoperative technical occurrences and process-related measurements (such as delays or incomplete surgical equipment).

Although the mantra for physicians since the time of Hippocrates more than 2,400 years ago has been "first, do no harm," objective and valid measures for safety remain lacking or are poorly developed. Standardized definitions are needed for safety surveillance in spine surgery. Reports of spine procedures show variations in safety that are unexplained by patient or study characteristics.[13,14] A brief list of consistently defined safety measures will greatly facilitate safety surveillance for spine surgery. Such a list could serve as a tool for the FDA to develop simplified public reports of safety of approved spinal surgery devices and standardized methods for postmarketing surveillance of spinal devices.

Adverse events occur frequently in patients undergoing spine surgery and have the potential to cause substantial harm. In the judgment of surgeons, many adverse events may be prevent-

Table 7

Incremental Increase in Risk of Complications With a Unit Increase in the Invasiveness Score[a]

Complication Category	Odds Ratio for Invasiveness Index (95% CI)	Model P-Value
Any adverse occurrence	1.073 (1.056, 1.091)	< 0.0001
Major adverse occurrence	1.082 (1.064, 1.101)	< 0.0001
Minor adverse occurrence	0.970 (0.949, 0.993)	0.0015
Cardiac complication	1.029 (1.004, 1.054)	< 0.0001
Hematologic complication	1.120 (1.084, 1.158)	< 0.0001
Neurologic complication	1.068 (1.041, 1.096)	< 0.0001
Respiratory complication	1.055 (1.026, 1.084)	< 0.0001
Iatrogenic injury	1.070 (1.042, 1.097)	0.0007
Wound problem	1.047 (1.021, 1.074)	< 0.0001
Technical complication	1.070 (1.031, 1.111)	0.1093
Anesthetic complication	0.996	0.0001
Gastrointestinal complication	0.372	0.2732
Urological complication	1.015	0.0002
Other life-threatening complication	1.018	< 0.0001
Death	1.043	< 0.0001

[a]Adjusted for age, sex, body mass index, smoking history, bleeding history, Charlson score, spinal diagnosis, revision surgery, neurologic deficit, and spinal level.

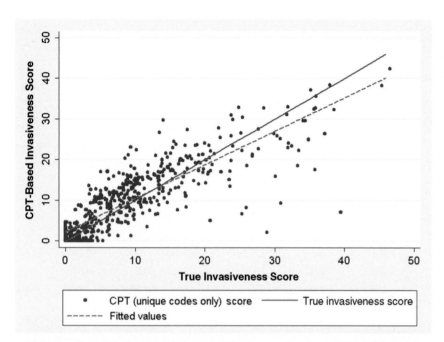

Figure 5 Scatter graph shows the strong association observed between the CPT-derived invasiveness index and the medical record-derived invasiveness index.

able. Systems of care must strive for an environment where conditions that increase the likelihood of adverse events are eliminated.[29-32] Reducing adverse events associated with surgical care requires a healthcare community that values error-free care, creates efficient surveillance systems to monitor the magnitude of the problem, and identifies contributing factors. Ultimately, such data can be used to link errors to outcomes and costs. Redesigning safety into the healthcare system begins by creating a culture of safety in healthcare organizations so that each member is valued for making contributions that improve safety.

Summary

Generalizable implementation lessons from the University of Washington experience described in this chapter are as follows: (1) integrating comprehensive surveillance for adverse events with routine care processes is feasible but difficult, expensive, and disruptive; (2) discrete data provided by busy

surgeons do not reliably capture the surgical complexity or the frequency of adverse events; (3) patients undergoing spinal surgery frequently experience adverse events; (4) the risk of adverse events is associated with surgical invasiveness; and (5) surgical invasiveness can be measured quantitatively from both surgical reports and surgical billing codes. The infrastructure required to implement the tools developed by this chapter's authors (a predefined list of adverse events, staff and training for multimodal ascertainment, and methods to measure the invasiveness of surgery) was prohibitively expensive to sustain without external support. The culture of safety surveillance among clinicians was not sufficient without a research staff that performed the core tasks of identifying and recording observed adverse events. Even then, members of the research staff were often viewed as interfering with clinical efficiency. The program faded through attrition after the research funding ended for nurses, coordinators, statisti-

cians, programmers, and computer systems. Future efforts to rigorously measure the safety of spinal surgery may be more successful if there is a focus on a few indicator adverse events that likely matter most to patients, such as infection, a new neurologic deficit, reoperation, readmission, and death. The last three indicators can be fully ascertained from administrative records, but infection and neurologic deficit require a review of medical records. Safety surveillance may benefit from the ability of electronic health records to capture discrete data, more specific descriptions provided by the ICD Version 10 codes, and unique implanted device identifiers.

Acknowledgments

The authors of this chapter express gratitude to all of the spine surgeons at the University of Washington for participating in the study. We thank Drs. Scott Barnhart, John Culver, Rick Goss, Eric Larson, and Tom Staiger for their support. We are grateful to Jan Bower, Michaela Galapon, Michelle Kelley, Chris Cooley, Louise Suhr, Virginia Arvold, and Jana Day for patient enrollment and data collection. We thank Dr. Noel Weiss for comments on earlier drafts of this manuscript.

References

1. Fenton JJ, Mirza SK, Lahad A, Stern BD, Deyo RA: Variation in reported safety of lumbar interbody fusion: Influence of industrial sponsorship and other study characteristics. *Spine (Phila Pa 1976)* 2007;32(4):471-480.

2. Pull ter Gunne AF, Hosman AJ, Cohen DB, et al: A methodological systematic review on surgical site infections following spinal surgery: Part 1. Risk factors. *Spine (Phila Pa 1976)* 2012;37(24): 2017-2033.

3. van Middendorp JJ, Pull ter Gunne AF, Schuetz M, et al: A methodological systematic review on surgical site infections following spinal surgery: Part 2. Prophylactic treatments. *Spine (Phila Pa 1976)* 2012;37(24): 2034-2045.

4. Smith JS, Fu K-M, Polly DW Jr, et al: Complication rates of three common spine procedures and rates of thromboembolism following spine surgery based on 108,419 procedures: A report from the Scoliosis Research Society Morbidity and Mortality Committee. *Spine (Phila Pa 1976)* 2010;35(24):2140-2149.

5. Cho K-J, Suk S-I, Park S-R, et al: Complications in posterior fusion and instrumentation for degenerative lumbar scoliosis. *Spine (Phila Pa 1976)* 2007;32(20):2232-2237.

6. Zheng F, Cammisa FP Jr, Sandhu HS, Girardi FP, Khan SN: Factors predicting hospital stay, operative time, blood loss, and transfusion in patients undergoing revision posterior lumbar spine decompression, fusion, and segmental instrumentation. *Spine (Phila Pa 1976)* 2002;27(8):818-824.

7. Street JT, Lenehan BJ, DiPaola CP, et al: A prospective cohort analysis of 942 consecutive patients. *Spine J* 2012;12(1):22-34.

8. Fritzell P, Hägg O, Nordwall A; Swedish Lumbar Spine Study Group: Complications in lumbar fusion surgery for chronic low back pain: Comparison of three surgical techniques used in a prospective randomized study. A report from the Swedish Lumbar Spine Study Group. *Eur Spine J* 2003;12(2):178-189.

9. Irwin ZN, Hilibrand A, Gustavel M, et al: Part I. Lumbar spine. *Spine (Phila Pa 1976)* 2005; 30(19):2208-2213.

10. Katz JN, Lipson SJ, Lew RA, et al: Lumbar laminectomy alone or with instrumented or noninstrumented arthrodesis in degenerative lumbar spinal stenosis: Patient selection, costs, and surgical outcomes. *Spine (Phila Pa 1976)* 1997;22(10):1123-1131.

11. Deyo RA, Mirza SK, Martin BI, Kreuter W, Goodman DC, Jarvik JG: Trends, major medical complications, and charges associated with surgery for lumbar spinal stenosis in older adults. *JAMA* 2010;303(13):1259-1265.

12. Deyo RA, Mirza SK, Martin BI: Error in trends, major medical complications, and charges associated with surgery for lumbar spinal stenosis in older adults. *JAMA* 2011;306(10):1088.

13. Martin BI, Mirza SK, Franklin GM, Lurie JD, MacKenzie TA, Deyo RA: Hospital and surgeon variation in complications and repeat surgery following incident lumbar fusion for common degenerative diagnoses. *Health Serv Res* 2013;48(1):1-25.

14. Martin BI, Mirza SK, Flum DR, et al: The quality implications of hospital and surgeon variation. *Spine J* 2012;12(2):89-97.

15. Mirza SK, Deyo RA: Systematic review of randomized trials comparing lumbar fusion surgery to nonoperative care for treatment of chronic back pain. *Spine (Phila Pa 1976)* 2007;32(7):816-823.

16. Deyo RA, Gray DT, Kreuter W, Mirza S, Martin BI: United States trends in lumbar fusion surgery for degenerative conditions. *Spine (Phila Pa 1976)* 2005;30(12): 1441-1445, discussion 1446-1447.

17. Mirza SK, Deyo RA, Heagerty PJ, Turner JA, Lee LA, Goodkin R: Towards standardized measurement of adverse events in spine surgery: Conceptual model and pilot evaluation. *BMC Musculoskelet Disord* 2006;7:53.

18. Mirza SK, Deyo RA, Heagerty PJ, et al: Development of an index to characterize the "invasiveness" of spine surgery: Validation by comparison to blood loss and operative time. *Spine (Phila Pa 1976)* 2008;33(24):2651-2661, discussion 2662.

19. Cizik AM, Lee MJ, Martin BI, et al: Using the spine surgical invasiveness index to identify risk of surgical site infection: A multivariate analysis. *J Bone Joint Surg Am* 2012;94(4):335-342.

20. Lee MJ, Konodi MA, Cizik AM, et al: A multivariate analysis of 582 patients. *Spine (Phila Pa 1976)* 2013;38(3):223-228.

21. Lee MJ, Hacquebord J, Varshney A, et al: A multivariate analysis of 767 patients. *Spine (Phila Pa 1976)* 2011;36(21):1801-1806.

22. Lee MJ, Konodi MA, Cizik AM, Bransford RJ, Bellabarba C, Chapman JR: Risk factors for medical complication after spine surgery: A multivariate analysis of 1,591 patients. *Spine J* 2012; 12(3):197-206.

23. Baker GA, Cizik AM, Bransford RJ, et al: A multivariate analysis. *Spine J* 2012;12(2):121-126.

24. US Department of Health & Human Services. Health Information Privacy. http://www.hhs.gov/ocr/privacy/. Accessed July 29, 2013.

25. International Classification of Diseases: Ninth Revision. http://www.cdc.gov/nchs/icd/icd9.htm. Accessed January 7, 2013.

26. Abraham M, Glenn RL, O'Heron MR: *CPT 2013 Professional Edition*. Chicago, IL, American Medical Association, 2012, pp 104-114, 331-340.

27. Maynard FM Jr, Bracken MB, Creasey G, et al: International Standards for Neurological and Functional Classification of Spinal Cord Injury. *Spinal Cord* 1997; 35(5):266-274.

28. Charlson ME, Pompei P, Ales KL, MacKenzie CR: A new method of classifying prognostic comorbidity

in longitudinal studies: Development and validation. *J Chronic Dis* 1987;40(5):373-383.

29. Kuo CC, Robb WJ III: Critical roles of orthopaedic surgeon leadership in healthcare systems to improve orthopaedic surgical patient safety. *Clin Orthop Relat Res* 2013;471(6):1792-1800.

30. Thomas L, Galla C: Building a culture of safety through team training and engagement. *BMJ Qual Saf.* 2012.

31. Gurses AP, Kim G, Martinez EA, et al: Identifying and categorising patient safety hazards in cardiovascular operating rooms using an interdisciplinary approach: A mul-

tisite study. *BMJ Qual Saf* 2012; 21(10):810-818.

32. Leape LL, Woods DD, Hatlie MJ, Kizer KW, Schroeder SA, Lundberg GD: Promoting patient safety by preventing medical error. *JAMA* 1998;280(16):1444-1447.

Adverse Events Recording and Reporting in Clinical Trials of Cervical Total Disk Replacement

Paul A. Anderson, MD
Robert A. Hart, MD

Abstract

Adverse events reporting in pivotal trials of new technologies, such as cervical total disk replacement, are essential to determine safety. Important questions concerning the adequacy of reporting about such new technologies in peer-reviewed publications have prompted this analysis to assess the safety of cervical disk replacement compared with fusion as presented in peer-reviewed publications and FDA summary reports. Identifying differences among these reports highlight the poor quality of adverse event reporting in the peer-reviewed literature. Nine peer-reviewed studies and five FDA summary reports documented excellent safety for both cervical fusion and disk arthroplasty. No differences in rates of adverse events were found to exist between the two treatments. The methods of recording and the actual reporting of adverse events were poor in peer-reviewed manuscripts, whereas they were comprehensive but difficult to clinically apply in the FDA summaries. Recommendations to improve documentation and reporting of adverse events are presented.

Instr Course Lect 2014;63:287-296.

New surgical technologies, such as cervical total disk replacement (TDR), must establish safety and efficacy before receiving FDA approval. This is a laborious process that begins with preclinical studies evaluating mechanical function, biocompatibility, neurotoxicity, and other factors. When a device has mobile-bearing surfaces, additional evaluation of wear testing is required. The FDA has produced guidance documents for the medical device industry that are intended to standardize this process.[1] If justified by preclinical data, a pivotal clinical trial intended to prove safety and efficacy is performed. In most instances, this clinical trial will be a randomized controlled trial (RCT) unless that is not feasible. Safety is primarily assessed based on the evaluation of adverse events in the pivotal trial.

Peer-reviewed publications of RCTs of cervical TDR include a description of the study methodology and reports of the outcomes of the primary and secondary variables, such as pain reduction, functional improvement, health-related quality of life, the ability to work, and pain medication use. The reporting of adverse events is also included, but it is often limited to a brief

Dr. Anderson or an immediate family member has received royalties from Pioneer Surgical and Stryker; serves as a paid consultant to or is an employee of Aesculap and Pioneer Surgical; serves as an unpaid consultant to Expanding Orthopedics, SI Bone, Spatatec, and Titan Surgical; has stock or stock options held in Expanding Orthopedics, Pioneer Surgical, SI Bone, Spartec, and Titan Surgical; and serves as a board member, owner, officer, or committee member of the American Academy of Orthopaedic Surgeons, the ASTM, the Lumbar Research Society, the North American Spine Society, the Spine Arthroplasty Society, and the American Association of Neurological Surgeons/Congress of Neurological Surgeons Joint Section on Disorders of the Spine and Peripheral Nerves. Dr. Hart or an immediate family member has received royalties from DePuy and SeaSpine; is a member of a speakers' bureau or has made paid presentations on behalf of DePuy, Kyphon, Medtronic, and Synthes; serves as a paid consultant to or is an employee of DePuy, Eli Lilly, and Medtronic; has stock or stock options held in Spine Connect; has received research or institutional support from DePuy, Medtronic, the Orthopaedic Research and Education Foundation, and Synthes; and serves as a board member, owner, officer, or committee member of the American Academy of Orthopaedic Surgeons, the American Orthopaedic Association, the Cervical Spine Research Society, the Lumbar Spine Research Society, the North American Spine Society, the Oregon Association of Orthopaedics, the Orthopaedic Research and Education Foundation, and the Scoliosis Research Society.

discussion contained in one paragraph or a single table. Adverse events may not be adequately reported in primary publications. To overcome the constraints of space limitations, some authors of cervical and lumbar TDR trials have reported adverse events in separate publications.[2,3]

As part of the approval process, the FDA reports a summary of safety and effectiveness data (SSED), which includes a detailed analysis of all adverse events in the pivotal trial, whether they were related to the procedure or not. In recent SSED reports of cervical TDRs, adverse events occurred in up to 85% of the patients, although most of the events were unrelated to the device or were insignificant.[4-7] Because clinical follow-ups of these trials have continued for up to 10 years, it likely that patients have experienced some medical problems that are unrelated to the initial surgical procedure.

Carragee et al[8] recently questioned whether adequate reporting of adverse events of new spinal technologies has occurred in peer-reviewed publications. The authors identified important differences between adverse events recorded in the SSED reports of pivotal trials and the peer-reviewed manuscripts of these same studies for bone morphogenetic protein. In some cases, it appeared that important adverse events associated with bone morphogenetic protein were not reported in the peer-reviewed literature.[8]

This chapter compares the adverse events of anterior cervical diskectomy and fusion (ACDF) with those of TDR. The adverse events reported in peer-reviewed RCTs of cervical TDRs are compared with those published in the FDA summaries. Distinctions are also drawn between methods followed in adverse events reporting for TDR trials compared with trials of bone morphogenetic protein. The goal of this chapter's authors is to make rec-

ommendations on how to report adverse events in RCTs so that surgeons and patients have better and more complete information on which to base decisions.

Methods

A literature search was conducted using the search terms of cervical disk replacement or cervical disk arthroplasty. Inclusion criteria included RCTs comparing ACDF and TDR for the treatment of radiculopathy and myelopathy, a minimum follow-up period of 1 year, adult patients, and reports using standard validated outcome measures. The FDA website also was searched for SSED reports of cervical TDRs.

Adverse event data were abstracted for each publication. When appropriate, data were pooled using statistical meta-analysis methods. A meta-analysis was performed using relative risk of having an adverse event in the TDR group compared with the ACDF control group. The pooled relative risk of having an adverse event of ACDF to TDR was calculated using Comprehensive Meta-Analysis software, version 2.2.050 (Biostat). A random effect model was chosen, and heterogeneity was assessed using the Q statistic. Confidence intervals (CIs) were set at 95%, and statistical significance was established at a P value of 0.05.

An overall score of the clarity of the methods to assess how adverse events were determined and reported was based on the presence or the absence of five factors, which were scored 0 or 1 and then summed. The criteria applied to how the adverse events were obtained, if definitions were provided, if the severity of the adverse event was graded, whether timing of the adverse event was stated, and whether statistical methods were stated a priori. The reporting of adverse events was similarly scored based on the sum of single

points given for whether adverse events were reported, categorized, timed, and statistically analyzed and if reoperations were evaluated.

Results
Study Description

Nine independent RCTs were identified[9-17] (**Table 1**). One manuscript also provided a separate report of adverse events for one of the RCTs.[2] Five of the studies were industry-sponsored trials. Five SSED reports on cervical TDRs were identified.[4-7,18] The overall number of randomized patients was 926 in the ACDF control group and 983 in the TDR group.

Quality of Adverse Event Acquisition Methodology and Reporting

The description of methods used to assess adverse events in the peer-reviewed publications was poor, with a mean score of 1.6 on a 5-point scale. Five studies did not report any of the methods used to obtain adverse events, whereas a score of 2 was obtained in three of the studies. Two studies, both using the same RCT data, scored 5 on the scale. All but one of the non–industry-funded studies did not identify any methods for reporting adverse events, whereas three of the four industry-sponsored trials did report these methods. In the SSED reports, the assessment for adverse event acquisition was substantially better, with two reports scoring 4 and three reports scoring 5. The reporting of adverse events in the peer-reviewed publications had a mean score of 2.0. All SSED reports included extensive reporting of adverse events and scored 5.

Overall Adverse Events

The rate of adverse events varied widely among studies, depending on definitions and the intensity of documentation. For example, Heller et al[12]

Table 1

Study Cohorts

Study (Year)	Device (Manufacturer)	Industry Funded	Number of Patients		Methods Clarity Score	Reporting Results Score
			ACDR	TDR	Range 0-5	Range 0-5
Peer-Reviewed Publications						
Porchet et al[16] (2004)	Prestige ST (Medtronic)	Yes	28	27	3	2
Mummaneni et al[13] (2007)	Prestige ST	Yes	265	276	2	2
Murrey et al[14] (2007)	ProDisc-C (Synthes)	Yes	106	103	2	4
Nabhan et al[15] (2007)	ProDisc-C	No	17	16	0	0
Anderson et al[2] (2008)	Bryan (Medtronic)	Yes	221	242	5	5
Heller et al[12] (2009)	Bryan	Yes	221	242	5	3
Cheng et al[10] (2009)	Bryan	No	34	31	0	0
Cheng et al[9] (2011)	Bryan	No	41	42	0	0
Coric et al[11] (2011)	Kineflex/C (Spinal Motion)	Yes	133	136	0	3
Zhang et al[17] (2012)	Bryan	No	53	56	0	1
FDA Summaries						
SSED[6]	Prestige ST	Yes	265	276	4	5
SSED[7]	ProDisc-C	Yes	106	103	4	5
SSED[5]	Bryan	Yes	221	242	5	5
SSED[4,a]	Secure C (Globus Medical)	Yes	144	148	5	5
SSED[18]	PCM (NuVasive)	Yes	190	214	5	5

[a]The study also reported 89 nonrandomized patients in the disk group.

SSED = summary of safety and effectiveness data, ACDF = anterior cervical disk fusion, TDR = total disk replacement.

reported only serious adverse events, whereas Murrey et al[14] reported only events attributable to the surgery or the device. Anderson et al[2] and Porchet and Metcalf[16] reported all adverse events, whether or not they appeared to be related to the spinal surgery. Three studies did not report adverse events. Rates of adverse events in the ACDF groups ranged from 2.9% to 67.9% compared with 2.9% to 63.0% in the TDR groups[2,9-17] (**Table 2**). Meta-analysis showed no significant difference between the ACDF and TDR groups, with a mean relative risk of 0.99 (**Figure 1**). The studies were consistent and homogeneous with a Q value of 5.4.

The SSED reports included all adverse events, most of which had no obvious relationship to the surgical procedure or device. The results were consistent among the five reports, with reported adverse event rates of 72.3% to 85.8%[4-7,18] (**Table 2**). The relative risk of TDR compared with ACDF was 0.99, which was not statistically significant. Homogeneity among the five reports was confirmed with a low Q value. The most common adverse events were neck and arm pain or a new neurologic symptom (including numbness); these events occurred any time in the 2- to 3-year postoperative period.

Surgery-Related Adverse Events

Surgery-related adverse events were those secondary to the procedure; these included medical and surgery-related events that occurred within 6 weeks of surgery. Episodes of pain, new cancers, or other surgeries not involving the cervical spine were excluded. Given the diversity between the studies in how adverse events were evaluated and reported, comparisons among devices were not performed.

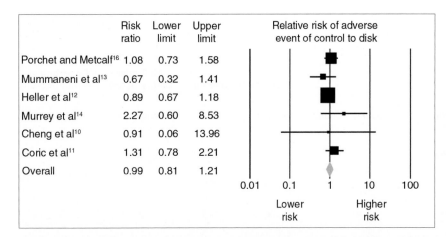

	Risk ratio	Lower limit	Upper limit
Porchet and Metcalf[16]	1.08	0.73	1.58
Mummaneni et al[13]	0.67	0.32	1.41
Heller et al[12]	0.89	0.67	1.18
Murrey et al[14]	2.27	0.60	8.53
Cheng et al[10]	0.91	0.06	13.96
Coric et al[11]	1.31	0.78	2.21
Overall	0.99	0.81	1.21

Figure 1 Forest plot of relative risk of adverse reactions in ACDF compared with disk arthroplasty in peer-reviewed publications.

However, ACDF and TDR were compared in each study using relative risk ratios[2,9-17] (**Table 3**). The pooled relative risk of ACDF to TDR in the peer-reviewed studies was 0.95, which was not significant. The SSED reports had a mean relative risk of 1.13, which indicates a higher rate of adverse events in the TDR group; however, this risk was not statistically significant.[4-7,18] Regarding safety, no differences between TDR and ACDF in surgery-related adverse events were demonstrated.

Types of Complications

The types of complications were analyzed from the SSED reports because these reports used similar reporting methods and were the most comprehensive[4-7,18] (**Table 4**). Complications were analyzed as medical or surgical, with inclusion of only those complications that appeared likely to be related to the surgical procedure or the device. Only those adverse events that occurred within 6 weeks of surgery were included, except for cancer and death, which were analyzed up to 5 years after surgery.

The most common medical events were nonwound infections and gastrointestinal problems, which occurred equally in both groups.[4-7,18] Cancer

occurred in 11 of the patients treated with TDR and 2 of the patients treated with ACDF. Given that the device designs are dissimilar and contain different metals, it is unlikely that this is a true effect but rather a random event. At the same time, eight deaths occurred in the ACDF group compared with three in the TDR group. All deaths were believed to be unrelated to the cervical spine condition or surgery. Again, it is likely that this difference results from random causes, not any biologic process related to spinal fusion.

The most common surgery-related adverse events were dysphagia and dysphonia, which were variably documented between studies but were similar between groups.[4-7,18] Superficial wound infections occurred in 7 of the ACDF patients and 18 of the TDR patients. Deep wound infection occurred in one patient in each group. The incidence of postoperative neurologic deficits was difficult to determine because exact definitions and reporting of methods were unclear. One criterion for success of the procedure was maintenance or improvement of neurologic function based on reflex, sensory, and motor examinations. However, this is not a useful metric to assess adverse

events because the status of reflexes has poor reliability, and changes do not indicate neurologic dysfunction, except (perhaps) in cases of hyperreflexia. In addition, transient sensory disturbances are common for most of the population, and any such symptom would be scored as an adverse neurologic event. The best estimate is that between 5% and 10% of the patients in both groups will have postoperative neurologic change within 6 weeks of surgery; most of these changes are expected to be mild in severity. One case of spinal cord injury was reported in a patient treated with ACDF.[2]

Reoperations

In peer-reviewed publications, considerable variations were found in the reported reoperation rates[2,9-17] (**Table 5**). In the ACDF group, reoperation rates ranged from 0% to 9.7% at the index spinal level and 13.5% if both index and adjacent levels are included. This compared with a range of 0% to 4.9% for index-level arthroplasty and 11.5% for both index- and adjacent-level arthroplasty in the TDR group. Mean reoperation rates at the index level were 6.2% versus 2.3% for the ACDF and TDR groups, respectively, and 3.9% versus 2.6% for adjacent segments, respectively. The relative risk of any cervical reoperation in the ACDF group compared with the TDR group was 2.06, which was not statistically significant (although it may represent a clinically significant difference).

In the five FDA summaries, the relative risk for reoperation was 1.87, which was significant.[4-7,18] Reoperation at adjacent segments was reported in only two studies and was not statistically different between the groups.[4,5]

In the ACDF group, index-level reoperations were almost always related to pseudarthrosis. Plate removal, if re-

Table 2
Adverse Events

Study (Year)	Incidence of Adverse Events (%)		Relative Risk of ACDF to TDR	95% CI	
	ACDF	TDR		ACDF	TDR
Peer-Reviewed Publications					
Porchet et al[16] (2004)	67.9	63.0	1.08	0.73	1.08
Mummaneni et al[13] (2007)	4.2	6.2	0.67	0.32	0.67
Murrey et al[14] (2007)	6.6	2.9	2.27	0.60	8.53
Nabhan et al[15] (2007)	NR	NR	-	-	-
Anderson et al[2] (2008)	30.2[a]	36.2[a]	0.85	0.65	1.12
Heller et al[12] (2009)	27.6[a]	31.0[a]	0.89	0.67	1.18
Cheng et al[10] (2009)	2.9	3.2	0.91	0.06	0.91
Cheng et al[9] (2011)	NR	NR	-	-	-
Coric et al[11] (2011)	9.8	4.4	1.31	0.78	1.31
Zhang et al[17] (2012)	NR	NR	-	-	-
Total	16.0	16.4	0.99	0.81	1.21
FDA Summaries (Device)					
SSED[6] (Prestige ST)	80.0	81.9	0.98	0.90	1.06
SSED[7] (ProDisc-C)	81.1	81.6	0.99	0.87	1.13
SSED[5] (Bryan)	78.7	83.9	0.94	0.86	1.02
SSED[4] (Secure C)	79.2	72.3	1.10	0.96	1.25
SSED[18] (PCM)	85.8	84.1	1.02	0.94	1.11
Total	80.9	81.4	0.99	0.95	1.04

[a]World Health Organization grade 3 and 4.
CI = confidence interval, NR = not reported, SSED = summary of safety and effectiveness data, ACDF = anterior cervical disk fusion, TDR = total disk replacement.

quired for an adjacent-level reoperation, was counted as an index-level reoperation in some studies, even if the purpose was to treat adjacent-segment disease. Thus, comparisons of revision at the index level for ACDF versus TDR patients will be biased in favor of TDR. Index-level reoperations in the TDR groups were for failure of resolution of initial symptoms and were usually a posterior fusion or foraminotomy. Mechanical failure and device expulsion were treated with removal and anterior interbody fusion and counted as index-level reoperations. Outcomes of patients having reoperations were not reported separately, thus it is unknown if revision strategies are effective.

Discussion

This chapter examines the recording and reporting of adverse events associated with cervical disk arthroplasty compared with fusion. It also attempts to understand if adverse events in SSED reports differed from those reported in the peer-reviewed literature. This chapter's authors found that TDR performed for single-level radiculopathy and myelopathy is as safe as ACDF. This conclusion is based on strong evidence that was derived from multiple RCTs having homogeneous results in both the peer-reviewed literature and the SSED reports.

The peer-reviewed literature and the SSED reports had similar statistical results when comparing treatment groups;[2,4-7,9-18] however, because the purposes of SSED reports and peer-reviewed publications are different, major differences exist in how adverse events are assessed and reported. The SSED reports use a broad definition of adverse events, which allow accumulation of data identifying unanticipated and systemic events that would not normally be considered surgical complications. Examples of such unanticipated adverse events from pharmaceutical trials are cardiac valve disease associated with weight loss medications or the risk of death from coronary artery disease from cyclooxygenase-2 inhibitors. In these cases, unexpected adverse events were

Table 3
Surgery-Related Adverse Events

Study (Year)	Adverse Events/Patients		Relative Risk ACDF to TDR	95% CI	
	ACDF	TDR		Lower	Upper
Peer-Reviewed Publications					
Porchet et al[16] (2004)	NR	NR	NR	NR	-
Mummaneni et al[13] (2007)	11/265	17/276	0.67	0.54	1.14
Murrey et al[14] (2007)	NR	NR	NR	NR	-
Nabhan et al[15] (2007)	NR	NR	NR	NR	-
Anderson et al[2] (2008)	64/221	82/242	0.85	0.65	1.12
Heller et al[12] (2009)	NR	NR	NR	NR	-
Cheng et al[10] (2009)	1/47	1/45	0.96	0.06	14.9
Cheng et al[9] (2011)	7/42	4/41	1.71	0.54	5.40
Coric et al[11] (2011)	13/133	7/136	1.90	0.78	4.61
Zhang et al[17] (2012)	NR	NR	NR	NR	-
Total	96/708	111/740	0.95	0.69	1.32
FDA Summaries (Device)					
SSED[6] (Prestige ST)	40/265	53/276	0.79	0.54	1.14
SSED[7] (ProDisc-C)	32/106	41/103	0.76	0.52	1.10
SSED[5] (Bryan)	50/221	55/242	1.00	0.71	1.39
SSED[4] (Secure C)	21/144	10/236	3.44	1.67	7.10
SSED[18] (PCM)	70/190	59/214	1.34	1.00	1.78
Total	143/736	159/857	1.13	0.78	1.63

CI = confidence interval, NR = not reported, SSED = summary of safety and effectiveness data, ACDF = anterior cervical disk fusion, TDR = total disk replacement.

related to the administration of the pharmaceutical agent.

An important difference in SSED report methodology between pharmaceutical and medical device research is that most of the reported events in device research are not associated with the surgical procedure and may give a false impression of a device being unsafe. The FDA also categorizes pain episodes as adverse events, which are concurrently measured and reported as a clinical outcome using standardized validation tools, such as the Neck Disability Index. Other systems to report adverse events recommend that events related to the disease or disease progression be excluded from the adverse events analysis.[19] Pain and other unre-lated events led to adverse event rates of up to 85%. In contrast, peer-reviewed publications are very diverse in recording and the reporting adverse events because some authors entirely ignore the events, whereas others include details similar to those reported in FDA summaries.

Mirza et al[20] identified important factors associated with the risk of adverse events in spine surgery, including demographics, medical comorbidities, severity of disease, and the intensity of treatment. To accurately quantify the risk and the effect of adverse events, a definition of these events needs to be established, the severity graded, and the timing of the events reported. The establishment of etiology and whether an adverse event is preventable should be incorporated into the definition so that quality improvement measures can ensue.

Quantification of the factors associated with adverse event risk is difficult, and there is little consistency in current practice. In the case of RCTs, proper randomization theoretically eliminates confounding caused by variables such as the intensity of treatment, medical comorbidities, and demographics. The effect of such variables can be established by using proper risk stratification techniques. Quantification of medical comorbidities is important to allow risk stratification and, in spinal research, is most commonly performed using the Charl-

Table 4
Adverse Event Type From Summary of Safety and Effectiveness Data

	Prestige ST		ProDisc-C		Bryan		Secure C		PCM	
	ACDF	TDR	ACDF	TDR	ACDF	TDR	ACDF	TDR	ACDF	TDR
Number	265	276	106	103	221	242	144	236	190	214
Medical Events										
Respiratory	2	3	NR	NR	4	4	NR	NR	0	3
Cardiac	2	2	1	0	1	0	1	1	3	4
Gastrointestinal	5	6	4	6	3	2	1	0	3	3
Genitourinary	0	0	0	1	0	0	0	0	3	3
Infection (nonwound)	7	10	1	0	5	2	1	0	5	3
Cancer	2	5	NR	NR	0	2	0	4	1[a]	NR
Death	3	0	3	2	1	0	1	1	1[a]	NR
Surgery-Related Events										
Dysphagia/dysphonia	21	18	4	2	19	28	9	4	11	13
Wound (superficial)	0	0	1	0	1	7	2	0	3	11
Wound (deep)	0	0	0	0	0	0	0	0	1	1
Neurologic	15	24	9	9	14	13	4	5	2	6
Wound issue (noninfections)	NR	NR	2	0	NR	NR	4	0	NR	NR
Technical difficulties	0	1	NR	NR	1	1	NR	NR	NR	NR
Vascular (intraoperative)	5	2	NR	NR	NR	NR	NR	NR	NR	NR
Dural tear	NR	NR	0	1	NR	NR	NR	NR	NR	NR

[a]One cancer-related death caused by recurrence. The treatment group was not mentioned.
NR = not reported, ACDF = anterior cervical disk fusion, TDR = total disk replacement.

son index.[21] Adverse event risk is dependent on the severity of the disease. For example, the chance of neurologic deterioration is substantially different between patients with cervical radiculopathy and those with severe multilevel stenosis and myelopathy. The risk of adverse events correlates with the intensity of treatment, that is, how much surgery was performed.[22]

Reoperation is an important metric to quantify the economic valuation of treatments because costs increase with secondary surgeries. Cost-effectiveness is substantially affected by a procedure's durability (avoiding reoperations). Reoperation rates in the SSED reports varied, with significantly higher rates for groups treated with ACDF in three studies and similar rates in two reports.[4-7,18] A high Q value for this analysis demonstrates heterogeneity. Because all of the

ACDF patients were treated with allograft and plate fixation and inclusion-exclusion criteria were similar among the investigations, it is unknown why these differences exist. The reoperation rates are similar to published studies,[23,24] although they were higher than reported in the retrospective study of Singh et al.[25] The authors suggested that surgeon bias in RCTs may lead to the avoidance of secondary surgery in experimental groups and an elevation of rates in ACDF groups, although limited evidence for this effect has been presented.

The methods, description, and the reporting of adverse events in peer-reviewed publications were generally inadequate because of a lack of standardized definitions, insufficient descriptions of how adverse events were obtained, the absence of classification, and poor reporting techniques. Only

two of the nine studies were comprehensive, one of which provided a separate report on adverse events.[2,16]

These shortcomings prevent readers from obtaining an adequate understanding of the safety of new technologies such as TDR. This lack of transparency and standardization in reporting adverse events in peer-reviewed publications has been widely debated in the case of recombinant human bone morphogenetic protein-2 (rhBMP-2).[8] The differences between the peer-reviewed publications and SSED reports in the study of TDRs are nearly identical to those in the rhBMP-2 reports and studies. As previously noted, the SSED report methodology includes all potentially related adverse events; this large quantity of data makes it difficult to gauge a real understanding of absolute product safety. The need for such recording

Table 5
Reoperations

Study (Year)	Index Level ACDF (%)	Index Level TDR (%)	Adjacent Level ACDF (%)	Adjacent Level TDR (%)	Relative Risk of ACDF to TDR (95% CI)[a]
Peer-Reviewed Publications					
Porchet et al[16] (2004)	NR	NR	NR	NR	—
Mummaneni et al[13] (2007)	8.7	1.8	3.4	0.8	4.17 (1.96, 8.8.7)
Murrey et al[14] (2007)	8.5	1.9	NR	NR	4.37 (0.97, 19.75)
Nabhan et al[15] (2007)	NR	NR	NR	NR	—
Anderson et al[2] (2008)	3.2	2.9	3.2	2.5	1.18 (0.57, 2.45)
Heller et al[12] (2009)	3.6	2.5	NR	NR	
Cheng et al[10] (2009)	NR	NR	NR	NR	—
Cheng et al[9] (2011)	NR	NR	NR	NR	—
Coric et al[11] (2011)	5.3	4.4	5.3	6.6	0.95 (0.48, 1.90)
Zhang et al[17] (2012)	1.9	0	5.7	1.8	4.23 (0.99, 4.28)
Total[b]	6.2	2.3	3.9	2.7	2.06 (0.99, 4.28)
FDA Summaries (Device)					
SSED[6] (Prestige ST)	9.1	3.3	NR	NR	2.78 (1.32, 5.86)
SSED[7] (ProDisc-C)	9.4	1.9	NR	NR	4.86 (1.09, 21.64)
SSED[5] (Bryan)	3.6	2.5	4.1	3.3	1.33 (0.67, 2.63)
SSED[4] (Secure C)	9.7	2.5	2.1	1.7	2.79 (1.31, 5.92)
SSED[18] (PCM)	7.4	8.7	NR	NR	0.85 (0.45, 1.60)
Total	8.9	3.3	3.3	2.7	1.87 (1.06, 3.3)

[a]Relative risk was calculated based on all reoperations, including index and adjacent level procedures.
[b]The study by Anderson was excluded from totals at the index level because it is duplicative of the study by Heller et al.[12]
CI = confidence interval, NR = not reported, SSED = summary of safety and effectiveness data, ACDF = anterior cervical disk fusion, TDR = total disk replacement.

procedures in pharmaceutical studies is different than in medical device studies, and this difference may have affected how authors in the rhBMP-2 trials reported adverse events in peer-reviewed publications. Despite this limitation, comparison with a control group is possible. In TDR procedures, many of the adverse events in SSED reports appear unrelated to the surgery or the device.

Recommendations of This Chapter's Authors

To improve understanding of adverse events in clinical investigations, studies reporting clinical outcomes should also analyze adverse events. This recommendation should be considered by journal editors during the peer-review process. In high-level studies, such as quality RCTs or studies reporting new technologies, a separate publication discussing only the adverse events would allow proper transparency. Two of the TDR trials used an independent safety board called a clinical event committee, which determined the seriousness of adverse events and judged their relationship to the device or surgery. A separate publication written by this type of committee (independent of the principal investigators and industry sponsor) would substantially improve transparency in adverse event reporting. There is a clear need for the development and adoption of validated, quantitative measures to deter-mine the effect and incidence of adverse events.

Documentation of Adverse Events

Important attributes regarding adverse events are type, timing, severity, whether they are preventable, etiology, and their effect on costs or the length of hospitalization. To evaluate the mortality and the morbidity of spinal surgery, Street et al[26] used the Spine Adverse Event Severity (SAVES) system to document the occurrence of an adverse event at the time of surgery, discharge, or later. This validated questionnaire documents the type, severity, and timing of the adverse event and the estimated effect of the event on the length of hospital stay. The questionnaire is not time consuming, has good reliability characteristics, and is available in both a paper and an electronic form. Street et al[26] concluded that a hospital database and self-reporting greatly underestimate the complexity of spine surgery compared with a prospective systematic approach, such as the SAVES system.

National and international efforts have produced paradigms to document adverse events in clinical trials. The purpose of the Consolidated Standards of Reporting Trials (CONSORT) initiative is to standardize methods used to report clinical trials, facilitate completeness and transparency in reporting, and aid in critical appraisal and interpretation. In 1996, CONSORT developed a checklist when reporting RCTs but later noted that harm was inadequately assessed.[27] By group consensus, 10 recommendations regarding adverse events were added to the checklist. The CONSORT recommendations are similar to the measures used to assess the quality of methods and reporting of adverse events described in this chapter and are the best method currently available in the opinion of this chapter's authors.

The National Cancer Institute and the World Health Organization have produced guidance documents for reporting harm in oncologic clinical trials; these guidelines can be modified for use in orthopaedic surgery trials.[19,28] The guidelines are comprehensive and include definitions, severity ratings, and recommendations on assessing and grading adverse events and provide criteria for the attribution of adverse events. These two systems are similar to those used in the SSED reports but require substantial resources. With modification, they would be an excellent pathway for reporting adverse events in clinical trials of medical devices.

Summary

Adverse events occur at similar rates in cervical TDR and ACDF. Reoperations rates may be greater in short-term follow-up after fusion, although the results are heterogeneous. Both procedures appear safe and have a low incidence of serious adverse events or significant neurologic injury. Because peer-reviewed publications lack adequate consistency in reporting adverse events, the importance of any conclusions presented in these reports is diminished. The SSED reports of the FDA are comprehensive and an excellent repository of data, but they are difficult to use in clinical applications and for drawing conclusions. Going forward, improvements in methods to collect, assess, and report adverse events are needed. Despite differences in methodology, it does not appear that clinically significant omissions or errors in peer-reviewed publications regarding cervical TDR have occurred.

References

1. Guidance for Industry and/or FDA Staff: Guidance Document for the Preparation of IDEs for Spinal Systems. Document issued on January 13, 2000. US Food and Drug Administration website. http://www.fda.gov/Medical Devices/DeviceRegulation andGuidance/Guidance Documents/ucm073771.htm. Accessed August 28, 2013.

2. Anderson PA, Sasso RC, Riew KD: Comparison of adverse events between the Bryan artificial cervical disc and anterior cervical arthrodesis. *Spine (Phila Pa 1976)* 2008;33(12):1305-1312.

3. Geisler FH, Blumenthal SL, Guyer RD, et al: Neurological complications of lumbar artificial disc replacement and comparison of clinical results with those related to lumbar arthrodesis in the literature: Results of a multicenter, prospective, randomized investigational device exemption study of Charité intervertebral disc. Invited submission from the Joint Section Meeting on Disorders of the Spine and Peripheral Nerves, March 2004. *J Neurosurg Spine* 2004; 1(2):143-154.

4. SECURE®-C Artificial Cervical Disc: P100003. Updated: October 2, 2013. US Food and Drug Administration website. http:// www.accessdata.fda.gov/scripts/ cdrh/cfdocs/cftopic/pma/ pma.cfm?num=p100003. Accessed August 28, 2013.

5. BRYAN® Cervical Disc: P060023. Updated May 27, 2009. US Food and Drug Administration website. http:// www.accessdata.fda.gov/scripts/ cdrh/cfdocs/cfTopic/pma/ pma.cfm?num=P060023. Accessed August 28, 2013.

6. PRESTIGE® Cervical Disc System: P060018. Updated: July 20, 2007. US Food and Drug Administration website. http:// www.accessdata.fda.gov/scripts/ cdrh/cfdocs/cfTopic/pma/ pma.cfm?num=P060018. Accessed August 28, 2013.

7. ProDisc™-C Total Disc Replacement: P070001. Updated: January 10, 2008. US Food and Drug Administration website. http:// www.accessdata.fda.gov/scripts/ cdrh/cfdocs/cftopic/pma/ pma.cfm?num=p070001. Accessed August 28, 2013.

8. Carragee EJ, Hurwitz EL, Weiner BK: A critical review of recombinant human bone morphogenetic protein-2 trials in spinal surgery: Emerging safety concerns and lessons learned. *Spine J* 2011; 11(6):471-491.

9. Cheng L, Nie L, Li M, Huo Y, Pan X: Superiority of the Bryan(®) disc prosthesis for cervical myelopathy: A randomized study with 3-year followup. *Clin Orthop Relat Res* 2011;469(12): 3408-3414.

10. Cheng L, Nie L, Zhang L, Hou Y: Fusion versus Bryan Cervical Disc in two-level cervical disc disease: A prospective, randomised study. *Int Orthop* 2009;33(5):1347-1351.

11. Coric D, Nunley PD, Guyer RD, et al: 269 patients from the Kineflex/C artificial disc investigational device exemption study with a minimum 2-year follow-up. Clinical article. *J Neurosurg Spine* 2011;15(4):348-358.

12. Heller JG, Sasso RC, Papadopoulos SM, et al: Comparison of BRYAN cervical disc arthroplasty with anterior cervical decompression and fusion: Clinical and radiographic results of a randomized, controlled, clinical trial. *Spine (Phila Pa 1976)* 2009;34(2):101-107.

13. Mummaneni PV, Burkus JK, Haid RW, Traynelis VC, Zdeblick TA: Clinical and radiographic analysis of cervical disc arthroplasty compared with allograft fusion: A randomized controlled clinical trial. *J Neurosurg Spine* 2007;6(3):198-209.

14. Murrey D, Janssen M, Delamarter R, et al: Results of the prospective, randomized, controlled multicenter Food and Drug Administration investigational device exemption study of the ProDisc-C total disc replacement versus anterior discectomy and fusion for the treatment of 1-level symptomatic cervical disc disease. *Spine J* 2009;9(4):275-286.

15. Nabhan A, Ahlhelm F, Pitzen T, et al: A prospective randomised and controlled radiographic and clinical study. *Eur Spine J* 2007;16(3):423-430.

16. Porchet F, Metcalf NH: Clinical outcomes with the Prestige II cervical disc: Preliminary results from a prospective randomized clinical trial. *Neurosurg Focus* 2004;17(3):E6.

17. Zhang X, Zhang X, Chen C, et al: Randomized, controlled, multicenter, clinical trial comparing BRYAN cervical disc arthroplasty with anterior cervical decompression and fusion in China. *Spine (Phila Pa 1976)* 2012;37(6):433-438.

18. PCM Cervical Disc System: P100012. Updated: November 8, 2012. US Food and Drug Administration website. http://www.accessdata.fda.gov/scripts/cdrh/cfdocs/cfTopic/pma/pma.cfm?num=P100012. Accessed August 28, 2013.

19. Protocol development: Common terminology criteria for adverse events (CTCAE). Updated: March 20, 2013. National Cancer Institute website. http://ctep.cancer.gov/protocolDevelopment/electronic_applications/ctc.htm. Accessed August 28, 2013.

20. Mirza SK, Deyo RA, Heagerty PJ, Turner JA, Lee LA, Goodkin R: Towards standardized measurement of adverse events in spine surgery: Conceptual model and pilot evaluation. *BMC Musculoskelet Disord* 2006;7:53.

21. Chitale R, Campbell PG, Yadla S, Whitmore RG, Maltenfort MG, Ratliff JK: International classification of disease clinical modification 9 modeling of a patient comorbidity score predicts incidence of perioperative complications in a nationwide inpatient sample assessment of complications in spine surgery. [Published online ahead of print September 6, 2012.] *J Spinal Disord Tech*. PMID: 22960417.

22. Cizik AM, Lee MJ, Martin BI, et al: Using the spine surgical invasiveness index to identify risk of surgical site infection: A multivariate analysis. *J Bone Joint Surg Am* 2012;94(4):335-342.

23. Saarinen T, Niemelä M, Kivisaari R, Pitkäniemi J, Pohjola J, Hernesniemi J: Early and late re-operation after anterior cervical decompression and fusion during an 11-year follow-up. *Acta Neurochir (Wien)* 2013;155:285-289.

24. Goffin J, Geusens E, Vantomme N, et al: Long-term follow-up after interbody fusion of the cervical spine. *J Spinal Disord Tech* 2004;17:79-85.

25. Singh K, Phillips FM, Park DK, Pelton MA, An HS, Goldberg EJ: Factors affecting reoperations after anterior cervical discectomy and fusion within and outside of a Federal Drug Administration investigational device exemption cervical disc replacement trial. *Spine J* 2012;12(5):372-378.

26. Street JT, Lenehan BJ, DiPaola CP: Morbidity and mortality of major adult spinal surgery: A prospective cohort analysis of 942 consecutive patients. *Spine J* 2012;12(1):22-24.

27. Ioannidis JP, Evans SJ, Gøtzsche PC, et al: Better reporting of harms in randomized trials: An extension of the CONSORT statement. *Ann Intern Med* 2004;141(10):781-788.

28. Chronic and late toxic effects, in *WHO Handbook for Reporting Results of Cancer Treatment: Geneva Switzerland.* 1979, p. 15. http://whqlibdoc.who.int/offset/WHO_OFFSET_48.pdf. Accessed August 28, 2013.

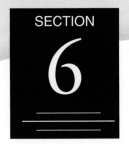

Pediatrics

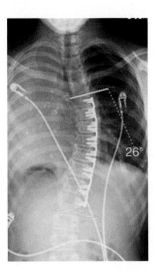

Fundamental Concepts of Developmental Dysplasia of the Hip

Stuart L. Weinstein, MD
Scott J. Mubarak, MD
Dennis R. Wenger, MD

Abstract

To provide the best possible care to patients with developmental dysplasia of the hip, it is helpful to understand the normal growth and development of the hip joint; the pathoanatomy, epidemiology, and diagnosis of the condition; and the natural history of a missed diagnosis of dislocation, subluxation, and dysplasia.

Instr Course Lect 2014;63:299-305.

A basic understanding of the normal growth and development of the hip joint, the pathoanatomy of developmental dysplasia of the hip (DDH) and dislocation, and the natural history of the spectrum of the condition is essential information for any physician making treatment decisions in children with DDH.

Normal Growth and Development of the Hip

The components of the hip joint—the femoral head and the acetabulum—develop from the same primitive mesenchymal cells. For normal hip joint growth and development to occur, there must be a balance of growth of the acetabular and triradiate cartilages (probably genetically determined) and a well-located and centered femoral head. Around the seventh intrauterine week of life, a cleft develops, defining the future femoral head and the acetabulum. The hip joint is fully formed by the 11th intrauterine week. This is the first time at which dislocation can occur.[1]

At birth, the proximal end of the femur has a single chondroepiphysis. The proximal femoral ossification center appears between the fourth and

seventh months of life. This bony centrum continues to enlarge, along with its cartilaginous anlage until adult life, when only a thin layer of articular cartilage remains. The proximal femur and the trochanter enlarge by appositional cartilage-cell proliferation.[2] The three main growth areas in the proximal femur are the physeal plate, the femoral neck isthmus, and the growth plate of the greater trochanter (**Figure 1**). It is the normal growth of these three physes that determine the shape of the adult proximal femur. Disturbances in growth in any of these three growth plates alter the shape of the proximal femur. The growth of the proximal femur is also affected by muscle pull, the forces transmitted across the hip joint by weight bearing, normal joint nutrition, circulation, and muscle tone.[3,4] Profound changes in the development of the proximal femur may occur with any alterations in these factors.[5] The proximal femoral physeal plate contributes approximately 30% of the growth of the overall length of the femur. Any disruption to the blood supply or damage to the proximal physeal plate results in a varus deformity caused by the contin-

Dr. Mubarak or an immediate family member has stock or stock options held in Rhino Pediatric Orthopedic Designs. Dr. Wenger or an immediate family member serves as a paid consultant to or is an employee of OrthoPediatrics and has stock or stock options held in Rhino Pediatric Orthopedic Designs. Neither Dr. Weinstein nor any immediate family member has received anything of value from or has stock or stock options held in a commercial company or institution related directly or indirectly to the subject of this chapter.

The material in this chapter is reprinted with minor changes from Weinsein SL, Mubarak SJ, Wenger DR: Developmental hip dysplasia and dislocation: Part I. Instr Course Lect 2004;53:523-530.

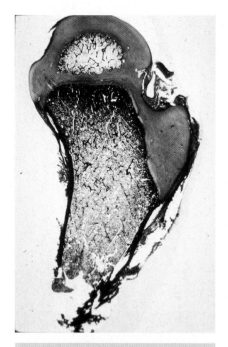

Figure 1 The proximal femur of the infant has three physeal plates: the growth plate of the greater trochanter, the proximal femoral physeal plate, and the growth plate of the femoral neck isthmus connecting the other two plates. (Reproduced with permission from Weinstein SL: Developmental hip dysplasia and dislocation, in Morrissy RT, Weinstein SL, eds: *Lovell and Winter's Pediatric Orthopaedics,* ed 5. Philadelphia, PA, Lippincott Williams and Wilkins, 2001, vol 2, pp 905-956.)

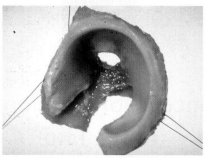

Figure 2 Lateral view of the normal acetabular cartilage complex of a 1-day-old infant show the cup-shaped acetabulum. The ilium, ischium, and pubis have been removed with a curet. (Reproduced from Ponseti IV: Growth and development of the acetabulum in the normal child: Anatomic, histological, and radiographic studies. *J Bone Joint Surg Am* 1978;60(5): 586-599.)

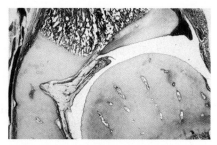

Figure 3 Coronal section through the center of the acetabulum in a full-term infant. Note the fibrocartilaginous edge of the acetabulum, the labrum, at the peripheral edge of the acetabular cartilage. The hip capsule inserts just above the labrum. (Reproduced with permission from Weinstein SL: Developmental hip dysplasia and dislocation, in Morrissy RT, Weinstein SL, eds: *Lovell and Winter's Pediatric Orthopaedics,* ed 5. Philadelphia, PA, Lippincott Williams and Wilkins, 2001, vol 2, pp 905-956.)

ued growth of the trochanter and the growth plate along the femoral neck.[6] Partial physeal arrest patterns may be caused by damage to portions of the proximal femoral physeal plate.

With respect to acetabular development, the acetabular cartilage complex is a three-dimensional structure, which is interposed between the ilium above, the ischium below, and the pubis in front.[7] The outer two thirds of the complex is called the acetabular cartilage; the medial one third, which is composed of a portion of the ilium, portions of the triradiate cartilage, and a portion of the ischium, is referred to as the nonarticular medial wall (**Fig-**

ure 2). Acetabular cartilage is very cellular hyaline cartilage. Articular cartilage covers the acetabular cartilage on the side that articulates with the femoral head; on the opposite side is a growth plate with its degenerating cells facing toward the ilium. The lateral portion of the acetabular cartilage is homologous with other epiphyseal cartilages of the skeleton. The fibrocartilaginous structure known as the labrum is located at the periphery of the acetabular cartilage. The capsule inserts just above the labrum (**Figure 3**).

The triradiate cartilage is the conjoined physeal plate of the three pelvic bones. Each side of each limb of the triradiate cartilage has a growth plate. Interstitial growth in the triradiate cartilage causes the acetabulum to expand during growth, determining the acetabular diameter. Differential rates of growth of the triradiate cartilage have been defined.[8]

It has been shown that the development of the acetabulum depends on the geometric pattern within during growth.[9] The concave shape of the hip

joint is determined by the presence of a spheric femoral head. This principle is important to remember because it is a predictor of acetabular shape in the dislocated hip or in the hip with injury to the proximal femoral growth centers resulting in deformity. Along with the presence of a spheric femoral head, acetabular depth is determined by several factors, including interstitial growth within the acetabular cartilage, appositional growth under the perichondrium, and the growth of adjacent bones (the ilium, the ischium, and the pubis). Because most of the shape of the acetabulum is developed by the age of 8 years, this is the watershed age for prognosis in many pediatric hip disorders. Other influencing factors include sex and skeletal maturity. Acetabular depth is further enhanced during the adolescent growth spurt by the development of three secondary ossification centers: the acetabular epiphysis, which is the secondary center of ossification of the ilium; the os acetabulum, which is the secondary ossification center of the pubis; and the unnamed, secondary ossification center of the ischium. Surgical interventions at the periphery of the acetabulum in the area of the groove of Ranvier or in the area of the development of the secondary centers of ossification have a profound potential to cause growth disturbances leading to dysplasia in adulthood.[10]

At maturity, it is ideal to have normal architecture radiographically, including a well-developed teardrop and intact Shenton line, a downsloping sourcil, and a Gothic arch (**Figure 4**).

Pathoanatomy of DDH

In the normal hip at birth, there is a tight fit between the femoral head and the acetabulum. The femoral head is held in the acetabulum by the surface tension created by the synovial fluid. In postmortem specimens, even after the capsule is sectioned, it is very difficult to dislocate a normal hip in an infant. In children with DDH, the tight fit is lost, and the femoral head can be made to glide into and out of the acetabulum with a palpable sensation (the Ortolani sign).[7,11,12]

In patients with DDH, most abnormalities are on the acetabular side. Femoral side changes are secondary to anteversion and pressure changes on the head from the acetabulum or ilium associated with subluxation or dislocation. With growth and development, acetabular growth is affected by the primary disease (abnormal acetabular cartilage either primary or secondary to pressure changes from the femoral head and neck) and any growth alterations incurred from secondary acetabular procedures. Proximal femoral anatomic abnormalities are generally secondary to growth disturbances resulting from treatment.

At birth, DDH pathology varies from mild capsular laxity to severe dysplastic changes.[13] The typical dysplastic hip will have a ridge in the superior

posterior and inferior aspect of the acetabulum. This ridge or neolimbus is composed of very cellular hyaline cartilage.[13] The femoral head glides in and out over this acetabular ridge to produce the palpable sensation known as the Ortolani sign. In most neonates with DDH, the labrum is everted. There is empiric evidence that these pathologic changes are reversible.

Epidemiology and Diagnosis

The etiology of DDH is multifactorial and includes both genetic and intrauterine environmental factors. DDH is detected at birth in most patients; however, despite newborn screening programs, some cases are missed.[14,15] Risk factors for DDH include any combination of the following factors: breech delivery, oligohydramnios, female sex, first born, positive family history or ethnic background (for example, Native American heritage), persistent hip asymmetry (for example, abducted hip on one side, adducted hip on the other), torticollis, and lower limb deformity.[10]

The terminology in DDH is somewhat confusing. The term dysplasia is used to describe a child with a positive Ortolani sign (the hip that can be provoked to dislocate or the hip is dislocated and can be relocated in the acetabulum). The term dislocation describes the presence of a negative Ortolani sign in a child who has secondary adaptive changes of shortening, decreased abduction and asymmetry of the folds, and a hip that cannot be reduced.

The Barlow maneuver is often referred to as the "click of exit" test. In this provocative maneuver, the hip is flexed and adducted, and the femoral head is palpated to exit the acetabulum partially or completely over a ridge of the acetabulum.[16] Many physicians refer to the Ortolani sign as the "click of entry," which is caused when the hip is

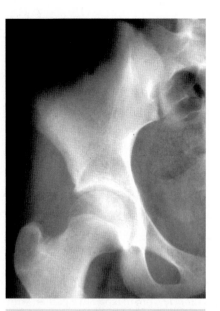

Figure 4 The ideal normal radiographic appearance of the hip at maturity is shown. Note the intact Shenton line (the continuous arch described by the obturator foramen and the femoral neck), a well-developed teardrop figure (the medial floor of the acetabulum), a downsloping sourcil (French for eyebrow [the radiodense arc of the acetabulum above the femoral head]), and well-developed Gothic arch (the two groups of trabeculae at the edge of the sourcil. The lateral one extends craniomedially, and the medial one extends craniolaterally. They meet above the sourcil to form an arch).

abducted, the trochanter is elevated, and the femoral head glides back into the acetabulum. Some physicians make treatment decisions on the basis of whether they believe the hip is Ortolani positive versus Barlow positive; it is thought that the Barlow-positive hip is more stable. In many centers, these classic diagnostic tests have been replaced by ultrasonography, which is used routinely in Europe but is rarely used as a screening tool in the United States.

If the diagnosis of DDH is missed at birth, the natural history of the disorder can follow one of four scenarios: the hip can become normal, it can go on to subluxation or partial contact, it can go on to complete dislocation, or the hip can remain located but retain dysplastic features.[17,18] Because the outcome of DDH cannot be predicted in the newborn, and because in the hands of experienced physicians the complications of treatment with a device such as a Pavlik harness are quite low, all newborn hip instability is treated to ensure the highest rate of normal outcomes.

If the diagnosis of DDH is not made in the newborn, the obstacles to reduction are different, treatment carries greater risks, and the results are considerably less predictable. In a patient with a late diagnosis of DDH, the physical findings include limb shortening; asymmetry of the gluteal, thigh, or labial folds; apparent shortening of the femur (Galeazzi sign); and limited hip abduction, the most reliable late diagnostic sign. In patients with bilateral DDH, the child may have a waddling gait and hyperlordosis.[10]

If DDH is diagnosed late, the extra-articular obstacles to reduction include the adductor longus and the iliopsoas. The intra-articular obstacles to reduction, in order of increasing importance are the anteromedial joint capsule, the ligamentum teres, the transverse acetabular ligament, and the neolimbus (which is rarely an obstacle to reduction).[19] With increasing age at detection (particularly in patients older than 6 months), the obstacles to reduction become increasingly difficult to overcome by nonsurgical methods, and restoration of normal acetabular development is less likely.[20-22]

Much of the older literature describes the limbus as an obstacle to reduction. A true limbus is a pathologic structure.[23] This chapter's authors believe that a true limbus occurs only in antenatal teratologic dislocations or after a failed closed reduction in which the tissue was forced into the acetabu-

lum.[13,24] This is an important distinction because the peripheral acetabular tissue in DDH may ossify differently from that in a normal patient. Accessory centers of ossification in the periphery of the acetabular cartilage may appear in up to two thirds of patients with DDH and may appear up to 2 to 3 years after reduction.[13,25-27] These accessory centers rarely occur in patients with normal hips (3.5%) and are rare before the age of 11 years. Patients with closed or open treatment for DDH should be evaluated for these centers of ossification because they must be taken into consideration when assessing acetabular development. These accessory centers of ossification are probably the result of damage to the peripheral acetabular cartilage that occurs secondary to pressure from the dislocated femoral head and/or neck pushing against the peripheral acetabular cartilage. This peripheral acetabular tissue or so-called neolimbus is never an obstacle to reduction and should never be excised.[19,28] Excision will lead to acetabular dysplasia. The apparent acetabular dysplasia in DDH is not truly a deficiency but a failure of ossification of the acetabulum. In young patients, this deficiency is usually anterior; however, in older patients with DDH, the deficiency may be anterior, posterior, or global.[29]

The ligamentum teres may be an obstacle to reduction because of its shear bulk and may require removal to obtain a reduction. The transverse acetabular ligament hypertrophies and narrows the inferior aspect of the acetabulum, thus making reduction difficult without excision. The most important intra-articular obstacle to reduction is the anteromedial joint capsule, which is markedly thickened in dislocated hips and becomes an increasingly severe obstacle to overcome the longer the hip is remains dislocated.[10,19]

Natural History in Untreated Patients

The natural history of untreated complete hip dislocations depends on two factors: bilaterality and the development or lack of development of a false acetabulum.[20,30] In bilateral, untreated, high dislocations without a false acetabulum, patients have good range of motion and no pain. Hyperlordosis and low back pain develop over time. If the complete dislocation articulates with the ilium and there is a false acetabulum, secondary degenerative arthritis will develop in the false acetabulum. In the unilateral untreated complete dislocation, the symptoms of pain are associated with the development or lack of development of a false acetabulum. Other associated problems include ipsilateral valgus knee deformity, with attenuation of the medial collateral ligament; lateral knee compartment degenerative changes; significant limb-length inequalities (up to 10 cm); gait disturbances; and secondary scoliosis.

It is necessary to define terms when discussing the natural history of dysplasia and subluxation in untreated adults. Dysplasia has an anatomic definition, which is inadequate development of the femoral head, the acetabulum, or both. The radiographic definition is determined by the presence or absence of an intact Shenton line. Radiographically, a patient with dysplasia has anatomic abnormalities of the femoral head and/or acetabulum (anatomic dysplasia) with an intact Shenton line. Radiographically, a patient with subluxation has anatomic abnormalities of the femoral head and/or acetabulum (anatomic dysplasia) and a disrupted Shenton line. The natural history of hip subluxation is clear; degenerative joint disease will develop in all patients, usually in the third to fourth decade of life. The nat-

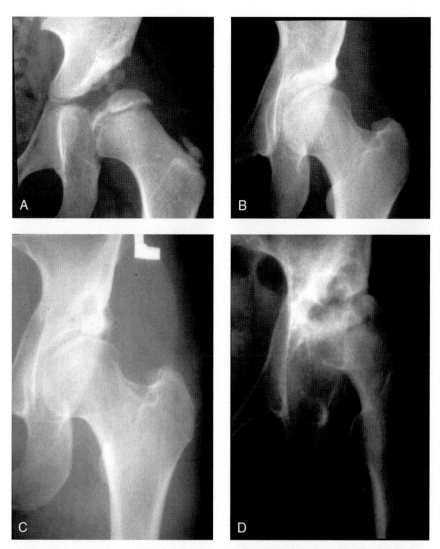

Figure 5 AP radiographs made after closed reduction of developmental dislocation of the hip that had been performed when the patient was 2 years and 4 months of age. **A,** Thirty-nine months after reduction, when the patient was 5 years and 7 months of age, the accessory centers of ossification are visible in the acetabular cartilage. **B,** Fifteen years after reduction, when the patient was 17 years of age, the Shenton line is intact, and there is mild acetabular dysplasia. **C,** Forty-two years after reduction, when the patient was 44 years of age, degenerative changes are present. **D,** Fifty-one years after reduction, when the patient was 53 years of age, the hip is subluxated and has severe degenerative changes (Iowa Hip Rating, 48 of 100 points). The patient subsequently underwent total hip replacement. (Reproduced with permission from Malvitz TA, Weinstein SL: Closed reduction for congenital dysplasia of the hip: Functional and radiographic results after an average of thirty years. *J Bone Joint Surg Am* 1994;76:1777-1792.)

ural history of untreated adults with dysplasia is more difficult to predict because the physical signs are usually lacking and patients present with dysplasia only as an incidental finding on radiographs or if they have symptoms.

However, there is good evidence that dysplasia, particularly in females, leads to degenerative joint disease in adults.[31-33]

The information on the natural history of dysplasia and subluxation in

untreated adults can be extrapolated to residual dysplasia and subluxation after treatment. In a study of 152 hips treated with closed reduction and followed for 31 years, the authors reported that the number of subluxations increased over time as dysplastic hips went on to subluxation and degenerative joint disease developed[22] (**Figure 5**).

The cause of degenerative changes in dysplastic hips is probably mechanical in nature and related to increased contact stress over time. There is a clear association between excessive contact stress and late degenerative joint diseases in other mechanical disorders, such as genu varum and genu valgum. This same correlation occurs in dysplastic hips with relation to the development of degenerative joint disease at long-term follow-up.[34,35]

The principles in the treatment of DDH include obtaining a reduction and maintaining that reduction to provide an optimum environment for acetabular and femoral head development. Intervention must be considered to alter an adverse natural history and treat residual subluxation and/or dysplasia. The only assurance of a normal hip in adult life is detection of DDH at birth.

Summary

Understanding normal hip joint growth and development, along with the pathoanatomy of DDH and its epidemiology, diagnosis, and natural history without treatment, are essential for making sound treatment decisions in children with DDH.

References

1. Watanabe RS: Embryology of the human hip. *Clin Orthop Relat Res* 1974;98:8-26.

2. Siffert RS: Patterns of deformity of the developing hip. *Clin Orthop Relat Res* 1981;160:14-29.

3. Gage JR, Cary JM: The effects of trochanteric epiphyseodesis on growth of the proximal end of the femur following necrosis of the capital femoral epiphysis. *J Bone Joint Surg Am* 1980;62(5): 785-794.

4. Osborne D, Effmann E, Broda K, Harrelson J: The development of the upper end of the femur, with special reference to its internal architecture. *Radiology* 1980; 137(1, pt 1):71-76.

5. Strayer LM: The embryology of the human hip joint. *Yale J Biol Med* 1943;16(1):13, 6.

6. Iwersen LJ, Kalen V, Eberle C: Relative trochanteric overgrowth after ischemic necrosis in congenital dislocation of the hip. *J Pediatr Orthop* 1989;9(4):381-385.

7. Ponseti IV: Growth and development of the acetabulum in the normal child: Anatomical, histological, and roentgenographic studies. *J Bone Joint Surg Am* 1978;60(5):575-585.

8. Portinaro NM, Murray DW, Benson MK: Microanatomy of the acetabular cavity and its relation to growth. *J Bone Joint Surg Br* 2001;83(3):377-383.

9. Coleman CR, Slager RF, Smith WS: The effect of environmental influence on acetabular development. *Surg Forum* 1958;9: 775-780.

10. Weinstein SL: *Lovell and Winter's Pediatric Orthopaedics,* ed 5. Philadelphia, PA, Lippincott Williams & Wilkins, 2001, pp 905-956.

11. Ortolani M: Congenital hip dysplasia in the light of early and very early diagnosis. *Clin Orthop Relat Res* 1976;119:6-10.

12. LeDamany P: *Etudes d'anatomie comparee d'anthropogenie normale et pathologique, deductions therapeutique.* Paris: Feliz Alcan, 1912.

13. Ponseti IV: Morphology of the acetabulum in congenital dislocation of the hip: Gross, histological and roentgenographic studies. *J Bone Joint Surg Am* 1978;60(5): 586-599.

14. Hadlow V: Neonatal screening for congenital dislocation of the hip: A prospective 21-year survey. *J Bone Joint Surg Br* 1988;70(5): 740-743.

15. Hansson G, Nachemson A, Palmén K: Screening of children with congenital dislocation of the hip joint on the maternity wards in Sweden. *J Pediatr Orthop* 1983; 3(3):271-279.

16. Barlow TG: Early diagnosis and treatment of congenital dislocation of the hip. *J Bone Joint Surg Br* 1962;44:292-301.

17. Coleman SS: Congenital dysplasia of the hip in the Navajo infant. *Clin Orthop Relat Res* 1968;56: 179-193.

18. Yamamuro T, Doi H: Diagnosis and treatment of congenital dislocation of the hip in newborns. *J Jpn Orthop Assoc* 1965;39:492.

19. Ishii Y, Weinstein SL, Ponseti IV: Correlation between arthrograms and operative findings in congenital dislocation of the hip. *Clin Orthop Relat Res* 1980;153: 138-145.

20. Weinstein SL: Natural history of congenital hip dislocation (CDH) and hip dysplasia. *Clin Orthop Relat Res* 1987;225:62-76.

21. Weinstein SL: Congenital hip dislocation: Long-range problems, residual signs, and symptoms after successful treatment. *Clin Orthop Relat Res* 1992;281:69-74.

22. Malvitz TA, Weinstein SL: Closed reduction for congenital dysplasia of the hip: Functional and radiographic results after an average of thirty years. *J Bone Joint Surg Am* 1994;76(12):1777-1792.

23. Leveuf J: Results of open reduction of true congenital luxation of the hip. *J Bone Joint Surg Am* 1948;30(4):875-882.

24. Weinstein SL, Ponseti IV: Congenital dislocation of the hip. *J Bone Joint Surg Am* 1979;61(1): 119-124.

25. Harris NH, Lloyd-Roberts GC, Gallien R: Acetabular development in congenital dislocation of the hip: With special reference to the indications for acetabuloplasty and pelvic or femoral realignment osteotomy. *J Bone Joint Surg Br* 1975;57(1):46-52.

26. Lindstrom JR, Ponseti IV, Wenger DR: Acetabular development after reduction in congenital dislocation of the hip. *J Bone Joint Surg Am* 1979;61(1):112-118.

27. Harris NH: Acetabular growth potential in congenital dislocation of the hip and some factors upon which it may depend. *Clin Orthop Relat Res* 1976;119:99-106.

28. Morcuende JA, Meyer MD, Dolan LA, Weinstein SL: Long-term outcome after open reduction through an anteromedial approach for congenital dislocation of the hip. *J Bone Joint Surg Am* 1997;79(6):810-817.

29. Millis MB, Murphy SB: Use of computed tomographic reconstruction in planning osteotomies of the hip. *Clin Orthop Relat Res* 1992;274:154-159.

30. Wedge JH, Wasylenko MJ: The natural history of congenital dislocation of the hip: A critical review. *Clin Orthop Relat Res* 1978;137: 154-162.

31. Schwend RM, Pratt WB, Fultz J: Untreated acetabular dysplasia of the hip in the Navajo: A 34 year case series followup. *Clin Orthop Relat Res* 1999;364:108-116.

32. Cooperman DR, Wallensten R, Stulberg SD: Acetabular dysplasia in the adult. *Clin Orthop Relat Res* 1983;175:79-85.

33. Harris WH: Etiology of osteoarthritis of the hip. *Clin Orthop Relat Res* 1986;213:20-33.

34. Hadley NA, Brown TD, Weinstein SL: The effects of contact

pressure elevations and aseptic necrosis on the long-term outcome of congenital hip dislocation. *J Orthop Res* 1990;8(4): 504-513.

35. Maxian TA, Brown TD, Weinstein SL: Chronic stress tolerance levels for human articular cartilage: Two nonuniform contact models applied to long-term follow-up of CDH. *J Biomech* 1995;28(2):159-166.

Developmental Dysplasia of the Hip: Diagnosis and Management to 18 Months

Nicholas M.P. Clarke, ChM, DM, FRCS, FRCS Ed

Abstract

Developmental dysplasia of the hip represents a spectrum of disease ranging from transient neonatal instability to established dislocation. It is accepted that female sex, breech presentation, and family history are risk factors for the disease. Early diagnosis by clinical examination or ultrasound imaging is emphasized, with splint treatment ideally commencing by 6 weeks of age. Treatment using the Pavlik harness is successful in up to 90% of patients. Ultrasound imaging is the gold standard for monitoring a patient during harness wear. Failed splintage or late presentation usually necessitates surgical intervention depending on the patient's age and the severity of the hip dysplasia and displacement.

Instr Course Lect 2014;63:307-311.

Congenital dislocation of the hip is defined as a congenital deformation of the hip joint in which the head of the femur is (or may be) partially or completely displaced from the acetabulum. The definition embraces secondary hip joint dysplasia, regardless of the persistence of instability or dislocation. To more precisely describe the condition in neonates, a more recent term—developmental dysplasia of the hip (DDH)—has been adopted.

Epidemiology

The incidence of neonatal hip instability is as high as 20 cases per 1,000 live births, but it varies according to the

clinical and ultrasound criteria applied. In most patients, DDH resolves spontaneously during the first weeks of life. The incidence of established dislocation in an untreated population is 1 to 2 cases per 1,000 live births; however, there are considerable geographic and cultural variations.

DDH occurs five times more frequently in girls than boys, possibly because of the effects of the hormone relaxin on the hip joint. First-born infants are affected twice as often as younger siblings. Instability is more common in the left hip, which probably reflects the most common intrauterine positioning. DDH occurs bi-

laterally in up to 20% of patients. Breech presentation, which has been reported in up to 32% of children with DDH, is also a risk factor.[1] The condition is also associated with a family history of DDH, torticollis, oligohydramnios, and, possibly, foot abnormalities. More recently, a resurgence of swaddling of the hips in extension has been implicated as a causative factor. More information on the etiology of DDH is available in *Instructional Course Lectures, Volume 63*, chapter 27 (Fundamental Concepts of Development Dysplasia of the Hip).

Pathology

The hip is cartilaginous at birth, and the acetabulum has a thin cartilaginous lateral rim. The femoral head is a chondroepiphysis, with the ossification center normally appearing after coalescence of the cartilage canal vasculature at approximately 6 months of age (although the appearance of the ossification center is characteristically delayed in patients with DDH). Hip instability and/or displacement deform the posterosuperior acetabulum, and local thickening produces the limbus, which may impede reduction. Hourglass capsular constriction also can impede reduction. Contractions develop

Neither Dr. Clarke nor any immediate family member has received anything of value from or has stock or stock options held in a commercial company or institution related directly or indirectly to the subject of this chapter.

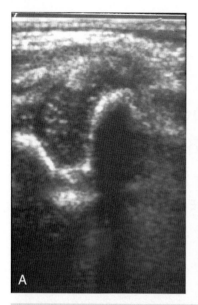
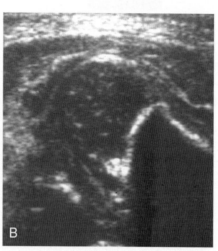

Figure 1 **A,** Static real-time ultrasonographic image of the hip joint of an infant. **B,** The femoral head is displaced with the application of transverse flexion stress. (Reproduced with permission from Clarke N, Castaneda P: Strategies to improve nonoperative childhood management. *Orthop Clin North Am* 2012;43[3]:281-289.)

in the adductors and psoas in the presence of dislocation. Persistent dislocation leads to abnormal acetabular development, a reduced depth-to-width ratio, and progressive obliquity. Inadequate femoral head coverage causes elevation and lateralization. The so-called teratologic dislocation is associated with syndromic or neurologic pathology and is excluded from this discussion.

Clinical Findings

Early diagnosis and treatment is critical in the management of DDH. All newborns should be clinically examined, with the Barlow maneuver and the Ortolani sign used in the evaluation. The Barlow maneuver is a provocative test that attempts to dislocate the hip by applying a gentle downward force. The Ortolani sign is positive if attempts to reduce a dislocated hip cause a palpable clunk. After the first few weeks of life, the tests are less sensitive because of the development of restriction of abduction and, in unilat-

eral presentations, limb-length asymmetry. Ultrasonography is also used in the diagnosis. After normal walking age, a limp or waddling gait is seen in patients with bilateral DDH.

Screening

Neonatal screening for DDH can be performed by clinical examination or ultrasonography,[2-6] although the need for screening remains controversial in the United States. Universal ultrasound screening is performed in some European countries, and selective ultrasound screening for at-risk infants is used in other countries. The current clinical practice guideline of the American Academy of Pediatrics recommends screening for hip dysplasia.[7] However, in 2006, the US Preventive Services Task Force concluded that "evidence is insufficient to recommend routine screening" because of a lack of clear scientific evidence.[8]

The result of the clinical examination is dependent on the examiner and is not 100% sensitive or specific.

Screening for DDH with ultrasonography was introduced in Austria by Graf,[9] who used angular measurements of static angles to classify the condition and dictate subsequent treatment. The incorporation of the real-time evaluation of stability during testing with a modified Barlow maneuver defines the dynamic method,[10] which may have a better correlation with clinical outcomes (**Figure 1**).

At the institution (Southampton General Hospital, England) of this chapter's author, a selective ultrasound screening protocol has been used for 20 years to detect DDH. Infants with clinically abnormal hips at birth undergo sonography at 2 weeks of age to allow transient instability to resolve. Infants with risk factors for DDH, such as breech presentation or family history, are examined at 6 weeks of age with ultrasonography. The results of this screening protocol have been confirmed by the program's efficacy and have been demonstrated by no false negative findings, a low treatment rate, and no instances of overtreatment (which can occur in some screening programs).[11]

Investigation

Radiographic imaging for hip dysplasia is useful only after the appearance of the proximal femoral ossific nucleus, which appears after 6 months of age. The acetabular index and the height of the dislocation are useful parameters. The center-edge angle of Wiberg can be used to evaluate older children. Dynamic arthrography is essential in the management of late presenting cases of hip dysplasia.

Management

The management of hip dysplasia is age dependant and can be divided into neonatal, early, and late groups.

Neonatal Management

Neonatal hip instability is ideally diagnosed early and treated appropriately. There is some debate about which clinically and sonographically abnormal hips should be treated and at what age. Because many hips have some degree of transient instability on ultrasonographic examination that corrects spontaneously, the neonate should be observed for 3 weeks without treatment. Observation is a permissible management approach for up to 6 weeks in patients with hip instability and subluxation and in those with sonographically detected acetabular growth retardation.

Treatment is indicated in hips that are clinically stable but at 6 weeks still have abnormal ultrasound findings. Treatment is also indicated for patients with a hip dislocation at birth. The use of an abduction device allows maintenance of hip location; the Pavlik harness has been established as the device of choice instead of rigid splints (**Figure 2**).

The Pavlik harness is used to treat hip instability in infants 2 to 6 weeks of age (preferably) and up to 3 months of age. Initially, the harness should be worn full time; a weaning program is commenced after the hip has been reduced for 6 weeks. Careful follow-up examinations with ultrasound monitoring and strap adjustment are mandatory. The success rate of harness treatment is 90%. Complications include femoral nerve palsy, which is caused by hip hyperflexion. Osteonecrosis is rare, with a reported incidence of less than 1%. After successful treatment, serial radiographic studies should continue for 5 years to monitor the acetabular index. Secondary surgical intervention is rare.[12] If ultrasound studies show that the hip is not responding to treatment within 3 weeks of application of the harness, the treatment should be discontinued, and the patient should undergo later assessment under anesthesia.

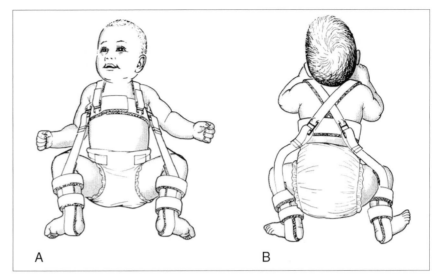

Figure 2   AP (**A**) and PA (**B**) illustrations of an infant in a Pavlik harness. (Courtesy of Southampton General Hospital, Southampton, UK.)

Early Management

Early management is instituted in patients between 3 and 18 months of age and includes patients who present late or in whom Pavlik harness treatment has failed. Surgical reduction is usually indicated. There is a correlation between residual dysplasia and the age at the time of reduction. To reduce the rate of osteonecrosis, some authors recommend that intervention should be delayed until the femoral ossification center appears, which coincides with mature anastomotic vascular circulation.[13]

Dynamic arthrography should be performed before attempting reduction in a patient at any age to establish whether the reduction is concentric or eccentric (requiring open reduction). Preoperative skin traction remains controversial, but it is often used. Adductor tenotomy increases the safe zone between full passive abduction and instability. Careful positioning in a hip spica cast is essential, with the use of the human position preferred to maintain the hips in 100° of flexion and controlled abduction. **Figure 3** illustrates the preferred treatment algorithm.

Most acetabular development is seen in the initial 6 months after closed reduction and continues for approximately 2 years; however, ultimately about 50% of all hips will require secondary surgery to address persistent dysplasia.[14]

Failure of closed reduction is synonymous with the need for open reduction, which is usually performed in patients older than 12 months. Staged procedures are used for patients with bilateral DDH. Several medial approaches have been described, but an anterior approach using a modified Smith-Petersen approach and a bikini incision is preferred. This approach allows excision and release of the constraining soft tissues without compromising the circumflex femoral vessels. The limbus should not be excised, but the hypertrophied adipose tissue (pulvinar) and ligamentum teres are excised. The transverse acetabular ligament is divided. Capsulorrhaphy, which is the critical step in maintaining hip reduction, is optimized through the anterior approach. Secure

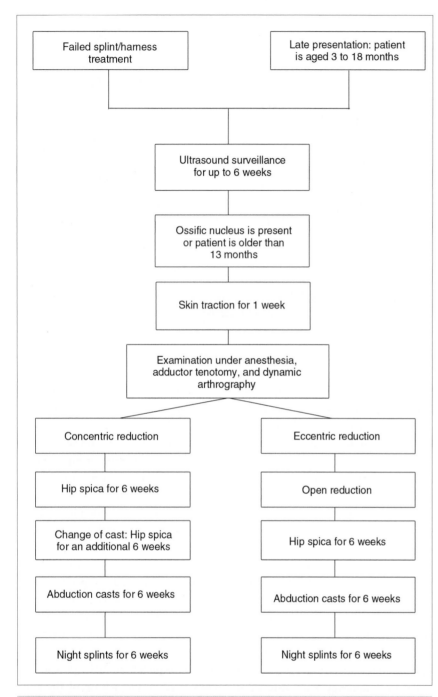

Figure 3 Algorithm used for the early management of infants with DDH or if splint/harness treatment has been unsuccessful.

tion on late treatment of DDH can be found in *Instructional Course Lectures, Volume 63,* chapter 30 (Diagnosis and Management of Developmental Dysplasia of the Hip from Triradiate Closure Through Young Adulthood).

Summary

DDH remains a substantial problem in terms of diagnosis and management. Early diagnosis allows simple treatment with a Pavlik harness, with a reported success rate of 90%. Screening for DDH with ultrasonography is becoming more prevalent. Late diagnosis of DDH necessitates surgical intervention, with careful anterior open reduction and capsulorrhaphy the key procedures.

References

1. Barlow TG: Early diagnosis and treatment of congenital dislocation of the hip. *Proc R Soc Med* 1963;56:804-806.

2. Sankar WN, Weiss J, Skaggs DL: Orthopaedic conditions in the newborn. *J Am Acad Orthop Surg* 2009;17(2):112-122.

3. Graf R: The diagnosis of congenital hip-joint dislocation by the ultrasonic Combound treatment. *Arch Orthop Trauma Surg* 1980; 97(2):117-133.

4. Graf R: Fundamentals of sonographic diagnosis of infant hip dysplasia. *J Pediatr Orthop* 1984; 4(6):735-740.

5. Boeree NR, Clarke NM: Ultrasound imaging and secondary screening for congenital dislocation of the hip. *J Bone Joint Surg Br* 1994;76(4):525-533.

6. Rosendahl K, Markestad T, Lie RT: Ultrasound screening for developmental dysplasia of the hip in the neonate: The effect on treatment rate and prevalence of late cases. *Pediatrics* 1994;94(1): 47-52.

7. American Academy of Pediatrics: Clinical practice guideline: Early

capsular plication contains the reduced femoral head. Open reduction can be augmented with an additional pelvic acetabuloplasty to encourage acetabular development and reduce the need for additional pelvic procedures.

Late Management

Late treatment, after the age of 18 months, introduces an additional degree of complexity and is beyond the scope of this chapter. More informa-

detection of developmental dysplasia of the hip. Committee on Quality Improvement, Subcommittee on Developmental Dysplasia of the Hip. *Pediatrics* 2000; 105(4, pt 1):896-905.

8. US Preventive Services Task Force: Screening for developmental dysplasia of the hip: Recommendation statement. *Pediatrics* 2006;117(3):898-902.

9. Graf R: New possibilities for the diagnosis of congenital hip joint dislocation by ultrasonography. *J Pediatr Orthop* 1983;3(3): 354-359.

10. Clarke NM, Harcke HT, McHugh P, Lee MS, Borns PF

, MacEwen GD: Real-time ultrasound in the diagnosis of congenital dislocation and dysplasia of the hip. *J Bone Joint Surg Br* 1985; 67(3):406-412.

11. Clarke NM, Reading IC, Corbin C, Taylor CC, Bochmann T: Twenty years experience of selective secondary ultrasound screening for congenital dislocation of the hip. *Arch Dis Child* 2012; 97(5):423-429.

12. Cashman JP, Round J, Taylor G, Clarke NM: The natural history of developmental dysplasia of the hip after early supervised treatment in the Pavlik harness: A prospective, longitudinal follow-up. *J Bone Joint Surg Br* 2002; 84(3):418-425.

13. Segal LS, Boal DK, Borthwick L, Clark MW, Localio AR, Schwentker EP: Avascular necrosis following treatment of DDH: The protective influence of the ossific nucleus. *J Pediatr Orthop* 1999; 19:177-184.

14. Bolland BJ, Wahed AK, Al-Hallao S, Culliford DJ, Clarke NM: Late reduction in congenital dislocation of the hip and the need for secondary surgery: Radiologic predictors and confounding variables. *J Pediatr Orthop* 2010; 30(7):676-682.

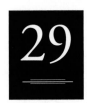

Surgical Treatment of Developmental Dysplasia of the Hip

Dennis R. Wenger, MD

Abstract

Ideally, developmental dysplasia of the hip is treated early in childhood by nonsurgical methods. If these methods are ineffective, surgical reduction in a nonambulating child is required. A young child (age 6 to 18 months) who requires surgical reduction can be treated by formal anterior open reduction or by the medial Ludloff approach to the hip. Additional bony procedures are usually not required in these young patients. Delayed diagnosis is still common, requiring surgical reduction for children of walking age. These older children usually require formal open reduction (anterior approach) plus an associated bony osteotomy (acetabular, proximal femoral, or, in some cases, both types of osteotomies) to better stabilize the hip. The addition of a proximal femoral derotational shortening osteotomy for open reduction in older children was first used in children older than 3 years, but now it is commonly used in children as young as 2 years. This osteotomy decreases the forces on the reduced hip and minimizes the chances for redislocation and osteonecrosis. In all surgical procedures for developmental dysplasia of the hip, the surgeon must avoid too great a focus on bony osteotomies because the management of soft-tissue abnormalities is critical in achieving a stable reduction.

Instr Course Lect 2014;63:313-323.

Despite great advances in the early diagnosis of developmental dysplasia of the hip (DDH), aided by the development of ultrasound, some children still require surgical treatment. These patients fall into two groups: children treated with a Pavlik harness or other brace in infancy in whom a stable reduction was not achieved and patients who did not benefit from early diagnosis and present after walking age with a dislocated hip. *Instructional Course Lectures Volume 63* chapter 28 (Developmental Dysplasia of the Hip: Diagnosis and Management to 18 Months) describes the management of infants in whom harness/brace treatment fails to obtain a stable reduction and who are then treated with closed reduction followed by spica cast immobilization.

Even in patients in this young age group (6 to 18 months), the success of a closed reduction is not always assured, and open reduction may be required.

Children Younger Than 18 Months

The need for a primary open reduction for DDH, without associated acetabular or femoral osteotomies, can be considered in children from approximately 3 to 18 months of age. However, for some children, such as those who are very small for their chronological age, the upper age limit may be 24 months. Children younger than 18 months can be scheduled for an attempted closed reduction, with open reduction performed under the same anesthesia if the closed reduction fails.

Methods for Open Reduction

Anteromedial (Ludloff) Approach: Age 6 to 18 Months

The important contributions by Mau et al[1] and Ferguson[2] repopularized the medial Ludloff approach to the hip for young children (younger than 24 months). The benefit of this approach is that it can be performed via a

Dr. Wenger or an immediate family member serves as a paid consultant to or is an employee of OrthoPediatrics and has stock or stock options held in Rhino Pediatric Orthopedic Designs.

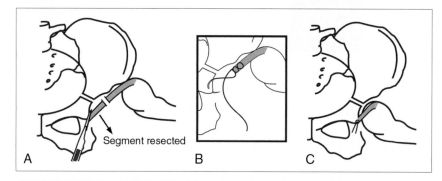

Figure 1 **A,** Illustration of the Ludloff medial approach shows the location of resection of the medial portion of the elongated ligamentum teres. **B,** A Bunnell-style suture in the ligamentum teres allows firm attachment for transfer. **C,** The shortened ligamentum teres is reattached to the periosteum at the anteroinferior acetabular margin. (Adapted with permission from Wenger Dr, Henderson PC: Ligamentum teres maintenance and transfer as a stabilizer in open reduction for pediatric hip dislocation: Surgical technique and early clinical results. *J Child Orthop* 2008;2:177-185.)

small cosmetic groin incision that allows exposure of the hip capsule; psoas lengthening; opening of the capsule; and gentle, atraumatic reduction of the femoral head.

Weinstein and Ponseti[3] described the medial approach of Mau et al[1] as an anteromedial variation of the Ludloff approach. This approach allows clear exposure of the acetabulum and the hip capsule as well as the overlying psoas tendon, which often restricts the capsule in an hourglass fashion. In most patients, the overlying psoas tendon is lengthened intramuscularly. After opening the capsule in a T fashion, the transverse acetabular ligament in the base of the acetabulum is sectioned to allow full reduction of the femoral head. Traditionally, the ligamentum teres was excised as part of the procedure because it is longer and thicker than normal and could impede a concentric reduction.

More recently Wenger et al[4] and Bache et al[5] described methods for maintaining the ligamentum teres by leaving it attached to the femoral head. The ligamentum teres is detached from its insertion near the transverse acetabular ligament and left attached to the femoral head. The ligamentum teres is used as a tether to pull the femoral head down into the acetabulum. The ligament is then shortened and sutured to the anteroinferior acetabular rim (**Figure 1**). This technique improves hip stability and minimizes the chance of having a hip that seems well reduced intraoperatively but then redislocates.

There are certain disadvantages to the Ludloff approach. The exposure is not familiar to many surgeons, and care must be taken to avoid the medial femoral circumflex vessel that encircles the psoas tendon within the confines of the approach. Also, a substantial capsulorrhaphy cannot be easily performed through the medial approach. Because no capsulorrhaphy is performed, the child is placed in the human position, with the hips hyperflexed and moderately abducted. As casting skills gradually diminish among orthopaedic surgeons in developed countries, a missing link in successful treatment of a child of this age can be the skill required for hip spica application because proper hip positioning and cast molding are critical for maintaining the reduction.

Anterior Approach: Age 6 to 18 Months

Because the surgical approach, handling of tissues, and application of the hip spica are somewhat demanding with an anteromedial Ludloff-type open reduction, many surgeons perform an open reduction via the anterior approach without associated osteotomies in children age 6 to 24 months. This approach allows excellent exposure and includes lengthening of the psoas tendon at the pelvic brim.

The capsule can be exposed superiorly and posteriorly where the pathologic capsular enlargement is located, allowing an appropriate capsulorrhaphy. This procedure, described in detail later in this chapter, decreases the volume of the pathologically enlarged capsule and allows internal rotation, which induces capsular repair, as described by Salter.[6,7]

Because the femur usually has increased anteversion in DDH, this capsulorrhaphy places the anteverted femur in internal rotation, modest flexion, and modest abduction, which improves stable reduction. Capsular sutures maintain this position, and the hip is carefully held in this position by the surgeon until a hip spica is applied. This spica includes the entire limb on the operated side and extends to above the knee on the contralateral side. Postoperative care includes maintaining the hip in this position for 6 weeks, followed by 4 to 6 additional weeks in a loosely applied single hip spica, again maintaining hip internal rotation.

After this type of reduction, the child should not be placed in a typical off-the-shelf hip abduction brace, which would encourage external hip rotation, because such a position would stress the anterior capsular repair. This chapter's author does not always use a postcasting brace; however, if one is needed, it should hold the hip in mod-

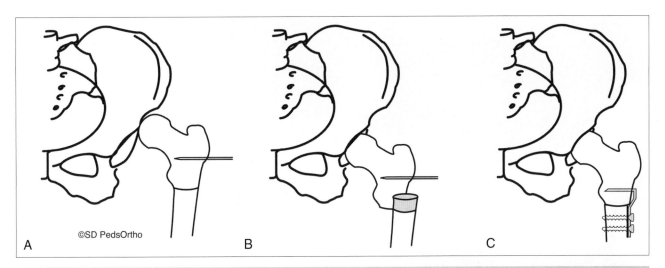

Figure 2 **A,** Illustration of the femoral head in the dislocated position, with a proximal femoral osteotomy performed. **B,** Femoral shortening with removal of a segment allows the femoral head to comfortably reduce in the acetabulum. **C,** Fixation with a blade plate device. (Copyright San Diego Pediatric Orthopedics, San Diego, CA.)

est abduction and substantial internal rotation and may need to be custom made. Great attention is needed to maintain the hip reduction in these young children because a derotational osteotomy has not been performed.

Surgical Treatment of the Child of Walking Age (18 Months and Older)

Prior to approximately 1980, older children with DDH were placed in preliminary skin traction or even skeletal traction for several weeks in an attempt to pull the femoral head down to the level of the acetabulum before performing a surgical procedure, which could include an open reduction alone or an open reduction plus a Salter procedure.[6,8]

In the mid-1970s, the work of Klisic and Jankovic[9] changed the North American viewpoint regarding the treatment of a completely dislocated hip in an older child. By derotating and shortening the proximal femur, preliminary traction was not required, and the risk for osteonecrosis could be reduced (**Figure 2**). This technique has proven effective in children from 2 to approximately 8 years of age. In children older than 8 years, the procedure

may not improve the natural history of this disorder regarding hip pain; therefore, the dislocated hip may be best left untreated. Some controversy remains regarding the cutoff age for treatment. A common standard is that children with a unilateral hip dislocation and a marked, unsightly limp should be treated with the Klisic and Jankovic[9] method up to the age of 8 years.

Patients with bilateral dislocations, particularly those who have a syndromic or teratologic component to their dislocations with a high, complete dislocation (femoral head not in contact with the acetabulum) likely should not be treated with surgical reduction after age 6 years.

Decisions regarding age limitations also can relate to when and if a total hip replacement would eventually be required for such patients. One argument for performing an open reduction in an older child is that the femoral head is positioned for a more predictable subsequent total hip reconstruction.

Comprehensive Surgical Approach to Reduction in the Older Child

For treating a child older than 2 years

with a completely dislocated hip, a comprehensive approach, including open reduction via an anterior approach, psoas tendon lengthening, a derotational shortening femoral osteotomy, and careful repair of the capsule, is recommended. The maldirected, deficient acetabulum is corrected by performing a Salter- or Dega-type acetabuloplasty.[7,10] This combined procedure gives the greatest chance for obtaining and maintaining a stable reduction in a child of walking age with DDH.[11]

Surgical Technique
Comprehensive Surgical Reduction
The patient is placed supine on a radiolucent operating table, with a sandbag under the shoulders (**Figure 3**). This positioning allows good skin preparation, with wide draping of the hip and excellent image intensifier views (placing a sandbag or other bolster behind the hip joint decreases image quality).

For a young child, a long curvilinear incision, which allows both reduction of the hip and shortening of the femur through the same incision, is recommended by some surgeons. This

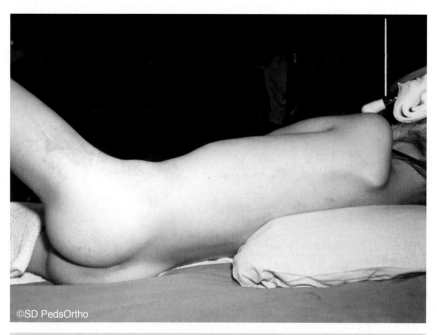

Figure 3 The patient is positioned supine on the operating table using the anterior approach to comprehensive corrective surgery for a dislocated hip. The sandbag bolster is placed under the shoulders to minimize any obstruction in image intensifier views. (Copyright San Diego Pediatric Orthopedics, San Diego, CA.)

chapter's author no longer uses this method because the curvilinear incision almost always stretches and widens over time, leaving an unsightly scar. Instead, anterior surgery is performed through a typical anterolateral Salter approach to the hip, with a separate lateral incision used for the femoral osteotomy. Adductor tenotomy is not routinely required because the femoral shortening reduces adductor tendon tightness.

Incision and Exposure

The anterolateral Salter incision has been described as being a bikini incision (a transverse incision following the Langer lines); however, in a child with a completely dislocated hip, a more longitudinal exposure improves visualization. The incision is made just below the iliac crest laterally and extended anteriorly and then distally for several centimeters to assure good visualization of the anterior and inferior hip capsule.[12]

The interval between the sartorius and tensor fascia muscles is identified anteriorly and then the iliac crest apophysis is split to allow good exposure of the wing of the ilium both medially (which facilitates psoas lengthening) and laterally (to allow proper exposure of the capsule). Because the iliac crest apophysis is a growth center, it is split carefully and later repaired anatomically to allow more normal subsequent iliac growth.

The direct and reflected heads of the rectus femoris tendon are detached from the anterior inferior spine area and retracted distally to provide anterolateral capsular exposure. Care is taken to avoid entering the hip capsule when the overlying tendon origins are separated from the capsule. It is important to note that in a dislocated hip, the neurovascular structures tend to be displaced laterally because of the lateral position of the femur. Thus, the femoral nerve, artery, and vein may be more readily encountered.

After the capsule is fully exposed anteriorly, the iliopsoas tendon is lengthened in an intramuscular fashion at the pelvic brim. This minimizes the hourglass constriction effect of the tendon as it crosses the hip capsule. Close attention is required in performing the tenotomy. The tendinous portion lies on the posterior part of the muscle, and it can be visualized by flexing and rotating the hip. The femoral nerve lies just anterior to the iliopsoas muscle. Care must be taken to be certain that the tendon is being lengthened and the femoral nerve is not being injured. The anesthesiologist should be asked to confirm that no muscle-paralyzing agents are being used before the surgeon touches the tendon with the electrocautery prior to performing the tenotomy. If the femoral nerve was mistakenly identified, a violent quadriceps contraction will occur.

Further lateral exposure of the femoral capsule is then undertaken. In a patient with DDH with a false acetabulum, the periosteum of the ilium and the distorted labrum, hip capsule, and abductor muscle fascia may have condensed into a tissue mass that can be difficult to separate from the overlying abductor muscles (**Figure 4**). Placing a scissors or hemostat in the space just above the hip capsule while dissecting downward in the subperiosteal space of the ilium will help improve the exposure. Eventually, these two spaces are joined with the abductor muscles pulled further laterally. A common cause of unintentional redislocation after surgery is the failure to adequately separate these muscles, which had become adherent to the capsule with the hip in its dislocated position. The posterior point of this capsule should extend to an area posterior to the true acetabulum to fully expose the posterior capsular sac into which the femoral head has dislocated. Failure to obliterate this sac is a common cause for failed surgical reduction.

Capsulotomy

This chapter's author performs a capsulotomy and a subsequent corrective capsulorrhaphy using a method similar to the method described by Salter.[7] The widely exposed capsule is opened with a scalpel in a T fashion, beginning with a cut made parallel to the acetabular rim. It is necessary to remain lateral enough to avoid damaging the acetabular labrum. Initially, this incision is relatively short, with the T incision (performed at right angles to the acetabular rim and paralleling the femoral neck) then performed. With the capsule now open, small Kocher clamps are used to retract the capsule. The initial cut at the acetabular rim then can be extended superiorly and posteriorly as well as distally and medially on the anterior capsule.

In most instances, the ligamentum teres is intact and is used as a guide to determine the depth of the true acetabulum. It is important to identify the true acetabulum because inexperienced surgeons have sometimes reduced a femoral head into what proved to be a false acetabulum. If needed, intraoperative imaging can be used to confirm that the level of the triradiate cartilage has been identified (which identifies the center of the true acetabulum).

The ligamentum teres is detached from the femoral head with a Kocher clamp attached and used as a guide to dissect anteriorly and medially to the distal margin of the true acetabulum. The ligamentum teres is excised, and the transverse acetabular ligament is sectioned. Any fatty (pulvinar) tissue that is within the acetabulum is cleared, with care taken to prevent the removal of any articular cartilage. The wound is packed, and the femoral osteotomy is started.

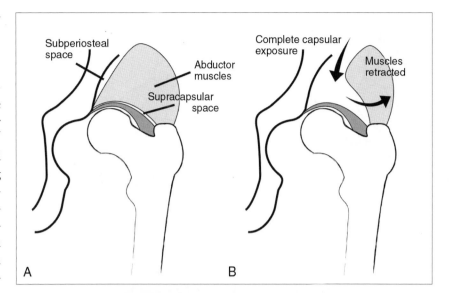

Figure 4   **A,** Illustration shows the development of the subperiosteal space for exposure of a dislocated hip in DDH. A plane is developed between the abductors and the wing of the ilium. The potential space is identified and expanded between the hip capsule and the abductors overlying the femoral head. **B,** Further extensive exposure separates the muscles from the capsule, both laterally and particularly posteriorly, where there is an expansile capsular sac.

Femoral Derotational and Shortening Osteotomy

A separate proximal lateral thigh incision is made, beginning at the tip of the greater trochanter and extending distally to allow adequate exposure of the proximal one quarter to one third of the femur. This incision allows careful palpation of the greater trochanter and palpation of the femoral neck axis, which helps in placing the Kirschner wires for planning an accurate derotation. To prepare for the derotation, the existing femoral anteversion is estimated by grasping the femur at the knee; the surgeon then places his or her finger on the anterolateral femoral neck. In most cases, the anteversion is 40° to 60°, and 30° to 40° of correction is planned.

Pins are placed both proximally and distally to guide the planned derotation in the femur to allow an accurate degree of derotation (**Figure 5**). Anteversion also can be determined by a preoperative CT and/or MRI analysis; however, this is usually not needed un-

less the child has had prior surgery, with complications such as scarring or osteonecrosis.

The neck shaft angle in a typical dislocated hip is normal, that is, approximately 130°. Therefore, no attempt is made to add varus correction to the osteotomy because it can lead to a deformity (excessive coxa vara) that may require later correction (**Figure 6**).

Proximal fixation is gained with the inserting chisel (traditional system) or by initial screw fixation (contemporary system), with the femur then transected using a power saw. The distal segment is externally rotated, and the estimated amount of bone required for femoral shortening is removed. The amount of femoral shortening can be assessed by reducing the femoral head in the acetabulum and assessing the degree of overlap required to produce a comfortable reduction. With experience, the surgeon can skip this step, knowing that children 2 to 3 years or younger need approximately 1.5 cm of

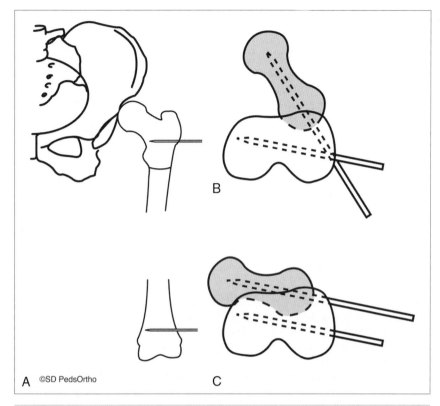

Figure 5 Illustrations showing the method for quantitating derotation of a proximal femoral osteotomy. **A,** Appropriate guide pins are placed proximally and distally. **B,** The planned derotation is noted, which in this case would be about 40°. Kirschner wires are used as guides. **C,** After derotation, the anteversion has been corrected to a more normal 10° to 15°. (Copyright San Diego Pediatric Orthopedics, San Diego, CA.)

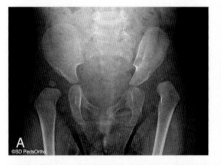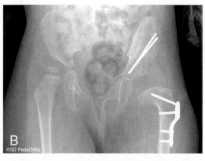

Figure 6 Preoperative (**A**) and postoperative (**B**) pelvic radiographs of a 2-year-old child with bilateral DDH. Treatment included comprehensive reduction, including the principles described in this chapter, but with too much varus added in the femoral osteotomy. The child now has a 90° neck-shaft angle, a significant limp, and will likely require correction with a subsequent valgus osteotomy. Most children with DDH do not have coxa valga but instead have significant anteversion. (Copyright San Diego Pediatric Orthopedics, San Diego, CA.)

shortening, and older children may need as much as 2 to 2.5 cm of shortening. Excessive shortening should be avoided because it can make the reduction less stable because there is a lack of good contact pressure between the femoral head and the redirected acetabulum. The osteotomy site is fixed with the appropriately sized blade plate or screw place device.

Occasionally, a derotational femoral osteotomy is needed for a very young child who has arthrogryposis or another syndrome.[12] A four-hole straight AO plate is placed anteriorly in the area just below the greater trochanter to allow fixation in a child who is too small for traditional blade plate systems (**Figure 7**).

After a stable femoral osteotomy correction is confirmed by imaging, the lateral wound is closed over a surgical drain. The lateral wound is completely closed at this point to minimize total blood loss.

Details of Capsular Management

The anterior wound is then reopened to allow for capsular repair and an acetabular osteotomy. To perform a Salter-type capsulorrhaphy, the superolateral flap of capsule that had been opened in a T shape is resected (**Figure 8**). This triangle of tissue is discarded. After this resection, the posterior incision can be continued parallel to the labrum, with further clearing of the posterior capsule from the overlying muscle. Often, the capsule is further excised. Finding and extinguishing the enlarged posterior capsular sac into which the femoral head has dislocated is essential to gain a stable reduction and minimize the chance for dislocation.

The capsular repair is then planned. Point A on the capsule, which is the distal extent of the T, which had been made anteriorly parallel to the femoral neck, is pulled proximally and medially by hip flexion and internal rotation. This maintains the femur in internal rotation and stabilizes the reduction. Traditionally, point B, which is the corner of the inferomedial flap as defined by Salter, was sewn to

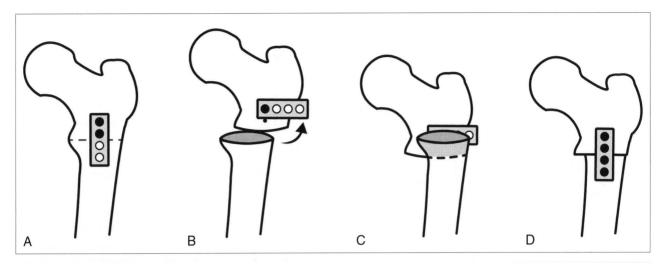

Figure 7 Illustrations of the method for performing femoral shortening in a very young child when the femoral head and neck may be too small for the insertion of a blade plate. In such patients, a small anterior plate is first attached to the proximal femur (**A**) and then rotated out of position (**B**). The femoral shortening is then performed. The plate is re-attached to the proximal segment (**C**) and then, after derotation and shortening, attached to the distal segment (**D**). (Copyright San Diego Pediatric Orthopedics, San Diego, CA.)

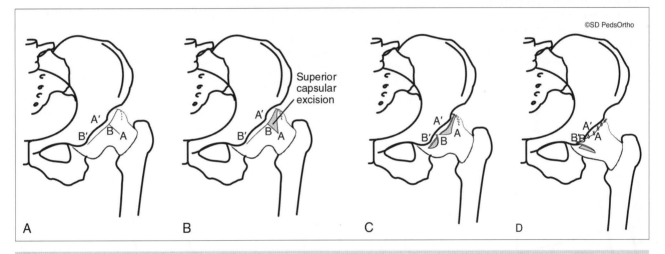

Figure 8 **A,** Illustrations show sequential capsular excision and repair using the principles described by Salter. **A,** The first cut is made parallel to the acetabulum, followed by a T-shaped incision formed by making a capsular cut at right angles to the first incision. The points A and A' and B and B' are noted. **B,** The shaded area shows the area of superior and posterior capsule that is excised. **C,** After excision of the capsule, an internal rotation maneuver is performed, bringing A to A' and later B to B'. **D,** Nonabsorbable No. 0 or No. 1 sutures are used to securely repair the capsule, in a manner similar to a hernia repair. (Copyright San Diego Pediatric Orthopedics, San Diego, CA.)

the periosteum of the pubis. Often, this medial and inferior capsular tissue is very redundant and requires excision, which lends credence to the view of some experts that a substantial portion of the capsule should be excised to gain a stable reduction (**Figure 9**).

There are multiple viewpoints regarding capsule management in DDH. Grudziak and Ward,[10] using the method of Dega, noted that much of the capsule requires excision. A method developed in Turkey includes a U-shaped flap, which differs from the method of Salter but provides similar stability.[13]

After the capsular reduction has been achieved, a series of nonabsorbable sutures are then placed, usually beginning with the suture in the capsule laterally and then advancing medially with 6- to 8-mm suture spacing, with the femur held in internal rotation. This ensures an internal rotation

Pediatrics

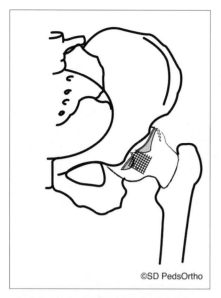

Figure 9 In older children with high hip dislocations, a portion of the inferior medial capsule often requires excision. The hatched area shows the region of the inferomedial capsule that may need to be excised. (Copyright San Diego Pediatric Orthopedics, San Diego, CA.)

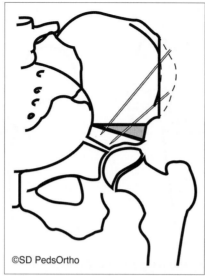

Figure 10 Illustration of a Salter innominate osteotomy. The acetabulum is redirected to improve anterolateral coverage of the femoral head. A triangular bone graft (shaded area) is taken from the adjacent ilium, placed in the osteotomy site, and fixed with two threaded Kirschner wires. (Copyright San Diego Pediatric Orthopedics, San Diego, CA.)

capsulorrhaphy with the hip stable in internal rotation.

Acetabuloplasty

This chapter's author believes that all patients older than 2 years who are treated with a formal anterior open reduction should have an acetabuloplasty performed, even though a femoral derotation osteotomy has been performed. Salter defined the importance of redirecting the acetabulum (correcting acetabular dysplasia that results from not having a femoral head within the acetabulum to allow normal development). The Salter osteotomy redirects the acetabulum but does not change its shape or the potential risk for changing acetabular volume (**Figure 10**). In general, the acetabulum is smaller than normal in children with DDH because of the lack of acetabular growth stimulated by the femoral head. A procedure that may reduce the size of the acetabulum is not recommended. Therefore, this chapter's author still advises using the Salter procedure in a typical case, although the Dega

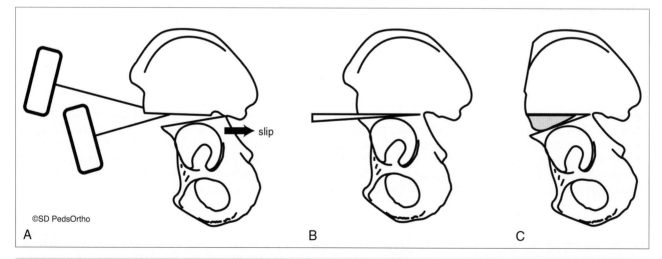

Figure 11 **A,** The typical method of cutting the Salter osteotomy with a Gigli saw completely separates the proximal and distal segments of the pelvis. This can allow a posterior slip and sometimes causes a surgeon to lose control of the distal segment, leading to improper pinning and placement of the graft and no improvement in acetabular coverage. **B,** A variation of the Salter technique performed by making the anterior two thirds of the cut with a power saw and the posterior one third carefully performed using an osteotome. The sciatic notch is not entered. **C,** The rotation is then performed, hinging on the intact posterior cortex near the sciatic notch. This allows a more stable construct without risk for subsequent displacement. (Copyright San Diego Pediatric Orthopedics, San Diego, CA.)

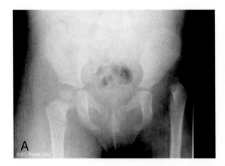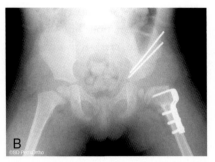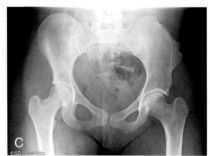

Figure 12   **A,** AP radiograph of the pelvis of a 20-month-old child with right DDH. **B,** AP radiograph after open reduction, femoral derotational shortening, capsulorrhaphy, and a Salter osteotomy. **C,** AP radiograph obtain 12 years later. The femoral head remains well covered and (in fact) may be slightly overcovered. (Copyright San Diego Pediatric Orthopedics, San Diego, CA.)

and Pemberton procedures are also commonly used.[10,14] A variation of the Salter procedure can be modified to maintain a posterior hinge to minimize inadvertent posterior slippage of the acetabular segment (**Figure 11**).

In the past, many experts have performed open reduction plus femoral derotation shortening without an acetabular procedure in children between 2 and 4 years of age; however, this chapter's author believes that an acetabular procedure should be routinely performed. Although an acetabuloplasty can be performed at a later date, a second procedure requires dissection through tissues that have been surgically altered. It seems more efficient to perform an acetabuloplasty at the time of the initial open reduction. Macnicol and Bertol[15] reported better results when acetabuloplasty was performed at the time of the primary open reduction.

Postoperative Care: Comprehensive Approach

After completing the single-stage procedure, suction drainage tubes are placed in both the proximal femoral and anterior hip wounds. The wounds are closed, including anatomic closure of the iliac crest apophysis, in a manner similar to that of a skin closure.

The child is placed in a one-and-a-half hip spica cast with the hip flexed 20°, abducted 20° to 25°, and moderately internally rotated. (If femoral derotation has not been performed and the Salter capsulorrhaphy is expected to maintain the reduction, the femur must be held in marked internal rotation.) With the child in the spica cast, a radiograph is obtained in the operating room to assure that stability has been maintained.

Despite the care taken intraoperatively, it is always possible that the hip will redislocate in children in this age group. In North America, advanced postoperative imaging with a fine-cut CT or MRI to confirm reduction has become the standard of care for children treated with open surgical reduction.[16]

The one-and-a-half hip spica cast is maintained for 6 weeks and then is changed (usually with the child under general anesthesia) to a loose-fitting single-hip spica cast, which is maintained for an additional 4 weeks. The second spica cast is removed 10 weeks after surgery, and no subsequent bracing is used because a typical abduction brace encourages external rotation, which could be damaging to the internal rotation–inducing capsulorrhaphy. If a brace is needed, the hip spica cast is retained at the time of removal and then used by an orthotist as a mold for a custom-made hip brace, which can be used for sleeping, with the hip held in modest flexion, abduction, and internal rotation.

Results

The results of open reduction and femoral shortening in children 2 to 6 years of age are generally excellent, with expected results more guarded in older children (up to 10 years of age)[11] (**Figure 12**).

Early complications can include hip redislocation or subluxation and osteonecrosis. The incidence of osteonecrosis ranges from 10% to 20% depending on the level of strictness in interpreting the grading scale. These patients require regular follow-up because subsequent procedures may be needed, including a procedure to correct residual dysplasia. In rare instances, excessive coverage gained by the procedure may require a subsequent hip preservation procedure to correct hip impingement caused by overcoverage of the femoral head.

Residual Hip Dysplasia in Children

A full discussion of the treatment of residual hip dysplasia is beyond the scope of this chapter, but a brief discussion of this complication is warranted because residual dysplasia is common despite the best possible primary treatment of DDH. Orthopaedic surgeons also encounter children with previously unrecognized hip dysplasia who present without symptoms (dysplasia found on an incidental radiograph) or who begin to have hip pain with activities, with subsequent imaging showing dysplasia.[17] The natural history of significant dysplasia leads to premature arthritis. Treatment in childhood is easier and achieves better results than treatment started in the teenage or young adult years.[18]

In most patients, mild to moderate residual hip dysplasia can be treated with an acetabular procedure alone. In patients with more severe dysplasia, an associated femoral osteotomy may be required. All corrective osteotomies in childhood are designed to improve the typical anterolateral deficiency of the acetabulum as described by Salter[7] and other authors. The prototype for such a correction is the Salter innominate osteotomy, which improves anterolateral coverage of the femoral head. The Pemberton acetabuloplasty gives similar improvement to the shape of the acetabulum and usually does not require internal fixation with Kirschner wires. The original Dega acetabuloplasty was described as being performed in association with primary open reduction of the hip, with associated femoral shortening. The bone removed from the femoral shortening was cut into two triangular pieces and used to hold the acetabular osteotomy open, providing coverage very similar to that achieved with the Salter and the Pemberton procedures. The Pemberton procedure and the original Dega procedure appear to be identical in biomechanical design, degree of coverage produced, and efficacy.[7,10] The only difference seems to be the type of bone graft used to hold open the acetabular osteotomy.

In a child older than 8 to 10 years, the pelvis becomes stiffer, and acetabular rotation becomes more difficult. Forcing a large triangular graft into the

acetabular osteotomy site can improve acetabular orientation but also may move the iliac crest upward, which lengthens the limb more than is desired. Such patients may be better treated with a triple innominate osteotomy, which completely frees the acetabular segment from the associated ilium and minimizes changes in limb length by allowing some upward displacement at the pubic cut and inward movement of the lower acetabulum near the ischial cut. This procedure is somewhat more difficult to perform.

Summary

Open reduction and stabilization of a dislocated hip in a child is a demanding orthopaedic procedure, but results can be satisfying if appropriate principles are applied. In children older than 2 years, a comprehensive approach is recommended, including open reduction of the hip, capsulorrhaphy, a femoral derotation shortening osteotomy, and an acetabuloplasty.

Residual hip dysplasia in childhood is common and is best treated by age 6 to 8 years by performing an acetabular corrective osteotomy, usually of the Salter, Pemberton, or Dega type. In the late juvenile and adolescent age groups, a triple pelvic osteotomy is often required to adequately mobilize the acetabulum.

References

1. Mau H, Dörr WM, Henkel L, Lutsche J: Open reduction of congenital dislocation of the hip by Ludloff's method. *J Bone Joint Surg Am* 1971;53(7):1281-1288.

2. Ferguson AB Jr: Primary open reduction of congenital dislocation of the hip using a median adductor approach. *J Bone Joint Surg Am* 1973;55(4):671-689.

3. Weinstein SL, Ponseti IV: Congenital dislocation of the hip. *J Bone Joint Surg Am* 1979;61(1):119-124.

4. Wenger DR, Mubarak SJ, Henderson PC, Miyanji F: Ligamentum teres maintenance and transfer as a stabilizer in open reduction for pediatric hip dislocation: Surgical technique and early clinical results. *J Child Orthop* 2008;2(3):177-185.

5. Bache CE, Graham HK, Dickens DR, et al: Ligamentum teres tenodesis in medial approach open reduction for developmental dislocation of the hip. *J Pediatr Orthop* 2008;28(6):607-613.

6. Salter RB, Dubos JP: The first fifteen year's personal experience with innominate osteotomy in the treatment of congenital dislocation and subluxation of the hip. *Clin Orthop Relat Res* 1974;98:72-103.

7. Salter RB: The classic: Innominate osteotomy in the treatment of congenital dislocation and subluxation of the hip by Robert B. Salter, J. Bone Joint Surg. (Brit) 43B:3:518, 1961. *Clin Orthop Relat Res* 1978;137:2-14.

8. Thomas SR, Wedge JH, Salter RB: Outcome at forty-five years after open reduction and innominate osteotomy for late-presenting developmental dislocation of the hip. *J Bone Joint Surg Am* 2007;89(11):2341-2350.

9. Klisic P, Jankovic L: Combined procedure of open reduction and shortening of the femur in treatment of congenital dislocation of the hips in older children. *Clin Orthop Relat Res* 1976;119:60-69.

10. Grudziak JS, Ward WT: Dega osteotomy for the treatment of congenital dysplasia of the hip. *J Bone Joint Surg Am* 2001;83(6):845-854.

11. Galpin RD, Roach JW, Wenger DR, Herring JA, Birch JG: One-stage treatment of congenital dislocation of the hip in older children, including femoral short-

ening. *J Bone Joint Surg Am* 1989;
71(5):734-741.

12. Weinstein SL, Mubarak SJ, Wenger DR: Developmental hip dysplasia and dislocation: Part II. *Instr Course Lect* 2004;53: 531-542.

13. Eren A, Altintaş F, Atay EF, Omeroğlu H: A new capsuloplasty technique in open reduction of developmental dislocation of the hip. *J Pediatr Orthop B* 2004;13(2):139-141.

14. Pemberton PA: Periacetabular osteotomy of the ilium for treatment of congenital subluxation and dislocation of the hip. *J Bone Joint Surg Am* 1965;47:65-86.

15. Macnicol MF, Bertol P: The Salter innominate osteotomy: Should it be combined with concurrent open reduction? *J Pediatr Orthop B* 2005;14(6):415-421.

16. Eberhardt O, Zieger M, Langendoerfer M, Wirth T, Fernandez FF: Determination of hip reduction in spica cast treatment for

DDH: A comparison of radiography and ultrasound. *J Child Orthop* 2009;3(4):313-318.

17. Wedge JH, Wasylenko MJ: The natural history of congenital dislocation of the hip: A critical review. *Clin Orthop Relat Res* 1978;137: 154-162.

18. Lalonde FD, Frick SL, Wenger DR: Surgical correction of residual hip dysplasia in two pediatric age-groups. *J Bone Joint Surg Am* 2002;84(7):1148-1156.

Diagnosis and Management of Developmental Dysplasia of the Hip From Triradiate Closure Through Young Adulthood

Klaus A. Siebenrock, MD
Simon D. Steppacher, MD
Christoph E. Albers, MD
Pascal C. Haefeli, MD
Moritz Tannast, MD

Abstract

The current treatment of painful hip dysplasia in the mature skeleton is based on acetabular reorientation. Reorientation procedures attempt to optimize the anatomic position of the hyaline cartilage of the femoral head and acetabulum in regard to mechanical loading. Because the Bernese periacetabular osteotomy is a versatile technique for acetabular reorientation, it is helpful to understand the approach and be familiar with the criteria for an optimal surgical correction. The femoral side bears stigmata of hip dysplasia that may require surgical correction. Improvement of the head-neck offset to avoid femoroacetabular impingement has become routine in many hips treated with periacetabular osteotomy. In addition, intertrochanteric osteotomies can help improve joint congruency and normalize the femoral neck orientation. Other new surgical techniques allow trimming or reducing a severely deformed head, performing a relative neck lengthening, and trimming or distalizing the greater trochanter.

An increasing number of studies have reported good long-term results after acetabular reorientation procedures, with expected joint preservation rates ranging from 80% to 90% at the 10-year follow-up and 60% to 70% at the 20-year follow-up. An ideal candidate is younger than 30 years, with no preoperative signs of osteoarthritis. Predicted joint preservation in these patients is approximately 90% at the 20-year follow-up. Recent evidence indicates that additional correction of an aspheric head may further improve results.

Instr Course Lect 2014;63:325-334.

None of the following authors or any immediate family member has received anything of value from or has stock or stock options held in a commercial company or institution related directly or indirectly to the subject of this chapter: Dr. Siebenrock, Dr. Steppacher, Dr. Albers, Dr. Haefeli, and Dr. Tannast.

Management of the Acetabular Side

Closure of the triradiate cartilage may occur as early as 8 to 10 years of age.[1] Typically, the pelvis of a very young teenager already is amenable to different kinds of juxta-acetabular osteotomies for the treatment of hip disorders. Treatment options for the dysplastic acetabulum can be divided into augmentation and reorientation procedures. Augmentation procedures include a Chiari osteotomy[2] or different techniques of shelf procedures[3] based on the principle of load reduction by distributing load through a larger surface area. However, the potentially damaged labrum and articular cartilage at the abnormally loaded acetabular rim[4] remain within the main weight-bearing zone with both of these surgical procedures. This may be one main cause of the inferior results reported with Chiari osteotomies in adolescents who are older than 14 years[5] or in patients with a torn labrum.[6] Currently, augmentation procedures are not commonly indicated in adolescents and young adults, but may be considered in acetabula with a very short roof or in hips in which the acetabular radius is smaller than the radius of the femoral head.

Three types of juxta-acetabular osteotomies for acetabular reorientation are currently in wider use. These osteotomies include (1) a spheric or rotational osteotomy, (2) a triple osteotomy, and (3) the Bernese periacetabular osteotomy. The principle of the spheric or rotational osteotomy was described by Wagner[7] in Europe and by Ninomiya and Tagawa[8] in Japan. The osteotomy is performed with a curved chisel close to the subchondral bone. The advantage is that it provides a mobile fragment. However, this osteotomy lacks the potential for medialization of the hip center and may become intraarticular in the caudal portion of the acetabulum.[9,10] Tönnis et al[11] popularized a triple osteotomy, with complete osteotomies of the iliac, ischial, and pubic bones. Initial fixation included osteosynthesis of the iliac and pubic bones. The recommended postoperative treatment was immobilization in a spica cast for several weeks. With the current technique, the ischial spine with the attached sacrospinal ligament remains attached to the pelvic segment, and fixation of the acetabular fragment has become easier without the need for postoperative cast immobilization. The Bernese periacetabular osteotomy was first performed in 1984 and was popularized in 1988 by Ganz et al.[12] This osteotomy has the advantage of creating a polygonal acetabular fragment while leaving the posterior column intact by an incomplete osteotomy of the ischium. There is immediate postoperative stability because the pelvic ring is not disrupted. There is no deformity of the true pelvis in young female patients, allowing for childbirth through vaginal delivery af-

ter surgical correction.[13] The mobile acetabular fragment allows adequate corrections, even for severe deformities, and has the potential for an optimal medialization of the acetabular center of rotation. Fixation of the osteotomized fragment can be done typically with screws only in the acetabular fragment, and postoperative care requires only partial weight bearing on crutches without the need for a cast. The Bernese periacetabular osteotomy has become the preferred treatment of this chapter's authors for correcting acetabular dysplasia in hips with a closed triradiate growth plate.

Treatment of the Abnormal Femoral Side

Developmental dysplasia of the hip also affects the femoral head side. There is a wide range of deformities of the proximal part of the femur from a subtle oval-shaped deformity of the femoral head to aberrant torsion or orientation of the femoral neck to more severe abnormalities of the entire proximal part of the femur.[14-16]

Additional Intertrochanteric Osteotomy

Generally, a concomitant intertrochanteric osteotomy is only indicated in approximately 10% of all patients treated with periacetabular osteotomy.[17] The most common indications for an additional intertrochanteric osteotomy are (1) an extreme valgus angulation of the femoral neck with a fovea alta, (2) joint incongruency after acetabular reorientation (typically seen with more severe femoral head deformities), and (3) restoration of a normal femoral neck-shaft angle after a previous varus osteotomy of the proximal part of the femur.

Extreme Valgus With Fovea Alta

In dysplastic hips, an abnormal valgus femoral neck configuration may be as-

sociated with a fovea alta,[18] with the fovea capitis femoris more cranial than in a normal hip joint and the ligamentum capitis femoris articulating with the weight-bearing area of the acetabular cartilage (**Figure 1**). A fovea alta further reduces the weight-bearing zone between the cartilaginous joint surfaces of the femoral head and the acetabulum, aggravating the underlying dysplastic pathomorphology.[18]

Joint Incongruency After Periacetabular Osteotomy

Primary or secondary deformity of the femoral head leads to numerous instantaneous centers of rotation that depend on the actual surface under stress, which varies with the relative position of the acetabulum and femur.[17] This can be seen on an abduction radiograph made either preoperatively or intraoperatively after periacetabular osteotomy. If the abduction radiograph shows improved hip congruency, a varus osteotomy should be considered[17] (**Figure 2**).

Femoral Neck-Shaft Realignment After a Previous Proximal Femoral Varus Osteotomy

If residual hip dysplasia after a previous proximal femoral varus osteotomy needs acetabular correction, a periacetabular osteotomy may lead to restricted hip abduction, flexion, and internal rotation. A corrective rotational valgus intertrochanteric osteotomy can then minimize anterolateral impingement and improve clinical abduction by advancing the greater trochanter distally and laterally (**Figure 3**).

Substantial (Perthes-Like) Femoral Head Deformities

Surgical correction of acetabular abnormalities associated with major femoral head deformities is complex. It is conceivable that hips with major fem-

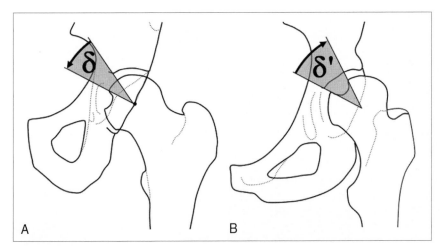

Figure 1   A, In a normal hip, the fovea capitis femoris is caudal to the weight-bearing area of the acetabulum. **B,** In dysplastic hips, because of the extreme valgus, the fovea can extend into the weight-bearing area, reducing the loaded articular cartilage surface. The fovea-acetabular angle is defined as the angle formed by a line from the femoral head center to the medial edge of the weight-bearing zone of the acetabulum (reference line) and a line from the femoral head center to the superior edge of the fovea capitis femoris. The value of the fovea-acetabular angle is positive if the superior edge of the fovea capitis femoris lies caudal to the medial edge of the weight-bearing zone of the acetabulum (**A**). It becomes negative if the superior edge of the fovea capitis femoris lies cranial to the medial edge of the weight-bearing zone of the acetabulum (**B**).

oral head deformities, such as Legg-Calvé-Perthes disease or slipped capital femoral epiphysis, should be treated with additional correction of the deformity of the proximal part of the femur. In severely deformed femoral heads, the femoral side needs to be addressed before the periacetabular osteotomy, at times with the technique of a surgical hip dislocation with or without an extended retinacular soft-tissue flap.[19] Surgical correction includes osteoplasty of a severely deformed femoral head, trimming of the greater trochanter, and relative lengthening of the femoral neck with distalization of the greater trochanter (**Figure 4**). In some patients, intertrochanteric flexion or extension osteotomies can be performed.

Prevention of Femoroacetabular Impingement

Hips with developmental dysplasia often have a decreased femoral head-

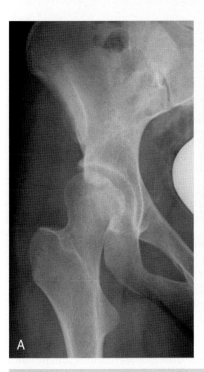
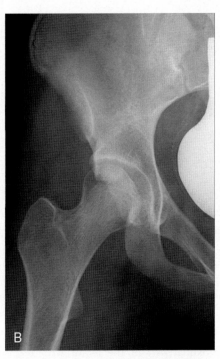
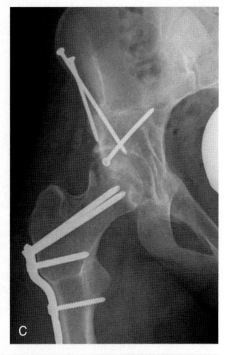

Figure 2   A 19-year-old woman presented with acetabular dysplasia, coxa valga, and a high fovea capitis femoris in the right hip. **A,** AP radiograph made at the time of presentation. **B,** The preoperative radiograph showed slight incongruence of the joint that resolved in the abduction view. **C,** Radiograph made after a periacetabular osteotomy with an intertrochanteric varus femoral osteotomy.

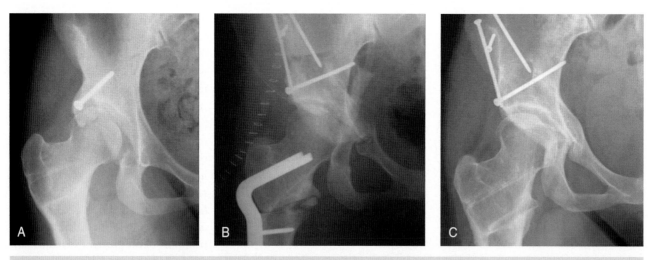

Figure 3 A 24-year-old man presented with residual dysplasia after a previous shelf acetabuloplasty and a varus femoral osteotomy of the right hip. **A,** Preoperative AP radiograph. **B,** AP radiograph made after a periacetabular osteotomy was performed with resection of the shelf acetabuloplasty and a concomitant intertrochanteric valgus femoral osteotomy. **C,** Radiograph of the hip made 10 years postoperatively showing an excellent clinical result.

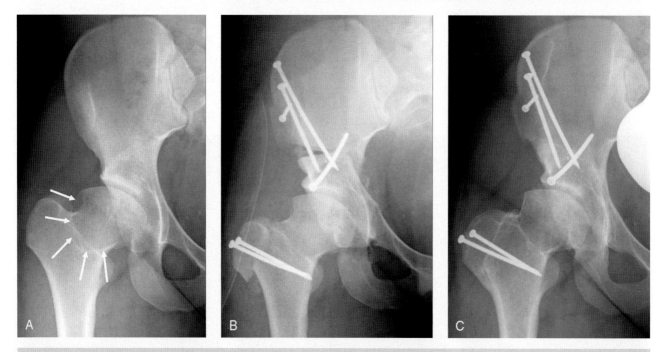

Figure 4 A 25-year-old woman presented with residual deformity after Legg-Calvé-Perthes disease in the right hip. **A,** AP radiograph made at the time of presentation shows acetabular dysplasia with asphericity of the femoral head and a high-riding greater trochanter. The arrows show the anterior extrusion of the aspheric portion of the femoral head. **B,** Radiograph made after a concomitant periacetabular osteotomy and surgical hip dislocation with trimming of the femoral head-neck junction and relative lengthening of the femoral neck. **C,** Radiograph made 10 years postoperatively shows excellent clinical results.

neck offset.[14] With the acetabular reorientation typically anterosuperior, head coverage will be increased, which potentially initiates painful femoroacetabular impingement against the proximal part of the femur with reduced femoral head-neck offset (**Figure 5**). Therefore, in hips with limited internal rotation (< 30°), the joint should be opened, visually inspected, and analyzed for impingement with the hip flexed and internally rotated.[20] The arthrotomy allows for inspection of the acetabular labrum and the assessment of the anatomy of the femo-

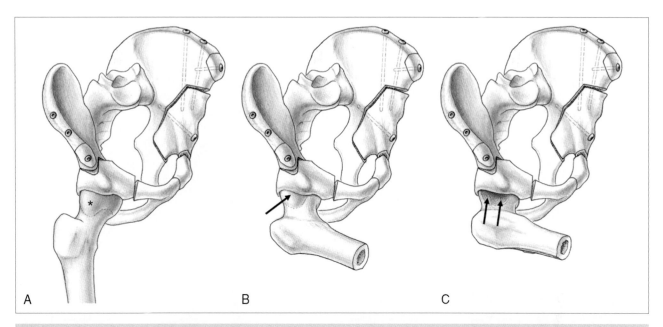

Figure 5   Illustrations showing the current technique of periacetabular osteotomy. **A,** Typically, dysplastic hips present with an aspheric femoral head (asterisk). Before periacetabular osteotomy, this decreased head-neck offset is compensated for by the diminished anterior acetabular coverage. **B,** After proper reorientation, femoroacetabular impingement may become apparent in deep flexion and internal rotation (arrow). Iatrogenic acetabular overcoverage can worsen this impingement. **C,** The femoroacetabular impingement can be assessed through an intraoperative arthrotomy. If necessary, a concomitant osteochondroplasty of the femoral neck can be performed (arrows). (Adapted with permission from Albers CE, Steppacher SD, Ganz R, Tannast M, Siebenrock KA: Impingement adversely affects 10-year survivorship after periacetabular osteotomy for DDH. *Clin Orthop Relat Res* 2013;471(5):1602-1614.)

ral head-neck junction. An osteochondroplasty with removal of the aspheric portion of the femoral head-neck junction should be done (**Figures 5** and **6**). To provide a rough guideline for the amount of bone to be resected, the goal of internal rotation of 30° in 90° of flexion seems appropriate.[21] Optionally, major unstable labral tears can be débrided or repaired with suture anchors.[15]

Surgical Considerations and the Preferred Technique of This Chapter's Authors

The patient is placed in a supine position with the hemipelvis and leg of the affected side sterilely prepared and draped. The skin incision is a shortened ilioinguinal incision. The incision starts laterally at the intersection between the medial and middle third of the iliac wing and extends approximately 5 cm medial to the anterior su-

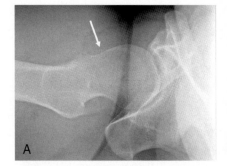
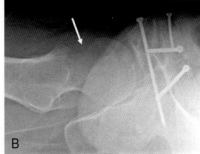

Figure 6   Axial cross-table radiographs of the proximal part of the femur in the right hip of a 29-year-old woman with developmental dysplasia of the hip. **A,** Preoperative radiograph shows a decreased femoral head-neck offset (arrow). **B,** Postoperative radiograph shows correction of the decreased offset through an arthrotomy (arrow).

perior iliac spine. The incision is placed approximately 2 cm distal to the iliac crest (**Figure 7, A**). This type of incision is cosmetically superior to the modified Smith-Petersen incision. The sartorius muscle (medial) is separated from the tensor fascia lata muscle (lateral), exposing the direct origin of the rectus femoris muscle from the an-

terior inferior iliac spine. The abdominal wall muscles are sharply dissected off the iliac crest, and the iliac muscle is mobilized from the iliac wing. The origin of the sartorius muscle together with the inguinal ligament is sharply dissected, mobilized, and medially retracted from the anterior superior iliac spine with the iliacus and psoas mus-

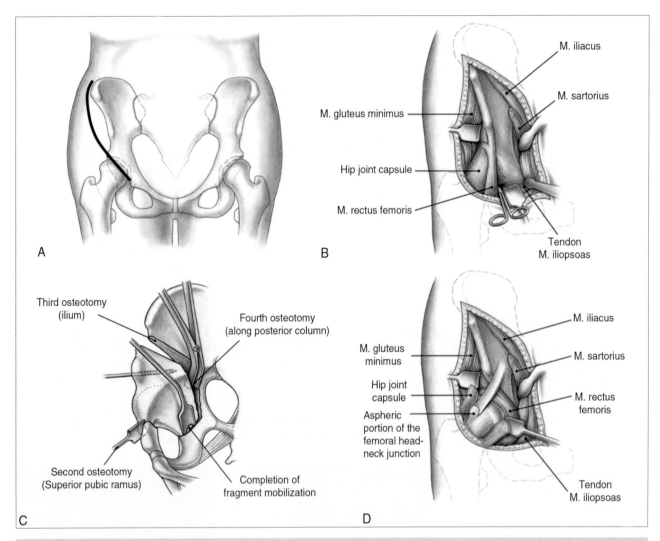

Figure 7 Illustrations showing the periacetabular osteotomy technique preferred by this chapter's authors. **A,** An ilio-inguinal incision is made. **B,** Intraoperative view after mobilization of the iliopsoas and the sartorius muscles. The first cut of the ischium is performed through the interval between the joint capsule and the rectus femoris muscle. **C,** The four periacetabular osteotomies are shown. **D,** Offset creation is performed with the rectus femoris muscle retracted medially through an H-shaped capsulotomy. M = muscle.

cles (**Figure 7, B**). As a further modification from the previously used technique, the two origins of the rectus femoris muscle are left intact and the interval between the rectus muscle (lateral) and the iliopsoas muscle (medial) is dissected and bluntly opened with scissors. The iliocapsularis muscle is sharply separated from the capsule laterally and mobilized medially, together with the iliopsoas muscle.[22] A Hohmann retractor is placed into the superior pubic ramus 2 to 3 cm medial to the pubic eminence. With use of scis-

sors, the infra-articular space is spread open strictly following the contour of the calcar directly on the intact capsule (**Figure 7, B**). With the tip of the scissors, the ischial bone can be palpated beneath the posterior horn. With a specially designed curved chisel, the first ischial osteotomy is done. The osteotomy of approximately 4 to 5 cm is an incomplete cut of the ischium. Next, two blunt retractors are placed around the superior aspect of the pubic bone to protect the soft tissues and perform the pubic osteotomy (**Fig-**

ure 7, C). At the level of the anterior superior iliac spine, partial elevation of the abductor muscles from the outside of the iliac wing is done to place a blunt retractor for protection of the abductor muscles. The periosteum and obturator internus muscles are bluntly dissected off the quadrilateral plate, and another blunt curved retractor is placed on the quadrilateral surface close to the ischial spine to further retract the soft tissues medially. With use of an oscillating saw, an oblique iliac osteotomy is performed at the level of the anterior superior iliac spine (**Figure 7, C**). This osteotomy ends 1 to 2 cm lateral to the pelvic rim. From there, an osteotomy is angled approximately 110° distally in regard to the previous horizontal cut of the ilium. This osteotomy is performed with straight and curved chisels and is directed to the ischial spine. A Schanz screw is inserted at the level of the anterior inferior iliac spine to do a controlled fracture of the remaining bone (**Figure 7, C**). A spreader inserted in the osteotomy gap of the iliac bone assists this maneuver. The controlled fracture can be aided by an additional cut with the specially designed curved chisel from the inside of the quadrilateral surface. Once the fragment is completely free, the acetabulum is oriented with the Schanz screw and Hohmann retractors. Preliminary fixation of the bone is done with use of 2.5-mm partially threaded pins.

An intraoperative radiograph is made with a radiographic plate slid underneath the patient, using a specially designed "sandwich" table, which eliminates the need to move the patient or the drapes. The evaluation criteria for an optimal correction are described in more detail in the following section of this chapter. The intraoperative decision for the need of an additional osteotomy on the femoral side may require additional abduction or adduction radiographs. Three 3.5-mm cortical screws are typically used to definitively fix the acetabular fragment. Internal rotation is evaluated with the hip flexed 90°. If there is less than 30° of internal rotation in the presence of decreased femoral head-neck offset on a lateral radiograph, an H-shaped capsulotomy is performed (**Figure 7, D**).

The rectus femoris muscle is retracted medially for the capsulotomy. The osseous contour of the anterosu-perior femoral head-neck contour is trimmed (a so-called offset correction) with a curved chisel and/or a high-speed burr[20] (**Figure 7, D**). This is best performed with the lower limb in 10° of flexion and various positions of rotation. The incision is closed with absorbable sutures, and a running suture is placed along the iliac crest to reattach the muscle sleeve and the inguinal ligament to the outer fascia of the pelvis and thigh. Postoperatively, a continuous passive motion machine is used and partial weight bearing of 15 to 20 kg is recommended for 6 to 8 weeks after surgery.

Intraoperative Evaluation

Intraoperative evaluation can most accurately and efficiently be done by examining an AP pelvic radiograph. The tube-to-film distance is approximately 1.2 m in the department of this chapter's authors. Recommendations for defining the so-called ideal correction parameters can only be given in ranges and not to the exact degree. The parameters and recommended goals are (1) a lateral center-edge angle between 20° and 35°, preferably between 25° and 30°; (2) an anterior center-edge angle between 0° and 10°, preferably in the upper range; (3) head medialization with a distance between the medial aspect of the femoral head and the ilioischial line of less than 10 mm; (4) restoration of the Shenton line; (5) a weight-bearing dome centered over the head; (6) anteversion of the acetabulum as defined by the absence of a crossover sign and the outlines of the anterior and posterior rim meeting at the lateral acetabular edge; and (7) restoration of hip joint congruency.[23]

Persistent joint incongruity after acetabular reorientation requires intraoperative functional radiographs made with the hip in abduction or adduction to decide whether an intertrochanteric osteotomy is necessary. After obtaining a satisfactory correction, the hip motion is judged, especially the flexion and the internal rotation. Although there is no agreement regarding the definition of decreased internal rotation, internal rotation that is only between 15° and 30° should lead to a further search for the cause. Exclusion of intra-articular femoroacetabular impingement or extra-articular impingement against the anterior inferior iliac spine is recommended.[24] In a recent series of 90 patients, a femoral head-neck offset correction was performed in 57% of the hips after acetabular reorientation through a periacetabular osteotomy.[25]

Review of the Literature

There is evidence that acetabular reorientation can decelerate joint degeneration.[26] The long-term results (10 to almost 30 years) for all three types of juxta-acetabular osteotomies are summarized in **Table 1**.[9,10,26-39] The survivorship of the hip has been reproducibly shown to be approximately 90% after 10 years and 60% to 70% after 20 years, independent of the reorientation technique. The long-term reports of the early series typically involved heterogeneous patient cohorts, including patients with advanced age and/or joint degeneration.[26-28] In a follow-up study with a more homogeneous patient cohort at the Inselspital, University of Bern, a good clinical result without progression of osteoarthritis was achieved in 90% of the patients at a minimum 10-year follow-up interval.[25] Follow-up studies that have shown survivorship of up to 100% typically have involved a nonconsecutive series of patients, exclusive of patients with previous surgical procedures on the hip, low numbers of patients, or a substantial percentage of patients lost to follow-up.[29-31] The natural history of hip dysplasia is not as good.[40]

Table 1

Minimum 10-Year Survivorship of the Hip After Surgical Treatment of Developmental Dysplasia With Conversion to Total Hip Arthroplasty as the End Point

Study (Year)	Technique	Duration of Follow-up[a] (Years)	No. of Hips	Age in Years[a]	Survival Rate (%)
Siebenrock et al[10] (1999)	Periacetabular	11.3 (10-14)	75	29 (13-56)	82
Kralj et al[27] (2005)	Periacetabular	12 (7-15)	26	34 (18-50)	85
Flecher et al[28] (2008)	Periacetabular	12 (2-19)	33	32 (18-47)	74
Steppacher et al[26] (2008)	Periacetabular	20.4 (19-23)	75	29.3 (13-56)	61
Matheney et al[36] (2009)	Periacetabular	9 ± 2.2	135	23 (10-44)	84
Ito et al[37] (2011)	Periacetabular	11 (5-20)	158	32 (12-56)	96
Nakamura et al[32] (1998)	Rotational	13 (10-23)	145	28 (11-52)	95
Takatori et al[38] (2000)	Rotational	13 (10-18)	28	33 (19-40)	96
Takatori et al[30] (2001)	Rotational	19.8 (15-22)	15	24.3 (20-28)	100
Nozawa et al[39] (2002)	Rotational	11.4 (10-15)	50	31.8 (13-53)	98
Yasunaga et al[35] (2004)	Rotational	11 (8-15)	61	35 (13-58)	100
Guille et al[31] (1992)	Triple	12 (10-16)	11	14 (11-16)	91
van Hellemondt et al[33] (2005)	Triple	15 (13-20)	51	28 (14-46)	88
Janssen et al[34] (2009)	Triple	12 (11-12)	35	39 (24-57)	85
Schramm et al[9] (2003)	Wagner spheric	23.9 (20-29)	22	24.4 ± 9.7	68
Zagra et al[29] (2007)	Wagner spheric	23.1 (21-27)	10	19.3 (17-27)	100

[a]Continuous data are expressed as the mean, with the range in parentheses if available, or the SD.

Several common negative predictors influencing the long-term outcome after acetabular reorientation for developmental dysplasia of the hip were identified. These include mainly demographic or independent preoperative factors such as advanced age, low preoperative functional hip scores, a body mass index of greater than 25 (kg/m²), preexisting early osteoarthritis, a preoperative limp, evidence of a labral tear with pain in flexion and internal rotation, and preoperative femoral head subluxation.[25-27,32-36,41-45]

Postoperative lateral acetabular undercoverage and excessive acetabular anteversion can lead to persistent static overload of the lateral and/or the anterior acetabular rim with subsequent degeneration.[25,46] Postoperative lateral overcoverage and acetabular retroversion have been associated with decreased hip survivorship because of

iatrogenic postoperative femoroacetabular impingement between the overcorrected acetabulum and the proximal part of the femur.[20,25,47] A previous femoral head-neck offset correction or, if necessary, an intraoperative offset correction in hips with an aspheric head-neck junction improves the 10-year survivorship.[25,48] Improper acetabular reorientation, specifically incorrect acetabular version and a concomitant persistence of an aspheric femoral head-neck junction, needs to be included as a risk factor for a less favorable outcome.[25]

Summary

The appropriate surgical treatment of hip dysplasia after closure of the triradiate cartilage is a reorientation of the entire acetabulum. Among the different surgical techniques for acetabular reorientation, periacetabular osteot-

omy has become the gold standard. It provides the largest reorientation potential with inherent stability because of its polygonal shape without changing the dimensions of the birth canal. There is increasing evidence that the natural degeneration in dysplastic hips can be decelerated by periacetabular osteotomy. The survival rate of the hip after acetabular reorientation is approximately 90% after 10 years and 60% to 70% after 20 years. Careful patient selection, an optimal acetabular reorientation, and a concomitant osteochondroplasty of an aspheric femoral head-neck junction may lead to improved long-term results.

Acknowledgment

The authors thank Joseph M. Schwab, MD, for assistance in the preparation of this manuscript.

References

1. Trousdale RT, Ganz R: Posttraumatic acetabular dysplasia. *Clin Orthop Relat Res* 1994;305:124-132.

2. Chiari K: [Pelvic osteotomy in hip arthroplasty]. *Wien Med Wochenschr* 1953;103(38):707-709.

3. Lance M: Consitution d'une butrée ostéoplastique dans les luxationes subluxations congénitales de la hanche. *Presse Med* 1925;33: 945-958.

4. Klaue K, Durnin CW, Ganz R: The acetabular rim syndrome: A clinical presentation of dysplasia of the hip. *J Bone Joint Surg Br* 1991;73(3):423-429.

5. Windhager R, Pongracz N, Schönecker W, Kotz R: Chiari osteotomy for congenital dislocation and subluxation of the hip: Results after 20 to 34 years followup. *J Bone Joint Surg Br* 1991; 73(6):890-895.

6. Nishina T, Saito S, Ohzono K, Shimizu N, Hosoya T, Ono K: Chiari pelvic osteotomy for osteoarthritis: The influence of the torn and detached acetabular labrum. *J Bone Joint Surg Br* 1990;72(5): 765-769.

7. Wagner H: Osteotomies for congenital hip dislocation, in *The Hip: Proceedings of the Fourth Open Scientific Meeting of the Hip Society*. St. Louis, MO, CV Mosby, 1976, pp 45-66.

8. Ninomiya S, Tagawa H: Rotational acetabular osteotomy for the dysplastic hip. *J Bone Joint Surg Am* 1984;66(3):430-436.

9. Schramm M, Hohmann D, Radespiel-Troger M, Pitto RP: Treatment of the dysplastic acetabulum with Wagner spherical osteotomy: A study of patients followed for a minimum of twenty years. *J Bone Joint Surg Am* 2003;85(5):808-814.

10. Siebenrock KA, Schöll E, Lottenbach M, Ganz R: Bernese periacetabular osteotomy. *Clin Orthop Relat Res* 1999;363:9-20.

11. Tönnis D, Behrens K, Tscharani F: A modified technique of the triple pelvic osteotomy: Early results. *J Pediatr Orthop* 1981;1(3): 241-249.

12. Ganz R, Klaue K, Vinh TS, Mast JW: A new periacetabular osteotomy for the treatment of hip dysplasias: Technique and preliminary results. *Clin Orthop Relat Res* 1988;232:26-36.

13. Leunig M, Siebenrock KA, Ganz R: Rationale of periacetabular osteotomy and background work. *Instr Course Lect* 2001;50: 229-238.

14. Steppacher SD, Tannast M, Werlen S, Siebenrock KA: Femoral morphology differs between deficient and excessive acetabular coverage. *Clin Orthop Relat Res* 2008; 466(4):782-790.

15. Clohisy JC, Barrett SE, Gordon JE, Delgado ED, Schoenecker PL: Periacetabular osteotomy in the treatment of severe acetabular dysplasia: Surgical technique. *J Bone Joint Surg Am* 2006; 88(suppl 1 pt 1):65-83.

16. Tannast M, Hanke M, Ecker TM, Murphy SB, Albers CE, Puls M: LCPD: Reduced range of motion resulting from extra- and intraarticular impingement. *Clin Orthop Relat Res* 2012;470(9):2431-2440.

17. Hersche O, Casillas M, Ganz R: Indications for intertrochanteric osteotomy after periacetabular osteotomy for adult hip dysplasia. *Clin Orthop Relat Res* 1998;347: 19-26.

18. Nötzli HP, Müller SM, Ganz R: [The relationship between fovea capitis femoris and weight bearing area in the normal and dysplastic hip in adults: A radiologic study] . *Z Orthop Ihre Grenzgeb* 2001; 139(6):502-506.

19. Ganz R, Huff TW, Leunig M: Extended retinacular soft-tissue flap for intra-articular hip surgery: Surgical technique, indications, and results of application. *Instr Course Lect* 2009;58:241-255.

20. Myers SR, Eijer H, Ganz R: Anterior femoroacetabular impingement after periacetabular osteotomy. *Clin Orthop Relat Res* 1999;363:93-99.

21. Siebenrock KA, Schoeniger R, Ganz R: Anterior femoroacetabular impingement due to acetabular retroversion: Treatment with periacetabular osteotomy. *J Bone Joint Surg Am* 2003;85(2): 278-286.

22. Babst D, Steppacher SD, Ganz R, Siebenrock KA, Tannast M: The iliocapsularis muscle: An important stabilizer in the dysplastic hip. *Clin Orthop Relat Res* 2011; 469(6):1728-1734.

23. Millis MB, Siebenrock KA; Session Participants: Report of breakout session: Defining parameters for correcting the acetabulum during a pelvic reorientation osteotomy. *Clin Orthop Relat Res* 2012;470(12):3453-3455.

24. Ziebarth K, Balakumar J, Domayer S, Kim YJ, Millis MB: Bernese periacetabular osteotomy in males: Is there an increased risk of femoroacetabular impingement (FAI) after Bernese periacetabular osteotomy? *Clin Orthop Relat Res* 2011;469(2):447-453.

25. Albers CE, Steppacher SD, Ganz R, Tannast M, Siebenrock KA: Impingement adversely impacts 10-year survivorship after periacetabular osteotomy for DDH. *Clin Orthop Relat Res* 2013; 471(5):1602-1614.

26. Steppacher SD, Tannast M, Ganz R, Siebenrock KA: Mean 20-year followup of Bernese periacetabular osteotomy. *Clin Orthop Relat Res* 2008;466(7):1633-1644.

27. Kralj M, Mavcic B, Antolic V, Iglic A, Kralj-Iglic V: The Bernese periacetabular osteotomy: Clinical, radiographic and mechanical 7-15-year follow-up of 26 hips. *Acta Orthop* 2005;76(6):833-840.

28. Flecher X, Casiraghi A, Aubaniac JM, Argenson JN: [Periacetabular osteotomy medium term survival in adult acetabular dysplasia]. *Rev Chir Orthop Reparatrice Appar Mot* 2008;94(4):336-345.

29. Zagra L, Corbella M, Giacometti Ceroni R: Wagner's spherical periacetabular osteotomy: Long term results. *Hip Int* 2007;17(suppl 5):S65-S71.

30. Takatori Y, Ninomiya S, Nakamura S, et al: Long-term results of rotational acetabular osteotomy in patients with slight narrowing of the joint space on preoperative radiographic findings. *J Orthop Sci* 2001;6(2):137-140.

31. Guille JT, Forlin E, Kumar SJ, MacEwen GD: Triple osteotomy of the innominate bone in treatment of developmental dysplasia of the hip. *J Pediatr Orthop* 1992; 12(6):718-721.

32. Nakamura S, Ninomiya S, Takatori Y, Morimoto S, Umeyama T: Long-term outcome of rotational acetabular osteotomy: 145 hips followed for 10-23 years. *Acta Orthop Scand* 1998;69(3):259-265.

33. van Hellemondt GG, Sonneveld H, Schreuder MH, Kooijman MA, de Kleuver M: Triple osteotomy of the pelvis for acetabular dysplasia: Results at a mean follow-up of 15 years. *J Bone Joint Surg Br* 2005;87(7):911-915.

34. Janssen D, Kalchschmidt K, Katthagen BD: Triple pelvic osteotomy as treatment for osteoarthritis secondary to developmental dysplasia of the hip. *Int Orthop* 2009;33(6):1555-1559.

35. Yasunaga Y, Ochi M, Shimogaki K, Yamamoto S, Iwamori H: Rotational acetabular osteotomy for hip dysplasia: 61 hips followed for 8-15 years. *Acta Orthop Scand* 2004;75(1):10-15.

36. Matheney T, Kim YJ, Zurakowski D, Matero C, Millis M: Intermediate to long-term results following the Bernese periacetabular osteotomy and predictors of clinical outcome. *J Bone Joint Surg Am* 2009;91(9):2113-2123.

37. Ito H, Tanino H, Yamanaka Y, Nakamura T, Minami A, Matsuno T: The Chiari pelvic osteotomy for patients with dysplastic hips and poor joint congruency: Long-term follow-up. *J Bone Joint Surg Br* 2011;93(6): 726-731.

38. Takatori Y, Ninomiya S, Nakamura S, Morimoto S, Moro T, Nagai I: Long-term results of rotational acetabular osteotomy in young patients with advanced osteoarthrosis of the hip. *J Orthop Sci* 2000;5(4):336-341.

39. Nozawa M, Shitoto K, Matsuda K, Maezawa K, Kurosawa H: Rotational acetabular osteotomy for acetabular dysplasia: A follow-up for more than ten years. *J Bone Joint Surg Br* 2002;84(1):59-65.

40. Murphy SB, Ganz R, Müller ME: The prognosis in untreated dysplasia of the hip: A study of radiographic factors that predict the outcome. *J Bone Joint Surg Am* 1995;77(7):985-989.

41. Murphy S, Deshmukh R: Periacetabular osteotomy: Preoperative radiographic predictors of outcome. *Clin Orthop Relat Res* 2002; 405:168-174.

42. de Kleuver M, Kooijman MA, Pavlov PW, Veth RP: Triple osteotomy of the pelvis for acetabular dysplasia: Results at 8 to 15 years. *J Bone Joint Surg Br* 1997; 79(2):225-229.

43. Trousdale RT, Ekkernkamp A, Ganz R, Wallrichs SL: Periacetabular and intertrochanteric osteotomy for the treatment of osteoarthrosis in dysplastic hips. *J Bone Joint Surg Am* 1995;77(1): 73-85.

44. Cunningham T, Jessel R, Zurakowski D, Millis MB, Kim YJ: Delayed gadolinium-enhanced magnetic resonance imaging of cartilage to predict early failure of Bernese periacetabular osteotomy for hip dysplasia. *J Bone Joint Surg Am* 2006;88(7):1540-1548.

45. Jessel RH, Zurakowski D, Zilkens C, Burstein D, Gray ML, Kim YJ: Radiographic and patient factors associated with pre-radiographic osteoarthritis in hip dysplasia. *J Bone Joint Surg Am* 2009;91(5): 1120-1129.

46. Sakai T, Nishii T, Takao M, Ohzono K, Sugano N: High survival of dome pelvic osteotomy in patients with early osteoarthritis from hip dysplasia. *Clin Orthop Relat Res* 2012;470(9):2573-2582.

47. Yasunaga Y, Yamasaki T, Matsuo T, Ishikawa M, Adachi N, Ochi M: Crossover sign after rotational acetabular osteotomy for dysplasia of the hip. *J Orthop Sci* 2010; 15(4):463-469.

48. Ohashi H, Hirohashi K, Yamano Y: Factors influencing the outcome of Chiari pelvic osteotomy: A long-term follow-up. *J Bone Joint Surg Br* 2000;82(4): 517-525.

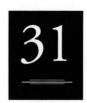

Surgical Aspects of Spinal Growth Modulation in Scoliosis Correction

Viral Jain, MD
Marios Lykissas, MD
Per Trobisch, MD
Eric J. Wall, MD
Peter O. Newton, MD
Peter F. Sturm, MD
Patrick J. Cahill, MD
Donita I. Bylski-Austrow, PhD

Abstract

Spine growth modulation for scoliosis correction is a technique for slowing growth on the convex side of the curve and enhancing growth on the concave side by using the Heuter-Volkmann principle; this results in gradual deformity correction. The theoretic advantages include speedier recovery because of the minimally invasive approach used, as well as motion preservation. Several devices have been used in humans, including vertebral body stapling, with either a flexible titanium clip or a nitinol staple, and anterior spinal tethering. Prerequisites for the use of these devices are a relatively flexible curve and sufficient remaining growth in the patient. Although vertebral body stapling is effective for moderate curves of less than 40°, anterior spinal tethering can be used for curves greater than 40°. The titanium clip and spinal tethers are used exclusively for thoracic scoliosis, whereas nitinol staples can be used for the thoracic spine or the lumbar spine.

The thoracoscopic technique is used for thoracic instrumentation, and the mini-open retroperitoneal technique is used for lumbar staple insertion. The insertion of a titanium clip and an anterior spinal tether requires sacrifice and mobilization of the segmental vessels, whereas nitinol staples can be inserted without such sacrifice. Single lung ventilation and CO_2 insufflation are used to improve visualization with the thoracoscope. The curve should be instrumented from an end vertebra to an end vertebra. Postoperative immobilization depends on the type of device used.

Most complications are approach related, such as atelectasis caused by a mucus plug, pain at the chest tube site, and pneumothorax. Device-related complications are rare. Overcorrection is a concern. In patients with early onset scoliosis, a hybrid construct with vertebral stapling and growing rods or a vertical expandable prosthetic titanium rib has been suggested. A failure of the spinal growth modulation procedure does not preclude spinal fusion. None of the devices for spine growth modulation have been approved by the FDA for human use and are still investigational. Early results are promising, and continued clinical studies are necessary.

Instr Course Lect 2014;63:335-344.

Scoliosis is a common disorder of the pediatric spine that results in a three-dimensional deformity. The etiology of scoliosis is largely unknown; however, genetic factors have been implicated. Biomechanical imbalance leading to asymmetric spinal growth has been postulated as the mechanism for progression. Among the various treatment methods used, only bracing and surgical fusion have been shown to change the natural history of the

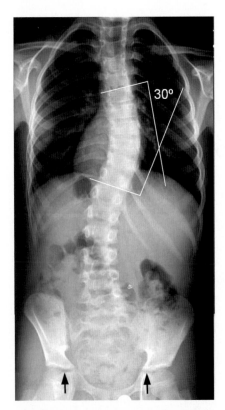

Figure 1 AP radiograph of an ideal scoliosis curve for growth modulation treatment with a flexible titanium clip. The triradiate cartilage is open (arrows).

disorder. Although spinal fusion with instrumentation for scoliosis correction has a high success rate and few complications, it is a very invasive procedure. Loss of motion after spinal fusion and the potential for adjacent segment degeneration is a long-term concern.

The concept of growth modulation correction in a growing child using staples for limb deformity, which was introduced by Blount and Clarke,[1] is well known to orthopaedic surgeons. It is presumed that staples inhibit growth according to the Heuter-Volkmann principle. More recently, a similar concept has been applied successfully to spinal growth modulation. These devices, which provide compressive forces on the convex side of the curve by using the Heuter-Volkmann principle, slow growth on the convex side of the curve and enhance growth on the concave side. This effect has been proven in animal models.[2] Motion is also preserved at the instrumented levels.[3] Radiographic and chemical analyses performed in animals have shown that disk function is maintained after the application of such device.[4]

This chapter discusses the clinical aspects of various spinal growth modulation techniques, including indications, contraindications, surgical principles and techniques, complications, alternative treatments, and salvage strategies. It should be noted that none of the devices described in this chapter are approved by the FDA for the purpose of spinal growth modulation and are considered investigational devices.

This chapter focuses on three such devices, which are already being used in humans in off-label applications. These include the flexible titanium clip, which is being studied prospectively in the United States in an FDA clinical trial; the nitinol staple, which has been studied in a retrospective manner; and the anterior spinal tether, which is being studied outside the United States.

Vertebral Body Stapling

Flexible Titanium Clip

Indications and Contraindications

Children with idiopathic scoliosis curves greater than 25° to 30° who are at the beginning of puberty and have not reached their peak height velocity (peak growth spurt) are at a nearly 100% risk of scoliosis progression to a 50° Cobb angle.[5,6] The best candidate for a flexible titanium clip is a child older than 8 years with a Cobb angle of 25° to 40°, a triradiate cartilage that is not closed, a Risser grade of 0, and an Atlas bone age younger than 13 years in girls and younger than 15 years in boys (**Figure 1**).

Children with a serious pulmonary or anatomic condition that would contraindicate an anterior endoscopic approach are unsuitable candidates. The use of clip-type devices is a relative contraindication in children with neu-

Dr. Jain or an immediate family member serves as a paid consultant to or is an employee of Medtronic Sofamor Danek. Dr. Wall or an immediate family member serves as a paid consultant to or is an employee of OrthoPediatrics; serves as an unpaid consultant to SpineForm and Stryker; has received nonincome support (such as equipment or services), commercially derived honoraria, or other non–research-related funding (such as paid travel) from SpineForm; and serves as a board member, owner, officer, or committee member of the Pediatric Orthopaedic Society of North America. Dr. Newton or an immediate family member has received royalties from DePuy; is a member of a speakers' bureau or has made paid presentations on behalf of DePuy; serves as a paid consultant to or is an employee of DePuy; has stock or stock options held in Nuvasive; has received research or institutional support from DePuy, Biospace Med, the Orthopaedic Research and Education Foundation, the Pediatric Orthopaedic Society of North America, the Scoliosis Research Society, the Harms Study Group Foundation, the Setting Scoliosis Straight Foundation, and the Children's Specialist Foundation; and serves as a board member, owner, officer, or committee member of the Pediatric Orthopaedic Society of North America, the Setting Scoliosis Straight Foundation, and the Children's Specialist Foundation. Dr. Sturm or an immediate family member serves as a paid consultant to or is an employee of DePuy; has stock or stock options held in Pioneer Surgical; has received research or institutional support from DePuy; and serves as a board member, owner, officer, or committee member of the Pediatric Orthopaedic Society of North America and the Scoliosis Research Society. Dr. Cahill or an immediate family member is a member of a speakers' bureau or has made paid presentations on behalf of DePuy Synthes Spine; serves as a paid consultant to or is an employee of DePuy Synthes Spine; has received research or institutional support from DePuy Synthes Spine; has received nonincome support (such as equipment or services), commercially derived honoraria, or other non–research-related funding (such as paid travel) from DePuy Synthes Spine; and serves as a board member, owner, officer, or committee member of the American Academy of Orthopaedic Surgeons, the Scoliosis Research Society, and the Pediatric Orthopaedic Society of North America. Dr. Bylski-Austrow or an immediate family member serves as an unpaid consultant to SpineForm and has received nonincome support (such as equipment or services), commercially derived honoraria, or other non–research-related funding (such as paid travel) from SpineForm and DePuy. Neither of the following authors nor any immediate family member has received anything of value from or has stock or stock options held in a commercial company or institution related directly or indirectly to the subject of this chapter: Dr. Lykissas and Dr. Trobisch.

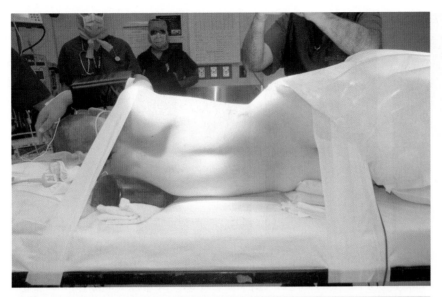

Figure 2   The patient is positioned in a true lateral position, with a large axillary roll and a high hip bump that allows the thorax to hang free and corrects the right-side curve.

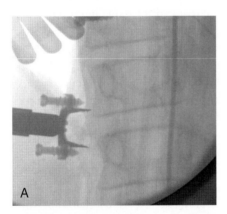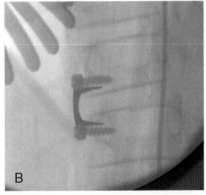

Figure 3   **A,** Positioning of the clip with the insertion tool. **B,** The angled internal surface of the clip tines gently compresses the convex side of the curve and mildly distracts the opposite side.

romuscular, congenital, and syndromic scoliosis because of an unpredictable vertebral growth plate response. Curves greater than 40° may be too large to correct with a flexible titanium clip device for growth modulation.

Surgical Technique

An anesthesiologist performs single lung ventilation after bronchoscopically inserting a double lumen tube and deflating the lung on the convex side of the child's thoracic curve. The patient is placed on a radiolucent table in a perfect lateral position with the main thoracic curve pointing upward. A padded axillary roll is placed just distal to the armpit, and a bump that elevates the hip allows the chest to hang freely so that it just barely contacts the table (**Figure 2**). The goal is to provide passive thoracic curve correction.

Via an endoscopic approach, the segmental vessels are cauterized with a har-monic scalpel. The titanium clips with preloaded screws are placed sequentially, starting at the most cranial level. After an acceptable position is confirmed with fluoroscopy (with the clip straddling the disk and growth plates in the midvertebral body on the lateral view), the clip is tamped into place, and the preloaded screws are advanced with a screwdriver (**Figure 3**). The clips are placed sequentially, cranially to caudally.

After placing a chest tube, the deflated lung is reexpanded under thoracoscopic visualization, and the opposite dependent lung is suctioned completely under bronchoscopic visualization before extubation to remove mucous plugs.

Postoperative Protocol

The patient must maintain aggressive pulmonary toilet with incentive spirometer, cough, and deep breathing. A brace is not used. The chest tube is removed when the output is less than 50 mL per 8-hour shift. Sports participation is restricted for 6 months, except for cardiovascular conditioning.

Pearls and Pitfalls

Patient positioning is critical to achieve gravity-assisted correction. The surgeon should stand anterior to the patient. The use of CO_2 gas insufflation helps to deflate the lung and improve endoscopic visualization. Bronchoscopic lavage and suction are used to clear mucus plugging from both lungs.

Results and Complications

In a phase I FDA study of six children with adolescent idiopathic scoliosis, the curve corrected from a mean of 34.5° preoperatively to 23° at 1 month postoperatively and 26° at 3 months postoperatively[7] (**Figure 4**). Procedure-related complications included atelectasis and mucous plugging on

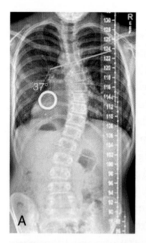
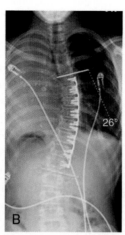
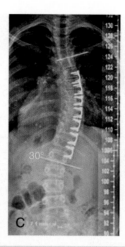
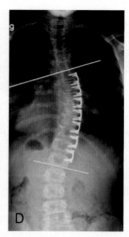
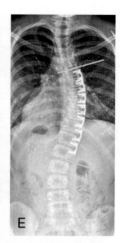

Figure 4 AP radiographs of the spine of a patient treated with a clip/staple device for a rapidly progressing scoliosis curve. **A,** The preoperative curve was 37°. **B,** The curve was 26° immediately after surgery. **C,** At 3 months after surgery, the curve was 30°. **D,** At 6 months after surgery, the curve was 30°. **E,** At 1 year after surgery, the curve was 32°.

the ventilated lung side (dependent lung). One patient had a chylous effusion that resolved with dietary restrictions and the insertion of a pigtail catheter. There were no device-related adverse events such as loosening or breakage.

Nitinol Staples

Indications

The ideal candidate for vertebral body stapling with a nitinol staple has remaining growth and moderate scoliosis with a significant risk for progression. The Sanders digital stage should be 4 or less. Patients are typically premenarchal and younger than 13 years in girls or younger than 14 years in boys.

Vertebral body stapling is limited to thoracic curves of 25° to 35° and lumbar curves of 25° to 40° that correct to less than 20° on bending radiographs. Larger curves are suitable for correction if extreme flexibility is present (bending to less than 10°). Vertebral body stapling is limited to vertebrae between T5 and L3.

Contraindications

The procedure is contraindicated in patients with congenital or high-risk neuromuscular scoliosis (Duchenne muscular dystrophy or spinal cord injury at a young age). Vertebral body stapling should be limited to children younger than 7 years.

Surgical Technique

Instrumentation is placed from end vertebra to end vertebra. If two curves have a leveled disk space in between, the space should remain uninstrumented. Thoracic curves are instrumented through a thoracoscopic approach. A mini-open retroperitoneal approach is used for lumbar curves.

The patient is positioned in a true lateral decubitus position, with the convex side facing upward. For the correction of lumbar curves, the up leg should be slightly flexed to take tension off the psoas muscle. The positioning should be confirmed with true AP and lateral fluoroscopic imaging. The upper and lower end vertebrae (AP view) and a line through the midportion of the vertebral bodies that will be instrumented (lateral view) are marked.

Two camera portals are typically required for vertebral body stapling of thoracic curves: one at 25% and one at 75% of the distance from the inferior end vertebra to the superior end vertebra, approximately in the anterior axillary line. Additional intercostal entries are required for staple insertion. After penetrating the chest wall, a switch should be made to single-lung ventilation. Insufflation with CO_2 will help keep the lung retracted (fan retractors are also used for lung retraction). Lumbar curves are approached via one small lateral oblique incision and blunt retroperitoneal dissection of the spine. The psoas muscle is retracted posteriorly.

A staple size is selected that will span the disk space but not insert more than 50% across the height of the vertebral body. A trial staple is placed above the disk space, and correct positioning is confirmed radiographically. The trial staple is impacted with a mallet to create pilot holes. The staple is inserted quickly because pilot holes usually bleed and disturb visualization.

Postoperative Protocol

The chest tube is removed when the 24-hour output is less than 20 mL. The use of an incentive spirometer is recommended. The patient may return to sports activities after 6 weeks. A thoracolumbosacral orthosis worn at night-

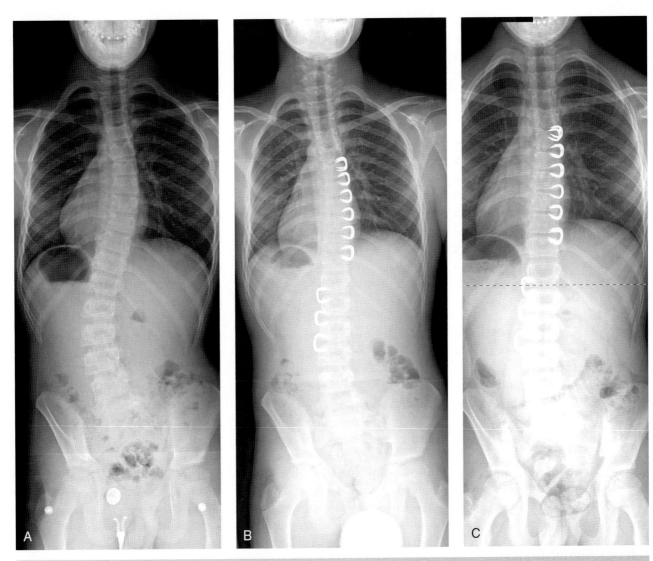

Figure 5   Radiographs of a 12-year-old boy with idiopathic scoliosis. **A,** Preoperative radiograph shows a lumbar curve measuring 33° and a thoracic curve measuring 25°. **B,** In the first erect postoperative standing radiograph, the thoracic curve was corrected to 11° and the lumbar curve to 7°. **C,** At 1 year postoperatively, the AP standing radiograph shows a thoracic curve measuring 0° and a lumbar curve still measuring 7°.

time may be considered for patients with a residual postoperative curve of more than 20° on upright radiographs.

Pearls and Pitfalls

Using the nitinol staple, segmental vessels are typically not mobilized. Bleeding can be controlled by pressure and cautery. Vaseline gauze is applied to the incision to maintain CO_2 pressure.

Results and Follow-Up

A retrospective data review included 28 patients (4 boys and 24 girls) with a mean age of 9.4 years who were treated with vertebral body stapling and followed for a minimum of 24 months postoperatively (mean, 3.2 years).[8] The patients had curves of 20° to 45°, were skeletally immature, and had a Risser grade of 0 or 1. A patient was evaluated based on the change in his or her Cobb angle (improvement equals > 10° decrease of Cobb angle; static equals < 10° decrease to < 10° increase; worsening equals > 10° increase). Success was defined as either static or improving curve development (**Figure 5**). The curve magnitude was 31° thoracic and 30° lumbar at the time of the index procedure. Although the success rate for thoracic curves of less than 35° was 78%, it was only 25% for curves greater than 35°. Very flexible curves that corrected to less than 20° on preoperative bending radiographs had a success rate of 86%. The success rate for lumbar curves was 86%.

Complications

The potential complications of vertebral body stapling with a nitinol staple are pneumothorax, staple displacement, curve progression, and overcorrection. Infections and neurologic complications are possible but have not yet been encountered.

Discussion

Bracing is the current standard of care for skeletally immature patients with moderate idiopathic scoliosis. However, a brace must be worn for up to 23 hours per day and may have a substantial effect on a patient's quality of life.[9] There is an ongoing debate regarding the effectiveness of brace treatment based on the results of various studies. Systematic reviews are often contradictory.[10,11] Patients and caregivers often request alternatives to brace treatment to prevent curve progression and the need for surgical fusion.

Based on the findings of this chapter's authors, vertebral body stapling represents an optional treatment for patients with a high risk of curve progression.[12,13] The invasiveness of the procedure as well as the lack of long-term results represent significant limitations that must be disclosed to the patient and family.

Anterior Spinal Tether

Indications

The indications for using an anterior spinal tether have not been well established. This technique will most likely benefit patients with enough growth remaining to substantially alter the shape of the spine. Two years or more of remaining growth is a conservative requirement in the early understanding of this technique. The presence of an open triradiate cartilage is a simple marker for adequate remaining growth. Ideally, only patients who would ultimately require spinal fusion if treated by other methods would be treated with spinal tethering because it is also a surgical intervention. Therefore, spinal tethering may be indicated

in patients with thoracic curves of 40° or greater. The upper limit of curvature is unknown at this time, but an arbitrary limit of 60° to 65° has been suggested.

The technique is most suited for primary thoracic curves with typical hypokyphotic apices. An anterior device that can limit anterior growth may induce kyphosis, aiding in the three-dimensional correction desired. The magnitude of proximal or lumbar curves that preclude the use of tethering also remains to be defined; however, using criteria similar to those used in choosing curves for selective thoracic fusion has been suggested. Flexible minor curves that are less than 75% of the magnitude of the thoracic curve are believed to be appropriate for selective thoracic tethering.

Contraindications

Anterior spinal tethering is contraindicated in patients with no remaining growth; those younger than 8 years; patients with curves less than 40° or more than 65°; and those with left-sided curves; pulmonary disease limiting single-lung ventilation; prior ipsilateral chest surgery; and poor bone quality, which may limit anterior vertebral fixation.

Surgical Technique

The selection of the levels to be tethered has generally followed the principles of anterior thoracic fusion. The instrumentation spans from the proximal end vertebra to the distal end vertebra. The approach is similar to anterior thoracic instrumented fusion, with open, mini-open, and endoscopic methods available. The thoracoscopic approach is preferred, with the use of single-lung ventilation and the patient in a lateral decubitus position. Screw trajectories in the coronal plane are marked using fluoroscopy, with planning for three posterior axillary line

15-mm portals for screw placement. An 11-mm anterior axillary line portal is used for endoscope placement. The pleura are opened longitudinally 1 cm anterior to the rib heads. The segmental vessels are coagulated, divided, and retracted anteriorly with sponges placed between the spine and the great vessels. Bicortical transverse vertebral body screws are placed through pronged washers using fluoroscopy to guide the screw trajectory. The tethering cord is introduced through a portal and captured with a set screw into the proximal vertebral body screw. The portals are adjusted to the appropriate interspace used to place the adjacent screw, and the long end of the tether is removed from the chest through that portal, allowing a tensioning device to take slack out of the tether as the next set screw is tightened. This sequence is repeated for each screw, with more or less compression applied as indicated based on the deformity (generally more compression at the apex and less to none at the ends). The tether is cut distally, and the pleura is closed over the device with the endoscopic suturing technique. A chest tube is placed, and the lungs are reinflated.

Postoperative Protocol

Postoperatively, the patient recovers in the hospital for 4 to 5 days. A thoracolumbosacral orthosis is recommended for 3 months after surgery. Noncontact activities can be resumed after 3 months.

Pearls and Pitfalls

Visualization is the key to a successful procedure. This requires complete deflation of the lung (double lumen endotracheal tube or a bronchial blocker) and a dry field (all bleeding is stopped). The surgeon directly looks down the 15-mm ports to help line up the vertebral screws. The prong staple position is verified before impacting it

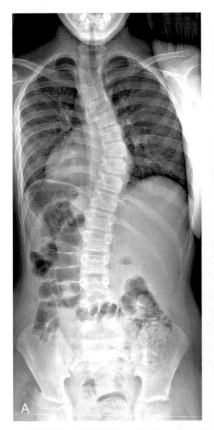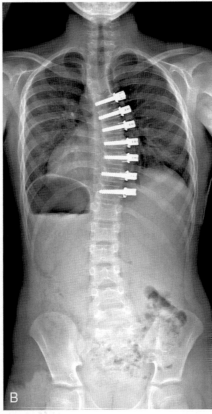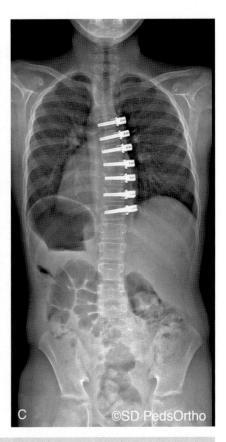

Figure 6 **A,** Preoperative PA view of the spine of a 10-year-old boy with a 45° curve and open triradiate cartilage (Risser 0). **B,** Radiograph taken 2 weeks postoperatively after treatment with anterior spinal tethering shows initial correction of the curve to 28°. **C,** The 18-month postoperative radiograph show curve correction to 11°. (Copyright J.D. Bomar, Children's Orthopedics, San Diego, CA.)

into place to ensure that the disk will not be impaled. To help prevent early overcorrection of the distal segments, it is important not to overtension the inferior levels where the disks are most flexible and the vertebral growth is greatest.

Results

To date, clinical results are limited (**Figure 6**). The longest follow-up study has been reported by Crawford and Lenke,[14] who reported scoliosis correction over several years. Anecdotal observations suggest immediate postoperative reductions of the curvature of approximately 20% to 60% depending on the flexibility and tension placed in the device. Subsequent correction varies based on a patient's growth. After 3 to 6 months, expected

angular changes are modest (roughly 10° to 15° per year). The efficiency of growth modulation created by tethering seems to be high enough that overcorrection is a real concern. This makes the need for a second procedure (for removal) also a concern; therefore, patients and parents should understand the possible need for additional surgery at the time of the initial implantation. Methods to track patients and monitor follow-up are critical because a patient lost to follow-up may have a substantial deformity because of overcorrection.

Complications

In addition to overcorrection, anterior spinal tethering is associated with all the potential complications associated with anterior spinal surgery. Parenchy-

mal injury to the lungs is a risk, particularly if an endoscopic procedure is attempted without complete lung deflation. Great vessel injury is a risk, both during the exposure and with regard to the aorta in a delayed fashion if the screws are long on the far side of the spine. Implant loosening and tether breakage remains a concern. In an animal study, the use of a staple or a pronged washer was found to limit screw migration.[15] The fate of the disk and the motion of the instrumented segments are unknown.

Hybrid Constructs and Salvage Techniques

Clinical studies in patients with adolescent idiopathic scoliosis and mild to moderate deformity have shown promising results after management

Table 1

Patient Demographics and Radiographic Data

Patient	Diagnosis	Age at Growth Modulation (Years)	Sex	Levels Stapled
1	Marfan syndrome	3	Male	T5-T12
2	Neuromuscular scoliosis	6.9	Female	T5-L1
3	Spinal cord injury	6.9	Male	T5-L3
4	Myelomeningocele	8.4	Female	T10-L4
5	Infantile idiopathic scoliosis	4.8	Male	T4-T11

with vertebral stapling.[16,17] However, when the efficacy of growth modulation was evaluated in patients with early onset scoliosis, most of the patients had further surgery at less than 2 years from the index procedure.[18] Possible etiologies for deformity progression after attempted growth modulation in patients who do not have adolescent idiopathic scoliosis curves include a deformity that is more likely to progress, a curve that is refractory to bracing, an underlying disease process that is fundamentally different from adolescent idiopathic scoliosis, a level of severity of vertebral rotation that introduces another factor that may be difficult to overcome with a correction method designed to work in only one plane and the treatment of younger patients because such patients tend to present with more significant deformities.

Only one study of the results of stapling in a population with early onset scoliosis exists in the literature.[18] The authors retrospectively reviewed 11 patients treated with open anterior vertebral stapling between August 2003 and August 2004. Data were collected on each patient's diagnosis, age at the time of surgery (stapling and hybrid instrumentation), Risser grade, maturity of the triradiate cartilage, and the length of the instrumentation. Radiographic analyses included Cobb angle measurements, translation of the apical vertebra (defined as the distance between the central sacral vertical line and the center of the apical vertebral body or disk), and concave length (measured from the apex of the T1 rib to the apex of the diaphragm on the concave side of the curve). Eleven patients with a non–adolescent idiopathic scoliosis curve were treated with an anterior vertebral stapling procedure via either a thoracotomy, a lateral lumbar retroperitoneal approach through a flank incision, or a combination of these approaches. In the 11 patients, 2 had infantile idiopathic scoliosis, 2 had juvenile idiopathic scoliosis, 1 had Marfan syndrome, 2 had neuromuscular scoliosis, 2 had a spinal cord injury, 1 had osteogenesis imperfecta, and 1 had myelomeningocele. The indication for surgery was unsuccessful nonsurgical treatment with a custom-made orthosis and curve progression of more than 10°. The average age at the time of the stapling procedure was 6 years (range, 3 to 8.4 years). The authors reported that the scoliosis Cobb angle improved from an average of 68° (range, 44° to 105°) to 45° (range, 25° to 87°) immediately after surgery and progressed to 69° (range, 51° to 107°) at the latest follow-up or before revision surgery. No significant residual deformity was recorded in three patients (27%), with an average curve magnitude of 47° (range, 38° to 53°) at final follow-up. Eight of the 11 patients (73%) had curve progression of more than 10° and required secondary surgeries, including growing rods placement (4 patients), vertical expandable prosthetic titanium rib (VEPTR) construct insertion (1 patient), and definitive spinal fusion (3 patients). In retrospect, the failure of this treatment method in this patient population could have been predicted. In this group of patients with large curves, stapling of the convex side could not overcome the continued pressure across the concave growth plate that led to continued curve progression.

Five of the 11 patients were followed and reported on after salvage surgery using a growing rod or VEPTR construct (P Gupta, MD, et al, Montreal, Canada, unpublished data presented at the International Congress on Early Onset Scoliosis and Growing Spine, 2008). The average age at the time of the salvage surgery was 7.86 years (range, 5.2 to 10.6 years) (**Table 1**). All five patients (3 boys and 2 girls) were skeletally immature, with a Risser grade of less than 2, and open triradiate cartilage. Three patients had dual rods placed, and one was treated with a single growing rod. No brace was used after surgery. The scoliosis Cobb angle showed a 33% improvement immediately after surgery and a 47% improvement at the last follow-up. Translation of the apical vertebra decreased from an average of 5 cm preoperatively to 2.8 cm immediately after surgery and 2.3 cm at the

Table 1 (Continued)

Patient Demographics and Radiographic Data

Preoperative Deformity	Postoperative Deformity	Presalvage Deformity	Salvage Procedure	Age at the Time of the Salvage Procedure (Years)	Follow-up (Months)
95°	88°	105°	Growing rods	5.2	50
70°	48°	80°	Growing rods	8.8	46
104°	37°	76°	Growing rod	8.6	44
74°	48°	80°	VEPTR	10.6	52
57°	57°	73°	Growing rods	6.1	40

VEPTR = vertical expandable prosthetic titanium rib.

last follow-up. Concave length increased by an average of 20% and 28% immediately after hybrid instrumentation and at the last follow-up, respectively. No failure of the growing rods or VEPTR implants requiring secondary procedures was recorded.

Based on these data, hybrid instrumentation can be effectively used as an adjunct to growth modulation in patients with severe non–adolescent idiopathic scoliosis curves that do not respond to vertebral stapling (**Figure 7**). Continued improvement occurs in both curve magnitude and concave length. Increased compressive forces in the concavity of severe curves may decrease or even inhibit the growth modulation potential.[18] An unloading effect of the hybrid construct on the concave side of the curve and, therefore, a synergistic action of the hybrid techniques with vertebral stapling for spinal deformity correction in skeletally immature patients with progressive early onset scoliosis may be possible. Simultaneous hybrid instrumentation and convex stapling in patients with adolescent idiopathic scoliosis with thoracic curves measuring 35° to 45° and nonbending curves less than 20° (the hybrid construct should be inserted first) have been used. No definitive results have been reported at this time. This technique should be considered as a possible option in the treatment armamentarium.

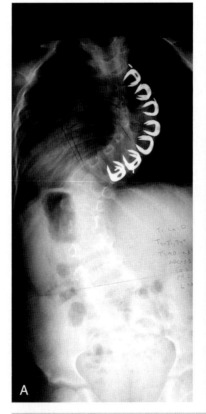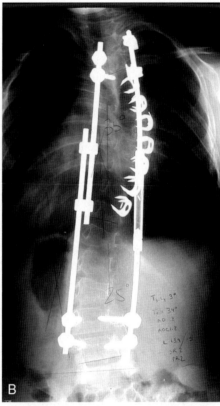

Figure 7 A 4.8-year-old boy with infantile idiopathic scoliosis. **A,** PA radiograph of the spine 16 months after T4-T11 anterior convex hemiepiphysiodesis shows curve progression from 57° to 73°. **B,** Two years after revision surgery with insertion of growing rod instrumentation, the curve measured 34°.

Early onset scoliosis represents a complex condition with limited treatment options. Both growing rods and VEPTR have been shown to be efficacious, but the complication rate remains high, and multiple surgeries are required.[19,20] Although growth modulation has a role in patients with ado-

lescent idiopathic scoliosis, its effect on malignant types of scoliosis remains unpredictable. Hybrid constructs may be a reliable salvage procedure after convex staple epiphysiodesis to control curve progression in patients with early onset scoliosis. Further studies are needed before considering these constructs as a primary treatment option.

Summary

The techniques of spine growth modulation for scoliosis correction use the Heuter-Volkmann principle. Flexible titanium clips, nitinol staples, and anterior spinal tethering have been used and studied in humans. Prerequisites for the use of these devices are a relatively flexible curve and sufficient remaining growth in the patient. Although flexible titanium clips and nitinol staples are effective for moderate curves of less than 40°, anterior spinal tethering can be used for curves greater than 40°. A minimally invasive thoracoscopic approach is commonly used. Most complications are related to the surgical approach. Overcorrection of the curve is a concern. Early onset scoliosis is less well studied and may require a hybrid posterior construct. The devices for spinal growth modulation are not yet approved by the FDA, but the early results are promising, and continued clinical studies are needed.

References

1. Blount WP, Clarke GR: Control of bone growth by epiphyseal stapling. *J Bone Joint Surg Am* 1949; 31(3):464-478.

2. Bylski-Austrow DI, Wall EJ, Glos DL, Ballard ET, Montgomery A, Crawford AH: Spinal hemiepiphysiodesis decreases the size of vertebral growth plate hypertrophic zone and cells. *J Bone Joint Surg Am* 2009;91(3):584-593.

3. Bylski-Austrow DI, Glos DL, Sauser FE, Jain VV, Wall EJ, Crawford AH: In vivo dynamic compressive stresses in the disc annulus: A pilot study of bilateral differences due to hemiepiphyseal implant in a quadruped model. *Spine (Phila Pa 1976)* 2012; 37(16):E949-E956.

4. Upasani VV, Farnsworth CL, Chambers RC, et al: Intervertebral disc health preservation after six months of spinal growth modulation. *J Bone Joint Surg Am* 2011;93(15):1408-1416.

5. Charles YP, Daures JP, de Rosa V, Diméglio A: Progression risk of idiopathic juvenile scoliosis during pubertal growth. *Spine (Phila Pa 1976)* 2006;31(17):1933-1942.

6. Sanders JO, Khoury JG, Kishan S, et al: A simplified classification during adolescence. *J Bone Joint Surg Am* 2008;90(3):540-553.

7. Evaluate initial safety of the HemiBridge System in guided spinal growth treatment of progressive idiopathic scoliosis. Clinical Trials.gov website. http://clinicaltrials.gov/show/NCT01465295. Accessed November 6, 2013.

8. Lavelle WF, Samdani AF, Cahill PJ, Betz RR: Clinical outcomes of nitinol staples for preventing curve progression in idiopathic scoliosis. *J Pediatr Orthop* 2011; 31(1):S107-S113.

9. Trobisch P, Suess O, Schwab F: Idiopathic scoliosis. *Dtsch Arztebl Int* 2010;107(49):875-883, quiz 884.

10. Dolan LA, Weinstein SL: Surgical rates after observation and bracing for adolescent idiopathic scoliosis: An evidence-based review. *Spine (Phila Pa 1976)* 2007;32(19):S91-S100.

11. Katz DE, Herring JA, Browne RH, Kelly DM, Birch JG: Brace wear control of curve progression in adolescent idiopathic scoliosis. *J Bone Joint Surg Am* 2010;92(6):1343-1352.

12. Betz RR, Ranade A, Samdani AF, et al: A fusionless treatment option for a growing child with moderate idiopathic scoliosis. *Spine (Phila Pa 1976)* 2010;35(2):169-176.

13. Trobisch PD, Samdani A, Cahill P, Betz RR: Vertebral body stapling as an alternative in the treatment of idiopathic scoliosis. *Oper Orthop Traumatol* 2011;23(3):227-231.

14. Crawford CH III, Lenke LG: Growth modulation by means of anterior tethering resulting in progressive correction of juvenile idiopathic scoliosis: A case report. *J Bone Joint Surg Am* 2010;92(1):202-209.

15. Snyder BD, Zaltz I, Hall JE, Emans JB: Predicting the integrity of vertebral bone screw fixation in anterior spinal instrumentation. *Spine (Phila Pa 1976)* 1995; 20(14):1568-1574.

16. Betz RR, D'Andrea LP, Mulcahey MJ, Chafetz RS: Vertebral body stapling procedure for the treatment of scoliosis in the growing child. *Clin Orthop Relat Res* 2005; 434:55-60.

17. Betz RR, Kim J, D'Andrea LP, Mulcahey MJ, Balsara RK, Clements DH: An innovative technique of vertebral body stapling for the treatment of patients with adolescent idiopathic scoliosis: A feasibility, safety, and utility study. *Spine (Phila Pa 1976)* 2003; 28(20):S255-S265.

18. O'leary PT, Sturm PF, Hammerberg KW, Lubicky JP, Mardjetko SM: Convex hemiepiphysiodesis: The limits of vertebral stapling. *Spine (Phila Pa 1976)* 2011; 36(19):1579-1583.

19. Akbarnia BA, Salari P: *The Growing Spine*. Berlin, Germany, Springer-Verlag, 2011.

20. Smith JT: Bilateral rib-to-pelvis technique for managing early-onset scoliosis. *Clin Orthop Relat Res* 2011;469(5):1349-1355.

Recurrent Spinal Deformity After Scoliosis Surgery in Children

Jaime A. Gomez, MD
Melvin C. Makhni, MD, MBA
Michael G. Vitale, MD, MPH

Abstract

The management of complex spinal deformities in the growing child continues to evolve. The implementation of new techniques and biomaterial constructs has improved outcomes of deformity correction procedures but has also led to unforeseen complications. After spinal alignment through posterior instrumentation and fusion, progressive global decompensation in the coronal and sagittal planes or local decompensation in the vertebral segments adjacent to the fusion have developed in some children. These complications can lead to poor cosmesis, function, and quality of life, and a higher risk for revision surgery. Although postoperative spinal imbalance develops in few children, diligent monitoring of patients with predisposing risk factors for decompensation will allow surgeons to better predict, manage, and potentially prevent these complications.

Instr Course Lect 2014;63:345-351.

The number of spinal deformity surgeries performed in pediatric patients has steadily increased over the past two decades. Fortunately, fewer than 10 in 100,000 children require spinal surgery for various indications.[1] Most of these children have good outcomes; however, depending on the diagnosis and procedure performed, complication rates have been reported to be from 4% to 200%.[2-6] The broad range of complications in children requiring further surgical interventions depends mainly on the type of scoliosis treated. Complication rates are lowest in corrections performed in patients with adolescent idiopathic scoliosis (AIS), increase in older patients with neurogenic and congenital scoliosis, and are highest in very young patients. The complication rate also depends on the procedure performed.

Although posterior spinal instrumentation and fusion techniques allow dramatic correction of three-dimensional spinal deformities, unintended outcomes in spinal alignment in both the coronal and sagittal planes can occur. The goals of posterior spinal instrumentation and fusion include aligning the head and trunk over the pelvis with level shoulders, positioning the C7 plumb line just behind the hip center, and maintaining these parameters over time. Despite powerful correction techniques, posterior fusion can result in suboptimal postoperative spinal balance. In contrast, decompensation is the continued loss of spinal balance over time. Fusion also can result in unintended reciprocal changes in the unfused segments above or below the level of the fusion.[7-9]

This chapter will focus on postoperative imbalance and decompensation after spinal fusion surgery. Although a relatively small percentage of children have postoperative complications, surgical planning and technique can positively affect postoperative outcomes.

Dr. Vitale or an immediate family member has received royalties from Biomet; serves as a paid consultant to or is an employee of Biomet and Stryker; has received research or institutional support from Synthes; and serves as a board member, owner, officer, or committee member of the Chest Wall and Spinal Deformity Study Group, the Scoliosis Research Society, the Pediatric Orthopaedic Society of North America, and the American Academy of Pediatrics-Orthopedic Section. Neither of the following authors nor any immediate family member has received anything of value from or has stock or stock options held in a commercial company or institution related directly or indirectly to the subject of this chapter: Dr. Gomez and Dr. Makhni.

Global Decompensation

Coronal Decompensation

Coronal decompensation is a recognized potential complication that can occur after the surgical correction of scoliosis. Despite the wide attention to the correction of coronal deformity in the literature, there is inconsistency in defining coronal decompensation and fully identifying its incidence and associated risk factors. Decompensation generally refers to the worsening of spinal alignment that develops over time after spinal fusion, and contrasts with spinal imbalance, which is a static measure of malalignment at any specific point in time.

Behensky et al[10] reported a coronal decompensation rate of 28% at a minimum 2-year postoperative follow-up in patients with Lenke type 3C curves. In a study of 86 immature patients, Roberto et al[11] reported that 28% of the patients had more than 10° in coronal curve progression after posterior spinal instrumentation and fusion for AIS, whereas 54% of patients with open triradiate cartilage had more than 10° in coronal curve progression.

Miller et al[12] analyzed 908 patients with AIS who had undergone fusion to determine risk factors for global decompensation. The authors found that patients with increased height or weight were at higher risk for coronal imbalance postoperatively, although Upasani et al[13] found no correlation between weight and global balance in patients with AIS before or after surgery. Miller et al[12] suggested that those patients in whom the lowest instrumented vertebra was in the thoracic region or those with higher preoperative major curve sizes were at substantially higher risk for coronal decompensation.

Gomez et al[14] reported that the rate of decompensation for all types of Lenke curves after posterior spinal instrumented fusion was 6.4% at 2 years. The analysis showed that risk factors for decompensation included a low preoperative Risser score and male gender. Adding vertebral levels can result in curve progression at adjacent unfused segments after corrective arthrodesis of AIS. Late extension of curvature into adjacent regions in the direction of the original curvature in patients with AIS has been shown to occur more often in patients with open triradiate cartilage versus closed triradiate cartilage (18% versus 8%, respectively), but the magnitude of curvature was similar between the groups.[15,16]

Surgeons who treat pediatric spinal deformity should be aware of these risk factors and consider delaying correction in younger male adolescents and should attempt adequate correction to prevent later decompensation when possible.

Sagittal Decompensation

Sagittal decompensation also can occur after spinal instrumentation and fusion for AIS and may lead to the need for revision surgery. A better understanding of the causes of sagittal decompensation may allow surgeons to better predict, monitor, manage, and prevent postoperative sagittal decompensation.

Global sagittal balance is described in terms of the sagittal vertebral axis or the plumb line from the middle of the C7 vertebral body to the posterior superior corner of the S1 body. This regional alignment can be defined as positive or negative, depending on whether the individual's plumb line is anterior or posterior to S1, respectively. Studies have reported on the effect of sagittal imbalance on the quality of life of patients with scoliosis.[17,18] Glassman et al[17] evaluated how radiographic parameters affected Scoliosis Research Society, Medical Outcomes Study Short Form 12-Item, and Os-

westry scores in 298 patients with scoliosis and found that positive sagittal balance was the most reliable predictor of clinical symptoms. The authors also reported that substantial coronal imbalance of more than 4 cm was associated with more pain and deterioration in functional scores.[17] Another study demonstrated that increasing the amount of positive sagittal alignment will negatively affect the health status of scoliosis patients.[18] More than 2 cm of positive sagittal alignment can be indicative of sagittal imbalance.[13]

In a study of 908 patients with AIS treated with spinal fusion, Miller et al[12] reported that sagittal decompensation was correlated with sagittal imbalance preoperatively (in either the positive or negative direction) as well as with pelvic obliquity (increased preoperative obliquity leads to greater positive sagittal alignment postoperatively). Of 1,053 patients with AIS who underwent posterior instrumentation and fusion, Gomez et al[19] reported that 46.5% had worsened sagittal balance at 2 years postoperatively. Patients with more than 50% coronal plane correction had significantly worsened sagittal alignment at the 2-year follow-up than those who underwent a lower degree of coronal correction.

Flatback syndrome can occur after thoracolumbar fusion in patients with AIS. Patients with AIS have inherent hypokyphosis; lumbar lordosis is believed to decrease with increasing age.[20-22] Fusion of the thoracic spine diminishes the natural thoracic kyphosis. To maintain initial sagittal balance, the lumbar spine compensates by progressively becoming even less lordotic to neutralize the artificial imbalance from the fusion. This decrease in lumbar lordosis and increase in pelvic tilt lead to global flatback syndrome in the sagittal plane.[20] A patient with severe deformity must flex his or her knees to maintain an upright posture. Biomechanical studies have suggested that this imbalance places disproportionate stress on the patient's erector spina musculature.[23] In adults, flatback deformity can lead to pain and decreased function.[20,24]

Recent analysis suggests a 68% correlation between postoperative decreased thoracic kyphosis and decreased lumbar lordosis.[25] Increased patient weight also correlates with decreasing postoperative lordosis. Direct vertebral derotation has been shown to improve rotational correction of vertebrae over conventional simple rod rotation; however, flatback deformity can be an unintended consequence because of increased thoracic kyphosis.[22] For patients with AIS, results of a 2-year follow-up study after fusion showed that multiple quality of life indicators were not substantially affected by flatback deformity; however, Scoliosis Research Society activity scores were significantly reduced.[25]

Smith-Peterson osteotomies or pedicle subtraction osteotomies have been proposed as methods to correct lumbar kyphosis or hypolordosis. Booth et al[24] treated 28 patients with flatback deformity, primarily with posterior osteotomies with anterior structural grafting. Substantially improved sagittal alignment was achieved. Patients self-reported outcomes regarding pain, function, and self-image were assessed with questionnaires derived from the Scoliosis Research Society and American Academy of Orthopaedic Surgeons Musculoskeletal Outcomes Data Evaluation and Management System (MODEMS) questionnaires. Patient dissatisfaction with their surgical reconstruction could be predicted by persistent postoperative positive sagittal balance, the presence of multiple medical comorbidities, and the development of coronal imbalance or pseudarthrosis.

The spinal alignment of some patients reverts to its state of balance before spinal fusion through flattening of the lumbar and cervical spine. With reduction in kyphosis of the thoracic spine after fusion in patients with AIS, the cervical spine has been found to lose lordosis and can become overtly kyphotic.[26,27] In a subset of AIS patients with Lenke type 1 and 2 curves treated with pedicle screw constructs, Hwang et al[27] found that the average thoracic kyphosis flattened from 45° to 25.6°. As a result, cervical lordosis of 13.8° progressed to eventual kyphosis of 10.5° by the end of the study period.

Regional Imbalance and Adjacent-Level Decompensation

Regional imbalance can occur across entire spinal segments or those locally adjacent to the instrumented vertebral levels, the latter of which are referred to as adjacent segment pathologies. The most commonly described adjacent segment pathologies that occur after the surgical correction of scoliosis are proximal junctional kyphosis and distal junctional kyphosis. Both of these adjacent deformities can influence sagittal alignment and lead to impaired cosmesis, function, and possibly even revision surgery to restore balance. The degree to which these pathologies occur and their risk factors are beginning to be understood; however, their clinical importance is inconclusive.

Proximal Junctional Kyphosis

Proximal junctional kyphosis refers to local kyphosis that is proximal to vertebral levels instrumented in spinal fusion procedures. Various definitions of proximal junctional kyphosis have appeared in the literature, each measuring spinal angulation in the sagittal plane relative to the upper instrument-ed vertebra. The most frequently used definition includes two components: (1) at least 10° of kyphosis between the lower vertebral end plate of the upper instrumented vertebra and the upper end plate of the vertebral body that is two segments proximal and (2) the Cobb angle at these segments must be at least 10° greater than the preoperative angulation.[4,28,29] Other definitions of proximal junctional kyphosis have required an increase in angulation between the upper instrumented vertebra and the adjacent vertebra of at least 15°.[30]

The risk for the development of proximal junctional kyphosis after fusion surgery in patients with AIS has been reported to be 27% and 28% at mean follow-ups of 2 and 3.5 years, respectively.[28,31] These rates can be compared with the risk of proximal junctional kyphosis in adults with idiopathic scoliosis, which has been reported in different populations to range from 17% to 39% at mean follow-ups of 4 and 7.8 years, respectively.[32,33]

The etiology of proximal junctional kyphosis is likely multifactorial.[28,31,34] There is little or no correlation between the development of proximal junctional kyphosis after fusion for AIS and age, sex, the number of fused vertebral levels, or the upper instrumented vertebra (the uppermost, most proximal instrumented vertebra).[28,31] Several radiographic, clinical, and surgical factors have been shown to correlate with an increased risk of proximal junctional kyphosis. Risk factors include thoracoplasty, the use of pedicle screws rather than hooks, a higher preoperative Cobb angle, patient obesity, and failure to appropriately incorporate sufficient proximal vertebrae.[28,30,31,35] In selecting the optimal upper instrumented vertebra level, enough levels must be included in the fusion construct (often including the upper end vertebra) to avoid the development of proximal junctional kyphosis; this must be done while concurrently minimizing the extent of the surgery and levels fused. In a study of patients with Scheuermann kyphosis at a mean age of 37 years, proximal junctional kyphosis was present in 30% of the patients. An increased risk of proximal junctional kyphosis was noted with disruption of the ligamentum flavum at the proximal end of the construct and without sufficient proximal extension of the construct.[35] Other factors, such as lower Risser grade and allograft implantation, may also increase the risk of proximal junctional kyphosis.[31]

Proximal junctional kyphosis manifests radiographically and can sometimes be noted at the time of the clinical examination; however, there has been little evidence to suggest that it has a deleterious effect on function. Kim et al[28] studied the effect of proximal junctional kyphosis on Scoliosis Research Society scores and quality of life and found no significant effect on pain, self-image, function, or patient satisfaction. A similar outcome analysis in adults also showed a lack of effect of proximal junctional kyphosis on patient-reported outcomes.[33] Progressive proximal junctional kyphosis may be of clinical importance, but further studies are needed to quantify the biomechanical, functional, and aesthetic consequences of this phenomenon.

Rhee et al[21] suggested that proximal junctional kyphosis could be decreased through an anterior rather than a posterior approach using thoracolumbar instrumentation; however, at a mean follow-up of 32 months, the decreased amount of proximal junctional kyphosis (9° versus 4°, $P = 0.03$) did not have clinical significance. None of the patients followed had resulting back pain or required revision surgery because of proximal junctional kyphosis. The use

of pedicle screws rather than hooks may also increase the risk of proximal junctional kyphosis.[28,30,31]

Biomechanical data from finite element analyses suggest that proximal junctional kyphosis may be prevented by using transition rods.[36] The mathematical model predicted that the transition rod extending one level proximal to the original instrumentation would avoid increased pressure on the disk nuclei and decrease stress from the implant.[36]

Distal Junctional Kyphosis

Surgical correction of adolescent deformity can lead to another form of adjacent-level sagittal plane misalignment known as distal junctional kyphosis.[13] This misalignment has been most commonly defined as at least 10° between the lower instrumented vertebra and the adjacent vertebra.[13,37] Sarlak et al[38] added the criteria that the change in kyphosis between T10 and L2 should also be at least 10°. Lowe et al[37] reported a 4.2% incidence of distal junctional kyphosis in patients with AIS and found that posterior instrumentation led to more than a twofold higher incidence in the condition compared with the group treated using anterior instrumentation at 2 years postoperatively. In their analysis, distal junctional kyphosis was defined as at least 10° between the lower instrumented vertebra and the adjacent distal vertebrae. Rates of distal junctional kyphosis after fusion are likely between 6.9% to 14.6%,[37,39] although rates have been reported as low as 1.5% and as high as 30.2% after Cotrel-Dubousset instrumentation.[37,39-41] In contrast to this finding, Rhee et al[21] studied magnitudes of distal junctional kyphosis after instrumentation and found no substantial difference in the amount of resulting distal junctional kyphosis after either anterior or posterior instrumentation.

The lower instrumented vertebra also significantly affects the incidence of distal junctional kyphosis. Distal junctional kyphosis resolved in patients if instrumentation encompassed the kyphotic vertebra, with an anterior level one level past the Cobb level and a posterior level two levels distal to the Cobb level. The study by Lowe et al[37] also showed that posterior instrumentation to one level distal to the lower Cobb vertebrae led to a significantly lower incidence of distal junctional kyphosis ($P = 0.0001$); this same trend was not seen in the anterior instrumentation group.

If the lowest instrumented vertebra is chosen at a level that has kyphosis preoperatively, a recent study by Vitale et al[42] reported a 33-fold higher risk of distal junctional kyphosis postoperatively. This reinforces the importance of capturing the adjacent kyphosis in the instrumentation. An increasing risk of distal junctional kyphosis was correlated with increasing patient weight and age at the time of surgery.[39] In a study of 645 patients with AIS, Vitale et al[42] reported an 11% rate of Lenke type 3 and 4 curves after instrumentation. If L1 was included distally in the fusion construct, the incidence of distal junctional kyphosis decreased dramatically, from nearly 30% when the fusion stopped at T11 to approximately 2% when the fusion was taken to L1. In general, proper selection of the lower instrumented vertebrae with incorporation of the first lordotic vertebrae into the fusion may help prevent the postoperative development of distal junctional kyphosis.[35,38] Anterior instrumentation may also reduce the incidence of distal junctional kyphosis, with a twofold increased risk associated with the posterior approach.[37]

Summary

Surgical techniques and indications for correcting pediatric spinal deformity are continuing to evolve, and new constructs are being developed for enhanced structural instrumentation of the spine. However, these advances place modified mechanical stresses on the vertebra and can lead to new types of complications. Some of these complications present challenges that benefit from revision surgery, and some can be minimized by good preoperative planning and recognition of the risk factors that predispose patients to poor outcomes. Awareness of these complications allows orthopaedic surgeons to provide closer follow-up and consideration of previously unforeseen complications, which should translate into better management of children with spinal deformities.

References

1. Boachie-Adjei O, Cunningham M: *Revision Spine Surgery in the Growing Child*. Berlin, Germany, Springer-Verlag, 2011.

2. Bess S, Akbarnia BA, Thompson GH, et al: Analysis of one hundred and forty patients. *J Bone Joint Surg Am* 2010;92(15):2533-2543.

3. Fu KM, Smith JS, Polly DW, et al: Morbidity and mortality associated with spinal surgery in children: A review of the Scoliosis Research Society morbidity and mortality database. *J Neurosurg Pediatr* 2011;7(1):37-41.

4. Kim YJ, Bridwell KH, Lenke LG, Kim J, Cho SK: Proximal junctional kyphosis in adolescent idiopathic scoliosis following segmental posterior spinal instrumentation and fusion: Minimum 5-year follow-up. *Spine (Phila Pa 1976)* 2005;30(18):2045-2050.

5. Kuklo TR, Potter BK, Lenke LG, Polly DW Jr, Bridwell KH: Surgical revision rates of hooks versus hybrid versus screws versus combined anteroposterior spinal fusion for adolescent idiopathic scoliosis. *Spine (Phila Pa 1976)* 2007; 32(20):2258-2264.

6. Sankar WN, Acevedo DC, Skaggs DL: Comparison of complications among growing spinal implants. *Spine (Phila Pa 1976)* 2010; 35(23):2091-2096.

7. Angevine PD, McCormick PC: The importance of sagittal balance: How good is the evidence? *J Neurosurg Spine* 2007;6(2):101-103, discussion 103.

8. Lenke LG, Betz RR, Bridwell KH, Harms J, Clements DH, Lowe TG: Spontaneous lumbar curve coronal correction after selective anterior or posterior thoracic fusion in adolescent idiopathic scoliosis. *Spine (Phila Pa 1976)* 1999; 24(16):1663-1671, discussion 1672.

9. Edwards CC II, Peelle M, Sides B, Rinella A, Bridwell KH: Selective thoracic fusion for adolescent idiopathic scoliosis with C modifier lumbar curves: 2- to 16-year radiographic and clinical results. *Spine (Phila Pa 1976)* 2004;29(5): 536-546.

10. Behensky H, Cole AA, Freeman BJ, Grevitt MP, Mehdian HS, Webb JK: Fixed lumbar apical vertebral rotation predicts spinal decompensation in Lenke type 3C adolescent idiopathic scoliosis after selective posterior thoracic correction and fusion. *Eur Spine J* 2007;16(10):1570-1578.

11. Roberto RF, Lonstein JE, Winter RB, Denis F: Curve progression in Risser stage 0 or 1 patients after posterior spinal fusion for idiopathic scoliosis. *J Pediatr Orthop* 1997;17(6):718-725.

12. Miller DJ, Jameel O, Matsumoto H, et al: Factors affecting distal end & global decompensation in coronal/sagittal planes 2 years after fusion. *Stud Health Technol Inform* 2010;158:141-146.

13. Upasani VV, Caltoum C, Petcharaporn M, et al: Does obesity affect surgical outcomes in adolescent idiopathic scoliosis? *Spine (Phila Pa 1976)* 2008;33(3): 295-300.

14. Gomez JA, Matsumoto H, Colacchio ND, et al: Poster No. P249. Risk factors for coronal decompensation following spinal fusion for adolescent idiopathic scoliosis. *AAOS 2012 Annual Meeting Proceedings*. CD-ROM. Rosemont, IL, American Academy of Orthopaedic Surgeons, 2012, p 835.

15. Sponseller PD, Betz R, Newton PO, et al: Differences in curve behavior after fusion in adolescent idiopathic scoliosis patients with open triradiate cartilages. *Spine (Phila Pa 1976)* 2009;34(8): 827-831.

16. Ericco TJ, Lonner BS, Moulton AW, eds: *Surgical Management of Spinal Deformities*. Philadelphia, PA, Elsevier, 2009.

17. Glassman SD, Berven S, Bridwell K, Horton W, Dimar JR: Correlation of radiographic parameters and clinical symptoms in adult scoliosis. *Spine (Phila Pa 1976)* 2005;30(6):682-688.

18. Glassman SD, Bridwell K, Dimar JR, Horton W, Berven S, Schwab F: The impact of positive sagittal balance in adult spinal deformity. *Spine (Phila Pa 1976)* 2005; 30(18):2024-2029.

19. Gomez JA, Matsumoto H, Colacchio ND, et al: Higher degrees of curve correction correlate with worsened sagittal balance. October 15, 2011. American Academy of Pediatrics website. https://aap.confex.com/aap/2011/webprogram/Paper14806.html. Accessed July 19, 2013.

20. Newton PO, Yaszay B, Upasani VV, et al: Preservation of thoracic kyphosis is critical to maintain lumbar lordosis in the surgical treatment of adolescent idiopathic scoliosis. *Spine (Phila Pa 1976)* 2010;35(14):1365-1370.

21. Rhee JM, Bridwell KH, Won DS, Lenke LG, Chotigavanichaya C,

Hanson DS: Sagittal plane analysis of adolescent idiopathic scoliosis: The effect of anterior versus posterior instrumentation. *Spine (Phila Pa 1976)* 2002;27(21):2350-2356.

22. Mladenov KV, Vaeterlein C, Stuecker R: Selective posterior thoracic fusion by means of direct vertebral derotation in adolescent idiopathic scoliosis: Effects on the sagittal alignment. *Eur Spine J* 2011;20(7):1114-1117.

23. Tveit P, Daggfeldt K, Hetland S, Thorstensson A: Erector spinae lever arm length variations with changes in spinal curvature. *Spine (Phila Pa 1976)* 1994;19(2):199-204.

24. Booth KC, Bridwell KH, Lenke LG, Baldus CR, Blanke KM: Complications and predictive factors for the successful treatment of flatback deformity (fixed sagittal imbalance). *Spine (Phila Pa 1976)* 1999;24(16):1712-1720.

25. Colacchio N, Matsumoto H, Schwab F, Lafage V, Roye D, Vitale M: Flatback revisited: Reciprocal loss of lumbar lordosis following selective thoracic fusion. American Orthopaedic Association 125th Annual Meeting: Scientific Poster Displays. http://www.aoassn.org/media/121602/aoa_scientific_poster_displays.pdf. Accessed July 19, 2013.

26. Hilibrand AS, Tannenbaum DA, Graziano GP, Loder RT, Hensinger RN: The sagittal alignment of the cervical spine in adolescent idiopathic scoliosis. *J Pediatr Orthop* 1995;15(5):627-632.

27. Hwang SW, Samdani AF, Tantorski M, et al: Cervical sagittal plane decompensation after surgery for adolescent idiopathic scoliosis: An effect imparted by postoperative thoracic hypokyphosis. *J Neurosurg Spine* 2011;15(5):491-496.

28. Kim YJ, Lenke LG, Bridwell KH, et al: Proximal junctional kyphosis in adolescent idiopathic scoliosis after 3 different types of posterior

segmental spinal instrumentation and fusions: Incidence and risk factor analysis of 410 cases. *Spine (Phila Pa 1976)* 2007;32(24):2731-2738.

29. Glattes RC, Bridwell KH, Lenke LG, Kim YJ, Rinella A, Edwards C II: Proximal junctional kyphosis in adult spinal deformity following long instrumented posterior spinal fusion: Incidence, outcomes, and risk factor analysis. *Spine (Phila Pa 1976)* 2005;30(14):1643-1649.

30. Helgeson MD, Shah SA, Newton PO, et al: Evaluation of proximal junctional kyphosis in adolescent idiopathic scoliosis following pedicle screw, hook, or hybrid instrumentation. *Spine (Phila Pa 1976)* 2010;35(2):177-181.

31. Wang J, Zhao Y, Shen B, Wang C, Li M: Risk factor analysis of proximal junctional kyphosis after posterior fusion in patients with idiopathic scoliosis. *Injury* 2010;41(4):415-420.

32. Kim HJ, Yagi M, Nyugen J, Cunningham ME, Boachie-Adjei O: Combined anterior-posterior surgery is the most important risk factor for developing proximal junctional kyphosis in idiopathic scoliosis. *Clin Orthop Relat Res* 2012;470(6):1633-1639.

33. Kim YJ, Bridwell KH, Lenke LG, Glattes CR, Rhim S, Cheh G: Proximal junctional kyphosis in adult spinal deformity after segmental posterior spinal instrumentation and fusion: Minimum five-year follow-up. *Spine (Phila Pa 1976)* 2008;33(20):2179-2184.

34. Kim HJ, Lenke LG, Shaffrey CI, Van Alstyne EM, Skelly AC: Proximal junctional kyphosis as a distinct form of adjacent segment pathology after spinal deformity surgery: A systematic review. *Spine (Phila Pa 1976)* 2012;37(22):S144-S164.

35. Denis F, Sun EC, Winter RB: Incidence and risk factors for

proximal and distal junctional kyphosis following surgical treatment for Scheuermann kyphosis: Minimum five-year follow-up. *Spine (Phila Pa 1976)* 2009;34(20):E729-E734.

36. Cahill PJ, Wang W, Asghar J, et al: The use of a transition rod may prevent proximal junctional kyphosis in the thoracic spine after scoliosis surgery: A finite element analysis. *Spine (Phila Pa 1976)* 2012;37(12):E687-E695.

37. Lowe TG, Lenke L, Betz R, et al: Distal junctional kyphosis of adolescent idiopathic thoracic curves following anterior or posterior instrumented fusion: Incidence, risk factors, and prevention. *Spine (Phila Pa 1976)* 2006;31(3):299-302.

38. Sarlak AY, Atmaca H, Kim WJ, Musaoğlu R, Tosun B: Radiographic features of the Lenke 1A curves to help to determine the optimum distal fusion level selection. *Spine (Phila Pa 1976)* 2011;36(19):1592-1599.

39. Ameri E, Behtash H, Mobini B, Ghandhari H, Vahid Tari H, Khakinahad M: The prevalence of distal junctional kyphosis following posterior instrumentation and arthrodesis for adolescent idiopathic scoliosis. *Acta Med Iran* 2011;49(6):357-363.

40. McCance SE, Denis F, Lonstein JE, Winter RB: Coronal and sagittal balance in surgically treated adolescent idiopathic scoliosis with the King II curve pattern: A review of 67 consecutive cases having selective thoracic arthrodesis. *Spine (Phila Pa 1976)* 1998;23(19):2063-2073.

41. Richards BS, Birch JG, Herring JA, Johnston CE, Roach JW: Frontal plane and sagittal plane balance following Cotrel-Dubousset instrumentation for idiopathic scoliosis. *Spine (Phila Pa 1976)* 1989;14(7):733-737.

42. Vitale MG, Roye DP, Miller DJ, Jameel OF, Schwab FJ: Paper No. 397. Factors affecting distal junctional kyphosis after spinal fusion for adolescent idiopathic scoliosis. *AAOS 2011 Annual Meeting Proceedings*. CD-ROM. Rosemont, IL, American Academy of Orthopaedic Surgeons, 2011, p 628.

Sports Medicine

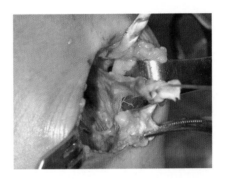

Sports Medicine

Patellofemoral Joint: From Instability to Arthritis

Elizabeth A. Arendt, MD
Diane L. Dahm, MD
David Dejour, MD
Donald C. Fithian, MD

Abstract

Disorders of the patellofemoral joint are commonly seen in musculoskeletal clinics. In recent years, the expansion of imaging techniques, improvements in correlative injury anatomy, and more focused physical examinations have resulted in new knowledge about patellofemoral disorders. To achieve optimal patient outcomes, it is helpful for orthopaedic surgeons who treat knee problems to review the management of patellar dislocations and isolated patellofemoral arthritis, including treatment algorithms.

Instr Course Lect 2014;63:355-368.

Patellofemoral disorders can be broadly divided into three categories: patella dislocations, patellofemoral arthritis, and anterior knee pain. These categories are not mutually exclusive, but their division can aid in the dissemination of information concerning patellofemoral disorders and their treatment. This chapter discusses patella dislocations and isolated patellofemoral arthritis, with an emphasis on a subgroup of surgical procedures used in the treatment algorithm for these conditions.

Patellar Dislocations (Anatomy of Lateral Patellar Dislocation)

For the purposes of this chapter, recurrent patellar dislocation is defined as intermittent transient lateral dislocation of the patella caused by deficient constraint of mediolateral patellar motion. Constraint of patellar motion results from the combination of trochlear engagement and competent capsular ligaments. Trochlear dysplasia, which is defined as a flat and sometimes shortened trochlear groove, is seen in a high proportion of patients presenting with recurrent patellar dislocation. A flat groove implies that the capsular restraints are taxed more heavily and frequently in restraining mediolateral patellar excursion, particularly in early flexion. This situation is more challenging in the setting of patella alta because the patella requires more knee flexion to engage the groove.

Normal Limits of Lateral Patellar Motion or Constraint

The two components of the knee extensor apparatus that primarily affect the limits of passive mediolateral patellar motion are (1) bony constraints resulting from the congruity between the patella and the femoral trochlea (bony buttress) and (2) soft-tissue tethers.

In a study of the complex articular geometry of the patellofemoral joint between 30° and 100° of knee flexion, Ahmad et al[1] reported that mediolateral patellar translation was controlled by the passive restraint provided by the

Dr. Arendt or an immediate family member serves as a paid consultant to or is an employee of Tornier and serves as a board member, owner, officer, or committee member of the American Academy of Orthopaedic Surgeons and the International Society of Arthroscopy, Knee Surgery, and Orthopaedic Sports Medicine. Dr. Dahm or an immediate family member has received royalties from Tenex Health; has stock or stock options held in Tenex Health; and serves as a board member, owner, officer, or committee member of the Arthroscopy Association of North America and the American Academy of Orthopaedic Surgeons. Dr. Dejour or an immediate family member has received royalties from Tornier and serves as a board member, owner, officer, or committee member of the French Society of Orthopaedic Surgery and Traumatology. Neither Dr. Fithian nor any immediate family member has received anything of value from or has stock or stock options held in a commercial company or institution related directly or indirectly to the subject of this chapter.

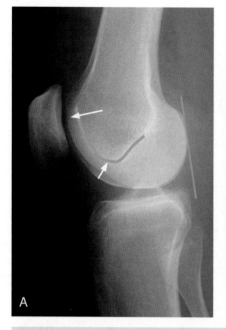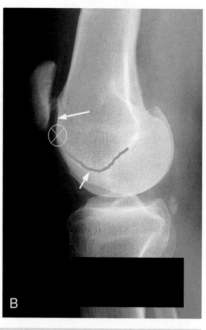

Figure 1 **A,** In the crossing sign, the sulcus line (short arrow) follows the Blumensaat line. In a normal knee, this line stays posterior to the condylar line (long arrow), representing a trochlea that is deep and congruent. **B,** In a knee with dysplasia, the crossing sign represents where the sulcus line (short arrow) crosses the lateral condylar line (long arrow) and represents a flat trochlea. X within the circle = the crossing sign.

topographic interaction of the patellofemoral contacting surfaces. Heegaard et al[2] and Senavongse et al[3] observed that constraint within the femoral groove was dominant over the stabilizing effect of the soft tissues through most of the range of motion in normal cadaver knees. At full extension, however, when there is little or no contact between the patella and the femur, the influence of the retinacula is greatest relative to the influence of the trochlea.[2-5] A shallow, short trochlear groove does not take on its stabilizing role as early in flexion as a normal trochlea; therefore, patella alta compounds this problem and results in greater loads on the capsular restraints through a greater range of early knee flexion.

The contribution of specific medial retinacular structures to restraint against lateral patellar displacement has been studied in normal cadaver knees using sequential cutting methods.[6-9] Ligamentous retinacular structures that may be relevant to lateral patellar translation include the superficial medial patellar retinaculum, the medial patellotibial ligament, the medial patellomeniscal ligament, and the medial patellofemoral ligament (MPFL).

In studies of human cadaver knees using selective cutting methods on medial retinacular tissues, the MPFL has consistently been shown to provide the primary restraint against lateral patellar displacement.[7,8] Interestingly, Desio et al[8] reported that isolated lateral release actually reduced resistance to lateral patella displacement. Hautamaa et al[6] observed that isolated release of the MPFL increased lateral patellar displacement 50% compared with intact knees. Repair of the MPFL alone restored lateral mobility to within normal values.[6,9] Repair of more superficial retinacular tissues, as typically occurs with medial reefing, was neither

necessary nor sufficient to restore stability.[6,9]

Although the vastus medialis obliquus is oriented to resist lateral patellar motion, by either active contraction or passive muscle resistance,[10-13] the effect of muscle forces on the patellar motion appears to be limited. With respect to resisting lateral patellar displacement, the orientation of the vastus medialis obliquus varies greatly during knee flexion. The line of pull of the vastus medialis obliquus most efficiently resists lateral patellar motion when the knee is in deep flexion because, at that time, the trochlear containment of the patella is quite independent of soft-tissue influences.[1,2,4] Farahmand et al[4] reported that lateral patellar force-displacement behavior was not affected by variations in simulated muscle forces at any flexion angle from 15° to 75°.

Anatomic Features of Acute Patellar Dislocators

It has long been appreciated that there are anatomic features that seem to be characteristic of patellar instability.[14-16] Several of these features can, either alone or in combination, reduce the containment of the patella within the trochlear groove, thus predisposing the patella to dislocation. A knee with one or more of these abnormalities is at risk for patellar dislocation.[17-21]

Dejour et al[22] defined the crossing sign as the intersection of the deepest part of the femoral groove with the most prominent aspect of the lateral femoral trochlear facet when viewed from a strict lateral projection on plain radiographs (**Figure 1**). The presence of the crossing sign has high diagnostic value in its association with recurrent patellar instability. The eminence represents the prominence of the trochlear end line in relation to the anterior cortex of the femur, which takes the shape of a beak or bump at the junction of the groove and the anterior femoral cortex.

A comparison of radiographs and CT scans of knees with objective patellar instability, contralateral asymptomatic knees, and control knees identified four relevant factors:[23] (1) Trochlear dysplasia, as defined by the crossing sign, was present in 96% of the patients with symptomatic patellar instability versus 3% of the patients in the control group. (2) Patellar tilt in extension of more than 20° on CT scans in patients with symptomatic patellar instability is correlated with trochlear dysplasia. (3) Patella alta, defined as a Caton-Deschamps index greater than or equal to 1.2, was present in 30% of patellar dislocators versus 0% of the patients in the control group. (4) The tibial tuberosity-trochlear groove (TT-TG) distance is defined as pathologic when greater than or equal to 20 mm. From these data, it was concluded that the etiology of recurrent patellar dislocation is multifactorial.

Patella alta is strongly associated with patellar dislocation and is the only one of the listed factors that directly reduces patellar constraint independent of the shape of the trochlea.[21,24-26] A high-riding patella may be seen in spastic neuromuscular disorders such as cerebral palsy, but it is idiopathic in most patients with patellar instability.[27] Geenen et al[28] reported that only minor trauma was required to produce a dislocation in patients with patella alta. The authors believed that patella alta was the only important contributing factor in patellar dislocation because a high-riding patella does not engage the trochlea in time to control the rotational and lateralizing forces produced by weight-bearing activities.[28] Ward et al[29] compared patellofemoral alignment on MRIs of normal knees and those with patella alta and found that individuals with patella alta had 20% more lateral patellar dis-

placement and 39% more lateral patellar tilt at 0° of flexion. In addition, individuals with patella alta had 19% less patellofemoral contact area from 0° to 60° of flexion.

A familial history of patellar dislocations has been reported to increase the risk of failed surgical stabilization.[30] At least some of the anatomic factors that contribute to patellar instability seem to be heritable.[31-33]

Acute lateral patellar dislocation may result in specific medial retinacular injuries.[34-38] Medial retinacular tenderness and bloody effusion have been used by authors to document the occurrence of a patellar dislocation.[39,40]

In a study using the MRI data of acute dislocators, Sillanpää et al[41] reported that 66% of MPFL ruptures were femoral, 21% midsubstance, and 13% patellar. After a mean follow-up of 7 years, 15 patients reported patellar instability (including painful subluxations and patellar redislocations). The authors concluded that an MPFL injury at the femoral attachment in primary traumatic patellar dislocations was predictive of subsequent patellar instability.

Medial retinacular injury is evident after a primary dislocation event in most patients when the retinaculum is inspected, and the injury usually involves the MPFL. Evidence suggests that residual laxity of the ligament is primarily responsible for patellar instability after the initial dislocation event. Injury to the MPFL can occur at more than one location along its length during the dislocation.[34,42,43] Controversy exists on whether the ligament must be repaired at the site of the injury for MPFL to function normally. After healing, it has not been determined if a rupture of the MPFL results in lengthening of the ligament, as is the case in medial collateral ligament injuries, or in an incompetent ligament, as occurs in anterior cruciate ligament injuries.

Reconstruction of the MPFL is an increasingly common surgical procedure for treatment of recurrent patellar dislocators. There is continued controversy regarding the use of this procedure in isolation. A radiographic workup with standard radiographic studies and MRI and CT slice imaging should be obtained to look for patella alta and excessive TT-TG distance in patients with recurrent patellar dislocation for whom MPFL reconstruction is being considered. Correction of patella alta has a direct stabilizing effect on the patella; correction of the TT-TG distance to 10 to 15 mm does not directly enhance patellar constraint, although it may reduce the loads on the medial ligamentous structures and graft. The algorithm in **Figure 2** may be helpful in evaluating and treating these patients. The goal of MPFL reconstruction is to reestablish check against lateral patellar motion and restore normal limits of passive patellar motion[37] (**Table 1**).

Patellar Alta as a Risk Factor for Lateral Patellar Dislocation

Patella alta is one of the documented risk factors for recurrent patellar dislocation.[44,45] The diagnosis of patella alta is confirmed with proper imaging studies.[46]

In the physical examination, the only sign that is specific for patella alta is the high position of the patella with the knee flexed more than 70°; the shape of the knee is modified from that of a normal knee. The apprehension sign is also highly positive because in extension the patella is above the trochlea and has only its soft-tissue constraints, including a lax or an insufficient MPFL.

Conventional Radiography

On the sagittal view at 30° flexion, the patella is measured using an index. The index choice can be surgeon specific,

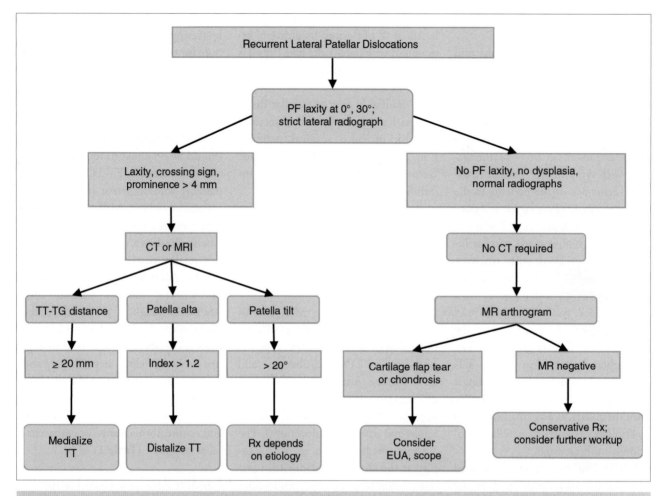

Figure 2   An algorithm for the workup and treatment of recurrent lateral patellar dislocations. PF = patellofemoral, MR = magnetic resonance, EUA = examination under anesthesia, Rx = treatment.

Table 1

The Limits of Patellar Motion

Type (No. of Subjects/Specimens)	Patella Displacement With 5 lb of Medially Directed Force	Patella Displacement With 5 lb of Laterally Directed Force
Normal (94)	9 mm ± 3 mm	10.7 mm ± 3 mm
Cadaver (17)	7.5 mm ± 3 mm	8.9 mm ± 2.5 mm

(Adapted with permission from Hautamaa PV, Fithian DC, Kaufman KR, Daniel DM, Pohlmeyer AM: Medial soft tissue restraints in lateral patellar instability and repair. *Clin Orthop Relat Res* 1998;349:174-182.)

but the Caton-Deschamps index is a reliable choice to provide precise guidelines to determine the amount of correction needed and avoid hypocorrection (patella infera). The Caton-Deschamps index is the ratio between the distance from the lower edge of the patellar articular surface to the antero-superior angle of the tibia outline (AT) and the length of the articular surface of the patella (ASP). An AT/ASP ratio of 0.6 and less determines patella infera, and a ratio greater than 1.2 indicates patella alta (**Figure 3**).

Slice Imaging

The patellar tendon length can be measured on sagittal MRIs or CT scans. It has been shown that the insertion of the patellar tendon is a constant value.[47] It is also interesting to examine functional engagement according to the patella-trochlear index[48] because this shows the relationship between the trochlea and the patella, which more precisely defines the engagement of the patella (**Figure 4**).

On an axial CT scan or an MRI, an easy indirect sign of patella alta is a patella that is not seen, or only the lowest part of it is visible (the empty trochlea sign), on the most proximal femoral slice that shows complete trochlear

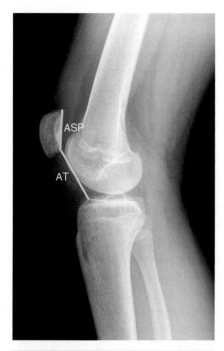

Figure 3 The Caton-Deschamps index is the ratio between the distance from the lower edge of the patellar articular surface to the anterosuperior angle of the tibia outline (AT) and the length of the articular surface of the patella (ASP). A true lateral radiograph of the knee shows the AT/ASP lines used to calculate the Caton-Deschamps index in this knee. AT/ASP = 42/27 = 1.5. A ratio greater than 1.2 indicates patella alta.

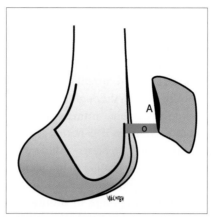

Figure 4 Illustration representing a sagittal MRI scan. Patella height can be measured by comparing the distal patella/superior trochlear overlap (O) to the length of the patella articular surface (A). A percentage value of less than 12.5% is considered patella alta.

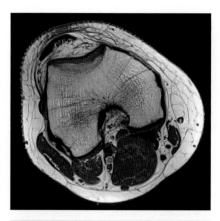

Figure 5 Axial MRI shows the empty sulcus sign. On the most proximal axial MRI or CT cut that has cartilage traversing the entire sulcus, the patella tendon occupies the groove. The bony patella remains above the sulcus because of patella alta. There is no functional engagement between the femoral sulcus and the patella in full extension.

cartilage (**Figure 5**). This finding means that the patella has no or low engagement in the trochlea.

Surgical Treatment of Patella Alta

The surgical technique of distalization osteotomy of the tibial tuberosity is straightforward, but a few pearls may aid in a favorable outcome. A large, 6-cm long tibial tuberosity osteotomy must be detached to avoid malunion or nonunion. Predrilling the anterior cortex of the tuberosity, with a 4.5-mm AO drill helps the compression effect, and widening of the holes assures that the screw heads will be flush and not interfere with kneeling. The amount of distalization should be measured and quantified with a ruler exactly to correlate with the use of Caton-Deschamps index. The desired ratio should be presurgically determined with precise objective measurements. If the desired end result is 1 and the ratio is 40:30, the amount of distalization will be 10 mm. After proper distalization, fixation is achieved with a strictly perpendicular insertion of two 4.5-mm AO bicortical screws placed using a compression technique. Any obliquity in the direction of the screws will lead to compression of the tuberosity fragment proximally and loss of the desired distalization. The surgeon should recognize that a distalization of 10 mm has an automatic medialization effect of approximately 4 mm because of the shape of the proximal tibia. When the patella returns to a normal height, the MPFL (medial constraint) must be restored according to the rules previously described.

In general, the recommendation was to use distalization when patella alta had a Caton-Deschamps index greater than 1.2.[45] In current practice, it is unclear when patella alta requires correction, particularly with the addition of the stabilizing factor of MPFL reconstruction. The indications for surgery as well as the choice of surgical stabilization methods must be individualized to the patient because the extent of bony and soft-tissue dysplasia is quite variable among patients with patella instability. It is clear that precise measurements must be made, and hypocorrection must be avoided. Optimal outcomes are best achieved with detailed and documented preoperative measurements; precise intraoperative measurements, which are recorded in the surgical notes; and follow-up measurements to assess the surgeon's technique.

Rehabilitation Protocol

The patient is allowed partial weight bearing with crutches until quadriceps strength returns. Full weight bearing, with the knee positioned in an extension brace for household ambulation, is allowed. The brace is removed for passive range of motion from 0° to

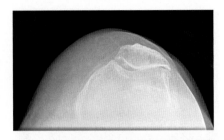

Figure 6 Axial radiograph of the patella showing pseudomalalignment. Excessive lateral tilt and/or translation on an axial radiograph are (in part) the result of grade IV chondral loss in the lateral patellofemoral compartment.

100°, which can be performed with the use of continuous passive motion machine twice daily, along with muscle strengthening (quadriceps sets, straight leg raises, and core) exercises. The brace is worn for the first 4 weeks postoperatively. Additional time in the brace depends on pain with weight bearing and radiographic imaging findings. In phase two (between 45 and 90 days postoperatively), physiotherapy work concentrates on closed kinetic chain muscle strengthening, core strengthening, and proprioception. In phase three of the rehabilitation regimen (approximately 90 days to 6 months postoperative), when complete bony union is achieved, the patient participates in global physical preparation before his or her return to full sport activities.

Discussion and Future Directions

Patellar dislocation usually occurs in knees with an identifiable anatomic predisposition; however, the initial dislocation event itself often results in injury to the medial ligaments responsible for restraining the patella. The central goal for current research is to determine which anatomic features play major roles in determining the risk of primary dislocation and recurrent instability and when these ana-

tomic features (such as patella alta) need to be surgically altered to effect successful patellar stabilization.[49]

The risk factors for primary patellar dislocation and recurrent dislocation are not the same. Although many clinical studies combine primary and recurrent dislocators, it is not clear that the two groups represent the same population. This chapter's authors believe that the failure to distinguish between these two groups of dislocators is partly responsible for the confusion surrounding the risk of lateral patellar dislocation.

Prospective clinical trials are needed to narrow the range of surgical approaches and compare success rates in specific clinical scenarios. The anatomic concepts presented in this chapter provide principles that could be used to design such studies.

Isolated Patellofemoral Arthritis

Osteoarthritis (OA) typically refers to full-thickness or near full-thickness loss of articular cartilage, with varying degrees of concomitant inflammation and pain. When OA involves the patellofemoral joint, varying degrees of extensor mechanism dysfunction typically accompany the clinical picture. End-stage patellofemoral OA is also characterized by radiographic findings, including patellofemoral joint space narrowing (typically lateral), periarticular osteophytes, and subchondral edema and cysts.

Independently or associated etiologic factors can be identified as risk factors for isolated patellofemoral arthritis.[50-53]

Extensor Mechanism Malalignment

Malalignment is a general term that describes active or passive malpositioning of the patella in the trochlear groove. Although this condition is rec-

ognized clinically, it is difficult to define objectively because it is the combination of patient symptoms and the findings of objective imaging parameters that suggest that symptoms are caused by malpositioning. No prospective study has proven that patients who have patellofemoral malalignment have a greater predisposition to arthritis, but patients who have patellofemoral arthritis often demonstrate malalignment.[51] However, in patients with patellofemoral arthritis, the malalignment is often pseudomalalignment, with lateral patella tilt and translation caused by a loss of cartilage height in the lateral patellofemoral joint (**Figure 6**). The greatest prevalence of chondral wear occurs on the lateral facet, suggesting that there is some degree of tilt or malalignment in the etiology of patellofemoral OA.[53,54]

Trochlea Dysplasia, Patella Alta, and Sex

Trochlea dysplasia (defined as a positive crossing sign on true lateral radiographs) is highly correlated with isolated patellofemoral arthritis, and patients with trochlear dysplasia are more likely to have patellofemoral OA.[51,55] Patella alta, as an isolated factor, was not found to be a predisposing factor to patellofemoral OA.[51] Although there are few studies that have evaluated sex as an independent risk factor, the available studies show an overwhelmingly female preponderance for the disease.[50-53]

Diagnosis of Isolated Patellofemoral OA

A patient with isolated patellofemoral OA will typically report anterior knee pain in bent-knee activities.[50,52] Walking on level ground is usually well tolerated. Sometimes, there is pseudolocking and giving way caused by the loss of surface gliding at the site of a kissing lesion.[50] The patient is often apprehensive about performing bent-knee activities, especially going down steps.

Routine radiographs are helpful in making the diagnosis.[56] Narrowing of the patellofemoral joint space seen on a lateral radiograph makes the diagnosis. The lateral radiograph also confirms the presence of trochlear dysplasia and can be used to measure patella height. A weight-bearing PA view eliminates tibiofemoral involvement, and narrowing of the lateral patellofemoral joint on an axial view confirms the diagnosis and allows for classification[55,57] (**Figure 7**). Clinicians should look for patellofemoral OA on routine radiographs because the disease is frequently missed as a source of knee pain.[58]

Although the relationship between cartilage wear (chondromalacia patellae) and patellofemoral OA has not been established, MRI can reveal subchondral edema and subchondral cysts, which are considered a prearthritic sign.[59] MRI also can help evaluate the tibiofemoral articulation.

Treatment
A thorough review of practical tips in the nonsurgical treatment of knee OA has been recently published.[60] Although no attempt was made to focus on unicompartmental arthritis, many of the recommendations can be included in the nonsurgical management of patellofemoral OA. There are several options for surgical management of a patient with clinically symptomatic patellofemoral OA (**Table 2**). An algorithm of clinical decision making is detailed in **Figure 8**. Two surgical procedures that can be used for the treatment of patellofemoral OA are partial lateral facetectomy and patellofemoral arthroplasty.

Partial Lateral Facetectomy
O'Donoghue[61] first described the technique of partial lateral facetectomy

in 1972 and collaborated with McCarroll et al[62] to publish the first results of the procedure in 57 patients. Since that time, a few studies with small sample sizes have reported encouraging results.[63-66] Partial lateral facetectomy is a simple intermediate treatment of isolated patellofemoral OA. If the technique is unsuccessful, the potential for a future total knee arthroplasty is not compromised. The patient has minimal restrictions for returning to functional activities.

A patient with documented isolated or near-isolated patellofemoral OA primarily involving the lateral patellofemoral joint in whom focused rehabilitation has been unsuccessful is a candidate for the procedure. The patient should have no (current) lateral patellofemoral dislocations. Midrange visual analog scale pain scores are ideal but not level 10 pain. Lateral to medial McConnell taping often gives short-term relief, depending on the relative mobility of the lateral tissues. These patients are not ideal candidates for a resurfacing procedure (partial or total) because of their young age and/or early tibiofemoral joint disease.

On examination, the patient will have lateral patellar facet tenderness with a negative medial patellar tilt test and reduced medial glide.[67] Axial imaging reveals isolated lateral Iwano stage III or IV patellofemoral arthritis and lateral patella tilt caused by a loss of lateral patellofemoral joint space. There is often a large trailing osteophyte that appears to trap the medial mobility of the patella.

The advantage of partial lateral facetectomy is its simplicity, with few temporal limitations imposed in the postoperative rehabilitation period. Partial facetectomy has been described combined with tibial tubercle medialization if the TT-TG distance is greater than 20 mm; however, this technique is not preferred by this chapter's au-

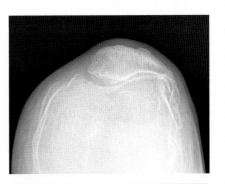

Figure 7 Axial radiograph of the patella showing narrowing of the lateral patellofemoral joint on the axial view confirms the diagnosis of patellofemoral arthritis and allows for classification.

thors because it imposes more stringent postoperative rehabilitation requirements.

The goal of the surgical procedure is to release or lengthen the lateral soft tissues and remove the lateral osteophyte, thereby allowing more medial and lateral mobility of the patella. An open technique is preferred over an arthroscopic technique to avoid a large joint effusion and allow for better control of the lengthened tissues. A lateral incision the approximate length of the patella is preferred, although a central incision is also possible and can be used for future knee surgeries. Because the cartilage wear pattern is usually bipolar and caused by OA, microfracture is not recommended. An MPFL reconstruction is never recommended.

Surgery is performed on a same-day outpatient basis. The patient is sent home with a straight leg knee immobilizer, and weight bearing as tolerated is allowed until normal gait pattern is achieved, usually at 1 to 2 weeks postoperatively. The knee immobilizer is removed for exercising, sitting quietly, and sleeping. Strengthening exercises emphasize core and proximal limb strengthening. The outcomes of partial lateral facetectomy are shown in **Table 2**.

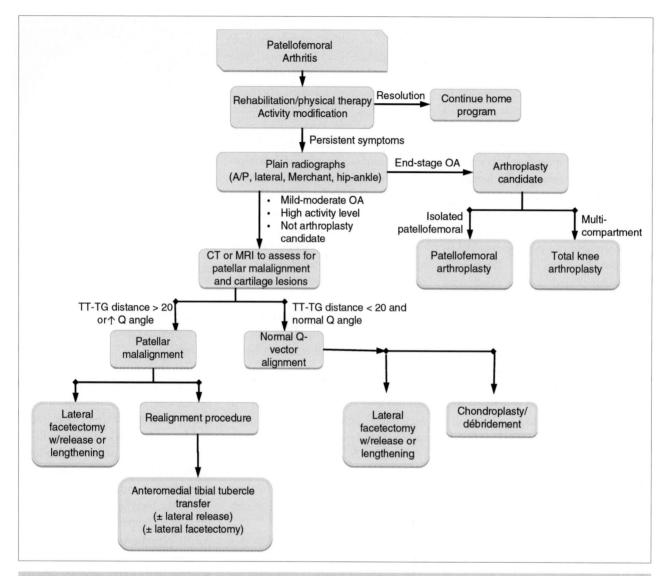

Figure 8   Algorithm for the workup and treatment of isolated patellofemoral arthritis.

Patellofemoral Arthroplasty

There has been renewed interest in surgical treatment options for advanced patellofemoral arthritis. Although patellectomy and patellar resurfacing have been described, these procedures have lost favor because of overall unsatisfactory results. Although total knee arthroplasty has been reported to provide pain relief and functional improvement in this patient population,[68,69] patellofemoral arthroplasty may allow for a more conservative alternative and may be a particularly attractive procedure for young,

more active patients.[70] Patellofemoral arthroplasty is indicated for patients with advanced, isolated patellofemoral degenerative arthritis or advanced posttraumatic patellofemoral arthritis in whom appropriate nonsurgical measures have been unsuccessful. Patients with a history of trochlear dysplasia and secondary patellofemoral degenerative arthritis may be particularly good candidates for patellofemoral arthroplasty because they exhibit less progression of tibiofemoral degenerative arthritis compared with patients who have idiopathic disease.[71] Contraindi-

cations include moderate to advanced tibiofemoral chondromalacia, severe malalignment or maltracking, and inflammatory arthritis. Relative contraindications include early tibiofemoral chondromalacia with marginal osteophyte formation, morbid obesity, and patella infera.[72]

Modern implant designs typically exhibit less constraint and greater proximal extension of the trochlear implant when compared with previous designs.[73] The surgical technique typically involves a medial peripatellar arthrotomy; however, a minimally inva-

Table 2

Surgical Procedures for Patients With Clinically Symptomatic Patellofemoral Osteoarthritis

	Indications	Contraindications	Other	(Study) Outcomes
	Realignment Procedures			
Lateral release	Intact medial patellar cartilage Lateral tilt Tight lateral retinaculum Abnormal (≤ 5 mm) patellar medial subluxation test	Medial patellar chondrosis Hypermobile patella Patellar instability	Must avoid cutting vastus lateralis tendon.	**(Aderinto and Cobb[76])** In patients with predominantly anterior knee pain, 80% had reduction in pain and 59% were satisfied or very satisfied. Average Oxford Knee Score = 27.
Anteromedialization of the tibial tubercle	TT-TG distance > 20 mm Lateral patellar tilt and subluxation with lateral facet degeneration Patellar arthrosis secondary to malalignment Lateral and/or distal patellar chondrosis with good medial cartilage	Skeletal immaturity Medial or proximal patellar chondrosis Complex regional pain syndrome Crush injury to proximal patella Central groove trochlear disease	May vary amount of anterior versus medial shift to accommodate specific location and degree of chondrosis.	**(Pidoriano et al[77])** 90% of patients with distal facet lesions and 85% with lateral facet lesions reported good or excellent outcomes. Only 56% of patients with medial facet lesions and 20% with proximal or diffuse lesions reported good or excellent outcomes. Overall, 63% of patients were satisfied with their level of sports activity, 72% thought their level of sports activity had improved after the procedure, and 92% would undergo the procedure again.
Lateral facetectomy with lateral release	Isolated lateral stage III or IV patellofemoral arthritis Late-stage lateral patellar compression syndrome Lateral patellar facet tenderness Negative passive patellar tilt test Excess lateral patellar tilt on radiographs Younger patients/not yet candidate for PFA arthroplasty or TKA	Moderate or advanced medial or lateral tibiofemoral DJD Medial or diffuse patellar chondrosis Patellar hypermobility	Good intermediate procedure to delay TKA	**(Paulos et al[78])** In 57 of 66 knees not progressing to TKA before follow-up, the mean Kujala patellofemoral score increased from 45.6 to 72.0 after the procedure, with 56% of patients very satisfied, 32% satisfied, and only 7% dissatisfied. **(Yercan et al[63])** In 11 patients with a minimum 3-year follow-up, average Knee Society knee and functional score significantly increased from 150 to 176. Good results were reported at a mean follow-up of 8 years. **(Martens and De Rycke[64])** Good results were reported in 18 of 20 patients (90%). **(Wetzels and Bellemans[65])** 50% of patients treated with partial lateral patellectomy were satisfied at 10-year follow-up.
	Preservation Procedures			
Chondroplasty/débridement	Small (< 1 cm) osteochondral fragments, or flaps Low-grade chondrosis Traumatic chondromalacia Chondral fibrillation	Untreated concomitant injuries, or malalignment, or instability		**(Federico and Reider[66])** In 36 patients undergoing arthroscopic débridement, the mean Fulkerson-Shea patellofemoral joint evaluation score increased from 51.9 to 75.3. 58% of patients with traumatic lesions and 41% with atraumatic lesions reported good or excellent results. **(Owens et al[79])** In a prospective analysis of 19 females undergoing mechanical débridement and 20 females undergoing nonablative radiofrequency débridement for isolated patellar chondral lesions, both groups showed improvement on the Fulkerson-Shea patellofemoral joint evaluation scores postoperatively, but radiofrequency débridement was superior at 1- and 2-year follow-ups.

TT-TG = tibial tuberosity-trochlear grove, TKA = total knee arthroplasty, PFA = patellofemoral arthroplasty, DJD = degenerative joint disease.

Table 2 (continued)

Surgical Procedures for Patients With Clinically Symptomatic Patellofemoral Osteoarthritis

	Indications	Contraindications	Other	(Study) Outcomes
Microfracture	Full-thickness articular cartilage defect Unstable cartilage overlying subchondral bone Traumatic chondral defects Satisfactory surrounding articular cartilage	Axial malalignment Partial-thickness articular defects Diffuse chondral wear Age older than 60 years (relative) Disease-induced arthritis	When combined with other procedures, microfracture should be performed last. No drains should be used.	**(Steadman et al[80])** After minimum 7-year follow-up in patients having microfracture for traumatic chondral defects, Lysholm score increased from 59 to 89, and 80% of patients rated themselves as improved. **(Miller et al[81])** In 81 patients with Outerbridge grade 4 degenerative chondral lesions, at minimum 2-year follow-up, the mean Lysholm score increased from 53.8 to 83.1, and the mean Tegner Activity Scale scores increased from 2.9 to 4.5.
		Replacement Procedures		
PFA	Isolated end-stage patellofemoral DJD Posttraumatic degenerative arthritis Advanced chondromalacia of patella, trochlea, or both Patellar or trochlear dysplasia Failed joint preservation with NSAIDs, weight loss, physical therapy, and repair or realignment procedures Isolated anterior retropatellar pain	Moderate or advanced medial or lateral tibiofemoral DJD Moderate to severe malalignment or maltracking Inflammatory arthritis Morbid obesity Normal patellofemoral joint space on plain radiographs (even if MRI shows patellofemoral chondromalacia) Idiopathic patellofemoral DJD (relative)	May be converted to TKA if necessary later.	**(Mont et al[82])** At mean follow-up of 7 years, 43 patellofemoral arthroplasties in 37 patients showed 95% survival; mean Knee Society objective and functional scores increased from 64 to 87 and 48 to 80, respectively. **(Ackroyd et al[75])** 5-year follow-up of patellofemoral arthroplasties with the Avon prosthesis showed 96% survival; median Oxford score increased from 18 to 39; 80% of patients had successful outcomes based on ≥ 20 points on the Bristol pain score; the main complication was radiographic progression of arthritis. **(Dahm et al[70])** PFA yielded equivalent clinical outcomes to TKA for isolated patellofemoral DJD with a mean Knee Society score of 89 for PFAs and 90 for TKAs and a mean Tegner score of 4.3 for PFAs and 2.6 for TKAs.
TKA	End-stage, multicompartment DJD Failed nonsurgical management Age older than 55 years (relative indication)	Active infection Younger patients (relative contraindication) High activity level (relative contraindication)	Good outcomes but controversy in younger patients.	**(Laskin and van Steijn[83])** In 48 knees treated with TKA for patellofemoral DJD, the mean knee score and pain score increased from 71 to 96 and 25 to 47, respectively. Patients had similar outcomes to patients undergoing TKA for multicompartment DJD. **(Mont et al[68])** At a mean follow-up of 81 months, 30 patients treated with TKA for patellofemoral DJD had 28 excellent, 1 good, and 1 poor result. **(Meding et al[84])** At a minimum 2-year follow-up, the mean Knee Society score improved from 49 preoperatively to 88 postoperatively. No or minimal pain was reported in 29 of 33 knees in patients younger than 60 years treated with TKA.

TT-TG = tibial tuberosity-trochlear groove, TKA = total knee arthroplasty, PFA = patellofemoral arthroplasty, DJD = degenerative joint disease.

sive subvastus or midvastus approach is often possible. The distal extent of the arthrotomy should be limited to avoid injury to the medial meniscus and/or intermeniscal ligament. The trochlea is prepared to receive the appropriately sized components so that the implant is flush distally with the articular cartilage both medially and laterally, and the proximal implant margin should not notch the anterior distal femur. The distal tip of the implant should be just above the roof of the notch to prevent impingement in extension. Internal rotation of the trochlear component should be avoided; however, excessive external rotation may compromise lateral patellar stability. Patellar preparation should attempt to recreate the original patellar thickness if possible. The patellar component may be slightly medialized as needed to improve patellar tracking. A lateral retinacular release is performed if necessary.

In general, the outcomes of patellofemoral arthroplasty using modern prostheses have been reported to be good to excellent in more than 80% of patients.[74] The most common cause for failure and/or revision is the progression of symptomatic tibiofemoral degenerative arthritis.[74,75] Patellofemoral complications, such as pain, snapping, and subluxation, can generally be avoided with careful attention to patient selection and surgical technique along with proper implant selection.[72,73] Patellofemoral arthroplasty represents an important option for salvage of the knee with symptomatic advanced isolated patellofemoral degenerative arthritis.

Summary

Interest in diseases and injuries of the patellofemoral joint have greatly increased because these disorders are a frequent reason for consultation with orthopaedic surgeons and other physi-

cians who treat knee problems. It is helpful to understand and review the anatomy and treatment options applicable to patella dislocations and patellofemoral arthritis to ensure that patients with these conditions have the best possible outcomes.

References

1. Ahmad CS, Stein BE, Matuz D, Henry JH: Immediate surgical repair of the medial patellar stabilizers for acute patellar dislocation: A review of eight cases. *Am J Sports Med* 2000;28(6):804-810.

2. Heegaard J, Leyvraz PF, Van Kampen A, Rakotomanana L, Rubin PJ, Blankevoort L: Influence of soft structures on patellar three-dimensional tracking. *Clin Orthop Relat Res* 1994;299: 235-243.

3. Senavongse W, Farahmand F, Jones J, Andersen H, Bull AM, Amis AA: Quantitative measurement of patellofemoral joint stability: Force-displacement behavior of the human patella in vitro. *J Orthop Res* 2003;21(5):780-786.

4. Farahmand F, Senavongse W, Amis AA: Quantitative study of the quadriceps muscles and trochlear groove geometry related to instability of the patellofemoral joint. *J Orthop Res* 1998;16(1): 136-143.

5. Farahmand F, Tahmasbi MN, Amis AA: Lateral force-displacement behaviour of the human patella and its variation with knee flexion: A biomechanical study in vitro. *J Biomech* 1998; 31(12):1147-1152.

6. Hautamaa PV, Fithian DC, Kaufman KR, Daniel DM, Pohlmeyer AM: Medial soft tissue restraints in lateral patellar instability and repair. *Clin Orthop Relat Res* 1998; 349:174-182.

7. Conlan T, Garth WP Jr, Lemons JE: Evaluation of the medial soft-tissue restraints of the extensor

mechanism of the knee. *J Bone Joint Surg Am* 1993;75(5): 682-693.

8. Desio SM, Burks RT, Bachus KN: Soft tissue restraints to lateral patellar translation in the human knee. *Am J Sports Med* 1998; 26(1):59-65.

9. Nomura E, Horiuchi Y, Kihara M: Medial patellofemoral ligament restraint in lateral patellar translation and reconstruction. *Knee* 2000;7(2):121-127.

10. Hughston JC: Subluxation of the patella. *J Bone Joint Surg Am* 1968;50(5):1003-1026.

11. Lieb FJ, Perry J: Quadriceps function: An anatomical and mechanical study using amputated limbs. *J Bone Joint Surg Am* 1968;50(8): 1535-1548.

12. Scharf W: Anatomical and mechanical studies of the extensor system of the knee joint. *Wien Klin Wochenschr Suppl* 1984;148: 1-20.

13. Scharf W, Weinstrabl R, Firbas W: Anatomic studies of the extensor system of the knee joint and its clinical relevance. *Unfallchirurg* 1986;89(10):456-462.

14. Albee FH: The bone graft wedge in the treatment of habitual dislocation of the patella. *Medical Record* 1915;88:257-259.

15. Brattstrom H: Shape of the intercondylar groove normally and in recurrent dislocation of patella: A clinical and x-ray anatomic investigation. *Acta Orthop Scand* 1964; 68(suppl 68):1-148.

16. Wiberg G: Roentgenographic and anatomic studies on the femoropatellar joint with special reference to chondromalacia patellae. *Acta Orthop Scand* 1941;12: 319-410.

17. Heywood AW: Recurrent dislocation of the patella: A study of its pathology and treatment in 106 knees. *J Bone Joint Surg Br* 1961;43(3):508-517.

18. Cash JD, Hughston JC: Treatment of acute patellar dislocation. *Am J Sports Med* 1988;16(3): 244-249.

19. Hawkins RJ, Bell RH, Anisette G: Acute patellar dislocations: The natural history. *Am J Sports Med* 1986;14(2):117-120.

20. Mäenpää H, Lehto MU: Patellar dislocation has predisposing factors: A roentgenographic study on lateral and tangential views in patients and healthy controls. *Knee Surg Sports Traumatol Arthrosc* 1996;4(4):212-216.

21. Larsen E, Lauridsen F: Conservative treatment of patellar dislocations: Influence of evident factors on the tendency to redislocation and the therapeutic result. *Clin Orthop Relat Res* 1982;171: 131-136.

22. Dejour H, Walch G, Neyret P, Adeleine P: Dysplasia of the femoral trochlea. *Rev Chir Orthop Reparatrice Appar Mot* 1990; 76(1):45-54.

23. Reynaud P: Les tracheoplasties: Cruesement. *Journées Lyonnaises de Chirurgie du Genou* 1995;1: 176-190.

24. Rünow A: The dislocating patella: Etiology and prognosis in relation to generalized joint laxity and anatomy of the patellar articulation. *Acta Orthop Scand Suppl* 1983;201:1-53.

25. Simmons EJ Jr, Cameron JC: Patella alta and recurrent dislocation of the patella. *Clin Orthop Relat Res* 1992;274:265-269.

26. Norman O, Egund N, Ekelund L, Rünow A: The vertical position of the patella. *Acta Orthop Scand* 1983;54(6):908-913.

27. Caton J, Mironneau A, Walch G, Levigne C, Michel CR: Idiopathic high patella in adolescents: Apropos of 61 surgical cases. *Rev Chir Orthop Reparatrice Appar Mot* 1990;76(4):253-260.

28. Geenen E, Molenaers G, Martens M: Patella alta in patellofemoral instability. *Acta Orthop Belg* 1989; 55(3):387-393.

29. Ward SR, Terk MR, Powers CM: Patella alta: Association with patellofemoral alignment and changes in contact area during weight-bearing. *J Bone Joint Surg Am* 2007;89(8):1749-1755.

30. Mäenpää H, Lehto MU: Surgery in acute patellar dislocation: Evaluation of the effect of injury mechanism and family occurrence on the outcome of treatment. *Br J Sports Med* 1995;29(4):239-241.

31. Beighton PH, Horan FT: Dominant inheritance in familial generalised articular hypermobility. *J Bone Joint Surg Br* 1970;52(1): 145-147.

32. Miller GF: Familial recurrent dislocation of the patella. *J Bone Joint Surg Br* 1978;60(2):203-204.

33. Rouvillain JL, Piquion N, Lepage-Lezin A, et al: A familial form of bilateral recurrent dislocation of the patella with major trochlea dysplasia. *Rev Chir Orthop Reparatrice Appar Mot* 1998;84(3): 285-291.

34. Sallay PI, Poggi J, Speer KP, Garrett WE: Acute dislocation of the patella: A correlative pathoanatomic study. *Am J Sports Med* 1996;24(1):52-60.

35. Spritzer CE, Courneya DL, Burk DL Jr, Garrett WE, Strong JA: Medial retinacular complex injury in acute patellar dislocation: MR findings and surgical implications. *AJR Am J Roentgenol* 1997;168(1): 117-122.

36. Feller JA, Feagin JA Jr, Garrett WE Jr: The medial patellofemoral ligament revisited: An anatomical study. *Knee Surg Sports Traumatol Arthrosc* 1993;1(3-4):184-186.

37. Bassett FH: Acute dislocation of the patella, osteochondral fractures, and injuries to the extensor mechanism of the knee. *Instr Course Lect* 1976;25:40-49.

38. Nomura E: Classification of lesions of the medial patello-femoral ligament in patellar dislocation. *Int Orthop* 1999;23(5): 260-263.

39. Vainionpää S, Laasonen E, Pätiälä H, Rusanen M, Rokkannen P: Acute dislocation of the patella: Clinical, radiographic and operative findings in 64 consecutive cases. *Acta Orthop Scand* 1986; 57(4):331-333.

40. Kirsch MD, Fitzgerald SW, Friedman H, Rogers LF: Transient lateral patellar dislocation: Diagnosis with MR imaging. *AJR Am J Roentgenol* 1993;161(1):109-113.

41. Sillanpää PJ, Peltola E, Mattila VM, Kiuru M, Visuri T, Pihlajamäki H: Femoral avulsion of the medial patellofemoral ligament after primary traumatic patellar dislocation predicts subsequent instability in men: A mean 7-year nonoperative follow-up study. *Am J Sports Med* 2009;37(8):1513-1521.

42. Burks RT, Desio SM, Bachus KN, Tyson L, Springer K: Biomechanical evaluation of lateral patellar dislocations. *Am J Knee Surg* 1998;11(1):24-31.

43. Marangi K, White LM, Brossman J, Resnick D, Fithian DC: Magnetic resonance imaging of the knee following acute lateral patellar dislocation. *American Academy of Orthopaedic Surgeons 1996 Annual Meeting Final Program*. Rosemont, IL, American Academy of Orthopaedic, Surgeons, 1996, p 221.

44. Brattström H: Patella alta in non-dislocating knee joints. *Acta Orthop Scand* 1970;41(5):578-588.

45. Dejour H, Walch G, Nove-Josserand L, Guier C: Factors of patellar instability: An anatomic radiographic study. *Knee Surg Sports Traumatol Arthrosc* 1994; 2(1):19-26.

46. Phillips CL, Silver DA, Schranz PJ, Mandalia V: The measurement of patellar height: A review of the methods of imaging. *J Bone*

Joint Surg Br 2010;92(8):1045-1053.

47. Neyret P, Robinson AH, Le Coultre B, Lapra C, Chambat P: Patellar tendon length: The factor in patellar instability? *Knee* 2002;9(1):3-6.

48. Biedert RM, Albrecht S: The patellotrochlear index: A new index for assessing patellar height. *Knee Surg Sports Traumatol Arthrosc* 2006;14(8):707-712.

49. Arendt EA, Dejour D: Patella instability: Building bridges across the ocean: A historic review. *Knee Surg Sports Traumatol Arthrosc* 2013;21(2):279-293.

50. Donell ST, Glasgow MM: Isolated patellofemoral osteoarthritis. *Knee* 2007;14(3):169-176.

51. Grelsamer RP, Dejour D, Gould J: The pathophysiology of patellofemoral arthritis. *Orthop Clin North Am* 2008;39(3):269-274, v.

52. Grelsamer RP, Stein DA: Patellofemoral arthritis. *J Bone Joint Surg Am* 2006;88(8):1849-1860.

53. Minkowitz RB, Bosco JA III: Patellofemoral arthritis. *Bull NYU Hosp Jt Dis* 2009;67(1):30-38.

54. Kalichman L, Zhang Y, Niu J, et al: The association between patellar alignment on magnetic resonance imaging and radiographic manifestations of knee osteoarthritis. *Arthritis Res Ther* 2007;9(2):R26.

55. Dejour D, Allain J: Histoire naturelle de l'arthrose fémoropatellaire isolée. *Rev Chir Orthop* 2004;90(suppl 5):IS69-IS129.

56. Bhattacharya R, Kumar V, Safawi E, Finn P, Hui AC: The knee skyline radiograph: Its usefulness in the diagnosis of patello-femoral osteoarthritis. *Int Orthop* 2007;31(2):247-252.

57. Iwano T, Kurosawa H, Tokuyama H, Hoshikawa Y: Roentgenographic and clinical findings of patellofemoral osteoarthrosis: With special reference to its relationship to femorotibial osteoarthrosis and etiologic factors. *Clin Orthop Relat Res* 1990;252:190-197.

58. McAlindon TE, Snow SW, Cooper C, Dieppe PA: Radiographic patterns of osteoarthritis of the knee joint in the community: The importance of the patellofemoral joint. *Ann Rheum Dis* 1992;51(7):844-849.

59. Luyten FP, Denti M, Filardo G, Kon E, Engebretsen L: Definition and classification of early osteoarthritis of the knee. *Knee Surg Sports Traumatol Arthrosc* 2012;20(3):401-406.

60. Barrett JR, Coleman BR, Arendt EA: Practical tips in the treatment of osteoarthritis of the knee. *Practical Pain Management* 2012;12:48-56.

61. O'Donoghue DH: Facetectomy. *South Med J* 1972;65(6):645-654.

62. McCarroll JR, O'Donoghue DH, Grana WA: The surgical treatment of chondromalacia of the patella. *Clin Orthop Relat Res* 1983;175:130-134.

63. Yercan HS, Ait Si Selmi T, Neyret P: The treatment of patellofemoral osteoarthritis with partial lateral facetectomy. *Clin Orthop Relat Res* 2005;436:14-19.

64. Martens M, De Rycke J: Facetectomy of the patella in patellofemoral osteoarthritis. *Acta Orthop Belg* 1990;56(3-4):563-567.

65. Wetzels T, Bellemans J: Patellofemoral osteoarthritis treated by partial lateral facetectomy: Results at long-term follow up. *Knee* 2012;19(4):411-415.

66. Federico DJ, Reider B: Results of isolated patellar debridement for patellofemoral pain in patients with normal patellar alignment. *Am J Sports Med* 1997;25(5):663-669.

67. Kolowich PA, Paulos LE, Rosenberg TD, Farnsworth S: Lateral release of the patella: Indications and contraindications. *Am J Sports Med* 1990;18(4):359-365.

68. Mont MA, Haas S, Mullick T, Hungerford DS: Total knee arthroplasty for patellofemoral arthritis. *J Bone Joint Surg Am* 2002;84(11):1977-1981.

69. Parvizi J, Stuart MJ, Pagnano MW, Hanssen AD: Total knee arthroplasty in patients with isolated patellofemoral arthritis. *Clin Orthop Relat Res* 2001;392:147-152.

70. Dahm DL, Al-Rayashi W, Dajani K, Shah JP, Levy BA, Stuart MJ: Patellofemoral arthroplasty versus total knee arthroplasty in patients with isolated patellofemoral osteoarthritis. *Am J Orthop (Belle Mead NJ)* 2010;39(10):487-491.

71. Nicol SG, Loveridge JM, Weale AE, Ackroyd CE, Newman JH: Arthritis progression after patellofemoral joint replacement. *Knee* 2006;13(4):290-295.

72. Leadbetter WB: Patellofemoral arthroplasty in the treatment of patellofemoral arthritis: Rationale and outcomes in younger patients. *Orthop Clin North Am* 2008;39(3):363-380, vii.

73. Lonner JH: Patellofemoral arthroplasty: Pros, cons, and design considerations. *Clin Orthop Relat Res* 2004;428:158-165.

74. Lustig S, Magnussen RA, Dahm DL, Parker D: Patellofemoral arthroplasty: Where are we today? *Knee Surg Sports Traumatol Arthrosc* 2012;20(7):1216-1226.

75. Ackroyd CE, Newman JH, Evans R, Eldridge JD, Joslin CC: The Avon patellofemoral arthroplasty: Five-year survivorship and functional results. *J Bone Joint Surg Br* 2007;89(3):310-315.

76. Aderinto J, Cobb AG: Lateral release for patellofemoral arthritis. *Arthroscopy* 2002;18(4):399-403.

77. Pidoriano AJ, Weinstein RN, Buuck DA, Fulkerson JP: Correlation of patellar articular lesions with results from anteromedial

tibial tubercle transfer. *Am J Sports Med* 1997;25(4):533-537.

78. Paulos LE, O'Connor DL, Karistinos A: Partial lateral patellar facetectomy for treatment of arthritis due to lateral patellar compression syndrome. *Arthroscopy* 2008;24(5):547-553.

79. Owens BD, Stickles BJ, Balikian P, Busconi BD: Prospective analysis of radiofrequency versus mechanical debridement of isolated patellar chondral lesions. *Arthroscopy* 2002;18(2):151-155.

80. Steadman JR, Briggs KK, Rodrigo JJ, Kocher MS, Gill TJ, Rodkey WG: Outcomes of microfracture for traumatic chondral defects of the knee: Average 11-year follow-up. *Arthroscopy* 2003;19(5): 477-484.

81. Miller BS, Steadman JR, Briggs KK, Rodrigo JJ, Rodkey WG: Patient satisfaction and outcome after microfracture of the degenerative knee. *J Knee Surg* 2004; 17(1):13-17.

82. Mont MA, Johnson AJ, Naziri Q, Kolisek FR, Leadbetter WB: Patellofemoral arthroplasty: 7-year mean follow-up. *J Arthroplasty* 2012;27(3):358-361.

83. Laskin RS, van Steijn M: Total knee replacement for patients with patellofemoral arthritis. *Clin Orthop Relat Res* 1999;367:89-95.

84. Meding JB, Wing JT, Keating EM, Ritter MA: Total knee arthroplasty for isolated patellofemoral arthritis in younger patients. *Clin Orthop Relat Res* 2007;464: 78-82.

85. Mehta VM, Inoue M, Nomura E, Fithian DC: An algorithm guiding the evaluation and treatment of acute primary patellar dislocations. *Sports Med Arthrosc* 2007; 15(2):78-81.

Video Reference

Arendt EA, Tompkins M: Video. Excerpt. Patella Distalization With Medial Patellofemoral Ligament Reconstrucion to Correct Patella Alta and Restore Medial Patella Support, from Fulkerson JP, ed: *Arthroscopic Surgical Techniques: Patella Instability and Arthrosis.* DVD. Rosemont, IL, Arthroscopy Association of North America and American Academy of Orthopaedic Surgeons, 2013.

Risks, Benefits, and Evidence-Based Recommendations for Improving Anterior Cruciate Ligament Outcomes

James H. Lubowitz, MD

Nikhil N. Verma, MD

John M. Tokish, MD

Vipool K. Goradia, MD

John W. McNeil II, BA

CDR Matthew T. Provencher, MD, MC, USN

Despite the fact that the study of anatomy dates back many centuries, our understanding of the surgical anatomy of the anterior cruciate ligament (ACL) continues to evolve. In the 21st century, the interest in ACL anatomy has, in a sense, been rediscovered. The science of ACL anatomy was deemphasized in the 1980s and 1990s because of the focus on endoscopic surgical techniques, including transtibial drilling of the femoral socket. Historically, the evolution from the two-incision technique, with outside-in drilling of a femoral tunnel, to a simpler single-incision endoscopic technique was elegant and less invasive but focused on graft isometry and avoiding impingement, not on achieving restoration of the anatomic footprint. The two-incision technique, by the very nature of the separate surgical

Abstract

Recently, injuries to the anterior cruciate ligament and subsequent surgical reconstructions have seen a great increase in interest from the perspectives of basic science, anatomy, mechanics, and clinical outcomes. Over the past few years, an emerging body of evidence has shown the importance of a more anatomic anterior cruciate ligament reconstruction, which uses sound anatomic and surgical principles, identifies an ideal graft for the patient, and ensures that all aspects of care (including postoperative rehabilitation) are fully addressed. It is helpful for orthopaedic surgeons to review the surgically relevant anatomy of the anterior cruciate ligament, graft choices, fixation techniques and constructs, and rehabilitation guidelines to optimize outcomes for their patients.

Instr Course Lect 2014;63:369-382.

Dr. Lubowitz or an immediate family member has received royalties from Arthrex; is a member of a speaker's bureau or has made paid presentations on behalf of Donor Services; serves as a paid consultant to or is an employee of Arthrex and Ivivi; has stock or stock options held in Ivivi; has received research or institutional support from Arthrex and MTF; has received nonincome support (such as equipment or services), commercially derived honoraria, or other non–research-related funding (such as paid travel) from Arthrex, Breg, Smith & Nephew, Ivivi, Tournier, Zimmer, and DJ Orthopaedics; and serves as a board member, owner, officer, or committee member of the Arthroscopy Association of North America; the American Orthopaedic Society for Sports Medicine; and the International Society of Arthroscopy, Knee Surgery, and Orthopaedic Sports Medicine. Dr. Verma or an immediate family member has received royalties from Smith & Nephew; serves as a paid consultant to or is an employee of Smith & Nephew and Arthrex; has stock or stock options held in Omeros; has received research or institutional support from Arthrex, Smith & Nephew, Athletico, ConMed Linvatec, Miomed, and Mitek; and serves as a board member, owner, officer, or committee member of the Arthroscopy Association Learning Center Committee. Dr. Goradia or an immediate family member has received royalties from Arthrex; serves as a paid consultant to or is an employee of Arthrex; has stock or stock options held in Pfizer; and serves as a board member, owner, officer, or committee member of the Arthroscopy Association of North America. Dr. Provencher serves as a paid consultant to or is an employee of Arthrex; has stock or stock options held in Pfizer; and serves as a board member, owner, officer, or committee member of the American Academy of Orthopaedic Surgeons; the American Orthopaedic Society for Sports Medicine; the American Shoulder and Elbow Surgeons; the Arthroscopy Association of North America, the International Society of Arthroscopy, Knee Surgery, and Orthopaedic Sports Medicine; the San Diego Shoulder Institute; and the Society of Military Orthopaedic Surgeons. Neither of the following authors nor any immediate family member has received anything of value from or has stock or stock options held in a commercial company or institution related directly or indirectly to the subject of this chapter: Dr. Tokish and Mr. McNeil.

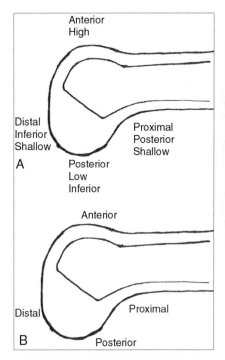

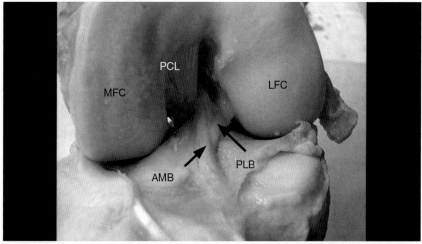

Figure 2 The ACL bundle anatomy. AMB = anteromedial bundle. PLB = posterolateral bundle. MFC = medial femoral condyle, LFC = lateral femoral condyle.

Figure 1 **A,** Sagittal section illustrating the lateral wall of the intercondylar notch of the right femur, labeled with various terms for describing the anatomy that create the potential for confusion. **B,** Recommended anatomic terminology to standardize reporting and minimize confusion.

approaches to the femoral and tibial sockets, provides more accurate representation and reconstruction of the ACL graft in terms of tunnel placement. Other alternative anatomic surgical techniques are also discussed in this chapter. The key point to remember is that transtibial creation of the ACL femoral socket poses a risk of nonanatomic placement of the ACL femoral socket, the tibial socket, or both.[1-3]

Anatomy of the ACL

Nomenclature

The anatomic nomenclature for ACL femoral positioning has been confused by the focus on endoscopic surgical techniques in which arthroscopy is typically performed with the knee flexed to 90°, rather than in the classic anatomic position.[4] Knee flexion tends

to change the femoral interpretation of the ACL femoral footprint. To ensure the anatomic femoral anatomy is well defined, it should be remembered that, regardless of the knee flexion angle, the femoral trochlea is anterior and the femoral articular cartilage is distal (**Figure 1**). With initial transtibial techniques, the most common endoscopic femoral socket malposition is too anterior and too proximal.[2] Further confusion results from the clockface description of the femoral ACL socket position (for example, 10-o'clock position or 2-o'clock position for a right or left knee, respectively), which is defined by convention with arthroscopic viewing of the posterior aspect of the lateral wall of the femoral intercondylar notch, with the knee at 90° flexion. This definition is quantitatively convenient but has been shown to be relatively imprecise.[5]

Gross Anatomy

The nonanatomic nature of endoscopic transtibial ACL techniques was recognized because of the renewed focus on the ACL anatomy, particularly the predominant two-bundle structure of the ligament (the anteromedial

[AM] and posterolateral [PL] bundles).[6] The bony ridges of the lateral wall of the intercondylar notch include a bifurcate ridge, which grossly runs anterior to posterior and separates the more proximal AM bundle from the more distal PL bundle, and a resident's ridge running grossly anterior to both bundles[7] (**Figure 2**).

With regard to arthroscopically measurable landmarks, the anatomic centrum of the ACL femoral footprint is, on average, in the sagittal plane and 43% of the distance from the proximal articular margin (the arthroscopically visualized osteochondral junction) to the distal articular margin on the lateral wall of the intercondylar notch. The anatomic centrum of the ACL femoral AM bundle footprint is 29.5% of the distance, and the anatomic centrum of the ACL femoral PL bundle footprint is 50% of the distance. In the axial plane, the anatomic centrum of the ACL femoral footprint is, on average, the socket radius plus 2.5 mm anterior to the posterior articular margin, with a 2.5-mm rim of bone between the posterior ACL fibers and the posterior articular cartilage margin. There are few published descriptions of the position of the femoral AM and PL bundles from the posterior cartilage[5] (**Figure 3**).

With regard to arthroscopically relevant landmarks, in the anterior-to-posterior plane, the anatomic centrum of the ACL tibial footprint as a whole is 15 mm anterior to the posterior cruciate ligament (PCL). The anatomic centrum of the AM bundle is 20 mm anterior to the PCL, and the anatomic centrum of the PL bundle is 11 mm anterior to the PCL (adjusted for patient size). The anatomic centrum of the ACL tibial footprint in the medial-to-lateral plane, as a whole, is two fifths of the medial-to-lateral width of the interspinous distance. The anatomic centrum of the AM bundle is one half of the medial-to-lateral width of the interspinous distance, and the anatomic centrum of the PL bundle is one fourth of the medial-to-lateral width of the interspinous distance (**Figure 4**).

Surgical Techniques: Clinical Alternatives and Limitations

The use of traditional cannulated femoral ACL endoscopic reamers can result in an improper femoral and tibial footprint anatomy.[2,4] Poorly positioned sockets are a primary cause of ACL graft failure.[8] The most common femoral malposition is too anterior and too proximal to the ideal ACL centroid. The most common tibial malposition is too posterior. Malpositioning of one or both ACL graft footprint centrums sometimes occurs dur-

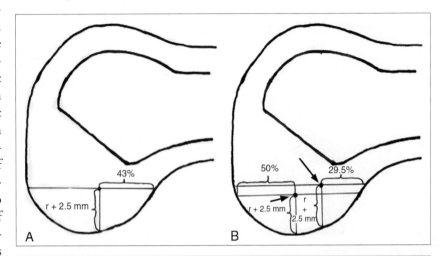

Figure 3 Sagittal section illustrations showing the lateral wall of the intercondylar notch of the right femur, with the mean anatomic centrum of the ACL femoral footprint. **A,** The anatomic centrum of the ACL femoral footprint is 43% of the proximal-to-distal length of the lateral femoral intercondylar notch wall and the femoral socket radius (r) plus 2.5 mm anterior to the posterior articular margin. **B,** The anatomic centrum of the ACL femoral footprint AM bundle (long arrow) is 29.5% of the proximal-to-distal length of the lateral femoral intercondylar notch wall. The anatomic centrum of the ACL femoral footprint PL bundle (short arrow) is 50% of the proximal-to-distal length of the lateral femoral intercondylar notch wall. From posterior to anterior, the AM bundle appears slightly anterior to the PL bundle. (Reproduced with permission from Piefer J, Pflugner T, Hwang M, Lubowitz J: Anterior cruciate ligament femoral footprint anatomy: Systematic review of the 21st century literature. *Arthroscopy* 2012;28(6):872-881.)

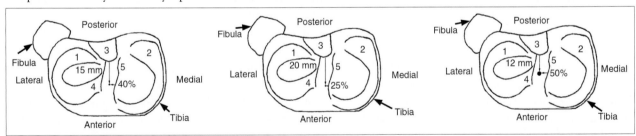

Figure 4 Axial, superior-to-inferior schematic view of the proximal tibia and fibula in a right knee. Illustrated on the proximal tibia are the lateral (1) and medial (2) menisci, as well as the PCL (3). Between the menisci, lines running from superior to inferior represent the lateral (4) and medial (5) intercondylar eminences (tibial spines). **A,** The black dot represents the centrum of the ACL tibial footprint as a whole, located approximately 15 mm anterior to the PCL and approximately two fifths of the interspinous distance from the medial to the lateral intercondylar eminence. **B,** The black dot represents the centrum of the ACL tibial AM bundle footprint, located approximately 20 mm anterior to the PCL and approximately one fourth of the interspinous distance from the medial to the lateral intercondylar eminence. **C,** The black dot marks the centrum of the ACL tibial PL bundle footprint, located approximately 12 mm anterior to the PCL and approximately one half of the interspinous distance from the medial to the lateral intercondylar eminence. (Reproduced with permission from Hwang MD, Piefer JW, Lubowitz JH: Anterior cruciate ligament tibial footprint anatomy: Systematic review of the 21st century literature. *Arthroscopy* 2012;28(5):728-734.)

Table 1
Properties of Common Grafts Used for ACL Reconstruction

Graft (Study)	Graft Type	Tensile Load (N)	Stiffness (N/mm)	Cross-sectional Area (mm²)
Native, intact ACL (Noyes et al[21])		1,725	182	44
Native, intact ACL (Woo et al[22])		2,160	242	44
BPTB (Markolf et al[17])	Autograft	3,057	455	35
Four-strand hamstring tendon graft (Hamner et al[23])	Autograft	4090	776	52.9
Quadriceps tendon (Harris et al[24])	Autograft	1,075	NA	
BPTB: frozen, nonirradiated (Fideler et al[25])	Allograft	2,552	633	NA
Tibialis anterior tendon (Haut Donahue et al[26])	Allograft	4,122	460	12

NA = Not available, BPTB = Bone-patellar tendon-bone.

ing transtibial drilling of the ACL femoral socket.[2,4]

New techniques are being developed to improve the anatomic positioning of the ACL tunnels on both the femur and the tibia. For example, anatomic transtibial drilling of the femoral socket in an anatomic position can be achieved by using flexible reamers. Other techniques that improve the anatomic positioning of the ACL tunnels include an accessory portal technique for creating the ACL femoral socket and a no-incision or all-inside technique (which has resulted after advances in retrograde socket drilling technology).[9-13]

A clinical limitation of current reconstruction techniques is that most of the techniques do not allow full coverage of the femoral or tibial footprints, because the ligament midsubstance has an hourglass morphology, not a cylindric morphology.[5,14] Microanatomic anisometric graft length changes occur during knee range of motion because the native ACL may have thousands

of individual fibers or fiber bundles (not just a double-bundle structure). Further research is needed to determine if anatomic ACL reconstruction can achieve improved clinical outcomes.[14-20]

Graft Selection
The ideal graft for use in ACL reconstruction has not yet been determined. The properties of such a graft would include high initial strength, rapid and reproducible biologic integration, good availability, cost-effectiveness, and limited comorbidities associated with graft harvesting. Because reproducible outcomes have been reported with many graft choices, graft selection should be individualized based on surgeon experience and host factors, including age, activity level, and prior surgeries. In most instances, the evaluation of the potential limitations or complications of each type of graft, including factors related to cosmesis, risk of rerupture, residual knee laxity, and anterior knee pain, will assist the sur-

geon and patient in making an informed decision.

Commonly used autograft options include bone-patellar tendon-bone (BPTB) or four-strand hamstring tendon. Common allograft choices include patellar tendon, Achilles tendon, and soft-tissue grafts (such as tibialis anterior allograft)[17,21-26] (**Table 1**). The routine use of synthetic grafts has fallen out of favor because of high complication rates, including synovitis, recurrent effusions, and early failure. Research continues in the field of ligament tissue engineering, with a goal of developing a biologically derived graft substitute.[27]

Biomechanically, all current commonly used grafts exceed the load to failure of the native ACL.[28] Four-strand hamstring autografts are the stiffest, whereas BPTB autografts most closely replicate native ACL properties, especially strength. From a fixation standpoint, BPTB grafts offer the most rigid time-zero fixation along

Table 1 (continued)

Properties of Common Grafts Used for ACL Reconstruction

Fixation	Healing	Advantages	Disadvantages
Interference screw	Bone to bone	Earlier rehabilitation and return to play	Risk of patellar fracture and rupture Anterior knee pain Extensor weakness
Variable	Soft tissue	Less donor site morbidity Stronger than BPTB	Superficial saphenous injury during harvest Hamstring weakness Slower rehabilitation depending on fixation
Interference screw	Combination	Stronger than BPTB	Risk of patellar fracture
Interference screw	Bone to bone	No donor site morbidity	Delayed allograft incorporation
Variable	Soft tissue	No donor site morbidity	Delayed allograft incorporation

NA = Not available, BPTB = Bone-patellar tendon-bone.

with the advantage of bone-to-bone healing.

BPTB Autografts

BPTB autograft has the longest available track record and reproducible clinical results.[28,29] Its rigid initial fixation and reproducible bone healing at the bone-tunnel interface allows for early aggressive rehabilitation and minimizes residual knee laxity after reconstruction.[28,29] Low rerupture rates have been reported.[30] Potential complications of BPTB autograft include persistent postoperative anterior knee pain, which has been reported to occur in 5% to 35% of patients, and extensor mechanism failure (tendon rupture or fracture).[31-33] Aggressive postoperative rehabilitation is required to minimize the risk of motion loss, flexion contracture, and patellar entrapment.[34,35] When using a BPTB graft, the surgeon should be prepared to deal with potential graft tunnel mismatch (for example, the graft is too long and cannot be adequately fixed in the tibial tunnel). Management options include recessing the femoral bone plug, shortening the tibial bone plug, or converting to an alternate fixation technique.[36-38]

Four-Strand Hamstring Autografts

The use of four-strand hamstring autograft has been gaining in popularity because of concerns about morbidity associated with BPTB harvesting. The advantages of four-strand hamstring grafts include low surgical morbidity, improved cosmesis, high initial graft strength, and decreased risk of anterior knee pain. Limitations include fixation strength, which is highly dependent on fixation choice; longer and less reproducible soft-tissue bone tunnel healing; and variable tensioning because of the graft's multiple strands.[39] During graft harvest, the surgeon must be careful to free any fibrous bands between the gracilis and semitendinous or the semitendinous and gastrocnemius, which can result in premature graft amputation and short graft length (**Figure 5**).

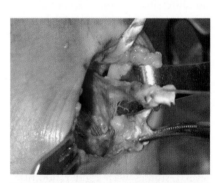

Figure 5 Fascial connections commonly observed between the gracilis, semitendinosus, and gastrocnemius during hamstring harvest. Connections must be released before passing the graft stripper to avoid premature graft amputation.

Outcome Comparisons: BPTB and Hamstring Autografts

Multiple studies have been performed to compare hamstring and patellar tendon autografts. A 2011 Cochrane database systematic review included randomized and quasirandomized comparative studies up to 2008.[39] In

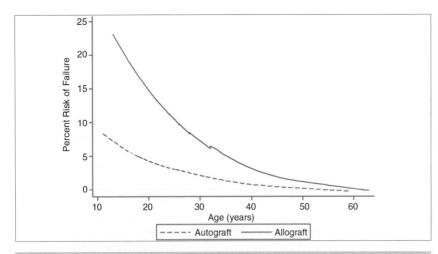

Figure 6 Graph comparing the probability of a retear for autograft versus allograft based on a patient's age. The graph clearly shows the inverse relationship between the risk of a retear and patient age for both graft types, but to a greater extent for allografts. (Reproduced with permission from Kaeding CC, Aros B, Pedroza A, et al: Allograft versus autograft anterior cruciate ligament reconstruction: Predictors of failure from a MOON prospective longitudinal cohort. *Sports Health* 2011;3(1):73-81.)

the 19 trials included by the authors, no difference in any functional outcome measure was found. The use of patellar tendon autograft resulted in a more statically stable construct but had an increased risk of anterior knee pain and extension strength deficit compared with an increased risk of knee flexion strength deficit with hamstring autograft. A systematic review by Reinhardt et al[31] reported on six level I studies with rigid randomization criteria. The authors noted a substantially increased risk of graft failure for hamstring autograft (15.8%) compared with BPTB autograft (7.2%). In a recent analysis, Magnussen et al[40] reported an increased risk of hamstring autograft failure associated with patients younger than 20 years and small graft size (< 8 mm diameter).

Allograft Considerations

Allografts have become an increasingly popular choice for ACL reconstruction because they eliminate graft harvest morbidity and reduce surgical time and the rehabilitation burden. However, allograft usage is potentially lim-

ited by the risk of disease transmission, delayed graft-tunnel healing, and ligamentization.[41-43] Improved donor screening protocols and terminal sterilization methods, including low-dose irradiation or proprietary secondary techniques, have substantially reduced the risk of disease transmission.

Currently, low-dose irradiation (1 to 1.5 Mrad) is the most common method for terminal sterilization and is effective against bacteria but not viruses. Unlike high-dose irradiation, low-dose irradiation for terminal sterilization has a negligible effect on initial graft biomechanics and subsequent graft healing.[42] It should be noted, however, that multiple animal studies have reported delayed soft-tissue and bone healing and graft remodeling with allografts compared with autografts, regardless of the sterilization technique used. This factor should be considered during graft selection and when considering return-to-sport criteria.[44,45]

Multiple factors, including initial biomechanics, fixation options, graft

cost and availability, and bone versus soft-tissue healing, should be considered when selecting an allograft. When using soft-tissue grafts, surgeons should consider alternate or supplemental fixation with interference screws based on limited initial fixation.[46]

Allograft Outcomes

Recent outcomes of allograft reconstruction have suggested higher rates of rerupture, most notably in younger, more active patients. Barrett et al[46] reported on allograft versus autograft patellar tendon reconstruction and found up to a 4.2 times increase in failure rates in patients with a high activity level. A 2011 multicenter prospective study of ACL reconstruction found younger age and a higher activity level to be important predictors of allograft failure and the need for revision surgery.[47] The authors reported a significantly increased failure rate in younger patients, with a marginal difference in failure rates in patients older than 40 years (**Figure 6**). Surgeons should consider these recent findings against the appeal of decreased surgical time and perioperative morbidity when recommending allograft use in younger, more active patients.

Fixation
ACL Fixation

Graft fixation is considered the weak link in ACL reconstruction during the early postoperative phase while the graft matures and incorporates into the bone tunnels.[48] The precise timing of the biologic incorporation of ACL grafts is unknown. Most studies have used animal models (rabbit, mouse, dog, and sheep) and different fixation methods, graft types, and activity restriction. These variables make it difficult to know precisely when the fixation is no longer the weakest part of the ACL reconstruction. Despite these limitations, it is generally believed that bone plugs heal within tunnels at 6 to 8 weeks, and soft-tissue grafts heal at 12 to 16 weeks after surgery.[29,44,49-53] The ligamentization process takes between 18 and 24 months. Stable fixation is important during the maturation period.

Ideal properties for a graft fixation device are listed in **Table 2**. The most important factors in determining a successful outcome after ACL reconstruction are whether the patient can resume activities of daily living and participate in a rehabilitation program. To achieve these goals, the graft fixation must be capable of withstanding repetitive forces until the graft incorporates into the tunnels. Noyes et al[21] estimated peak ACL forces of 454 N during the performance of activities of daily living. More sophisticated computer modeling has shown peak ACL forces of 303 N during the single stance phase of gait.[54] Isokinetic and isometric knee extension results in peak forces of 0.55 N × body weight at knee flexion angles of 35° to 40°.[55] Electromyography has demonstrated that one-leg squats result in peak ACL forces between 0° and 40° of knee flexion (59 N ± 52 N at 30°), and minimal forces occur during two-leg wall squats.[56] These findings support the use of closed-chain, rather than open-chain, strengthening exercises during rehabilitation after ACL reconstruction.

Fixation of BPTB Grafts

Biomechanical studies comparing bioabsorbable and titanium interference screws have shown similar ultimate failure strengths and responses to cyclic loading.[57,58] A meta-analysis of 10 level I and II studies reported similar clinical outcomes but higher rates of postoperative effusions and tunnel widening with bioabsorbable screws compared with metal interference

screws.[59] Advantages of interference screws include joint line fixation with high strength and stiffness. The principle disadvantage is that the interference screw is inserted along one side of the bone plug, which prevents circumferential healing of the plug within the bone tunnel. Because biocomposite interference screws are osteoconductive, future studies may show that they promote circumferential bone-to-bone incorporation of the graft plugs.

For femoral fixation, other options include cortical buttons and cross pins (**Figure 7**). Cortical buttons (for example, EndoButton, Smith & Nephew) provide similar strength but less stiffness and more displacement under cyclic loading compared with interference screws.[60] The main disadvantage of cross pins is bone plug fracture, which is more likely if the plug diameter is small or if the cross pin is not properly centered in the plug.

Fixation of Soft-Tissue Grafts

The gold standard for soft-tissue graft fixation has not been determined. Milano et al[61] provided a useful method for categorizing the various soft-tissue femoral fixation devices (**Figure 7** and **Table 3**). The authors showed that cortical-cancellous transcondylar fixation devices (such as graft wraps around cross pins) had the best properties in terms of graft elongation, strength, and stiffness, whereas interference screws had the lowest strength and greatest elongation. Expansion devices (pin-pierced grafts) had more than 2 mm elongation after cyclic loading, and the properties of the cortical suspension devices (such as buttons) correlated with their contact surface area. In contrast, a biomechanical study showed no difference in graft motion between cortical suspension, cortical-cancellous transcondylar fixation, and aperture fixation.[60] One important point of distinction for the

two types of cross pins is that more slippage occurs when pins go through the graft fibers compared with those in which the tendon graft wraps around (or over) the pin.[62]

It is difficult to design a clinical study isolating the fixation device as the only evaluated variable. A recent level I study randomized 120 patients to the following fixation methods: (1) corticocancellous transcondylar femoral and tibia screw/sheath, (2) corticocancellous transcondylar femoral and tibial bioabsorbable interference screws, (3) femoral bioabsorbable interference screws and tibial screw/sheath, or (4) bioabsorbable interference screw in both tunnels.[63] The authors reported no clinical differences between groups at a minimum follow-up of 2 years.

Animal studies have suggested inferior tibial graft incorporation compared with femoral tunnel healing in a rabbit model, whereas no difference was seen in a sheep model.[49,64] Biomechanically, a screw within a sheath, a long spiked washer, tandem standard spiked washers, and bioabsorbable interference screws all have strengths greater than 600 N; however, after 1,500 loading cycles, the screw within the sheath showed the least displacement.[57]

Because of concerns regarding tibial fixation, supplementary fixation has been suggested. Although biomechani-

Table 2
Properties of an Ideal ACL Fixation Device
Securely fixes graft until it attaches to bone allowing rehabilitation
Easy to use and insert
Allows postoperative MRI (if needed)
Permits revision
Does not cause biologic problems
Does not cause adverse symptoms in the patient

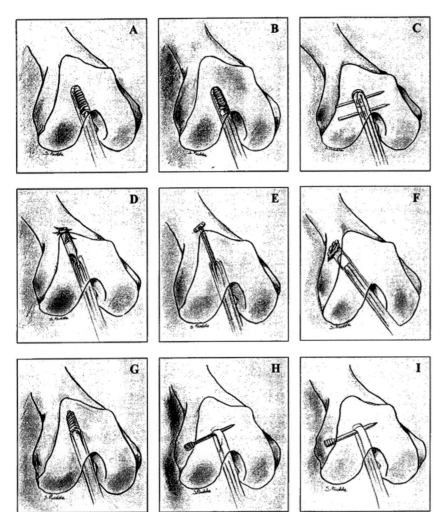

Figure 7 Illustrations of femoral fixation devices for soft-tissue grafts. **A** and **B**, Metal and bioabsorbable interference screws. **C**, Expansion fixation. **D** through **F**, Cortical suspension. **G**, Cancellous suspension. **H** and **I**, Metal and bioabsorbable corticocancellous transcondylar suspension. (Reproduced with permission from Milano G, Mulas PD, Ziranu F, Piras S, Manunta A, Fabbriciani C: Comparison between different femoral fixation devices for ACL reconstruction with doubled hamstring tendon graft: A biomechanical analysis. *Arthroscopy* 2006;22(6):660-668.)

cal studies do not provide clear evidence to support supplemental fixation, surgeons should consider supplemental fixation based on the perceived security of the fixation and the patient's bone quality.

Clinical studies have not shown clear superiority of one soft-tissue graft fixation device over another. Even though interference screw fixation is biomechanically weaker than other devices for soft-tissue fixation, a level I study comparing tibial interference screws and staples with a centrally placed screw within a sheath showed no clinical differences at 2-year follow-up.[65]

Postoperative Rehabilitation and Return to Play

Successful outcomes after ACL reconstruction require a comprehensive team approach consisting of the patient, the surgeon, and the rehabilita-tion specialist. Several studies have shown that ACL grafts weaken over time, with strengths 25% to 40% of normal at 1 year, long after return to play is often allowed.[49,66,67] It is important to remember the ACL exists within a framework of dynamic muscular stabilizers, all of which are affected by the injury and the postoperative rehabilitation program. Simultaneous protection of the reconstruction and mobilization of the dynamic stabilizers are the most important considerations in the postoperative period. These dynamic stabilizers are not just specific to the knee. Postural stability, proprioception, balance, and fatigue loading are all measures of dynamic stabilization and are part of the greater kinetic chain. Failure to appreciate the role of dynamic stabilizers in postoperative rehabilitation may risk graft rerupture and limit the patient's ability to return to sports participation.[68]

Getting Started: Baseline Criteria

Certain baseline criteria should be met before returning to sports activities after ACL reconstruction (**Table 4**). It should be noted that there are no specific time-based guidelines because factors such as associated procedures, access to care, and patient motivation contribute to wide variations in the rate of rehabilitation progression.

Static Phase Rehabilitation

The hallmark of the static phase of rehabilitation is that one leg remains in contact with the ground throughout the exercises. Core strengthening, postural stability, and aerobic fitness must be regained to return the knee to its proper role in the kinetic chain. The primary exercises for the first phase of ACL rehabilitation are the single-leg squat and lunge (**Figures 8** and **9**). These exercises force the patient to use

Table 3

Fixation Mechanisms for Soft-Tissue Grafts

Mechanism	Description	Forces
Compressive	Interference screws	Loads are transverse to longitudinal axis of graft
Expansion	One or more cross pins go through graft	Centrifugal force from bulging of graft caused by volume of pins
Cortical suspension	Cortical implant (for example, button) and suture material suspends graft	Forces are in line with graft and focused on the surface area of fixation on the cortex
Cancellous suspension	Graft suspended by screw inserted in cancellous bone	Strength dependent on fixation of screw within cancellous bone
Corticocancellous	Graft wraps around a transverse pin that is secured in cortical and cancellous bone	Forces are perpendicular to pin and strength is based on pin fixation within bone

(Adapted from Milano G, Mulas PD, Ziranu F, Piras S, Manunta A, Fabbriciani C: Comparison between different femoral fixation devices for ACL reconstruction with doubled hamstring tendon graft: A biomechanical analysis. *Arthroscopy* 2006; 22(6):660-668.)

Table 4

General Rehabilitation Criteria to Consider Before the Commencement of Sport-Specific Rehabilitation

Baseline Criteria for Consideration of Return to Sport Progression
Lysholm knee score > 75
Single assessment numeric evaluation score > 75
No sense of instability
Normal performance of activities of daily living

Objective Examination Findings
Complete wound healing
No effusion
Quadriceps atrophy < 2 cm
No more than 3 mm on Lachman or trace pivot shift test

Performance Measures
Knee extension, flexion > 70% of normal value
Single-leg lunge full, with good balance
Single-leg squat > 60°

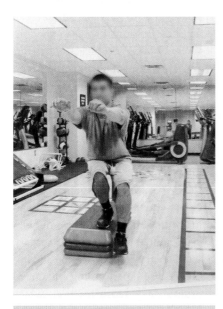

Figure 8   Static phase of postoperative rehabilitation with patient engaged in single-leg squat.

Figure 9   Static phase of postoperative rehabilitation with patient engaged in single-leg lunge.

the leg within the context of the kinetic chain, firing dynamic stabilizers and cocontracting muscle groups in functional patterns that simulate athletic motion. The initial goal should be achieving 60° of knee flexion in a controlled manner for 5 seconds. The athlete is ready to progress when this position can be held with good postural core stability, excellent balance, and no quiver throughout the exercise.

Method of Progression

Progression is based on a ramped approach. Loading of the joint begins low and increases, and speed begins slow and gets faster. In early rehabilitation, the platform can be a stable floor,

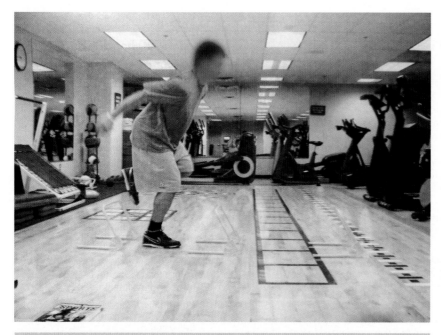

Figure 10 Dynamic phase of postoperative rehabilitation showing patient engaged in a single-leg multiplanar jumping and landing maneuver.

with progression to a less stable surface to encourage better dynamic stabilization. Exercise repetitions are increased to improve stamina. The rehabilitation specialist directly supervises these activities because breakdowns in core and balance are frequent and often unrecognized by the athlete.[69,70] Breakdowns must be recognized so progression can be delayed and the athlete returned to a level at which exercises can be properly performed. This progression-based approach is different from traditional approaches that allow activity advancement based on the time elapsed from surgery.

Dynamic Phase Progression

Progression to the dynamic phase of the rehabilitation regimen is marked by the incorporation of jumping and landing maneuvers. This phase begins with the athlete standing on two feet in a single plane. The athlete progresses to single-leg, uniplanar, vertical, and horizontal jumps and finally to multiplanar jumps and landings from progressive heights (**Figure 10**).

The rehabilitation specialist should monitor the landing to ensure that there is not too little knee flexion or valgus positioning because both are risk factors for ACL injury.[71,72] As the athlete becomes proficient in these maneuvers, perturbations in heights, speeds, and planes are added to introduce complexity to the activity. Timed tests give the athlete performance-based feedback and can identify subtle defects in postural core stability that must be corrected before return to competition. Performance-based tests, such as the triple hop, are used near the end of the dynamic phase. Normalization to within 10% to 15% of the uninjured side is a good indicator that functional strength has returned.

Ballistic Progression and Return to Sports

By the completion of the dynamic phase, the athlete should have achieved essential normalcy in static and dynamic activities. The ballistic phase simulates sport-specific activities in a controlled environment. This is the specialty area of the athletic trainer, who is familiar with the drills and requirements specific to the athlete's sport. For a basketball player, activities may include defensive slide drills or rebounding from a squatted position. For the football player, drills may include changing direction from a back pedal to a break on the ball at full speed. The rehabilitation specialist should watch for breakdowns in core kinetics, which may indicate the need to decelerate the pace of the program. With adequate performance in these drills, the athlete should be able to return to controlled competition, the final phase before return to play. The athlete is allowed to participate in full competition but in limited scenarios and with a limited number of repetitions to allow the return of endurance and confidence. The rehabilitation specialist should have the authority to limit these sessions based on the athlete's symptoms or objective performance. With gradual progression based on objective performance criteria, return to sports after ACL reconstruction can be achieved.

Summary

A thorough understanding of patient factors, ACL anatomy, graft selection options, and postoperative rehabilitation are important to achieve the best possible outcomes after ACL surgery. There is renewed emphasis on the importance of performing a near-anatomic ACL reconstruction, which more closely replicates the complex biomechanic properties of the ACL. The type of graft chosen (autograft or allograft), fixation techniques, and postoperative rehabilitation all play an important role in the patient's outcomes. A careful assessment of patient factors, surgical techniques, graft selection, and rehabilitation will likely provide meaningful improvements in the care of patients with ACL injuries.

References

1. Howell SM: Principles for placing the tibial tunnel and avoiding roof impingement during reconstruction of a torn anterior cruciate ligament. *Knee Surg Sports Traumatol Arthrosc* 1998;6(suppl 1):S49-S55.

2. Marchant BG, Noyes FR, Barber-Westin SD, Fleckenstein C: Prevalence of nonanatomical graft placement in a series of failed anterior cruciate ligament reconstructions. *Am J Sports Med* 2010;38(10):1987-1996.

3. Abebe ES, Moorman CT III, Dziedzic TS, et al: An in vivo imaging analysis comparing transtibial and 2-incision tibial tunnel-independent techniques. *Am J Sports Med* 2009;37(10):1904-1911.

4. Kaseta MK, DeFrate LE, Charnock BL, Sullivan RT, Garrett WE Jr: Reconstruction technique affects femoral tunnel placement in ACL reconstruction. *Clin Orthop Relat Res* 2008;466(6):1467-1474.

5. Piefer JW, Pflugner TR, Hwang MD, Lubowitz JH: Anterior cruciate ligament femoral footprint anatomy: Systematic review of the 21st century literature. *Arthroscopy* 2012;28(6):872-881.

6. Chhabra A, Starman JS, Ferretti M, Vidal AF, Zantop T, Fu FH: Anatomic, radiographic, biomechanical, and kinematic evaluation of the anterior cruciate ligament and its two functional bundles. *J Bone Joint Surg Am* 2006;88(suppl 4):2-10.

7. Ferretti M, Ekdahl M, Shen W, Fu FH: Osseous landmarks of the femoral attachment of the anterior cruciate ligament: An anatomic study. *Arthroscopy* 2007;23(11):1218-1225.

8. Andersson D, Samuelsson K, Karlsson J: Treatment of anterior cruciate ligament injuries with special reference to surgical technique and rehabilitation: An assessment of randomized controlled trials. *Arthroscopy* 2009;25(6):653-685.

9. Steiner ME, Smart LR: Flexible instruments outperform rigid instruments to place anatomic anterior cruciate ligament femoral tunnels without hyperflexion. *Arthroscopy* 2012;28(6):835-843.

10. Lubowitz JH: Anteromedial portal technique for the anterior cruciate ligament femoral socket: Pitfalls and solutions. *Arthroscopy* 2009;25(1):95-101.

11. Lubowitz JH, Ahmad CS, Anderson K: All-inside anterior cruciate ligament graft-link technique: Second-generation, no-incision anterior cruciate ligament reconstruction. *Arthroscopy* 2011;27(5):717-727.

12. Smith PA, Schwartzberg RS, Lubowitz JH: No tunnel 2-socket technique: All-inside anterior cruciate ligament double-bundle retroconstruction. *Arthroscopy* 2008;24(10):1184-1189.

13. Lubowitz JH: No-tunnel anterior cruciate ligament reconstruction: The transtibial all-inside technique. *Arthroscopy* 2006;22(8):e1-e11.

14. Hwang MD, Piefer JW, Lubowitz JH: Anterior cruciate ligament tibial footprint anatomy: Systematic review of the 21st century literature. *Arthroscopy* 2012;28(5):728-734.

15. Lubowitz JH, Poehling GG: Techniques in double-bundle anterior cruciate ligament reconstruction: As simple as ABC, or putting the cart before the horse? *Arthroscopy* 2008;24(10):1089-1091.

16. Ho JY, Gardiner A, Shah V, Steiner ME: Equal kinematics between central anatomic single-bundle and double-bundle anterior cruciate ligament reconstructions. *Arthroscopy* 2009;25(5):464-472.

17. Markolf KL, Park S, Jackson SR, McAllister DR: Anterior-posterior and rotatory stability of single and double-bundle anterior cruciate ligament reconstructions. *J Bone Joint Surg Am* 2009;91(1):107-118.

18. Meredick RB, Vance KJ, Appleby D, Lubowitz JH: Outcome of single-bundle versus double-bundle reconstruction of the anterior cruciate ligament: A meta-analysis. *Am J Sports Med* 2008;36(7):1414-1421.

19. Irrgang JJ, Bost JE, Fu FH: Re: Outcome of single-bundle versus double-bundle reconstruction of the anterior cruciate ligament. A meta-analysis. *Am J Sports Med* 2009;37(2):421-422, author reply 422.

20. Lubowitz JH, Poehling GG: Watch your footprint: Anatomic ACL reconstruction. *Arthroscopy* 2009;25(10):1059-1060.

21. Noyes FR, Butler DL, Grood ES, Zernicke RF, Hefzy MS: Biomechanical analysis of human ligament grafts used in knee-ligament repairs and reconstructions. *J Bone Joint Surg Am* 1984;66(3):344-352.

22. Woo SL, Debski RE, Withrow JD, Janaushek MA: Biomechanics of knee ligaments. *Am J Sports Med* 1999;27(4):533-543.

23. Hamner DL, Brwon CH Jr, Steiner ME, Hecker AT, Hayes WC: Hamstring tendon grafts for reconstruction of the anterior cruciate ligament: Biomechanical evaluation of the use of multiple strands and tensioning techniques. *J Bone Joint Surg Am* 1999;81(4):549-557.

24. Harris NL, Smith DA, Lamoreaux L, Purnell M: Central quadriceps tendon for anterior cruciate ligament reconstruction: Part 1. Morphometric and biomechanical evaluation. *Am J Sports Med* 1997;25(1):23-28.

25. Fideler BM, Vangsness CT Jr, Lu B, Orlando C, Moore T: Gamma irradiation: Effect on biomechanical properties of hu-

man bone-patellar tendon-bone allografts. *Am J Sports Med* 1995; 23(5):643-646.

26. Haut Donahue TL, Howell SM, Hull ML, Gregersen C: A Biomechanical evaluation of anterior and posterior tibialis tendons as suitable single-loop anterior cruciate ligament grafts. *Arthroscopy* 2002;18(6):589-597.

27. Legnani C, Ventura A, Terzaghi C, Borgo E, Albisetti W: Anterior cruciate ligament reconstruction with synthetic grafts: A review of literature. *Int Orthop* 2010;34(4): 465-471.

28. West RV, Harner CD: Graft selection in anterior cruciate ligament reconstruction. *J Am Acad Orthop Surg* 2005;13(3):197-207.

29. Rodeo SA, Arnoczky SP, Torzilli PA, Hidaka C, Warren RF: Tendon-healing in a bone tunnel: A biomechanical and histological study in the dog. *J Bone Joint Surg Am* 1993;75(12):1795-1803.

30. Shelton WR, Papendick L, Dukes AD: Autograft versus allograft anterior cruciate ligament reconstruction. *Arthroscopy* 1997;13(4): 446-449.

31. Reinhardt KR, Hetsroni I, Marx RG: Graft selection for anterior cruciate ligament reconstruction: A level I systematic review comparing failure rates and functional outcomes. *Orthop Clin North Am* 2010;41(2):249-262.

32. Ibrahim SA, Al-Kussary IM, Al-Misfer AR, Al-Mutairi HQ, Ghafar SA, El Noor TA: Clinical evaluation of arthroscopically assisted anterior cruciate ligament reconstruction: Patellar tendon versus gracilis and semitendinosus autograft. *Arthroscopy* 2005;21(4): 412-417.

33. Roe J, Pinczewski LA, Russell VJ, Salmon LJ, Kawamata T, Chew M: A 7-year follow-up of patellar tendon and hamstring tendon grafts for arthroscopic anterior cruciate ligament reconstruction:

34. Stein DA, Hunt SA, Rosen JE, Sherman OH: The incidence and outcome of patella fractures after anterior cruciate ligament reconstruction. *Arthroscopy* 2002;18(6): 578-583.

35. Bonamo JJ, Krinick RM, Sporn AA: Rupture of the patellar ligament after use of its central third for anterior cruciate ligament reconstruction. *J Bone Joint Surg Am* 1984;66:1294-1297.

36. Taylor DE, Dervin GF, Keene GC: Femoral bone plug recession in endoscopic anterior cruciate ligament reconstruction. *Arthroscopy* 1996;12(4):513-515.

37. Augé WK II, Yifan K: A technique for resolution of graft-tunnel length mismatch in central third bone-patellar tendon-bone anterior cruciate ligament reconstruction. *Arthroscopy* 1999;15(8): 877-881.

38. Risinger RJ, Verma NN, Bach BR: Graft fixation alternatives. *Tech Orthop* 2005;20(4):382-390.

39. Mohtadi NG, Chan DS, Dainty KN, Whelan DB: Patellar tendon versus hamstring tendon autograft for anterior cruciate ligament rupture in adults. *Cochrane Database Syst Rev* 2011;9:CD005960.

40. Magnussen RA, Lawrence JT, West RL, Toth AP, Taylor DC, Garrett WE: Graft size and patient age are predictors of early revision after anterior cruciate ligament reconstruction with hamstring autograft. *Arthroscopy* 2012;28(4):526-531.

41. Buck BE, Malinin TI, Brown MD: Bone transplantation and human immunodeficiency virus: An estimate of risk of acquired immunodeficiency syndrome (AIDS). *Clin Orthop Relat Res* 1989;240:129-136.

42. Bhatia S, Bell R, Frank RM, et al: Bony incorporation of soft tissue

anterior cruciate ligament grafts in an animal model: Autograft versus allograft with low-dose gamma irradiation. *Am J Sports Med* 2012;40(8):1789-1798.

43. Scheffler SU, Schmidt T, Gangéy I, Dustmann M, Unterhauser F, Weiler A: Fresh-frozen free-tendon allografts versus autografts in anterior cruciate ligament reconstruction: Delayed remodeling and inferior mechanical function during long-term healing in sheep. *Arthroscopy* 2008;24(4): 448-458.

44. Jackson DW, Grood ES, Goldstein JD, et al: A comparison of patellar tendon autograft and allograft used for anterior cruciate ligament reconstruction in the goat model. *Am J Sports Med* 1993;21(2):176-185.

45. Park DK, Fogel HA, Bhatia S, et al: Comparison of 1-, 2-, and 4-stranded constructs. *Am J Sports Med* 2009;37(8):1531-1538.

46. Barrett GR, Luber K, Replogle WH, Manley JL: Allograft anterior cruciate ligament reconstruction in the young, active patient: Tegner activity level and failure rate. *Arthroscopy* 2010;26(12): 1593-1601.

47. Kaeding CC, Aros B, Pedroza A, et al: Predictors of failure from a MOON prospective longitudinal cohort. *Sports Health* 2011;3(1): 73-81.

48. Ekdahl M, Wang JH, Ronga M, Fu FH: Graft healing in anterior cruciate ligament reconstruction. *Knee Surg Sports Traumatol Arthrosc* 2008;16(10):935-947.

49. Goradia VK, Rochat MC, Grana WA, Rohrer MD, Prasad HS: Tendon-to-bone healing of a semitendinosus tendon autograft used for ACL reconstruction in a sheep model. *Am J Knee Surg* 2000;13(3):143-151.

50. Butler DL, Grood ES, Noyes FR, et al: Mechanical properties of primate vascularized vs. nonvascu-

larized patellar tendon grafts; changes over time. *J Orthop Res* 1989;7(1):68-79.

51. Tomita F, Yasuda K, Mikami S, Sakai T, Yamazaki S, Tohyama H: Comparisons of intraosseous graft healing between the doubled flexor tendon graft and the bone-patellar tendon-bone graft in anterior cruciate ligament reconstruction. *Arthroscopy* 2001;17(5): 461-476.

52. Weiler A, Hoffmann RF, Bail HJ, Rehm O, Südkamp NP: Tendon healing in a bone tunnel: Part II. Histologic analysis after biodegradable interference fit fixation in a model of anterior cruciate ligament reconstruction in sheep. *Arthroscopy* 2002;18(2):124-135.

53. Zantop T, Weimann A, Wolle K, Musahl V, Langer M, Petersen W: Initial and 6 weeks postoperative structural properties of soft tissue anterior cruciate ligament reconstructions with cross-pin or interference screw fixation: An in vivo study in sheep. *Arthroscopy* 2007; 23(1):14-20.

54. Shelburne KB, Pandy MG, Anderson FC, Torry MR: Pattern of anterior cruciate ligament force in normal walking. *J Biomech* 2004; 37(6):797-805.

55. Toutoungi DE, Lu TW, Leardini A, Catani F, O'Connor JJ: Cruciate ligament forces in the human knee during rehabilitation exercises. *Clin Biomech (Bristol, Avon)* 2000;15(3):176-187.

56. Escamilla RF, Zheng N, Imamura R, et al: Cruciate ligament force during the wall squat and the one-leg squat. *Med Sci Sports Exerc* 2009;41(2):408-417.

57. Kousa P, Järvinen TL, Kannus P, Järvinen M: Initial fixation strength of bioabsorbable and titanium interference screws in anterior cruciate ligament reconstruction: Biomechanical evaluation by single cycle and cyclic loading. *Am J Sports Med* 2001; 29(4):420-425.

58. Weiler A, Windhagen HJ, Raschke MJ, Laumeyer A, Hoffmann RF: Biodegradable interference screw fixation exhibits pull-out force and stiffness similar to titanium screws. *Am J Sports Med* 1998;26(1):119-126.

59. Shen C, Jiang SD, Jiang LS, Dai LY: Bioabsorbable versus metallic interference screw fixation in anterior cruciate ligament reconstruction: A meta-analysis of randomized controlled trials. *Arthroscopy* 2010;26(5):705-713.

60. Brown CH Jr, Wilson DR, Hecker AT, Ferragamo M: Graft-bone motion and tensile properties of hamstring and patellar tendon anterior cruciate ligament femoral graft fixation under cyclic loading. *Arthroscopy* 2004;20(9): 922-935.

61. Milano G, Mulas PD, Ziranu F, Piras S, Manunta A, Fabbriciani C: Comparison between different femoral fixation devices for ACL reconstruction with doubled hamstring tendon graft: A biomechanical analysis. *Arthroscopy* 2006;22(6):660-668.

62. Ahmad CS, Gardner TR, Groh M, Arnouk J, Levine WN: Mechanical properties of soft tissue femoral fixation devices for anterior cruciate ligament reconstruction. *Am J Sports Med* 2004; 32(3):635-640.

63. Harilainen A, Sandelin J: A prospective comparison of 3 hamstring ACL fixation devices—Rigidfix, BioScrew, and Intrafix: Randomized into 4 groups with 2 years of follow-up. *Am J Sports Med* 2009;37(4):699-706.

64. Wen C-Y, Qin L, Lee K-M, Wong MW, Chan K-M: Grafted tendon healing in tibial tunnel is inferior to healing in femoral tunnel after anterior cruciate ligament reconstruction: A histomorphometric study in rabbits. *Arthroscopy* 2010;26(1):58-66.

65. De Wall M, Scholes CJ, Patel S, Coolican MR, Parker DA: Tibial

fixation in anterior cruciate ligament reconstruction: A prospective randomized study comparing metal interference screw and staples with a centrally placed polyethylene screw and sheath. *Am J Sports Med* 2011;39(9):1858-1864.

66. Jackson DW, Grood ES, Arnoczky SP, Butler DL, Simon TM: Cruciate reconstruction using freeze dried anterior cruciate ligament allograft and a ligament augmentation device (LAD): An experimental study in a goat model. *Am J Sports Med* 1987; 15(6):528-538.

67. Shino K, Horibe S: Experimental ligament reconstruction by allogeneic tendon graft in a canine model. *Acta Orthop Belg* 1991; 57(suppl 2):44-53.

68. Salmon L, Russell V, Musgrove T, Pinczewski L, Refshauge K: Incidence and risk factors for graft rupture and contralateral rupture after anterior cruciate ligament reconstruction. *Arthroscopy* 2005; 21(8):948-957.

69. Ageberg E, Zätterström R, Moritz U, Fridén T: Influence of supervised and nonsupervised training on postural control after an acute anterior cruciate ligament rupture: A three-year longitudinal prospective study. *J Orthop Sports Phys Ther* 2001;31(11):632-644.

70. Zätterström R, Fridén T, Lindstrand A, Moritz U: The effect of physiotherapy on standing balance in chronic anterior cruciate ligament insufficiency. *Am J Sports Med* 1994;22(4):531-536.

71. Chappell JD, Creighton RA, Giuliani C, Yu B, Garrett WE: Kinematics and electromyography of landing preparation in vertical stop-jump: Risks for noncontact anterior cruciate ligament injury. *Am J Sports Med* 2007;35(2): 235-241.

72. Hewett TE, Myer GD, Ford KR, et al: Biomechanical measures of neuromuscular control and valgus loading of the knee predict anterior cruciate ligament injury risk in female athletes: A prospective study. *Am J Sports Med* 2005; 33(4):492-501.

Video Reference

Provencher MT, Gross DJ: Video. *Failed ACL Surgery: Technical Pearls.* Boston, MA.

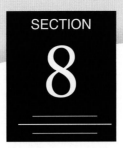

SECTION

8

Orthopaedic Medicine

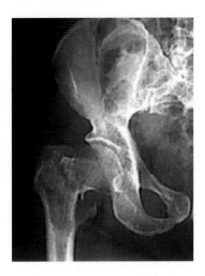

Bacterial Biofilms and Periprosthetic Infections

William V. Arnold, MD, PhD
Mark E. Shirtliff, PhD
Paul Stoodley, PhD

Abstract

In the past, diagnosing and treating periprosthetic infections in joint arthroplasty have often been challenging for orthopaedic surgeons. Certain diagnostic criteria and different treatment strategies can be better directed if these infections are placed in the context of microbial biofilms. An understanding of the biofilm mode of microbial infection can help explain the phenomenon of culture-negative infection and provide an understanding of why certain treatment modalities often fail. Continued basic research into the role of biofilms in infection will likely provide improved strategies for the clinical diagnosis and treatment of periprosthetic joint infections.

Instr Course Lect 2014;63:385-391.

The diagnosis and treatment of periprosthetic infections after joint arthroplasty are often challenging for an orthopaedic surgeon. The application of certain diagnostic criteria and different treatment strategies can be better directed if these infections are placed in the context of microbial biofilms. An understanding of this biofilm mode of microbial infection can help explain the phenomenon of culture-negative infection as well as provide an understanding of why certain treatment modalities often fail. Continued basic research into the role of biofilms in infection will likely provide improved strategies for the clinical diagnosis and treatment of periprosthetic infection.

Periprosthetic infection is a devastating complication of joint arthroplasty with substantial morbid sequelae. In even the best scenarios, patients routinely experience a prolonged period of lost function, lost employment, and lost time that often culminates in a compromised result. Contributing to these poor outcomes is the difficulty of making a proper diagnosis early and providing the proper treatment. A basic understanding of the pathology of these infections may help direct both the diagnosis and the treatment of periprosthetic infections and provide a framework from which current data may be understood.

In most medical settings, the current standard of diagnosing infection continues to rely on a variation of Koch's postulates, which were formulated in 1884.[1,2] In practice, this involves the isolation of an infecting organism from tissue or fluid that is cultured in a specialized broth or on solid growth media. Once isolated, the pathogen can be identified, and the sensitivity of the pathogen to various

Dr. Arnold or an immediate family member is an employee of Merck and URL Pharma; has stock or stock options held in Merck and URL Pharma, and has received research or institutional support from Stryker. Dr. Shirtliff or an immediate family member serves as a paid consultant to Mead and Johnson, Dentsply, Twin Star Medical, the National Institutes of Health (NIAMS & NICHD), and Stryker, and has stock or stock options held in Difusion. Dr. Stoodley or an immediate family member is a member of a speakers' bureau or has made paid presentations on behalf of Philips Oral Healthcare and has received research or institutional support from Philips Oral Healthcare.

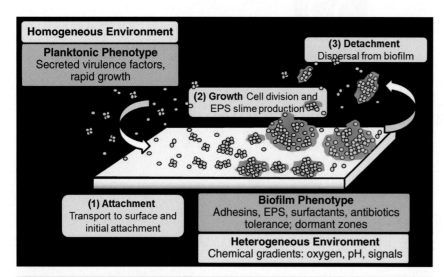

Figure 1 Schematic drawing showing salient features of biofilm formation in a staphylococcal biofilm model based on studies by Boles and Horswill,[5] Otto,[6] and Resch et al.[7] The blue boxes show the main processes in biofilm formation, the yellow boxes show the chemical environment, and the red boxes show the phenotype. In planktonic cells, expression of the accessory gene regulator system results in the production of secreted virulence factors, reduced attachment, and suppression of biofilm accumulation by increasing dispersal. EPS = extracellular polymeric substances.

antimicrobial agents can be determined. This simple paradigm has formed the basis of infectious disease treatment for decades, and its effectiveness in most cases is indisputable. The problem, however, is that most bacteria do not grow naturally as simple colonies on agar plates, as do their microbiologic laboratory counterparts. Most bacteria in nature grow as biofilms.

The biofilm theory of microbiologic growth has been thoroughly studied and has a firm scientific foundation.[3,4] The biofilm theory has been well accepted in areas such as marine fouling, water treatment, and the food industry. By this theory, bacteria grow and exist using two different modalities[5-7] (**Figure 1**). In one form, these unicellular bacteria can survive and grow in a complex biofilm matrix that has a structure and function analogous to the extracellular matrix that is the hallmark of higher-order multicellular organisms.[8] As with the extracellular matrix, the biofilm matrix is produced by cells but, in this case,

bacterial cells. This biofilm matrix offers protection and provides an organizing scaffold, which can facilitate metabolic activity and even communication between its members within. Bacteria can also exist in a planktonic form, in which they act as more traditionally viewed unicellular organisms. In the planktonic phenotype, there is no structural organization between the individual cells and no development of chemical gradients and accompanying microniches.

The state of the bacteria as either the planktonic form or the biofilm form has major implications for the treatment of bacterial infections. Bacteria in the planktonic form allow for the spread of infection because free bacteria can spread to or infect other sites (bacteremia and/or sepsis); but, at the same time, these bacteria are more susceptible to attack by the immune system and antimicrobial agents. On the other hand, bacteria in the biofilm form may not have the same freedom to roam, but they are nonetheless bet-

ter protected from immune system attack and are less susceptible to antibiotics. It is important to realize that fungal infections, such as *Candida*, can also exist as biofilms.

The Biology of Infection

It is useful to dissect the course of infection to identify areas that may be exploited for its treatment and prevention. This will be reviewed as it applies to bacterial infections. To initiate infection, an inoculum of bacteria must first become established at a favorable site of infection. This may seem obvious, but it should be remembered that humans routinely coexist with the staphylococci that normally inhabit their skin. It is generally only when these bacteria breach the natural barriers of the dermis, such as in surgery, that they become pathogens. Bacteria that initially enter via the transcutaneous route to initiate localized infection are generally believed to be in the planktonic state. After entry, these bacteria must then adhere to the periprosthetic tissue or the implant surface.[9] The molecular mechanisms of bacterial adhesion are becoming better elucidated. In the case of staphylococci, for example, adhesins belonging to the MSCRAMM (microbial surface components recognizing adhesive matrix molecules) protein family facilitate the binding of these bacteria to a variety of extracellular matrix proteins.[10] *Staphylococcus aureus* has more than 20 genes encoding such adhesins. Furthermore, the adhesins that bind to fibronectin in the extracellular matrix also seem to mediate the internalization of these *S aureus* bacteria into human cells, where they can even replicate inside the host cell.[11]

After the bacteria have adhered to a site, they will then go through a replication phase. It is during this planktonic initiation phase that the bacteria are perhaps most vulnerable. As with any infection in an immunocompetent host, the course of the infection is ultimately dependent on the ability of the host's immune system to clear the infection. Antimicrobial agents alone will not eliminate infection, but they can certainly tip the balance in favor of the host. Likewise, any mechanism that helps the infecting bacteria to evade or counteract the action of antimicrobial agents or the host's immune system will provide an advantage to the pathogen. The establishment of a biofilm confers just such an advantage to the bacterium. Once adhered to a surface, *S aureus* will enter a phase of growth and colonization. In the course of this process, *S aureus* will also release virulence factors that are toxic to the host. The entire process is an extremely well-coordinated system, in which specific bacteria genes are turned on and off in response to growth and environmental cues.[10] Furthermore, a tightly regulated system of communication, called quorum sensing, has been discovered to occur between these bacteria.[12,13] This quorum sensing, perhaps akin to the paracrine hormonal system of communication in multicellular organisms, may help organize the overall growth of the colony as well as coordinate biofilm formation. The production of certain proteins, such as Aap in *Staphylococcus epidermidis* and SasG in *S aureus,* appears to play a role in intercellular adhesion.[10] Ultimately, bacteria will become embedded in a matrix composed of polysaccharides, glycoproteins, and extracellular DNA (eDNA) that form the bacterial biofilm. Evidence suggests that *S aureus* controls the release of eDNA into the biofilm matrix from the regulated lysis of cells controlled by the *cidA* gene.[14]

Bacteria growing in biofilms are fundamentally different from their planktonic counterparts. The former can be thought of as a different phenotype of the latter, although they share

the same genotype. In a biofilm, bacteria can be tolerant to antibiotics at concentrations that are several hundredfold greater than that needed to kill planktonic bacteria. Biofilm bacteria are also much more resistant to the toxic effects of human immunity, although leukocytes likely still penetrate biofilm layers. Biofilms also facilitate the exchange of nutrients and provide a continual source of bacteria that can detach from the biofilm, either as released planktonic cells or as biofilm fragments, which can then go on to infect other sites or cause acute systemic infection. In biofilms, bacteria seem to exist in a more quiescent, less virulent state. However, these biofilms can still elicit a host inflammatory response that contributes to continual adjacent tissue destruction that results, ultimately, in the clinical symptoms of pain and implant loosening seen in long-standing chronic periprosthetic infections. Bacterial biofilms have been directly identified on a variety of medical implant devices, including peritoneal catheters, vascular catheters, contact lenses, orthopaedic devices, and joint replacement implants.[15-19] Biofilms have also been identified in a variety of medically important non–implant-related chronic infections, such as prostatitis, cystic fibrosis, endocarditis, otitis media, and osteomyelitis.[20-25]

Diagnosis of Periprosthetic Infection in the Context of Biofilms

The diagnosis of chronic periprosthetic infection can be difficult and frustrating for both the patient and the practitioner. Often, chronic periprosthetic infection must be diagnosed using indirect methods, such as the erythrocyte sedimentation rate, C-reactive protein levels, the synovial fluid cell count, and the synovial fluid neutrophil percentage.[26] Newer studies have also used the anal-

ysis of leukocyte esterase levels in aspirated fluid.[27] All of these diagnostic criteria are basically measures of the native immune response to periprosthetic infection rather than a direct identification of an infecting organism. With this difficulty in mind, both the Musculoskeletal Infection Society and the American Academy of Orthopaedic Surgeons have published criteria and pathways for diagnosing periprosthetic infection.[28,29]

The failure to isolate an infecting organism from the aspiration of suspicious joints is not unusual in cases of chronic periprosthetic infection. These difficulties can be better understood when the infection is placed in the context of biofilms. Planktonic bacteria can be isolated and grown with traditional hospital microbiologic culture techniques. Biofilm bacteria generally do not culture well using these techniques.[30] Therefore, chronic infections, which are present mostly in a biofilm state, will be difficult to positively identify with these traditional techniques. Some newer methods have used molecular biologic techniques to diagnose periprosthetic infections. This includes the use of polymerase chain reaction methodologies. One recent use of such techniques was able to positively identify the presence of bacteria by ultimately detecting the presence of bacteria-specific ribosomal RNA.[31] A positive test in this case confirms the presence of bacteria, but further tests are required to identify the specific bacterial strain. This requires the design of polymerase chain reaction primers unique to these specific strains.

A recent promising technology, called the Ibis technology, which combines the techniques of polymerase chain reaction and mass spectrometry, has been introduced for the identification of infecting organisms.[30] The Ibis technology was recently used to diagnose the presence of *Bacillus cereus* in two orthopaedic implant-related infections.[32] Ibis technology was also recently successful in identifying organisms in culture-negative periprosthetic infection as well as in cases of revision arthroplasty believed to be caused by aseptic loosening.[33] The latter is especially concerning because 50 of 57 revisions that were not thought to be related to infection may have involved an unrecognized, subclinical infection. This adds to the suspicion, which has been previously suggested, that many aseptic failures of arthroplasty components may actually involve low-grade chronic infections.[34] Such new molecular techniques may provide value both in the initial diagnosis of periprosthetic infections as well as helping to confirm the clearance of infection when planning a reimplantation. The utility of using molecular techniques for the diagnosis of biofilm-dominated infections has already been proven. In chronic otitis media, molecular techniques have been used to identify a pathogen in 80% to 100% of cases, in which traditional culture provided only 20% to 30% positive results.[23] A similar improvement in diagnosis using molecular techniques has been demonstrated in a pilot study for cases of infective endocarditis.[35]

Treatment of Periprosthetic Infection in the Context of Biofilms

Great effort has been made to define treatment paradigms for periprosthetic infection. As part of these paradigms, periprosthetic infections are often classified as acute or chronic. By one such classification scheme, early postoperative periprosthetic infection occurs within 4 weeks after the index procedure and late chronic infection occurs more than 4 weeks postoperatively.[36] Early infection is usually accompanied by pain, poor healing, erythema, and

prolonged wound drainage. Another category of this type of periprosthetic infection includes an acute infection at the site of a previously well-functioning joint replacement, often years after surgery. These infections are often thought to result secondarily from the hematogenous spread of an infection somewhere else in the body and are accompanied by an acute onset of pain accompanied by erythema and joint effusion, such as septic arthritis in a native joint. Chronic periprosthetic infections are often more indolent and may simply present as chronic pain, which may be the only clinical symptom.

The type of infection, acute or chronic, has implications for its treatment. Acute infections have been treated surgically with a variety of techniques, including irrigation and débridement with component retention; irrigation and débridement with removal of the prosthetic components and the immediate placement of new components (a single-stage exchange); and irrigation and débridement with removal of the prosthetic components, placement of an interim antibiotic cement spacer, and placement of new prosthetic components usually weeks to months later (a two-stage exchange). Chronic infections are treated surgically with either a single-stage exchange or a two-stage exchange. Simple irrigation and débridement with component retention as the treatment for a chronic infection has an unacceptably high failure rate.[36]

There are conflicting data regarding the merits of simple irrigation and débridement with component retention as the treatment of choice in patients with acute periprosthetic infections. The success rates of this treatment vary considerably. In a recent review of the literature for periprosthetic infection after total knee arthroplasty, the average failure rate of irrigation and débridement with component retention

to clear the infection was 68% (range, 61% to 82%).[37] One explanation for these varying results is that the success of the procedure may be related to the virulence of the infecting organism. For example, irrigation and débridement with component retention as a treatment for infections involving methicillin-resistant bacteria has had very poor results, with a failure rate reported to be as high as 84% at a minimum 2-year follow-up period.[38] However, another recent study has suggested that irrigation and débridement with component retention has a high failure rate regardless of the infecting organism.[39]

For the treatment of chronic infection, two-stage exchange procedures have generally been considered the gold standard, with a success rate reported to be between 80% and 100% when used to treat periprosthetic infection after knee arthroplasty.[37] Similar excellent results have been reported for treating periprosthetic infection after hip arthroplasty.[40,41] Comparable success rates have also been noted for single-stage exchange procedures for the treatment of periprosthetic infection after both knee and hip arthroplasty.[42-44]

Some of the controversy in these treatment procedures can be reconciled by placing them in the framework of biofilm eradication. Simply stated, any surgical treatment will ultimately fail if that treatment does not adequately remove the biofilm at the infection site. With this in mind, the varying success of these surgical treatments can be clarified. A simple irrigation and débridement with component retention can be successful if the infection is treated quickly enough so that a biofilm either has not been established on the prosthesis or the biofilm is adequately removed from the prosthesis. This also assumes that other infected tissue has been adequately débrided. Likewise with a chronic infection, a single-stage exchange can be successful if it adequately removes the biofilm at the infection site. This may require a more thorough débridement because a chronic, well-established infection may be established as a biofilm in the osseous tissue adjacent to the prosthesis. Although the bacteria in a quickly treated acute infection may not have established a biofilm, it must be assumed that all chronic infections involve biofilms and so must be treated with this in mind. Although a two-stage exchange may seem more reliable, it will also ultimately fail if a biofilm is left behind at the treatment site. The single-stage and two-stage procedures, by virtue of the removal of the arthroplasty components (and any biofilms contained on their surfaces) and allowing access to infected tissue around the removed components, simply allow for a better opportunity for removing the infecting biofilm at the site of the infection.

Future Directions

Future goals involve exploiting the fundamental processes that contribute to bacterial infection and biofilm formation. An obvious first step is to prevent bacterial adhesion. One strategy in this regard has been to design implant surfaces that are unattractive to bacteria. A specific example of this would be the use of antiadhesive silicone rubber surfaces in voice prostheses.[45] Although an obvious area for future research, this is also perhaps one of the most challenging as well because any surface modification of cementless arthroplasty components would have to also allow for osseointegration. Another approach has involved the application of antibiotic coatings to implant surfaces. This has been studied for hydroxyapatite materials with some promising in vitro results.[46] Other studies have involved vancomycin that is covalently linked to

the implant surface.[47] Recent studies in a sheep model have shown such an implant to be effective in inhibiting *S aureus* infection while still promoting bone healing.[48] Although promising, these approaches using antibiotic coatings are still susceptible to the remarkable capacity of bacteria to develop antimicrobial resistance.

Another strategy to inhibit bacterial adhesion involves the use of biosurfactants.[49,50] These are amphiphilic compounds that can be adsorbed onto surfaces. Some of these occur naturally and are actually produced by certain bacteria such as lactobacilli. These compounds may be applicable for coating silicone surfaces. It is unknown if such compounds will find an application in orthopaedic devices. Other materials may prove to be more useful. Recent studies have used farnesol, a citrus-derived alcohol that inhibits quorum sensing, and have shown that it can inhibit *S aureus* biofilm formation on titanium alloy disks.[51] Although some materials may not be appropriate for coating implant surfaces, they may still find an application in the removal or disruption of biofilms. Such effective materials could be used to complement the usual débridement performed in surgical treatments of periprosthetic infections.

Interfering with the phenomenon of quorum sensing presents another area for possible therapeutic treatment. As the molecular details of quorum sensing become better understood, strategies for disrupting this bacterial crosstalk become more realistic. For example, researchers have found that they can prevent graft-associated infections by a variety of *Staphylococcus* species, including methicillin-resistant species, by using the quorum-sensing inhibitor ribonucleic-acid-III-inhibiting peptide.[52] The ultimate goal is to find such inhibitors that may be active across several bacterial species and are not

unique to preventing only very specific infections.

Other research has focused on the idea of developing a vaccination against common pathogens such as *S aureus*. In a rabbit model of chronic *S aureus* osteomyelitis, researchers were able to develop a vaccination against specific biofilm antigens. This vaccination in combination with vancomycin treatment significantly reduced the infections in this model and even showed efficacy against methicillin-resistant *S aureus* biofilm infections.[53] This model also highlighted the important phenotypic differences between planktonic and biofilm bacteria because vancomycin treatment was necessary to eliminate the former, and vaccination treatment was necessary to eliminate the latter. Treatment with vancomycin or vaccination alone was not as effective as dual treatment in eliminating these infections. The isolation of specific antigens and the subsequent production of antibodies may find a valuable application in the diagnosis and treatment of biofilm infections. Antibody and/or antigen-derived molecular technologies have been used to great effect in cancer diagnosis and treatment. It is certainly reasonable to conjecture that such technologies could be applied to the treatment of periprosthetic infection.

Summary

Many of the frustrations encountered in the diagnosis and treatment of chronic periprosthetic infection can be understood if placed in the context of biofilms. Basic research will continue to provide insights into the biology of biofilms that should provide opportunities for the improved diagnosis and treatment of these chronic infections. One specific challenge will be to develop strategies that are applicable for the treatment of a broad spectrum of pathogens and are not simply unique to a single bacterial or fungal strain.

References

1. Koch R: Die Aetiologie der tuberkulose. *Mitt Kaiser Gesundh* 1884;2:1-88.

2. Inglis TJ: Principia aetiologica: Taking causality beyond Koch's postulates. *J Med Microbiol* 2007; 56(pt 11):1419-1422.

3. Costerton JW: *The Biofilm Primer*. Berlin, Germany, Springer-Verlag, 2007.

4. Hall-Stoodley L, Stoodley P, Kathju S, et al: Towards diagnostic guidelines for biofilm-associated infections. *FEMS Immunol Med Microbiol* 2012;65(2): 127-145.

5. Boles BR, Horswill AR: Agr-mediated dispersal of Staphylococcus aureus biofilms. *PLoS Pathog* 2008;4(4):e1000052.

6. Otto M: Staphylococcus epidermidis: The 'accidental' pathogen. *Nat Rev Microbiol* 2009;7(8): 555-567.

7. Resch A, Rosenstein R, Nerz C, Götz F: Differential gene expression profiling of Staphylococcus aureus cultivated under biofilm and planktonic conditions. *Appl Environ Microbiol* 2005;71(5): 2663-2676.

8. Flemming HC, Wingender J: The biofilm matrix. *Nat Rev Microbiol* 2010;8(9):623-633.

9. Darouiche RO: Device-associated infections: A macroproblem that starts with microadherence. *Clin Infect Dis* 2001;33(9):1567-1572.

10. Heilman C: Adhesion mechanisms of staphylococci, in Linke D, Golman A, eds: *Bacterial Adhesion*. Dordrecht, The Netherlands, Springer, 2011, pp 105-123.

11. Sinha B, Herrmann M: Mechanism and consequences of invasion of endothelial cells by Staphylococcus aureus. *Thromb Haemost* 2005;94(2):266-277.

12. Givskov M, Rasmussen TB, Ren D, Balaban N: Bacterial cell-to-cell communication (quorum sensing), in Balaban N, ed: *Control of Biofilm Infections by Signal Manipulation*. Berlin, Germany, Springer-Verlag, 2008, pp 13-38.

13. Rumbaugh KP: *Quorum Sensing*. New York, NY, Springer, 2011.

14. Mann EE, Rice KC, Boles BR, et al: Modulation of eDNA release and degradation affects Staphylococcus aureus biofilm maturation. *PLoS One* 2009;4(6):e5822.

15. Oasgupta MK, Bettcher KB, Ulan RA, et al: Relationship of adherent bacterial biofilms to peritonitis in chronic ambulatory peritoneal dialysis. *Perit Dial Int* 1987; 7(3):168-173.

16. Kowalewska-Grochowska K, Richards R, Moysa GL, Lam K, Costerton JW, King EG: Guidewire catheter change in central venous catheter biofilm formation in a burn population. *Chest* 1991; 100(4):1090-1095.

17. Feldman GL, Krezanoski JZ, Ellis BD, Lam K, Costerton JW: Control of bacterial biofilms on rigid gas permeable lenses. *CL Spectrum* 1992;7(10):36-39.

18. Gristina AG, Costerton JW, McGanity PL: Bacteria-laden biofilms: A hazard to orthopedic prostheses. *Infect Surg* 1984;3: 655-662.

19. Stoodley P, Nistico L, Johnson S, et al: Direct demonstration of viable Staphylococcus aureus biofilms in an infected total joint arthroplasty: A case report. *J Bone Joint Surg Am* 2008;90(8):1751-1758.

20. Nickel JC, Costerton JW, McLean RJ, Olson M: Bacterial biofilms: Influence on the pathogenesis, diagnosis and treatment of urinary tract infections. *J Antimicrob Chemother* 1994; 33(suppl A):31-41.

21. Lam J, Chan R, Lam K, Costerton JW: Production of mucoid microcolonies by Pseudomonas aeruginosa within infected lungs in cystic fibrosis. *Infect Immun* 1980;28(2):546-556.

22. Sullam PM, Drake TA, Sande MA: Pathogenesis of endocarditis. *Am J Med* 1985;78(6B):110-115.

23. Hall-Stoodley L, Hu FZ, Gieseke A, et al: Direct detection of bacterial biofilms on the middle-ear mucosa of children with chronic otitis media. *JAMA* 2006;296(2): 202-211.

24. Mayberry-Carson KJ, Tober-Meyer B, Smith JK, Lambe DW Jr, Costerton JW: Bacterial adherence and glycocalyx formation in osteomyelitis experimentally induced with Staphylococcus aureus. *Infect Immun* 1984;43(3): 825-833.

25. Brady RA, Leid JG, Calhoun JH, Costerton JW, Shirtliff ME: Osteomyelitis and the role of biofilms in chronic infection. *FEMS Immunol Med Microbiol* 2008; 52(1):13-22.

26. Parvizi J, Adeli B, Zmistowski B, Restrepo C, Greenwald AS: Management of periprosthetic joint infection: The current knowledge. AAOS exhibit selection. *J Bone Joint Surg Am* 2012;94(14):e104.

27. Parvizi J, Jacovides C, Antoci V, Ghanem E: Diagnosis of periprosthetic joint infection: The utility of a simple yet unappreciated enzyme. *J Bone Joint Surg Am* 2011; 93(24):2242-2248.

28. Parvizi J, Zmistowski B, Berbari EF, et al: From the Workgroup of the Musculoskeletal Infection Society. *Clin Orthop Relat Res* 2011;469(11):2992-2994.

29. Della Valle C, Parvizi J, Bauer TW, et al: American Academy of Orthopaedic Surgeons clinical practice guideline on: The diagnosis of periprosthetic joint infections of the hip and knee. *J Bone Joint Surg Am* 2011;93(14):1355-1357.

30. Costerton JW, Post JC, Ehrlich GD, et al: New methods for the

detection of orthopedic and other biofilm infections. *FEMS Immunol Med Microbiol* 2011;61(2): 133-140.

31. Bergin PF, Doppelt JD, Hamilton WG, et al: Detection of periprosthetic infections with use of ribosomal RNA-based polymerase chain reaction. *J Bone Joint Surg Am* 2010;92(3):654-663.

32. Gallo PH, Melton-Kreft R, Nistico L, et al: Demonstration of Bacillus cereus in orthopaedic-implant-related infection with use of a multi-primer polymerase chain reaction-mass spectrometric assay: Report of two cases. *J Bone Joint Surg Am* 2011;93(15):e85.

33. Jacovides CL, Kreft R, Adeli B, Hozack B, Ehrlich GD, Parvizi J: Successful identification of pathogens by polymerase chain reaction (PCR)-based electron spray ionization time-of-flight mass spectrometry (ESI-TOF-MS) in culture-negative periprosthetic joint infection. *J Bone Joint Surg Am* 2012;94(24):2247-2254.

34. Nelson CL, McLaren AC, McLaren SG, Johnson JW, Smeltzer MS: Is aseptic loosening truly aseptic? *Clin Orthop Relat Res* 2005;437:25-30.

35. Mallmann C, Siemoneit S, Schmiedel D, et al: A pilot study. *Clin Microbiol Infect* 2010;16(6): 767-773.

36. Segawa H, Tsukayama DT, Kyle RF, Becker DA, Gustilo RB: Infection after total knee arthroplasty: A retrospective study of the treatment of eighty-one infections. *J Bone Joint Surg Am* 1999; 81(10):1434-1445.

37. Sherrell JC, Fehring TK, Odum S, et al: Fate of two-stage reimplantation after failed irrigation and débridement for periprosthetic knee infection. *Clin Orthop Relat Res* 2011;469(1):18-25.

38. Bradbury T, Fehring TK, Taunton M, et al: The fate of acute methicillin-resistant Staphylococcus aureus periprosthetic knee infections treated by open debridement and retention of components. *J Arthroplasty* 2009; 24(6):101-104.

39. Odum SM, Fehring TK, Lombardi AV, et al: Irrigation and debridement for periprosthetic infections: Does the organism matter? *J Arthroplasty* 2011;26(6): 114-118.

40. Kraay MJ, Goldberg VM, Fitzgerald SJ, Salata MJ: Cementless two-staged total hip arthroplasty for deep periprosthetic infection. *Clin Orthop Relat Res* 2005;441: 243-249.

41. Hofmann AA, Goldberg TD, Tanner AM, Cook TM: Ten-year experience using an articulating antibiotic cement hip spacer for the treatment of chronically infected total hip. *J Arthroplasty* 2005;20(7):874-879.

42. Silva M, Tharani R, Schmalzried TP: Results of direct exchange or debridement of the infected total knee arthroplasty. *Clin Orthop Relat Res* 2002;404:125-131.

43. Buechel FF, Femino FP, D'Alessio J: Primary exchange revision arthroplasty for infected total knee replacement: A long-term study. *Am J Orthop (Belle Mead NJ)* 2004;33(4):190-198, discussion 198.

44. Oussedik SI, Dodd MB, Haddad FS: Outcomes of revision total hip replacement for infection after grading according to a standard protocol. *J Bone Joint Surg Br* 2010;92(9):1222-1226.

45. Rodrigues LR, Banat IM, Teixeira JA, Oliveira R: Strategies for the prevention of microbial biofilm formation on silicone rubber voice prostheses. *J Biomed Mater Res B Appl Biomater* 2007;81(2):358-370.

46. Teller M, Gopp U, Neumann HG, Kühn KD: Release of gentamicin from bone regenerative materials: An in vitro study. *J Biomed Mater Res B Appl Biomater* 2007;81(1):23-29.

47. Shapiro IM, Hickok NJ, Parvizi J, Stewart S, Schaer TP: Molecular engineering of an orthopaedic implant: From bench to bedside. *Eur Cell Mater* 2012;23:362-370.

48. Stewart S, Barr S, Engiles J, et al: Vancomycin-modified implant surface inhibits biofilm formation and supports bone-healing in an infected osteotomy model in sheep: A proof-of-concept study. *J Bone Joint Surg Am* 2012; 94(15):1406-1415.

49. Rodrigues L, Banat IM, Teixeira J, Oliveira R: Biosurfactants: Potential applications in medicine. *J Antimicrob Chemother* 2006; 57(4):609-618.

50. Rodrigues L: Inhibition of bacterial adhesion on medical devices, in Linke D, Golman A, eds: *Bacterial Adhesion*. Dordrecht, The Netherlands, Springer, 2011, pp 351-367.

51. Unnanuntana A, Bonsignore L, Shirtliff ME, Greenfield EM: The effects of farnesol on Staphylococcus aureus biofilms and osteoblasts: An in vitro study. *J Bone Joint Surg Am* 2009;91(11):2683-2692.

52. Balaban N, Stoodley P, Fux CA, Wilson S, Costerton JW, Dell'Acqua G: Prevention of staphylococcal biofilm-associated infections by the quorum sensing inhibitor RIP. *Clin Orthop Relat Res* 2005;437:48-54.

53. Brady RA, O'May GA, Leid JG, Prior ML, Costerton JW, Shirtliff ME: Resolution of Staphylococcus aureus biofilm infection using vaccination and antibiotic treatment. *Infect Immun* 2011;79(4): 1797-1803.

The Effects of Nutritional Deficiencies, Smoking, and Systemic Disease on Orthopaedic Outcomes

Byron F. Stephens, MD
G. Andrew Murphy, MD
William M. Mihalko, MD, PhD

Abstract

Most patients are evaluated by an internist for medical clearance before undergoing an elective orthopaedic procedure. Internists and anesthesiologists evaluate a patient's risk for morbidity or mortality from a procedure, whereas orthopaedic surgeons are often primarily concerned with a patient's risk for a poor outcome. Nutritional and systemic comorbidities can increase the risks for surgical site infections and poor outcomes. Knowing how to handle and identify these issues before surgery can have a substantial effect on improving the likelihood of good outcomes from elective orthopaedic procedures.

Instr Course Lect 2014;63:393-399.

Many patients undergoing elective orthopaedic procedures have multiple comorbidities and nutritional deficiencies. During the preoperative medical assessment, several correctable factors important to the surgical outcome may be overlooked because of a focus on the risk of heart attack, stroke, and death from surgery. These overlooked risk factors can have a clinically important effect on the orthopaedic procedure. As Medicare and other third-party payers begin the shift toward a so-called pay-for-performance model, orthopaedic surgeons need to be more aware of these modifiable risk factors that can alter outcomes.

Nutritional Deficiencies

Albumin has been long recognized as an important harbinger of overall nutritional status and wound-healing capacity. Produced in the liver, albumin is the most abundant protein in human plasma and provides 75% to 80% of the plasma oncotic pressure.[1] When albumin concentrations decrease, the serum colloid oncotic pressure no longer counterbalances the hydrostatic pressure of the vascular system, resulting in extracellular collection of fluids. In addition, albumin is a transporter protein for fatty acids, bilirubin, metals, hormones, and exogenous drugs. When albumin levels decrease, the effective concentration of drugs in human serum can increase or the hepatic metabolism of the drug can increase, or both can occur. Alterations in albumin also have been associated with platelet dysfunction and lower levels of transferrin. Of note, the precursor protein prealbumin much more accurately portrays current nutritional status because its half-life of 2 to 3 days is substantially shorter than that of albumin (20 days). In patients undergoing hip and knee arthroplasty, Lavernia et al[2] demonstrated that those with albumin levels of less than 3.4 g/dL had 32.7% higher hospital charges ($50,108 versus $33,720; $P < 0.006$), significantly higher medical severity of

Dr. Murphy or an immediate family member serves as an unpaid consultant to Wright Medical Technology; has received research or institutional support from Biomimetic, Smith & Nephew, Allostem, and Arthrex; and serves as a board member, owner, officer, or committee member of the American Academy of Orthopaedic Surgeons. Dr. Mihalko or an immediate family member has received royalties from Aesculap/B. Braun; is a member of a speakers' bureau or has made paid presentations on behalf of Aesculap/B. Braun; serves as a paid consultant to Aesculap/B. Braun and Medtronic; has received research or institutional support from Aesculap/B. Braun; and serves as a board member, owner, officer, or committee member of the American Orthopaedic Association and ASTM International. Neither Dr. Stephens nor any immediate family member has received anything of value from or has stock or stock options held in a commercial company or institution related directly or indirectly to the subject of this chapter.

illness ($P = 0.03$), and a longer hospital stay (5.7 versus 5.4 days; $P = 0.004$). Greene et al[3] reviewed the cases of 217 patients who had a primary hip or knee arthroplasty and reported that those with major wound complications had an average preoperative albumin level of 3.1 g/dL. Having a preoperative albumin level of less than 3.5 g/dL resulted in a sevenfold increase in the risk of a major wound complication.

Zinc is an integral component of many enzymes involved in wound healing, and patients deficient in zinc have a higher risk for the development of wound complications. Only 2 to 3 g of zinc are stored in the human body and are readily consumed. Fortunately, zinc is ubiquitous in soil, and nutritional deficiency is rare in well-nourished patients. If a patient's nutritional status is questionable, the surgeon should consider counseling the patient regarding the importance of taking a zinc-containing multivitamin. Zorrilla et al[4] reported that patients with serum zinc levels of less than 95 μg/dL had 11.76 times the risk for postoperative wound problems. The study also showed that serum zinc levels were predictive of delayed wound healing in patients undergoing hip hemiarthroplasty for fracture.

The active form of vitamin D, 1,25-dihydroxyvitamin D_3, is essential for normal calcium metabolism and homeostasis and, therefore, for bone growth, maintenance, and repair. In addition, active vitamin D is responsible for maintaining normal levels of plasma calcium and phosphorus. More than 50 genes, expressed in tissues throughout the body, are regulated by 1,25-dihydroxyvitamin D_3, and the vitamin-D receptor has been identified in almost every cell in the human body. Vitamin D deficiency leads to impaired calcium absorption, which in turn leads to the increased release of parathyroid hormone, causing the release of calcium stores from the skeleton. The optimal range for 1,25-dihydroxyvitamin D_3 measured in serum is wide and has been reported as 25 to 80 ng/mL.[5] Deficiency and insufficiency have been defined as 20 ng/mL and 30 ng/mL, respectively.[5] Adults in temperate latitudes require a vitamin D dietary intake of 800 to 1,000 IU to achieve serum levels in the optimal range.[5]

Many clinical studies have demonstrated the prevalence of hypovitaminosis D and emphasized the importance of avoiding vitamin D deficiency in patients with orthopaedic disorders. Bogunovic et al[6] assessed the prevalence of vitamin D insufficiency (< 32 ng/mL) and deficiency (< 20 ng/mL) in 723 orthopaedic patients. The prevalence of vitamin D insufficiency varied by orthopaedic specialty, with 66.1% of trauma patients, 52.3% of sports medicine patients, 40% of hand fracture patients, 34% of patients with foot and ankle injuries, and 23% of patients with metabolic bone disease having inadequate levels.[6] Hypovitaminosis D was more prevalent in men ($P = 0.006$). Patients with darker skin tones (blacks and Hispanics) were 5.5 times more likely to have low vitamin-D levels compared with patients with lighter skin color (Asians and whites) ($P < 0.001$). After total hip arthroplasty, patients with hypovitaminosis D had lower preoperative and postoperative Harris hip scores ($P = 0.018$) and were less likely to have an excellent outcome ($P = 0.038$).[7] In a study involving 37 patients with nonunion of an appendicular fracture or fracture of the pubic rami and/or sacral ala, despite adequate reduction and stabilization, endocrinologic evaluation identified vitamin D deficiency in 68%.[8] Up to 83% of patients with idiopathic chronic axial back pain had abnormally low levels of vitamin D, and clinical improvement occurred in all patients treated with vitamin D supplementation.[9]

Clearly, the nutritional status of patients with orthopaedic disorders and those undergoing orthopaedic procedures has an effect on outcomes and complication rates. Fortunately, there are a few simple ways to determine a patient's overall nutritional status. The Mini-Nutritional Assessment form is a short, six-category screening questionnaire that is useful for identifying elderly orthopaedic patients at risk of malnutrition.[10] The Rainey-MacDonald nutritional index is another useful screening formula that quantifies nutritional deficiency.[11] When the formula ([1.2 × serum albumin] + [0.013 × serum transferrin] − 6.43) is used, a sum of 0 or less indicates nutritional depletion and an increased risk for perioperative and postoperative complications. Another simple yet accurate tool used to quantify the overall nutritional status of elderly patients is the Geriatric Nutritional Risk Index (GNRI), which is calculated by the formula GNRI = (1.489 × albumin [g/dL]) + (41.7 × body weight/ideal body weight).[12] GNRI scores correlate inversely with the risk of complications and 6-month mortality. A GNRI score of less than 92 has been suggested as a cutoff for moderate risk of nutritional deficiency and should serve as an indicator for the need for nutritional supplementation and support.[13]

Smoking and Nicotine

Despite their long known and highly publicized deleterious health effects, smoking and nicotine use enjoy great popularity in the United States, with approximately 19.3% of US citizens being regular smokers in 2010.[14] Although the use of cigarette tobacco products by young adults decreased from 24.4% to 20.1% from 2005 to 2010,[15] smokeless tobacco use is increasing in many areas of the country, as is the dual use of cigarettes and smokeless tobacco.[16] Smokeless tobacco use varies greatly by location, with Wyoming, West Virginia, and Mississippi having rates of smokeless tobacco use up to seven times higher than California.[16]

The deleterious effects of smoking and nicotine use on human physiology are numerous and well documented. Nicotine, one of the more than 4,000 chemicals present in cigarette smoke, attaches to nicotinic acetylcholine receptors in the central nervous system that amplify the release of dopamine, which ultimately results in a physical addiction similar to that seen in heroin addicts. Peripherally, nicotine causes vasoconstriction (and thus hypoxia); increased platelet adhesion (resulting in microvascular thrombosis); and reduced proliferation of keratinocytes, erythrocytes, macrophages, and fibroblasts.[17] Animal studies have confirmed the deleterious effects of nicotine on wound and fracture healing.[18-20]

The hypoxic effects of cigarette smoking are exemplified by van Adrichem et al,[21] who found a 23.8% reduction ($P = 0.03$) in peripheral blood flow to the thumbs of patients after smoking one cigarette. In addition, smokers have substantially decreased neutrophil and monocyte oxidative burst activity, which may account for increased infections seen in smokers postoperatively.[22] All of these physiologic consequences of smoking and nicotine consumption work in a synergistic manner to negatively affect wound healing.

Multiple clinical studies have documented the detrimental effects of smoking on postoperative results and complications. A single institution retrospective study of 811 consecutive patients undergoing arthroplasty of the hip or knee found that smoking was the single most important risk factor for a postoperative complication, including wound healing issues, cardiopulmonary complications, and the need for admission to an intensive care unit.[17] In a prospective cohort study of 906 patients with ankle fractures, smokers had a significantly increased prevalence of overall postoperative complications compared with nonsmokers (30.1% versus 20.3%; $P = 0.005$) and deep wound infections (4.9% versus 0.8%; $P < 0.001$).[23] In another prospective cohort study, Moghaddam et al[24] reported that smokers and former smokers with tibial shaft fractures had a significantly increased risk of delayed union or nonunion, increased time to union, and increased time off work compared with nonsmokers. Smokers also have an increased risk of deep vein thrombosis, with a hazard ratio of 1.32 to 1.52, although the risk of former smokers was reduced to a level approaching that of patients who never smoked.[25] The Lower Extremity Assessment Project found that smokers with open tibial fractures had a 37% increased risk of nonunion, a 3.7 times higher risk for the development of osteomyelitis, and twice the risk for the development of acute postoperative infection.[26]

Patients with spine disorders also have worse outcomes with cigarette use. Patients who smoked and had surgery for lumbar spinal stenosis had less improvement in walking ability, higher dissatisfaction rates, and a higher rate of analgesic use compared with nonsmokers.[27] Smokers with thoracolumbar spinal fractures were 11% less satisfied and 13% more disabled than nonsmokers.[28] Both short- and long-term outcomes are better in nonsmokers after anterior cervical decompression and arthrodesis.[29] Lumbar spine arthrodesis also is affected by smoking status, with tobacco use increasing the risk of nonunion 2.01 to 3.03 times.[30] It is not surprising that smoking has been shown to have a significant effect on infection after all surgical procedures on the spine.[31]

Smoking cessation can make an important difference in the outcomes and complication rates following orthopaedic procedures. Two recent meta-analyses concluded that preoperative smoking cessation reduces both pulmonary and wound-related complications.[32,33] Although smoking cessation of any time period is beneficial, each additional week of cessation decreases the magnitude of the effect of smoking by approximately 19%.[34] A randomized clinical trial involving 120 patients with hip or knee arthroplasty compared smoking intervention (counseling, nicotine replacement therapy, and either smoking cessation or a 50% reduction) with a control group of smokers and demonstrated a significant reduction in overall complications (18% versus 52%, respectively) and wound complications (5% versus 31%, respectively).[35] Despite the short-term success in perioperative complication reduction, a long-term review of the same patients reported that only 22% of the study group had continued to be tobacco free at 1 year.[36]

Many orthopaedic surgeons believe that counseling patients on smoking cessation is the responsibility of the primary care physician; however, the orthopaedic surgeon's ability to express the importance of quitting tobacco use can have a profound effect on the patient's ability to successfully quit. This is best exemplified by a study of more than 10,000 spine patients that demonstrated a 35.6% quit rate in patients whose surgeons placed a "high priority" on tobacco cessation compared with a 19.5% quit rate in the "low priority" group.[37] There are several tools that orthopaedic surgeons should have at their disposal when counseling patients on preoperative smoking cessation. So-called cold-turkey or unassisted methods have a reported 10-month success rate of 7.3%;[38] however, physician advice to quit can increase abstinence rates up to 10.2%.[39] Personal counseling programs with more than eight sessions of so-called high intensity interventions (counseling sessions lasting more than 10 minutes) achieve a 24.7% quit rate.[39] The US government offers free programs (1-800-QUIT-NOW and http://www.smokefree.gov) that offer access to specialized tobacco cessation counselors. When a patient dials the QUIT-NOW phone number, he or she is set up with a quit coach, a professional tobacco cessation counselor in his or her state who answers questions and helps the patient develop a plan to quit smoking. The government-sponsored smoking cessation website offers a "SmokefreeTXT" program that provides free text message data with occasional words of encouragement, advice, and tips to successfully quit smoking.

Pharmaceutical assistance can be an effective tool for helping patients to quit smoking. Stead et al[40] reported nicotine replacement therapy increases tobacco cessation by 50% to 70% compared with placebo. Nicotine replacement therapy can be offered in the form of gum, a transdermal patch, a nasal spray, an inhaler, and sublingual tablets or lozenges. The antidepressant bupropion is an atypical antidepressant that is approved by the FDA to reduce the severity of nicotine cravings and withdrawal symptoms. Varenicline tartrate (Chantix; Pfizer) is a partial agonist of the nicotinic acetylcholine receptor that has been demonstrated in a meta-analysis (funded by Pfizer) to be more efficacious (absti-

nence rate of 33.2%) than nicotine replacement therapy or bupropion.[41] However, recent concern has been raised regarding the safety of varenicline, with reports of severe adverse cardiovascular and neuropsychiatric side effects.[42,43] More recently, electronic cigarettes (e-cigarettes or the electronic nicotine delivery system [ENDS]) have been touted as safer or with so-called harm reduction compared with conventional cigarettes. These devices produce aerosol by heating a humectant (usually propylene glycol) containing nicotine and flavoring without actually burning tobacco. When inhaled, the aerosol delivers nicotine to the user. Although the ENDS is effective in reducing nicotine consumption,[44] its long-term health effects are unknown. Recent studies have been contradictory concerning the physiologic effects of the aerosol components, flavorings, and nicotine in ENDS,[45-52] and future research should focus on the health effects of long-term ENDS use.

Systemic Disease

Pulmonary disease is common and can have a profound effect on outcomes after orthopaedic procedures. A Hospital for Special Surgery review of the Nationwide Inpatient Sample database involving more than 1 million arthroplasties of lower extremity joints revealed that patients with a preoperative diagnosis of pulmonary hypertension had a 4.0- to 4.5-fold increased risk of mortality after hip and knee arthroplasty, respectively.[53] Obstructive sleep apnea, a disease affecting up to one in five Americans, is a common pulmonary process that is both potentially correctable and deleterious to outcomes in orthopaedic patients.[54] Patients with obstructive sleep apnea have higher rates of perioperative complications associated with ambulatory surgery.[55] Despite the use of regional

anesthesia, orthopaedic patients with sleep apnea have a 34% rate of hypoxemia postoperatively.[56] The STOP-BANG (snoring, tiredness during daytime, observed apnea, and high blood pressure-body mass index, age, neck circumference, and gender) questionnaire is a useful mnemonic and screening tool to identify patients at risk for obstructive sleep apnea.[57] Patients with chronic obstructive pulmonary disease often regularly use a glucocorticoid inhaler, which can contribute to osteoporosis. A study by Regan et al[58] found that chronic obstructive pulmonary disease was noted in 47% of all the hip fracture patients, and chronic obstructive pulmonary disease severity correlated with the overall complication rate and mortality at 1 year. Of note, modifiable risk factors that were associated with outcomes were current smoking status, the use of general anesthesia, and the timing of surgery.[58]

Summary

Although primary care physicians and anesthesiologists are sometimes concerned more with the risk of life-threatening comorbidities and whether a patient can have a reasonable risk of surviving an elective or semielective orthopaedic procedure, orthopaedic surgeons generally are more concerned with factors that affect a patient's functional outcome. Nutritional status and smoking status are two important factors influencing outcome, and both should be investigated and managed before elective orthopaedic surgery.

Acknowledgment

The authors thank Kay Daugherty, the Campbell Foundation Medical Editor, for her help in preparing this manuscript.

References

1. Fanali G, di Masi A, Trezza V, Marino M, Fasano M, Ascenzi P: Human serum albumin: From bench to bedside. *Mol Aspects Med* 2012;33(3):209-290.

2. Lavernia CJ, Sierra RJ, Baerga L: Nutritional parameters and short term outcome in arthroplasty. *J Am Coll Nutr* 1999;18(3): 274-278.

3. Greene KA, Wilde AH, Stulberg BN: Preoperative nutritional status of total joint patients: Relationship to postoperative wound complications. *J Arthroplasty* 1991;6(4):321-325.

4. Zorrilla P, Salido JA, López-Alonso A, Silva A: Serum zinc as a prognostic tool for wound healing in hip hemiarthroplasty. *Clin Orthop Relat Res* 2004;420:304-308.

5. Kennel KA, Drake MT, Hurley DL: Vitamin D deficiency in adults: When to test and how to treat. *Mayo Clin Proc* 2010;85(8): 752-757, quiz 757-758.

6. Bogunovic L, Kim AD, Beamer BS, Nguyen J, Lane JM: Hypovitaminosis D in patients scheduled to undergo orthopaedic surgery: A single-center analysis. *J Bone Joint Surg Am* 2010;92(13):2300-2304.

7. Nawabi DH, Chin KF, Keen RW, Haddad FS: Vitamin D deficiency in patients with osteoarthritis undergoing total hip replacement: A cause for concern? *J Bone Joint Surg Br* 2010;92(4):496-499.

8. Brinker MR, O'Connor DP, Monla YT, Earthman TP: Metabolic and endocrine abnormalities in patients with nonunions. *J Orthop Trauma* 2007;21(8): 557-570.

9. Al Faraj S, Al Mutairi K: Vitamin D deficiency and chronic low back pain in Saudi Arabia. *Spine (Phila Pa 1976)* 2003;28(2): 177-179.

10. Murphy MC, Brooks CN, New SA, Lumbers ML: The use of the Mini-Nutritional Assessment (MNA) tool in elderly orthopaedic patients. *Eur J Clin Nutr* 2000;54(7):555-562.

11. Guo JJ, Yang H, Qian H, Huang L, Guo Z, Tang T: The effects of different nutritional measurements on delayed wound healing after hip fracture in the elderly. *J Surg Res* 2010;159(1):503-508.

12. Bouillanne O, Morineau G, Dupont C, et al: A new index for evaluating at-risk elderly medical patients. *Am J Clin Nutr* 2005; 82(4):777-783.

13. Cereda E, Pedrolli C: The Geriatric Nutritional Risk Index. *Curr Opin Clin Nutr Metab Care* 2009; 12(1):1-7.

14. Centers for Disease Control and Prevention (CDC): Table: Percentage of persons aged ≥ 18 years who were current cigarette smokers, by selected characteristics: National Health Interview Survey, United States, 2005 and 2010. *MMWR Morb Mortal Wkly Rep* 2011;60(35):1216. http://www.cdc.gov/mmwr/pdf/wk/mm6035.pdf#page=21. Accessed October 2, 2013.

15. Centers for Disease Control and Prevention (CDC): Vital signs: Current cigarette smoking among adults aged ≥18 years: United States, 2005-2010. *MMWR Morb Mortal Wkly Rep* 2011;60(35): 1207-1212.

16. Centers for Disease Control and Prevention (CDC): State-specific prevalence of cigarette smoking and smokeless tobacco use among adults: United States, 2009. *MMWR Morb Mortal Wkly Rep* 2010;59(43):1400-1406.

17. Møller AM, Pedersen T, Villebro N, Munksgaard A: Effect of smoking on early complications after elective orthopaedic surgery. *J Bone Joint Surg Br* 2003;85(2): 178-181.

18. de Almeida TF, Romana-Souza B, Machado S, Abreu-Villaça Y, Monte-Alto-Costa A: Nicotine affects cutaneous wound healing in stressed mice. *Exp Dermatol* 2013;22(8):524-529.

19. Donigan JA, Fredericks DC, Nepola JV, Smucker JD: The effect of transdermal nicotine on fracture healing in a rabbit model. *J Orthop Trauma* 2012;26(12): 724-727.

20. Raikin SM, Landsman JC, Alexander VA, Froimson MI, Plaxton NA: Effect of nicotine on the rate and strength of long bone fracture healing. *Clin Orthop Relat Res* 1998;353:231-237.

21. van Adrichem LN, Hovius SE, van Strik R, van der Meulen JC: Acute effects of cigarette smoking on microcirculation of the thumb. *Br J Plast Surg* 1992;45(1):9-11.

22. Sørensen LT, Nielsen HB, Kharazmi A, Gottrup F: Effect of smoking and abstention on oxidative burst and reactivity of neutrophils and monocytes. *Surgery* 2004;136(5):1047-1053.

23. Nåsell H, Ottosson C, Törnqvist H, Lindé J, Ponzer S: The impact of smoking on complications after operatively treated ankle fractures: A follow-up study of 906 patients. *J Orthop Trauma* 2011;25(12): 748-755.

24. Moghaddam A, Zimmermann G, Hammer K, Bruckner T, Grützner PA, von Recum J: Cigarette smoking influences the clinical and occupational outcome of patients with tibial shaft fractures. *Injury* 2011;42(12):1435-1442.

25. Severinsen MT, Kristensen SR, Johnsen SP, Dethlefsen C, Tjønneland A, Overvad K: Smoking and venous thromboembolism: A Danish follow-up study. *J Thromb Haemost* 2009;7(8):1297-1303.

26. Castillo RC, Bosse MJ, MacKenzie EJ, Patterson BM; LEAP Study Group: Impact of smoking on fracture healing and risk of complications in limb-threatening open tibia fractures. *J Orthop Trauma* 2005;19(3):151-157.

27. Sandén B, Försth P, Michaëlsson K: Smokers show less improvement than nonsmokers two years after surgery for lumbar spinal stenosis: A study of 4555 patients from the Swedish spine register. *Spine (Phila Pa 1976)* 2011; 36(13):1059-1064.

28. Vorlat P, Leirs G, Tajdar F, Hulsmans H, De Boeck H, Vaes P: Predictors of recovery after conservative treatment of AO-type A thoracolumbar spine fractures without neurological deficit. [Published online ahead of print August 23, 2010.] *Spine (Phila Pa 1976)*. PMID: 20736893.

29. Peolsson A, Peolsson M: Predictive factors for long-term outcome of anterior cervical decompression and fusion: A multivariate data analysis. *Eur Spine J* 2008;17(3): 406-414.

30. Andersen T, Christensen FB, Laursen M, Høy K, Hansen ES, Bünger C: Smoking as a predictor of negative outcome in lumbar spinal fusion. *Spine (Phila Pa 1976)* 2001;26(23):2623-2628.

31. Veeravagu A, Patil CG, Lad SP, Boakye M: Risk factors for postoperative spinal wound infections after spinal decompression and fusion surgeries. *Spine (Phila Pa 1976)* 2009;34(17):1869-1872.

32. Wong J, Lam DP, Abrishami A, Chan MT, Chung F: Short-term preoperative smoking cessation and postoperative complications: A systematic review and meta-analysis. *Can J Anaesth* 2012; 59(3):268-279.

33. Sørensen LT: Wound healing and infection in surgery: The clinical impact of smoking and smoking cessation. A systematic review and meta-analysis. *Arch Surg* 2012; 147(4):373-383.

34. Mills E, Eyawo O, Lockhart I, Kelly S, Wu P, Ebbert JO: Smoking cessation reduces postoperative complications: A systematic review and meta-analysis. *Am J Med* 2011;124(2):144-154, e8.

35. Møller AM, Villebro N, Pedersen T, Tønnesen H: Effect of preoperative smoking intervention on postoperative complications: A randomised clinical trial. *Lancet* 2002;359(9301):114-117.

36. Villebro NM, Pedersen T, Møller AM, Tønnesen H: Long-term effects of a preoperative smoking cessation programme. *Clin Respir J* 2008;2(3):175-182.

37. Rechtine GR II, Frawley W, Castellvi A, Gowski A, Chrin AM: Effect of the spine practitioner on patient smoking status. *Spine (Phila Pa 1976)* 2000;25(17): 2229-2233.

38. Baillie AJ, Mattick RP, Hall W: Quitting smoking: Estimation by meta-analysis of the rate of unaided smoking cessation. *Aust J Public Health* 1995;19(2): 129-131.

39. 2008 PHS Guideline Update Panel, Liaisons, and Staff: Treating tobacco use and dependence: 2008 update U.S. Public Health Service Clinical Practice Guideline executive summary. *Respir Care* 2008;53(9):1217-1222.

40. Stead LF, Perera R, Bullen C, Mant D, Lancaster T: Nicotine replacement therapy for smoking cessation. *Cochrane Database Syst Rev* 2008;1:CD000146.

41. Mills EJ, Wu P, Spurden D, Ebbert JO, Wilson K: Efficacy of pharmacotherapies for short-term smoking abstinence: A systematic review and meta-analysis. *Harm Reduct J* 2009;6:25.

42. Singh S, Loke YK, Spangler JG, Furberg CD: Risk of serious adverse cardiovascular events associated with varenicline: A systematic review and meta-analysis. *CMAJ* 2011;183(12):1359-1366.

43. Medicines and Healthcare Products Regulatory Agency. Drug safety update. Varenicline: Suicidal thoughts and behavior. July 2008. http://www.mhra.gov.uk/home/groups/pl-p/documents/

publication/con020567.pdf. Accessed October 2, 2013.

44. Polosa R, Morjaria JB, Caponnetto P, et al: A 24-month prospective observational study. [Published online ahead of print. July 20, 2013.] *Intern Emerg Med.* PMID: 23873169.

45. Bahl V, Lin S, Xu N, Davis B, Wang YH, Talbot P: Comparison of electronic cigarette refill fluid cytotoxicity using embryonic and adult models. *Reprod Toxicol* 2012;34(4):529-537.

46. Flouris AD, Chorti MS, Poulianiti KP, et al: Acute impact of active and passive electronic cigarette smoking on serum cotinine and lung function. *Inhal Toxicol* 2013; 25(2):91-101.

47. Goniewicz ML, Knysak J, Gawron M, et al: Levels of selected carcinogens and toxicants in vapour from electronic cigarettes. [Published online ahead of print. March 6, 2013.] *Tob Control* PMID: 23467656.

48. Miura N, Yuki D, Minami N, Kakehi A, Onozawa M: Pharmacokinetic analysis of nicotine when using non-combustion inhaler type of tobacco product in Japanese adult male smokers. *Regul Toxicol Pharmacol* 2013; 67(2):198-205.

49. Romagna G, Allifranchini E, Bocchietto E, Todeschi S, Esposito M, Farsalinos KE: Cytotoxicity evaluation of electronic cigarette vapor extract on cultured mammalian fibroblasts (ClearStream-LIFE): Comparison with tobacco cigarette smoke extract. *Inhal Toxicol* 2013;25(6):354-361.

50. Vardavas CI, Anagnostopoulos N, Kougias M, Evangelopoulou V, Connolly GN, Behrakis PK: Short-term pulmonary effects of using an electronic cigarette: Impact on respiratory flow resistance, impedance, and exhaled nitric oxide. *Chest* 2012;141(6):1400-1406.

51. Wagener TL, Siegel M, Borrelli B: Electronic cigarettes: Achieving a balanced perspective. *Addiction* 2012;107(9):1545-1548.

52. Williams M, Villarreal A, Bozhilov K, Lin S, Talbot P: Metal and silicate particles including nanoparticles are present in electronic cigarette cartomizer fluid and aerosol. *PLoS One* 2013; 8(3):e57987.

53. Memtsoudis SG, Ma Y, Chiu YL, Walz JM, Voswinckel R, Mazumdar M: Perioperative mortality in patients with pulmonary hypertension undergoing major joint replacement. *Anesth Analg* 2010; 111(5):1110-1116.

54. Shamsuzzaman AS, Gersh BJ, Somers VK: Obstructive sleep apnea: Implications for cardiac and vascular disease. *JAMA* 2003; 290(14):1906-1914.

55. Stierer TL, Wright C, George A, Thompson RE, Wu CL, Collop N: Risk assessment of obstructive sleep apnea in a population of patients undergoing ambulatory surgery. *J Clin Sleep Med* 2010; 6(5):467-472.

56. Liu SS, Chisholm MF, John RS, Ngeow J, Ma Y, Memtsoudis SG: Risk of postoperative hypoxemia in ambulatory orthopedic surgery patients with diagnosis of obstructive sleep apnea: A retrospective observational study. *Patient Saf Surg* 2010;4(1):9.

57. Chung F, Yang Y, Liao P: Predictive performance of the STOP-Bang score for identifying obstructive sleep apnea in obese patients. *Obes Surg* 2013;23(12): 2050-2057.

58. Regan EA, Radcliff TA, Henderson WG, et al: Improving hip fractures outcomes for COPD patients. *COPD* 2013;10(1): 11-19.

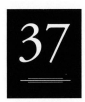

Differentiating Cervical Spine and Shoulder Pathology: Common Disorders and Key Points of Evaluation and Treatment

Thomas (Quin) Throckmorton, MD
Paul Kraemer, MD
John E. Kuhn, MD, MS
Rick C. Sasso, MD

Abstract

Accurately diagnosing patients with self-described pain in the shoulder or cervical spine (neck) remains a challenge for the orthopaedic surgeon. The overlapping presentations of shoulder disorders with those of the cervical spine, along with a lack of precision in physical examination testing, can create a confusing clinical picture and may result in disorganized or ineffective diagnostic and treatment regimens. A careful physical examination combined with judicious use of adjunctive tests, including selective corticosteroid injections, may help clarify the diagnosis. A high index of suspicion for the presence of cervical spine pathology is recommended in patients presenting with shoulder pain and vice versa.

Instr Course Lect 2014;63:401-408.

Disorders of both the neck and the shoulder can refer pain to anatomic sites not commonly associated with the location of the problem causing the pain. For example, an injection of hypertonic saline into the acromioclavicular joint can result in neck pain, whereas the same injection in the subacromial space can cause posterior shoulder pain; either presentation of pain can be interpreted as cervical radiculopathy.[1] Subacromial pain also can be referred to the trapezial area or neck.[2] A thorough understanding of physical examination testing for shoulder and cervical spine disorders is necessary to identify the pathologic process.

Shoulder Evaluation

The physical examination of the shoulder starts at the neck. Because of the anatomic proximity of the neck and shoulder and the overlapping innervations of the involved structures, an understanding that disorders can exist individually or in combination (the Venn diagram concept) is vital to achieving an accurate diagnosis and selecting the proper treatment (**Figure 1**).

History

A careful patient history that characterizes the type of pain and any exacerbating and relieving activities is an important initial diagnostic step. Pain that is burning or tingling often indicates a neuropathic lesion, whereas aching or sharp pain points the exam-

Dr. Throckmorton or an immediate family member is a member of a speakers' bureau or has made paid presentations on behalf of Biomet; serves as a paid consultant to Biomet and Zimmer; has received research or institutional support from Biomet; and serves as a board member, owner, officer, or committee member of the American Academy of Orthopaedic Surgeons and the Mid-American Orthopaedic Association. Dr. Kraemer or an immediate family member is a member of a speakers' bureau or has made paid presentations on behalf of Synthes. Dr. Kuhn or an immediate family member has stock or stock options held in Pfizer; has received research or institutional support from Arthrex; and serves as a board member, owner, officer, or committee member of the American Orthopaedic Society for Sports Medicine and the American Shoulder and Elbow Surgeons. Dr. Sasso or an immediate family member has received royalties from Medtronic; has stock or stock options held in Biomet; has received research or institutional support from Cerapedics, Medtronic, Smith & Nephew, and Stryker; and serves as a board member, owner, officer, or committee member of the Cervical Spine Research Society.

iner toward shoulder pathology. Pain that is worse with active use of the arm and/or worse at night is often seen in shoulder disorders. Conversely, patients who report symptom relief with shoulder abduction are more likely to have a disorder of the cervical spine.

The location of pain is also helpful for differentiating between shoulder and neck pathology. Pain that radiates from the neck to the medial scapula or distally to the elbow should direct the examiner toward the diagnosis of a neck disorder. Pain in the subdeltoid region may indicate rotator cuff pathology, whereas anterior shoulder pain distal to the acromion suggests a biceps tendon disorder. Superior shoulder pain with a trapezial or periscapular component can occur in several disorders and often indicates overlapping or multiple disorders (**Figure 2**).

Cervical Spine Examination (For the Shoulder Surgeon)

A brief series of maneuvers can allow the shoulder surgeon to detect pathology of the cervical spine. Range-of-motion testing, including flexion, extension, rotation, and lateral bending, can alert the examiner to any stiffness or motion loss. A myotomal and dermatomal examination of strength and sensation can isolate affected nerve roots. The Lhermitte sign, the reproduction of radicular symptoms with passive neck flexion, has been described.[3] The Spurling test, the repro-

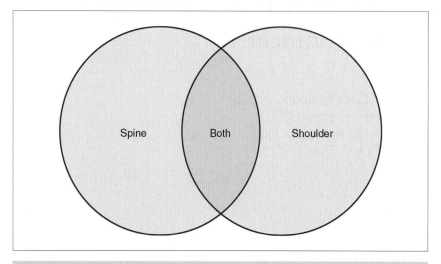

Figure 1 Understanding that shoulder and cervical spine disorders can exist individually or concurrently is critical to the accurate diagnosis and treatment of these often overlapping disorders.

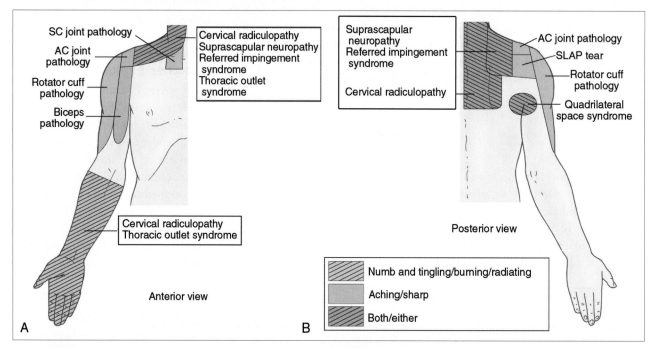

Figure 2 Anterior (**A**) and posterior (**B**) views of the upper extremity showing characteristic locations of referred pain in certain shoulder and cervical spine disorders. Because areas of referred pain can often overlap, confirmatory testing is helpful in clarifying the diagnosis. SC = sternoclavicular, AC = acromioclavicular, SLAP = superior labrum anterior to posterior.

duction of radicular signs with passive neck extension and compression of the foramen on the affected side, is also used. This test has varying levels of sensitivity but high specificity value as a confirmatory maneuver.[4,5]

Physical Examination of the Shoulder

The initial examination of the shoulder should include active and passive range-of-motion testing in forward elevation and internal and external rotation. Passive range of motion is usually preserved in disorders of the cervical spine but may be limited in some shoulder conditions such as adhesive capsulitis or glenohumeral arthritis. Weakness detected in strength testing can point the examiner toward rotator cuff tears or neurologic disorders.

Testing for subacromial impingement is traditionally done with the Hawkins and Neer maneuvers. The Hawkins sign is elicited with internal rotation of the glenohumeral joint while in abduction. Seventy-nine percent sensitivity and 59% specificity for impingement has been reported with this maneuver.[6] The Neer impingement test is performed by passively elevating the shoulder while in internal rotation. Sensitivity and specificity for subacromial impingement with this test have been reported at 79% and 53%, respectively.[4] High rates of intraobserver and interobserver agreement have been reported.[7] A recent systematic review found that both the Neer and Hawkins maneuvers have sensitivity but low specificity for diagnosing impingement.[8]

Tenderness along the long head of the biceps is commonly described as an indicator of symptomatic biceps pathology and has approximately 50% sensitivity and specificity for diagnosing partial tears of the tendon.[9] The Speed test, performed by resisting forward elevation with the shoulder exter-

nally rotated while in adduction, is also a commonly cited test but is not specific for any one disorder.[10]

The physical examination of labral pathology has been well documented; however, many studies have reported only equivocal accuracy for many maneuvers. The O'Brien test is fairly unreliable for diagnosing superior labrum anterior to posterior lesions.[11] Other evaluation methods include the Speed, the active compression, the crank, and the anterior slide tests. All of these tests have been studied in a meta-analysis, and none was found to be independently diagnostic of labral tears.[12] Cheung and O'Driscoll[13] described the dynamic labral shear test in which the arm is placed in abduction and external rotation and passively moved through a range of elevation. Posterior pain reproduced between 90° to 120° of abduction is suggestive of a symptomatic superior labrum anterior to posterior tear; the test has reported high sensitivity and specificity.

Acromioclavicular pathology is typically diagnosed by tenderness at the acromioclavicular joint and/or pain with passive cross-adduction testing. No published studies have reported on the diagnostic accuracy of these maneuvers.

Scapular dyskinesis is a disorder caused by alterations in the position of the scapula and the patterns of scapular motion in relationship to the thoracic cage.[14] Scapular dyskinesis often occurs in throwing athletes and weightlifters and often manifests with impingement symptoms. The disorder is characterized by subtle scapular winging and coracoid tenderness caused by pectoralis minor tightness secondary to scapular protraction. Kibler and McMullen[14] described the scapular assistance and scapular retraction tests, which are positive if the patient's impingement symptoms are relieved.

Imaging and Other Testing

A standard series of three shoulder radiographic views is useful in the initial patient evaluation. Osteophytes in the inferior humeral head or degenerative changes in the acromioclavicular joint can suggest glenohumeral arthritis or acromioclavicular arthrosis. Rounding and sclerosis of the greater tuberosity is often seen in chronic rotator cuff disorders. Superior subluxation of the humeral head resulting in articulation with the acromion suggests a chronic, massive rotator cuff tear.

MRI of the shoulder is also a valuable tool for characterizing tendon and other soft-tissue disorders. Although rotator cuff tendinopathy, biceps tendon degeneration, and labral fraying are commonly seen on MRI, they are often incidental findings; therefore, correlating the study with the physical examination is critical for an accurate diagnosis. Full-thickness rotator cuff tears, with or without associated muscle atrophy, can be identified and characterized. The presence of subacromial spurs, perilabral cysts, and the condition of the glenohumeral cartilage also can be assessed.

Other tests can include CT, if better visualization of the bony architecture is needed, and electromyography (EMG), if neurologic disorders are suspected. Selective injections of the shoulder complex to isolate pain-generating structures also can be considered. In patients with pathology of the cervical spine, radiographs of the neck are indicated, with possible adjunctive MRI to isolate sites of neurologic compression.

Cervical Spine (Neck) Evaluation

History and Examination

A thorough patient history is essential in differentiating the cervical spine from the shoulder as the primary source of pain. Knowledge of any inciting injury can be helpful in making the diagnosis. The examiner should focus on the position of the neck during repetitive motions or the most painful motions. Any distal symptoms, no matter how trivial and despite any previous diagnosis, should be thoroughly investigated because related problems can be manifestations of radiculopathy or myelopathy.

All associated symptoms in the affected extremity are important; however, patients may not voluntarily mention symptoms that they believe to be unrelated. Numbness, coordination problems, altered reflexes, or spastic motions may be signs of spinal cord compression. These problems should be verified on physical examination, which should also include a thorough evaluation of reflexes, repetitive hand motions, and the ability to perform simple fine-motor tasks, such as buttoning a shirt.

Imaging and Other Tests

Although routine radiographic studies of the cervical spine are recommended, there are no special views that reliably differentiate spinal and shoulder disorders. MRI continues to be a mainstay for evaluating the cervical spine. CT can be particularly helpful in delineating facet disease, and, in conjunction with myelography, can provide valuable details about neurologic compression. EMG and nerve conduction velocity tests are commonly used to evaluate upper extremity pain. Although negative EMG and nerve conduction velocity tests are not able to differentiate the source of the pathology (shoulder or cervical spine), a positive tests indicating radiculopathy indicates that the cervical spine is likely part of the symptom complex.

Selective nerve root blocks are an interventional procedure commonly performed by specialists in pain management or physical medicine. These procedures entail some risks (particularly to the vertebral artery) if particulate steroid preparations are used; therefore, injection with local anesthetic only is preferred. Selective nerve root blocks, however, are ideal for testing the hypothesis of a specific nerve root as a pain generator. If the patient experiences excellent analgesia, including some numbness in the blocked distribution, the pain generator is confirmed, and surgical decompression can offer substantial pain relief.

This chapter's authors recommend caution when considering and interpreting selective nerve root injections. A selective nerve root block should be performed only if surgery will be possible at that cervical level if pain relief is achieved. False-positive results can result from patient expectations or from downstream pain relief within the neurologic distribution of the selective nerve root block. For example, a patient with biceps tendinitis and shoulder pain may respond well to a C5 block because the biceps is within the C5 distribution. In this way, an upstream block may hide downstream pathology. A thorough physical examination and close attention to important imaging pathology at the blocked level is recommended to avoid this diagnostic pitfall.

Shoulder Disorders That Present With Pain in the Cervical Spine

Parsonage-Turner Syndrome

Acute brachial plexitis was first described in 1887 and later characterized by Parsonage and Turner.[15] Idiopathic brachial plexus neuropathy occurs at a rate of 2 in 100,000 people per year, usually in the third and seventh decades of life.[16] Males are more commonly affected than females, and the syndrome may be preceded by a viral illness, shoulder surgery, or pregnancy. Parsonage-Turner syndrome is char-

acterized by the rapid onset of severe, burning, upper extremity pain; more than one third of patients describe pain radiating from the neck down the arm. Motor weakness occurs in approximately one third of patients but does not follow a myotomal pattern.[16] Trophic changes of autonomic dysfunction may be seen. This syndrome can be distinguished from cervical radiculopathy by asking the patient to perform the Valsalva maneuver. Where cervical radicular pain is often worsened with the Valsalva maneuver, it is typically unchanged in brachial plexitis.

Additional testing includes chest radiography to evaluate for Pancoast tumor. MRI of the shoulder may show fatty infiltration of the rotator cuff and other involved muscles. MRI of the brachial plexus is often unhelpful despite its common use. EMG will localize the lesion to the brachial plexus and typically shows changes of acute denervation at 3 weeks. Repeat studies 3 to 4 months after symptom onset may show chronic denervation and early reinnervation.

Treatment is primarily supportive, with the use of corticosteroids, nonsteroidal anti-inflammatory drugs, and opioid analgesics. Physical therapy may be instituted after pain begins to subside. Resolution of symptoms can be expected in 3 to 4 years in 80% to 90% of patients.[17]

Suprascapular Neuropathy

Compression neuropathy of the suprascapular nerve may occur at the suprascapular or spinoglenoid notches (**Figure 3**). Mechanisms of injury include traction injuries from rotator cuff tears, direct compression from the transverse scapular ligament at the scapular notch, or a spinoglenoid notch cyst.[18,19]

The clinical presentation is often protean, with dull, poorly localized neck and/or shoulder pain and weak-

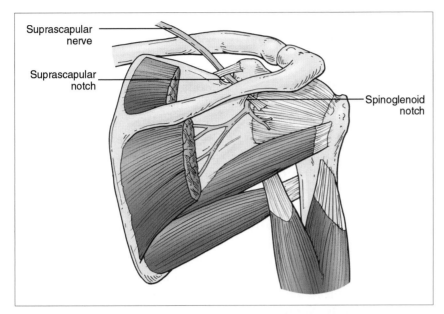

Figure 3 The suprascapular nerve is most commonly compressed at either the suprascapular notch or the spinoglenoid notch. Although treatment is initially conservative, surgical release has been described for recalcitrant cases.

ness in external rotation. Wasting of the supraspinatus and infraspinatus muscles (if the injury is at the scapular notch) or infraspinatus muscle only (if the injury is at the spinoglenoid notch) may occur in chronic cases. Physical examination signs are usually nonspecific.[20]

EMG may show decreased amplitude and increased latency of the suprascapular nerve, but it often cannot precisely localize the lesion. MRI will show muscle atrophy of the involved muscles and space-occupying lesions.[20] Sagittal cuts that visualize the course of the suprascapular nerve may occasionally localize the site of compression.

Noncompressive lesions are typically treated nonsurgically and involve an extended course of rehabilitation; some lesions take more than 1 year to resolve. Compression at the scapular notch can be treated with open or arthroscopic release of the transverse scapular ligament. Similarly, compression at the spinoglenoid notch can be treated with open or arthroscopic decompression.[21]

Thoracic Outlet Syndrome

Although the etiology of thoracic outlet syndrome is usually neurogenic, arterial and venous etiologies have been described. A traumatic onset, often with a whiplash-type neck hyperextension injury, is common. Other predisposing factors include cervical ribs, anomalous first ribs, and narrow scalene triangles.

Symptoms of thoracic outlet syndrome mimic those of cervical radiculopathy. Radiating pain, paresthesias, and weakness in the arm or hand are often seen. Accompanying neck or trapezial pain may be present. The physical examination evaluation includes the upper limb tension test and the abduction/external rotation tests; however, these tests have not been proven to be specific for the diagnosis. Confirmatory tests include EMG, ultrasound, and CT.

Most patients with thoracic outlet syndrome have resolution with conservative therapy, including physical therapy for postural correction and periscapular strengthening. Neck traction and resistive strengthening may exacerbate symptoms. When conservative treatment fails, surgical decompression of the brachial plexus, including first rib resection or scalene muscle excision, is an option.[22]

Scapular Dyskinesis

Abnormal scapular kinematics caused by trauma, overuse, repetitive microtrauma, or fatigue can result in uncontrolled scapular protraction, which manifests as periscapular pain or clinical findings consistent with shoulder impingement. The superior and medial border of the scapula and, possibly, the trapezial area may be prominent and tender. The coracoid may also be tender because of adaptive tightening of the pectoralis minor.

Physical therapy is the mainstay of treatment for scapular dyskinesis and includes closed chain cocontracture exercises that progress to open chain movements.[14] Core strengthening is also a key component in restoring the kinetic chain. Therapy to preserve or restore full glenohumeral range of motion is essential, particularly in overhead athletes who may have a glenohumeral internal rotation deficit.

Atraumatic Sternoclavicular Disorders

Pain from sternoclavicular joint disease may localize precisely to the sternoclavicular joint but often may radiate more diffusely around the anterior neck. The differential diagnoses include osteoarthritis, septic arthritis, crystal deposition, hyperostosis, condensing osteitis, and osteonecrosis of the medial clavicle (Friedrich disease). The clinical evaluation may show sternoclavicular joint instability, tenderness, or fluctuance. Laboratory work for inflammatory disorders and infection is indicated.[23]

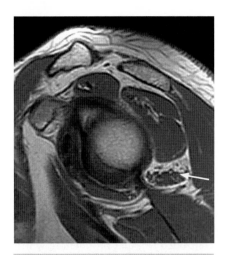

Figure 4 MRI showing isolated fatty infiltration (arrow) of the teres minor that is characteristic of quadrilateral space syndrome.

Treatment is usually nonsurgical, but excision of the medial clavicle may be considered in patients with septic arthritis or refractory pain.[23] Care must be taken to preserve the sternoclavicular ligaments to prevent postoperative instability. Extreme caution should be taken to prevent retrosternal injury; thoracic surgical back-up is recommended as a precaution.

Quadrilateral Space Syndrome

Compression of the axillary nerve as it passes through the quadrilateral space may cause posterior shoulder pain that can mimic cervical radiculopathy. Patients may have tenderness over the quadrilateral space, but symptoms are often vague and involve a protracted course of treatment. EMG findings are often negative, but MRI will show inflammation or fatty infiltration of the teres minor (**Figure 4**). When conservative treatment fails, surgical decompression of the quadrilateral space through a posterior approach has been proven effective.[24]

Cervical Spinal Disorders That Present With Shoulder Pain

Cervical Radiculopathy

Cervical radiculopathy is a common disorder characterized by cervical nerve root inflammation, compression, and dysfunction. Although the classic pain patterns follow the neurologic dermatomes or sensory patterns of a particular nerve into the arm, there is considerable overlap in shoulder and more proximal musculature. It may be difficult to identify an individual nerve root as the cause of radiculopathy based on the patient history or by evaluating only shoulder symptoms. More distal symptoms, even if not bothersome, may clarify the nerve root pattern. Classic patterns may stop more proximally, and distal symptoms may be absent, making the shoulder and neck the only site of pain. In such instances, it is difficult to distinguish cervical radiculopathy from a primary shoulder disorder. Less common radicular patterns may result in a shoulder diagnosis in the presence of a primary spinal disorder.

The C2 and C3 nerve roots do not refer pain to the upper extremity, rendering these levels extremely uncommon as a cause of shoulder pain. However, the C4 nerve root resides in the C3-4 foramen and can be compressed by disk or facet pathology at that level. The C4 dermatome includes the dorsal and lateral neck extending to approximately the clavicle anteriorly, the acromion distally, and the trapezius posteriorly (including the medial scapular border). Because of the relative lack of light touch sensory nerve endings in this region, numbness or tingling is an uncommon symptom.[25] C4 radiculopathy is characterized primarily by unilateral neck and shoulder pain without arm symptoms. There is no reliable C4 reflex, and manual motor testing is not helpful because all the affected muscles have concomitant innervation by the C5 nerve root.

The C5 nerve root is affected in the foramen by the C4-5 disk/facet complex. Because C5 is largely a motor nerve, numbness and tingling may not be a major source of reported symptoms.[26] Weakness in the innervated rotator cuff muscles, deltoid, and biceps is easily confused with shoulder pathology. Although neurologic weakness may be painless and consistent, shoulder girdle weakness from rotator cuff pathology is often painful and break-away. The dermatomal pattern extends from the neck to the deltoid and anterior arm along the course of the biceps, but rarely below the elbow. As a result, this pattern may also mimic rotator cuff pathology.

C6 and C7 nerve roots are affected in the C5-6 and C6-7 foramen, respectively. Both are commonly affected roots with classic distributions that largely affect the arms, and are by themselves rarely confused with shoulder disorders. However, there are atypical patterns, including dorsal scapular nerve root distributions (from C6 and C7) along the medial border of the scapula (mimicking scapular disorders) or pectoralis pain from C6 (mimicking subscapularis or other shoulder pain). There may not be substantial symptoms distal to the elbow or even past the shoulder; this may lead the practitioner to quickly remove radiculopathy from the differential diagnosis. In some instances, EMG can be helpful in clarifying these diagnoses.

Cervical Spondylotic Myelopathy

Cervical spondylotic myelopathy refers to spinal cord compression and upper motor neuron disease, not nerve root compression and lower motor neuron disease. It is common for one or both shoulders to be affected, and pain may be isolated or at least most severe in the shoulder. Pain is commonly exacerbated with extension of the neck. Patterns of pain and weakness tend to be much more diffuse and will not follow a discrete radicular pattern. Hyperreflexia and pathologic reflexes, such as the Hoffmann reflex, are also common. All symptoms may affect both the upper and the lower extremities.

Facet Arthrosis and Discogenic Disease

Although cervical disk disease is highly prevalent in patients older than 40 years, degenerative cervical disks are usually not a major source of pain. Patterns of pain are not well understood but tend to be central and symmetric in the neck and generally should not be confused with shoulder pain. Structural deformity associated with degenerative disks, particularly kyphosis, may be a pain generator, and may extend into the shoulders because of trapezial spasm or fatigue. Facet arthrosis can affect any level of the subaxial cervical spine and tends to coexist with degenerative disk disease because they are both manifestations of motion segment degeneration.

Reflex Sympathetic Dystrophy

Complex regional pain syndrome, previously known as reflex sympathetic dystrophy or causalgia, is a chronic pain condition that may affect the arms and shoulders, producing substantial pain and dysesthesia. This syndrome is believed to be a hypersensitivity response of the central or peripheral nervous system that is out of proportion to the initial injury. It may follow trauma or even benign interventions such as a tourniquet. Symptoms include warmth, redness, swelling, skin changes, and substantial pain. Complex regional pain syndrome does not typically follow a specific dermatomal pattern.

Musculoskeletal Not-Otherwise-Specified Disorders

Many neck and shoulder pains do not have a single identifiable anatomic cause and are often transient. Pain that is persistent or recurrent warrants medical evaluation. Although included in the original differential diagnosis, syndromes (such as myofascial pain, fibromyalgia, or nonorganic pathology) should be considered a final diagnosis of exclusion only when all other sources of pain in the shoulder and neck have been rigorously ruled out with appropriate testing.

Summary

The overlapping patterns of cervical spine and shoulder pathology continue to present a confusing and often conflicting clinical presentation. Understanding the common disorders that often coexist, along with a focused and thorough physical examination, can help clarify the diagnosis. Appropriate use of advanced imaging studies and other tests such as EMG can assist in confirming the diagnosis. An understanding of the differential diagnoses of disorders that can mimic shoulder and/or neck disorders can also help direct treatment.

References

1. Gerber C, Galantay RV, Hersche O: The pattern of pain produced by irritation of the acromioclavicular joint and the subacromial space. *J Shoulder Elbow Surg* 1998;7(4):352-355.

2. Gorski JM, Schwartz LH: Shoulder impingement presenting as neck pain. *J Bone Joint Surg Am* 2003;85(4):635-638.

3. Malanga GA, Landes P, Nadler SF: Provocative tests in cervical spine examination: Historical basis and scientific analyses. *Pain Physician* 2003;6(2):199-205.

4. Tong HC, Haig AJ, Yamakawa K: The Spurling test and cervical radiculopathy. *Spine (Phila Pa 1976)* 2002;27(2):156-159.

5. Bridwell KH, Anderson PA, Boden SD, Vaccaro AR, Wang JC: What's new in spine surgery. *J Bone Joint Surg Am* 2012; 94(12):1140-1146.

6. Hegedus EJ, Goode A, Campbell S, et al: A systematic review with meta-analysis of individual tests. *Br J Sports Med* 2008;42(2): 80-92.

7. Johansson K, Ivarson S: Intra- and interexaminer reliability of four manual shoulder maneuvers used to identify subacromial pain. *Man Ther* 2009;14(2):231-239.

8. Beaudreuil J, Nizard R, Thomas T, et al: A systematic literature review. *Joint Bone Spine* 2009; 76(1):15-19.

9. Gill HS, El Rassi G, Bahk MS, Castillo RC, McFarland EG: Physical examination for partial tears of the biceps tendon. *Am J Sports Med* 2007;35(8):1334-1340.

10. Holtby R, Razmjou H: Accuracy of the Speed's and Yergason's tests in detecting biceps pathology and SLAP lesions: Comparison with arthroscopic findings. *Arthroscopy* 2004;20(3):231-236.

11. Cook C, Beaty S, Kissenberth MJ, Siffri P, Pill SG, Hawkins RJ: Diagnostic accuracy of five orthopedic clinical tests for diagnosis of superior labrum anterior posterior (SLAP) lesions. *J Shoulder Elbow Surg* 2012;21(1):13-22.

12. Karlsson J: Physical examination tests are not valid for diagnosing SLAP tears: A review. *Clin J Sport Med* 2010;20(2):134-135.

13. Cheung EV, O'Driscoll S: Abstract: Dynamic labral shear test for superior labral anterior posterior tears of the shoulder. *74th Annual Meeting Proceedings*. Rosemont, IL, American Academy of

Orthopaedic Surgeons, 2007, p 574.

14. Kibler WB, McMullen J: Scapular dyskinesis and its relation to shoulder pain. *J Am Acad Orthop Surg* 2003;11(2):142-151.

15. Parsonage MJ, Turner JW: Neuralgic amyotrophy: The shoulder-girdle syndrome. *Lancet* 1948; 1(6513):973-978.

16. Tjoumakaris FP, Anakwenze OA, Kancherla V, Pulos N: Neuralgic amyotrophy (Parsonage-Turner syndrome). *J Am Acad Orthop Surg* 2012;20(7):443-449.

17. Tsairis P, Dyck PJ, Mulder DW: Natural history of brachial plexus neuropathy: Report on 99 patients. *Arch Neurol* 1972;27(2): 109-117.

18. Freehill MT, Shi LL, Tompson JD, Warner JJ: Suprascapular neuropathy: Diagnosis and management. *Phys Sportsmed* 2012;40(1): 72-83.

19. Moen TC, Babatunde OM, Hsu SH, Ahmad CS, Levine WN: Suprascapular neuropathy: What does the literature show? *J Shoulder Elbow Surg* 2012;21(6):835-846.

20. Boykin RE, Friedman DJ, Higgins LD, Warner JJ: Suprascapular neuropathy. *J Bone Joint Surg Am* 2010;92(13):2348-2364.

21. Piasecki DP, Romeo AA, Bach BR Jr, Nicholson GP: Suprascapular neuropathy. *J Am Acad Orthop Surg* 2009;17(11):665-676.

22. Nichols AW: Diagnosis and management of thoracic outlet syndrome. *Curr Sports Med Rep* 2009; 8(5):240-249.

23. Higginbotham TO, Kuhn JE: Atraumatic disorders of the sternoclavicular joint. *J Am Acad Orthop Surg* 2005;13(2):138-145.

24. McAdams TR, Dillingham MF: Surgical decompression of the quadrilateral space in overhead athletes. *Am J Sports Med* 2008; 36(3):528-532.

25. Alberstone CD, Steinmetz MP, Najm IM, Benzel EC: *Anatomic Basis of Neurologic Disorders*. New York, NY, Thieme Medical Publishers, 2009, p 129.

26. Wood GW II, in Canale ST, Beaty JH, eds: *Campbell's Operative Orthopaedics*, ed 12. Maryland Heights, MO, Mosby, 2012, pp 1524-1551.

38

Prophylaxis for Thromboembolic Disease and Evaluation for Thrombophilia

Geoffrey H. Westrich, MD
Jeffrey S. Dlott, MD
Fred D. Cushner, MD
Norman A. Johanson, MD
Allison V. Ruel, BA

Abstract

Patients treated with total hip or knee arthroplasty are at risk for venous thromboembolic disease. Laboratory evaluation of thrombophilia can help to better identify patients at higher risk for venous thromboembolic disease, and newer methods that test for genetic factors continue to evolve; however, more research is needed to justify routine testing for thrombophilia.

Research studies have yielded differing results in determining the most appropriate prophylactic regimen. Both pharmaceutical and mechanical treatments are commonly used for prophylaxis. New pharmacologic prophylaxes include the Xa inhibitor rivaroxaban and the thrombin inhibitor dabigatran etexilate. The newest mechanical device used to prevent venous thromboembolism is a miniature, mobile, battery-operated pneumatic system called Continuous Enhanced Circulation Therapy. The American College of Chest Physicians guidelines and the American Academy of Orthopaedic Surgeons clinical guideline were reviewed to directly compare specific agents and balance the risks of venous thromboembolism. Future studies for venous thromboembolic prophylaxis will continue to evaluate new oral agents, improved pneumatic compression devices, and improved methods to decrease bleeding in the immediate postoperative period.

Instr Course Lect 2014;63:409-419.

Dr. Westrich or an immediate family member has received royalties from Exactech; serves as a paid consultant to DJ Orthopaedics, Exactech, and Stryker; has received research or institutional support from DJ Orthopaedics, Exactech, and Stryker; and serves as a board member, owner, officer, or committee member of the Eastern Orthopedic Association. Dr. Cushner or an immediate family member has received royalties from Smith & Nephew; is a member of a speakers' bureau or has made paid presentations on behalf of Medtronic and Smith & Nephew; and serves as a paid consultant to Angiotech, Smith & Nephew, Aperion, Alter G, Medtronic, and Allergan. None of the following authors nor any immediate family member has received anything of value from or has stock or stock options held in a commercial company or institution related directly or indirectly to the subject of this chapter: Dr. Dlott, Dr. Johanson, and Ms. Ruel.

Venous thromboembolic disease continues to pose a major threat to patients treated with total hip arthroplasty (THA) and total knee arthroplasty (TKA). Despite substantial research, there is controversy concerning the best prophylactic regimen. This chapter reviews the various methods of mechanical and pharmacologic prophylaxis, reviews the current laboratory evaluation and risk factors for thrombophilia, and describes the role of biomarkers in determining the duration of anticoagulation therapy. The pros and cons of the guidelines of the American Academy of Orthopaedic Surgeons (AAOS) and the American College of Chest Physicians (ACCP) are described. This chapter's authors outline their approaches to preventing venous thromboembolism and focus on new advances in and approaches to prophylaxis.

Prophylactic Modalities
Mechanical Prophylaxis
Mechanical devices help prevent venous thromboembolic disease by increasing fibrinolysis and decreasing

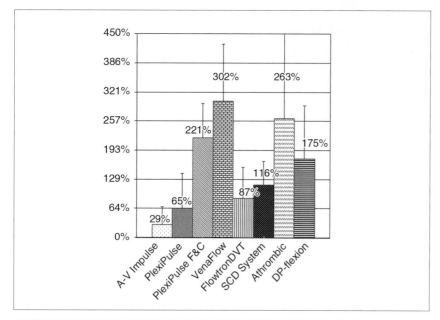

Figure 1 Comparison of increases in peak venous velocity for seven pneumatic compression devices. DP-flexion = active dorsal to plantar flexion.

stasis with accelerated venous emptying. Research on these devices has been less extensive than that on pharmacologic agents. The three major types of mechanical prophylactic devices are foot pumps, calf pumps, and calf-thigh pumps. The type of pneumatic compression varies: standard, sequential, or rapid inflation compression may be used. Although these compression devices are associated with extremely low complication rates, compliance issues may decrease their effectiveness. A study by Pitto et al[1] to assess patient compliance reported very satisfactory compliance rates, with 86% of the patients randomized to a foot pump using the device. In a study at the Hospital for Special Surgery, 90.1% of the patients were compliant in using a compression device.[2] At some hospitals, protocols have been instituted for nurses, physical therapists, and patients to increase the likelihood of compliance. When a patients returns from the bathroom or a physical therapy session, there is a risk that the compression device will not be reapplied. To reduce this risk, nurses and physical therapists are trained to properly reapply the devices. Patients are also instructed about the importance of pneumatic compression in preventing thromboembolic disease and are asked to remind medical staff to reapply the devices expeditiously.

The hemodynamics of mechanical compression devices in patients treated with THA or TKA have been examined.[3,4] In one study of patients treated with THA, three designs of calf-thigh pumps, two designs of foot pumps, one type of foot-calf pump, and one type of calf pump were tested.[3] The greatest increase in peak venous velocity occurred with pulsatile calf and calf-foot pneumatic compression with a rapid inflation time. A second crossover study performed by Westrich et al[4] on 10 patients treated with TKA evaluated the hemodynamic effect of active dorsal to plantar flexion and evaluated several pneumatic compression devices. The devices differed in the length and the location of the sleeve and bladder, the frequency and duration of activation, the rate of pressure rise, and the maximum pressure

achieved. The increase in peak venous velocity for active dorsal to plantar flexion was 175%. **Figure 1** shows the increase in peak venous velocity for seven different pneumatic compression devices: two foot pumps (A-V Impulse System [Covidien] and Plexi-Pulse [KCI]), one foot-calf pump (PlexiPulse F&C), one calf pump (VenaFlow [DJO Global]), and three calf-thigh pumps (Flowtron DVT [Huntleigh], SCD System [Covidien], and Athrombic [Jobst]).[3] Based on these results, this chapter's authors transition from a standard sequential compression device to a high flow, rapid inflation device.

A new, miniature, mobile, battery-operated pneumatic system called Continuous Enhanced Circulation Therapy (CECT; Medical Compression Systems) combined with low-dose aspirin was compared with enoxaparin in a study by Gelfer et al.[5] Patients treated with THA or TKA were randomized into two groups. One group (61 patients) received CECT for the length of their hospital stay (8.8 ± 1.9 days) and low-dose aspirin therapy, and the other group (60 patients) received 40 mg daily of enoxaparin. Bilateral venograms were assessed on the fifth postoperative day. Deep vein thrombosis was diagnosed in 17 of 60 patients in the enoxaparin group and 4 of 61 patients who received CECT ($P = 0.002$). The results showed that the combination of CECT and low-dose aspirin is more effective than enoxaparin in preventing deep vein thrombosis after joint arthroplasty.

Colwell et al[6] compared a CECT device worn for 10 days and low-molecular-weight heparin (LMWH) in 410 THA patients (414 hips). The rate of major bleeding events was 0% in the compression group and 6% in the group receiving LMWH. A major bleeding event was defined as bleeding that required rehospitalization (prolonged hospitalization), required an intervention (such as surgery), endangered critical organs, or was life threatening. The rates of distal and proximal deep vein thrombosis were 3% and 2%, respectively, in the compression group compared with 3% and 1%, respectively, in the LMWH group, which was not statistically different. Similarly, the rates of pulmonary embolism were 1% in the compression group and 1% in the LMWH group, and there were no fatal pulmonary emboli.

The concern with portable pneumatic compression devices is the potentially low increase in peak venous velocity compared with high-flow, rapid inflation devices. Some physicians have expressed concern regarding the cost of using CECT. Using data reported by Botteman[7] et al and Ollendorf et al,[8] it can be shown that CECT can save up to $2,628 in hospital costs per patient. Cost analyses must evaluate not only the cost of the device or medication but also the costs of treating deep vein thrombosis and rehospitalization. Further study of CECT devices is necessary to fully appreciate their effectiveness, although the small size and portability of the unit are attractive features.

New Pharmacologic Prophylaxis

Rivaroxaban is a direct Xa inhibitor that is orally administered once daily. For THA and TKA patients, the proposed dose is 10 mg daily, starting 6 to 8 hours postoperatively. The FDA reviewed this drug in July 2009 and requested additional analysis. Rivaroxaban has been studied in patients treated with THA or TKA in four pivotal studies and one meta-analysis.[9-13] Compared with enoxaparin, rivaroxaban demonstrated superiority in primary efficacy outcomes, the prevention of total venous thromboembolic events, secondary efficacy outcomes, and the prevention of major venous thromboembolisms. There was no important difference in the primary safety outcome of major bleeding compared with enoxaparin. Major bleeding occurred in 0.3% to 1.3% of the patients given daily doses of 10 mg or less of rivaroxaban. Major bleeding was defined as bleeding that started after the first postoperative drug dose and no later than 2 days after that dose. This included bleeding that was fatal; bleeding into critical organs; and bleeding that required reoperation, warranted cessation of treatment, resulted in a 2 g/dL or more drop in hemoglobin level, or required a transfusion of greater than 2 units of blood.

When any bleeding event was considered, rivaroxaban had a 6.23% rate in the RECORD1 and RECORD2 hip studies and an 8% rate in the RECORD3 and RECORD4 knee studies.[9-13] Enoxaparin showed a 5.76% overall bleeding rate for the THA studies and a 7.35% rate for the TKA studies, suggesting no difference in the risk of bleeding events. When only major bleeding was considered, rivaroxaban showed a 0.2% rate in the THA studies versus a 0.09% rate for enoxaparin, and a 0.62% rate in the TKA studies versus a 0.36% rate for enoxaparin. Although a small increased bleeding rate was noted in these studies, rivaroxaban appeared efficacious in preventing symptomatic venous thromboembolisms. For example, in the RECORD3 study, 10 mg of rivaroxaban daily had a 0.7% symptomatic thromboembolic event rate versus 2% for 40 mg of enoxaparin daily (the European dose). The US study of nearly 2,000 patients had a symptomatic venous thromboembolism rate of 0.7% with 10 mg of rivaroxaban daily versus 1.2% for 30 mg of enoxaparin dosed twice daily.[9-13]

Rivaroxaban has a rapid onset, high oral bioavailability, and predictable pharmacokinetic properties; however, there is no specific antidote or reversal agent for rivaroxaban, and it is not expected to be dialyzable. It can be taken orally with no required coagulation monitoring and given without dose adjustment. Phase II studies show it to be well tolerated and effective in preventing thromboembolic disease after orthopaedic surgery.[14] A Phase III study of patients treated with TKA showed it to be significantly superior to enoxaparin in terms of efficacy ($P = 0.01$), with a similar risk of bleeding. Questions are still being raised regarding the need to better understand bleeding reports, possible liver toxicity, and adverse cardiovascular events after cessation of the drug. In dosing studies, bleeding complications increased with drug exposure.[14]

Dabigatran etexilate is an oral prodrug that is rapidly converted by a serum esterase to a potent direct thrombin inhibitor. It has a serum half-life of 12 to 17 hours and does not require regular monitoring. In a multicenter double-blind study, approximately 2,000 patients treated with THA or TKA were randomized to receive either 6 to 10 days of oral dabigatran etexilate starting 1 to 4 hours after surgery or 40 mg daily of enoxaparin starting 12 hours after surgery.[15] Compared with enoxaparin, the rate of venous thromboembolism (measured symptomatically or by bilateral venography) within 12 hours of the last drug dose was significantly lower in patients receiving dabigatran etexilate 150 mg twice daily ($P = 0.04$), 300 mg once daily ($P = 0.02$), or 225 mg twice daily ($P = 0.0007$). The rate of venous thromboembolism was higher in patients receiving a 50 mg dose of dabigatran etexilate twice daily compared with enoxaparin, but this was not significant ($P = 0.57$). Major bleeding was defined as clinically overt bleeding associated with a 20 g/L or more decrease in hemoglobin, which lead to transfusion of 2 or more units of packed cells or whole blood; fatal, retroperitoneal, intraocular, or intraspinal bleeding; or bleeding warranting the cessation of treatment or reoperation. These major bleeding complications were significantly lower ($P = 0.047$) in the group receiving 50 mg dabigatran etexilate twice daily but were elevated in patients treated with the higher dosing regimens.

The approved dose of dabigatran etexilate for venous thromboembolic treatment and the prevention of stroke is 150 mg twice a day, whereas the dose for venous thromboembolism prophylaxis is 150 mg daily. The anticoagulant effect of the drug is immediate after dosing and peaks with 2 to 3 hours. Dabigatran etexilate is 80% renally excreted and should not be used in patients with renal failure. In patients with normal renal function, discontinuation of dabigatran etexilate for 24 hours reduces levels to 25% of the steady state trough, whereas holding for 36 and 48 hours lowers levels 12% to 15% and 5% to 10% of the trough, respectively. It should be used only with extreme caution and with dosing adjustments in patients with renal insufficiency, although it is not generally recommended in that patient population. Dabigatran etexilate has no known antidote. Although there are no clear guidelines, dabigatran etexilate should generally be withheld for 5 days before surgery to ensure that normal hemostasis has been restored, especially if regional anesthesia will be used.

AAOS and ACCP Guidelines

The recently released AAOS and ACCP guidelines on preventing venous thromboembolic disease in patients treated with elective THA or TKA used different quantitative methodologies.[16-21] The AAOS used network meta-analysis, which facilitated the comparison of agents that may not have been formally compared in head-to-head trials. The ACCP relied on the grade profile strategy, which synthesized event rates pooled from the literature versus a calculated baseline risk (no prophylaxis) of either symptomatic deep vein thrombosis or pulmonary embolism (2.8%). The resulting graphic display of important parameters, relative risk reflecting rates of asymptomatic deep vein thrombosis (%), absolute risk for symptomatic venous thromboembolism (events/1,000) less than baseline, and bleeding risk (events/1,000) can be used to directly compare specific agents and balance risks.

Both guidelines recommend against routine Doppler ultrasound screening for venous thromboembolism because it is unreliable for clinical decision making. Instead, both guidelines either suggest (AAOS) or recommend (ACCP) starting a prophylactic regimen and continuing it for 10 to 14 days (ACCP; grade 1B recommendation) or a full 35-day period (ACCP; grade 2B recommendation). Rather than a prescribed period of prophylaxis, the AAOS recommends discussion with the patient to arrive at a decision. This process is in full accord with the ACCP's support for decisions made in consideration of patient values and preferences.

The AAOS does not specifically recommend any particular prophylactic strategy over another because data do not suggest that any one agent is more effective at preventing symptomatic thromboembolism, mortality from pulmonary embolism, and all-cause mortality. The ACCP gives a suggested preference of LMWH, although this is a weak grade 2C/B recommendation, and recommends starting it at or more than 12 hours postoperatively. In-hospital use of an intermittent pneumatic compression device, in addition to pharmacologic agents, is suggested by both guidelines. Neither guideline suggests or recommends any specific risk-stratification strategy for venous thromboembolism other than the procedure-specific risk. Both guidelines suggest using an intermittent pneumatic compression device only (no pharmacologic prophylaxis) for patients with an increased risk of bleeding.

These guidelines should not substitute for clinical judgment. It is better to focus on the absolute benefit versus risk for interventions. Future research on standardized definitions for major bleeding and surgical site bleeding complications are needed as well as an evidence-based system for baseline risk assessment for venous thromboembolism and bleeding. AAOS and ACCP guidelines no longer conflict; however, more collaboration and refinement could further improve the guidelines.

Laboratory Evaluation of Thrombophilia and Risk Factors

Traditional Testing

Venous thromboembolic disease is a multifactorial disorder resulting from the interaction of genetic, acquired (such as antibodies), and environmental (such as prolonged immobility, surgery, or trauma) risk factors.[22] Suspicion for inherited thrombophilia is heightened when there is a clinical history of a first venous thromboembolism in a patient younger than 40 years, a strong family history of venous thromboembolic disease or a venous thromboembolism in a first-degree relative with thrombosis at a young age, a spontaneous or unprovoked venous thromboembolism, or a venous thromboembolism at an unusual site (such as hepatic or mesen-

Table 1

Inherited Thrombophilia Risk Factors

Condition	Healthy (%)	Venous Thrombo-embolism (%)	Relative Risk of Thrombosis (%)
Activated protein C resistance/factor V Leiden mutation	5	21	3-7
Antithrombin deficiency	0.02-0.17	1	15-40
Protein C deficiency	0.3	3	5-12
Protein S deficiency	0.7	2	4-10
Prothrombin (FII) G20210A mutation	2	6	2-3
Factor VIII excess	11	25	6
Hyperhomocysteinemia > 18.5 µmol/L	5-10	10-25	3-4

teric vein thrombosis).[23] The prevalence of inherited thrombophilia and the associated relative risk of thrombosis are summarized in **Table 1**. The relative risk is the percentage risk of general thrombosis given the condition stated versus the absolute risk of venous thromboembolism.

Possessing more than one hereditary risk factor or homozygosity in the case of genetic risk factors (such as factor V Leiden or prothrombin G20210A mutation) generally imparts a greater risk of recurrent thromboembolism.[24,25] Elevated factor VIII activity and hyperhomocysteinemia have hereditary and environmental influences.[26] Antibody-mediated thrombosis, a form of acquired thrombophilia, may occur in association with autoimmune disease or may be idiopathic. Antiphospholipid antibody syndrome is a clinical pathologic syndrome that includes a history of thrombosis and the presence of persistently positive antibodies (immunoglobulin G [IgG] or immunoglobulin M [IgM] anticardiolipin antibodies > 40 µg of IgG antibody/microgram of IgM antibody, positive IgG or IgM antibeta-2 glycoprotein I antibodies, or a lupus anticoagulant).[27] Patients with antiphospholipid antibody syndrome are also at increased risk for recurrent venous thromboembolic events.[27]

Thrombophilia evaluation in orthopaedic surgery has been studied to a limited extent. In a case-controlled retrospective analysis of 96 patients treated with THA, Salvati et al[28] reported that the development of venous thromboembolism was more likely in a patient with a deficiency of antithrombin III or protein C or in those with one or two copies of the prothrombin G20210A mutation; the control population lacked any risk factors for thrombophilia. In a series of 86 patients treated with THA or TKA receiving prolonged LMWH prophylaxis, Szücs et al[29] identified thrombophilia risk factors in 18 of 33 patients with venous thromboembolic events compared with 12 of 53 patients in whom a thromboembolic event did not develop. Risk factors included factor V Leiden, the prothrombin G20210A mutation, and lupus anticoagulant. Combined thrombophilia (more that one risk factor for thrombophilia) was reported in seven patients with venous thromboembolic complications and in two patients without complications. Although both studies reported a statistical difference between symptomatic and asymptomatic patients, larger prospective studies will likely be required to justify routine testing.[28,29] In general, thrombophilia testing should be done only if the re-

sults are likely to change medical management.[23]

Clinical Score Cards

Clinical scoring systems, such as $CHADS_2$, Padua, and Caprini, are used to stratify the risk of venous thromboembolic events in both medical and nonorthopaedic surgical settings.[30,31] The Padua and Caprini risk scores incorporate known thrombophilia as an important weighted variable, implying that thrombophilia screening should be selectively applied.[30,31] The perioperative section of the ninth ACCP supplement on anticoagulants described a new risk classification system that addresses the perioperative management of patients receiving vitamin K antagonists or antiplatelet drugs (such as aspirin or clopidogrel) who elect surgical or other invasive procedures.[32] High risk is classified as the presence of a venous thromboembolism within 3 months of planned surgery or having severe thrombophilia (deficiency of protein C, protein S, or antithrombin). Moderate risk is classified as the occurrence of venous thromboembolism from within 3 to 12 months of the planned surgery, the presence of nonsevere thrombophilia (heterozygous factor V Leiden or prothrombin G20210A mutations), the presence of recurrent ve-

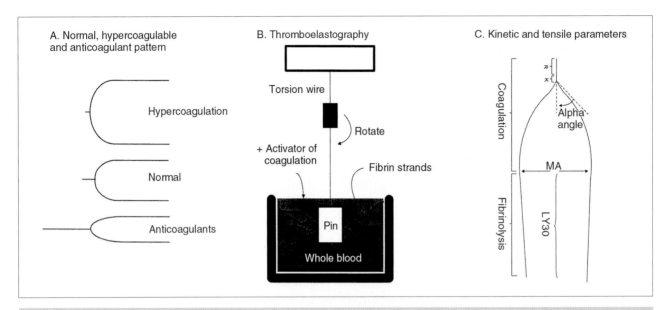

A. Normal, hypercoagulable and anticoagulant pattern

Hypercoagulation

Normal

Anticoagulants

B. Thromboelastography

Torsion wire

Rotate

+ Activator of coagulation

Fibrin strands

Pin

Whole blood

C. Kinetic and tensile parameters

Coagulation

Alpha angle

MA

Fibrinolysis

LY30

Figure 2   Thromboelastography is a global coagulation assay that measures the kinetics of clot formation, retraction, and lysis.

nous thromboembolism, or the presence of cancer (treated within 6 months or palliative). Low risk is defined as having a prior, single, venous thromboembolism more than 12 months before planned surgery or no other risk factors. The role of this risk stratification model in personalizing the duration or intensity of anticoagulant therapy has not yet been determined.[32]

Global Assays

Activated Partial Thromboplastin Time

Global coagulation assays provide a more overarching snapshot of hemostasis. The most basic and readily available assay is routine activated partial thromboplastin time (aPTT). New insights in screening coagulopathies are now being drawn in the context of recurrent venous thromboembolism. Zakai et al[33] reported that a single, shortened aPTT (27.7 seconds versus 28.9 seconds; $P < 0.001$) below the median increased the risk of recurrent venous thromboembolism in patients with a history of venous thromboembolic events compared with controls. A

second prospective study of patients with idiopathic venous thromboembolisms reported that an abnormally short aPTT was associated with an increased risk of venous thromboembolism after oral anticoagulation therapy withdrawal.[34] The venous thromboembolism recurrence rate was 17.5% in patients with aPTT in the lower quartile (ratio ≤ 0.9) versus 7.5% in the upper quartile (ratio > 1.05).

Recurrence risk was more than twofold higher in patients with a ratio of 0.9 or less versus the reference category. The studies were adjusted for elevations of prothrombotic clotting factors or other thrombophilia conditions. It was concluded that the aPTT predictive value was independent of these alterations.[33,34] Abnormally short aPTT values are associated with a substantially increased risk of venous thromboembolism recurrence.[33,34]

Thromboelastography

Thromboelastography is a global coagulation assay performed with fresh blood and requires interpretation by trained personnel. This test measures

the kinetics of clot formation, retraction, and lysis (**Figure 2**). One particular parameter, the maximum amplitude, measures the tensile strength of the clot. Blood with increased maximum amplitude is interpreted as being hypercoagulable. Different parameters are used to guide selective transfusion therapy.[35] Although several studies have used thromboelastography in the postoperative period to monitor prolonged hypercoagulability, the literature is limited regarding its use in orthopaedic surgery.[36,37]

Thrombin Generation Test

The thrombin generation test is a promising new platform that is primarily used as a research tool but may be a potential test option in the future as so-called personalized medicine continues to evolve. The generation of thrombin from its precursor prothrombin is a tightly regulated and localized process (occurring in the affected vascular bed). Dysfunctional thrombin generation is the common denominator for many thrombophilic disorders, and it conversely may be the underlying defect in some bleeding disorders such as hemophilia. **Figure 3** illustrates typical thrombin generation, which has been likened to a match striking a matchbox, igniting, reaching a maximum flame height, and then extinguishing. As with thromboelastography, multiple parameters, including kinetics, maximum peak, and the area under the curve are interpreted, and conclusions are made concerning the overall hemostatic condition (normal, hypercoagulable, or hypocoagulable) of the patient. One report comparing rivaroxaban with dalteparin showed more postoperative consistency in patients treated with rivaroxaban and a greater decrease in the thrombin generation test than with dalteparin.[38]

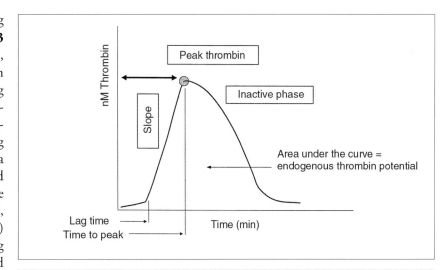

Figure 3   Illustration of a typical thrombin generation assay process, which has been likened to a match striking a matchbox, igniting, reaching a maximum flame height, and then extinguishing.

Biomarkers for Duration of Anticoagulant Therapy

Indirect markers of thrombin generation (prothrombin fragment 1.2, thrombin-antithrombin, and D-dimer) have been shown to rise in patients treated with THA or TKA.[39] The general availability of D-dimer has resulted in its rise in prominence as a surrogate marker for assessing the duration of anticoagulant therapy in patients with idiopathic venous thromboembolism. Palareti et al[40] studied patients who were negative for D-dimer at the end of treatment and another group who were D-dimer positive. Patients in the positive D-dimer group were randomized to continued anticoagulant therapy or cessation of treatment. Patients with an abnormal D-dimer 1 month after the discontinuation of anticoagulant therapy had a substantial incidence of recurrent venous thromboembolism, which was then reduced by the resumption of therapy.[41] Some of the challenges in using D-dimer as a biomarker are the selection of the optimal cut-off value and the myriad of conditions associated with elevated levels (such as systemic inflammatory condi-

tions, positive rheumatoid factor, severe infections, and pregnancy).

Elevated factor VIIIa is a risk factor for both primary and recurrent venous thromboembolism.[42,43] The basal level of a patient is in part inherited, although the genetic factors are not known and are influenced by ABO blood types and inflammation.[43] In one study, patients with factor VIII levels above the 90th percentile (234%) had a 37% likelihood of recurrence of a thromboembolic event within 2 years.[42] In comparison, Shrivastava et al[43] reported a risk of thromboembolism recurrence for factor VIIIa greater than 150%. The difference between the studies may have resulted from differing methodologies. Guidelines for treatment, frequency of testing, and methodology have not yet been determined.

Thrombophilia baseline testing should be used only for select populations and when results are likely to change medical management. In the future, new technologies may provide insights to a personalized anticoagulant strategy, but well-powered pro-

spective studies and assay standardization are needed before this technology can be translated into clinical reality.

Multifactorial Approach

This chapter's authors advocate a multifactorial approach to prevent venous thromboembolism.[44-48] The protocol includes a combination of preoperative, intraoperative, and postoperative prophylactic techniques. Preoperative assessment involves a full medical evaluation of the patient with attention paid to coagulation risk factors such as a current malignant tumor; a history of pulmonary embolism or deep vein thrombosis; and the use of estrogen therapy, oral contraceptives, or tobacco. Patients must discontinue procoagulant medications before admission. Using regional anesthesia decreases blood loss and the rate of deep vein thrombosis, and intraoperative pneumatic compression decreases venous stasis and the risk of clotting.[49-51] Standard inpatient postoperative prophylaxis includes pneumatic compression combined with pharmacologic prophylaxis (usually warfarin or aspirin). The dosing regimen continues for 6 weeks starting the night of surgery, with a daily evening dose with an International Normalized Ratio of 1.8 to 2.3. It is important for prophylaxis to continue after discharge from the hospital and for the patient to be aware of the symptoms of venous thromboembolism.

González Della Valle et al[47] reported that a multimodal approach of preoperative and intraoperative measures combined with pneumatic compression, knee-high elastic stockings, early mobilization, and chemoprophylaxis with acetylsalicylic acid (83% of the study patients) or warfarin (17% of the study patients) for 4 to 6 weeks after THA was safe and efficacious. The study included 1,947 consecutive patients (2,032 THAs) who were observed prospectively for 3 months. The first 171 patients had a 6.4% prevalence of asymptomatic deep vein thrombosis as assessed with routine ultrasound examination, and the other 1,776 patients had a 2.5% prevalence of symptomatic deep vein thrombosis. Nonfatal symptomatic pulmonary embolism occurred in 12 of the 1,947 patients (0.6%). The low rates of thromboembolic complications in this population provide evidence that routine anticoagulant therapy with potent chemoprophylactic agents is unnecessary.

The Future of Thromboembolic Disease Prophylaxis

Although LMWH is commonly used in some institutions for deep vein thrombosis chemoprophylaxis, newer oral agents may slowly replace LMWH because of ease of use. However, there is a growing trend to use less potent anticoagulants to avoid the bleeding risk associated with more potent agents. Both the AAOS and ACCP guidelines recommend aspirin as an appropriate alternative agent.

Although the benefits of LMWH have been well described, the main drawbacks are the subcutaneous route of administration, the risk of thrombocytopenia, and the increased risk of surgical site bleeding. It is believed that venous thromboembolic events originate at the time of surgery. It is known that earlier dosing may decrease the rate of venous thromboembolism but perhaps at the cost of increased bleeding. Fitzgerald et al[52] evaluated enoxaparin dosing at 8 hours rather than the 12- to 24-hour dosing prescribed on the product label. Venous thromboembolism was defined as deep vein thrombosis documented by contrast venography, symptomatic deep vein thrombosis documented by ultrasound of the lower extremity, or symptomatic pulmonary embolism confirmed by a positive lung scan. The result was near elimination of proximal deep vein thrombosis (2% versus 11%; $P = 0.002$) and a substantial decrease in the occurrence of total venous thromboembolic events (25% versus 45%; $P = 0.0001$); however, an increased trend toward bleeding was noted.

Many bleeding events may not be reported because several different definitions of bleeding are described in the literature.[53] Often major bleeding includes intracranial or retroperitoneal bleeding but excludes surgical site bleeding. Many studies are not reporting bleeding events that are clinically relevant to orthopaedic surgeons (such as increased hemarthrosis at the site of the joint arthroplasty or prolonged surgical site bleeding). Although many factors play a role in surgical site bleeding, such events are often attributed to the agent used for venous thromboembolic prophylaxis. This complicates issues because it is well recognized that the causes of bleeding are multifactorial. Although the perception of postoperative bleeding relates to venous

thromboembolic prophylaxis, it should be noted that bleeding events occur at a rate of 2% to 4% regardless of the agent used. This baseline bleeding rate may be more closely related to the procedure itself rather than the prophylactic agent.

Patel et al[54] reviewed factors associated with prolonged postoperative drainage in patients treated with THA or TKA. Although venous thromboembolic prophylaxis played a role in the drainage, the most important predictive factor was the amount of drainage (measured by the volume of discharge from a closed suction drain reservoir) that occurred in the immediate postoperative period. More drainage in the recovery room led to more drainage on days 2, 3, 4, and 5 after surgery. It is possible that more emphasis should be placed on controlling bleeding in the immediate postoperative period, which occurs well before the administration of prophylactic agents. At the Hospital for Special Surgery, the immediate use of continuous passive motion has been eliminated, and immediate wound hemostasis has become the focus.

Some surgeons are using a lidocaine and epinephrine injection along the arthrotomy site. This technique combined with a smaller parapatellar incision leads to a substantial decrease in postoperative blood loss and safely provides excellent pain control and functional recovery.[55] Other intraoperative measures include the use of tranexamic acid, which is an antifibrinolytic agent that helps stop the breaking of fibrinogen. A 10 mg/kg dosing is used for high-risk patients. However, the role of tranexamic acid is expanding and is now routinely used in some joint replacement centers.[56] Combining modalities may improve wound appearance and reduce surgical site bleeding complications.

Summary

The goal of venous thromboembolic prophylaxis is to protect patients from symptomatic venous thromboembolism while avoiding bleeding complications. Future studies on venous thromboembolic prophylaxis will continue to evaluate new oral agents, improved pneumatic compression devices, and improved methods to decrease bleeding in the immediate postoperative period. As new agents are becoming available, there is hope that combining prophylactic modalities will decrease the rate of venous thromboembolism, reduce bleeding complications, improve wound appearance, and, perhaps, reduce the overall infection rate by minimizing surgical site complications.

References

1. Pitto RP, Hamer H, Heiss-Dunlop W, Kuehle J: Mechanical prophylaxis of deep-vein thrombosis after total hip replacement: A randomised clinical trial. *J Bone Joint Surg Br* 2004;86(5):639-642.

2. Westrich GH, Jhon PH, Sanchez PM: Compliance in using a pneumatic compression device after total knee arthroplasty. *Am J Orthop* 2003;32(3):135-140.

3. Westrich GH, Specht LM, Sharrock NE, et al: Evaluation of active dorsal to plantar flexion and several mechanical compression devices. *J Bone Joint Surg Br* 1998;80(6):1057-1066.

4. Westrich GH, Specht LM, Sharrock NE, et al: Pneumatic compression hemodynamics in total hip arthroplasty. *Clin Orthop Relat Res* 2000;372:180-191.

5. Gelfer Y, Tavor H, Oron A, Peer A, Halperin N, Robinson D: Deep vein thrombosis prevention in joint arthroplasties: Continuous enhanced circulation therapy vs low molecular weight heparin.

6. Colwell CW Jr, Froimson MI, Mont MA, et al: A prospective, randomized trial comparing a mobile compression device with low-molecular-weight heparin. *J Bone Joint Surg Am* 2010;92(3):527-535.

7. Botteman MF, Caprini J, Stephens JM, et al: Results of an economic model to assess the cost-effectiveness of enoxaparin, a low-molecular-weight heparin, versus warfarin for the prophylaxis of deep vein thrombosis and associated long-term complications in total hip replacement surgery in the United States. *Clin Ther* 2002;24(11):1960-1986.

8. Ollendorf DA, Vera-Llonch M, Oster G: Cost of venous thromboembolism following major orthopedic surgery in hospitalized patients. *Am J Health Syst Pharm* 2002;59(18):1750-1754.

9. Eriksson BI, Borris LC, Friedman RJ, et al: Rivaroxaban versus enoxaparin for thromboprophylaxis after hip arthroplasty. *N Engl J Med* 2008;358(26):2765-2775.

10. Kakkar AK, Brenner B, Dahl OE, et al: Extended duration rivaroxaban versus short-term enoxaparin for the prevention of venous thromboembolism after total hip arthroplasty: A double-blind, randomised controlled trial. *Lancet* 2008;372(9632):31-39.

11. Lassen MR, Ageno W, Borris LC, et al: Rivaroxaban versus enoxaparin for thromboprophylaxis after total knee arthroplasty. *N Engl J Med* 2008;358(26):2776-2786.

12. Turpie AG, Lassen MR, Davidson BL, et al: Rivaroxaban versus enoxaparin for thromboprophylaxis after total knee arthroplasty (RECORD4): A randomised trial. *Lancet* 2009;373(9676):1673-1680.

13. Fisher WD, Eriksson BI, Bauer KA, et al: Pooled analysis of two studies. *Thromb Haemost* 2007;97(6):931-937.

14. Perzborn E, Kubitza D, Misselwitz F: Rivaroxaban: A novel, oral, direct factor Xa inhibitor in clinical development for the prevention and treatment of thromboembolic disorders. *Hamostaseologie* 2007;27(4):282-289.

15. Eriksson BI, Dahl OE, Büller HR, et al: A new oral direct thrombin inhibitor, dabigatran etexilate, compared with enoxaparin for prevention of thromboembolic events following total hip or knee replacement: The BISTRO II randomized trial. *J Thromb Haemost* 2005;3(1):103-111.

16. Johanson NA, Lachiewicz PF, Lieberman JR, et al: American Academy of Orthopaedic Surgeons clinical practice guideline on prevention of symptomatic pulmonary embolism in patients undergoing total hip or knee arthroplasty. *J Bone Joint Surg Am* 2009;91(7):1756-1757.

17. Eikelboom JW, Karthikeyan G, Fagel N, Hirsh J: American Association of Orthopedic Surgeons and American College of Chest Physicians guidelines for venous thromboembolism prevention in hip and knee arthroplasty differ: What are the implications for clinicians and patients? *Chest* 2009;135(2):513-520.

18. Jennings HR, Miller EC, Williams TS, Tichenor SS, Woods EA: Reducing anticoagulant medication adverse events and avoidable patient harm. *Jt Comm J Qual Patient Saf* 2008;34(4):196-200.

19. Geerts WH, Bergqvist D, Pineo GF, et al: Prevention of venous thromboembolism: American College of Chest Physicians evidence-based clinical practice guidelines (8th edition). *Chest* 2008;133(6):381S-453S.

20. Mont MA, Jacobs JJ, Boggio LN, et al: Preventing venous thromboembolic disease in patients undergoing elective hip and knee arthroplasty. *J Am Acad Orthop Surg* 2011;19(12):768-776.

21. Falck-Ytter Y, Francis CW, Johanson NA, et al: Prevention of VTE in orthopedic surgery patients: Antithrombotic Therapy and Prevention of Thrombosis, 9th ed. American College of Chest Physicians Evidence-Based Clinical Practice Guidelines. *Chest* 2012; 141(2):e278S-e325S.

22. Rosendaal FR: Venous thrombosis: A multicausal disease. *Lancet* 1999;353(9159):1167-1173.

23. Heit JA: Thrombophilia: Common questions on laboratory assessment and management. *Hematology Am Soc Hematol Educ Program* 2007;127-135.

24. Heit JA, Cunningham JM, Petterson TM, Armasu SM, Rider DN, de Andrade M: Genetic variation within the anticoagulant, procoagulant, fibrinolytic and innate immunity pathways as risk factors for venous thromboembolism. *J Thromb Haemost* 2011;9(6): 1133-1142.

25. Cushman M: Inherited risk factors for venous thrombosis. *Hematology Am Soc Hematol Educ Program* 2005;452-457.

26. Bauer KA: Duration of anticoagulation: Applying the guidelines and beyond. *Hematology Am Soc Hematol Educ Program* 2010; 2010:210-215.

27. Miyakis S, Lockshin MD, Atsumi T, et al: International consensus statement on an update of the classification criteria for definite antiphospholipid syndrome (APS). *J Thromb Haemost* 2006; 4(2):295-306.

28. Salvati EA, Della Valle AG, Westrich GH, et al: Heritable thrombophilia and development of thromboembolic disease after

total hip arthroplasty. *Clin Orthop Relat Res* 2005;441:40-55.

29. Szücs G, Ajzner E, Muszbek L, Simon T, Szepesi K, Fülesdi B: Assessment of thrombotic risk factors predisposing to thromboembolic complications in prosthetic orthopedic surgery. *J Orthop Sci* 2009;14(5):484-490.

30. Kahn SR, Lim W, Dunn AS, et al: Prevention of VTE in nonsurgical patients: Antithrombotic Therapy and Prevention of Thrombosis, 9th ed. American College of Chest Physicians Evidence-Based Clinical Practice Guidelines. *Chest* 2012;141(2): e195S-e226S.

31. Gould MK, Garcia DA, Wren SM, et al: Prevention of VTE in nonorthopedic surgical patients: Antithrombotic Therapy and Prevention of Thrombosis, 9th ed. American College of Chest Physicians Evidence-Based Clinical Practice Guidelines. *Chest* 2012; 141(2):e227S-e277S.

32. Douketis JD, Spyropoulos AC, Spencer FA, et al: Perioperative management of antithrombotic therapy: Antithrombotic therapy and prevention. American College of Chest Physicians Evidence-Based Clinical Practice Guidelines (9th edition). *Chest* 2012;141(2): e326S-e350S.

33. Zakai NA, Ohira T, White R, Folsom AR, Cushman M: Activated partial thromboplastin time and risk of future venous thromboembolism. *Am J Med* 2008; 121(3):231-238.

34. Legnani C, Mattarozzi S, Cini M, Cosmi B, Favaretto E, Palareti G: Abnormally short activated partial thromboplastin time values are associated with increased risk of recurrence of venous thromboembolism after oral anticoagulation withdrawal. *Br J Haematol* 2006; 134(2):227-232.

35. Shore-Lesserson L, Manspeizer HE, DePerio M, Francis S, Vela-Cantos F, Ergin MA:

Thromboelastography-guided transfusion algorithm reduces transfusions in complex cardiac surgery. *Anesth Analg* 1999;88(2): 312-319.

36. Mahla E, Lang T, Vicenzi MN, et al: Thromboelastography for monitoring prolonged hypercoagulability after major abdominal surgery. *Anesth Analg* 2001;92(3): 572-577.

37. McCrath DJ, Cerboni E, Frumento RJ, Hirsh AL, Bennett-Guerrero E: Thromboelastography maximum amplitude predicts postoperative thrombotic complications including myocardial infarction. *Anesth Analg* 2005; 100(6):1576-1583.

38. Klein SM, Slaughter TF, Vail PT, et al: Thromboelastography as a perioperative measure of anticoagulation resulting from low molecular weight heparin: A comparison with anti-Xa concentrations. *Anesth Analg* 2000;91(5):1091-1095.

39. Su EP, Chatzoudis N, Sioros V, Go G, Sharrock NE: Markers of thrombin generation during resurfacing and noncemented total hip arthroplasty: A pilot study. *Clin Orthop Relat Res* 2011;469(2): 535-540.

40. Palareti G, Cosmi B, Legnani C, et al: D-dimer testing to determine the duration of anticoagulation therapy. *N Engl J Med* 2006; 355(17):1780-1789.

41. Koster T, Blann AD, Briët E, Vandenbroucke JP, Rosendaal FR: Role of clotting factor VIII in effect of von Willebrand factor on occurrence of deep-vein thrombosis. *Lancet* 1995;345(8943): 152-155.

42. Kyrle PA, Minar E, Hirschl M, et al: High plasma levels of factor VIII and the risk of recurrent venous thromboembolism. *N Engl J Med* 2000;343(7):457-462.

43. Shrivastava S, Ridker PM, Glynn RJ, et al: D-dimer, factor VIII

coagulant activity, low-intensity warfarin and the risk of recurrent venous thromboembolism. *J Thromb Haemost* 2006;4(6): 1208-1214.

44. Westrich GH, Bottner F, Windsor RE, Laskin RS, Haas SB, Sculco TP: VenaFlow plus Lovenox vs VenaFlow plus aspirin for thromboembolic disease prophylaxis in total knee arthroplasty. *J Arthroplasty* 2006;21(6):139-143.

45. Boscainos PJ, McLardy-Smith P, Jinnah RH: Deep vein thrombosis prophylaxis after total-knee arthroplasty. *Curr Opin Orthop* 2006;17:60-7.

46. Westrich GH, Haas SB, Mosca P, Peterson M: Meta-analysis of thromboembolic prophylaxis after total knee arthroplasty. *J Bone Joint Surg Br* 2000;82(6): 795-800.

47. González Della Valle A, Serota A, Go G, et al: Venous thromboembolism is rare with a multimodal prophylaxis protocol after total hip arthroplasty. *Clin Orthop Relat Res* 2006;444:146-153.

48. Westrich GH, Rana AJ, Terry MA, Taveras NA, Kapoor K, Helfet DL: Thromboembolic disease prophylaxis in patients with hip fracture: A multimodal approach. *J Orthop Trauma* 2005; 19(4):234-240.

49. Lieberman JR, Huo MM, Hanway J, Salvati EA, Sculco TP, Sharrock NE: The prevalence of deep venous thrombosis after total hip arthroplasty with hypotensive epidural anesthesia. *J Bone Joint Surg Am* 1994;76(3):341-348.

50. Miric A, Lombardi P, Sculco TP: Deep vein thrombosis prophylaxis: A comprehensive approach for total hip and total knee arthroplasty patient populations. *Am J Orthop (Belle Mead NJ)* 2000; 29(4):269-274.

51. Westrich GH, Farrell C, Bono JV, Ranawat CS, Salvati EA, Sculco TP: The incidence of venous thromboembolism after total hip arthroplasty: A specific hypotensive epidural anesthesia protocol. *J Arthroplasty* 1999;14(4): 456-463.

52. Fitzgerald RH Jr, Spiro TE, Trowbridge AA, et al: Prevention of venous thromboembolic disease following primary total knee arthroplasty: A randomized, multicenter, open-label, parallel-group comparison of enoxaparin and warfarin. *J Bone Joint Surg Am* 2001;83(6):900-906.

53. Hull RD, Yusen RD, Bergqvist D: State-of-the-art review: Assessing the safety profiles of new anticoagulants for major orthopedic surgery thromboprophylaxis. *Clin Appl Thromb Hemost* 2009;15(4): 377-388.

54. Patel VP, Walsh M, Sehgal B, Preston C, DeWal H, Di Cesare PE: Factors associated with prolonged wound drainage after primary total hip and knee arthroplasty. *J Bone Joint Surg Am* 2007; 89(1):33-38.

55. Parvataneni HK, Shah VP, Howard H, Cole N, Ranawat AS, Ranawat CS: Controlling pain after total hip and knee arthroplasty using a multimodal protocol with local periarticular injections: A prospective randomized study. *J Arthroplasty* 2007;22(6): 33-38.

56. Gillette BP, DeSimone LJ, Trousdale RT, Pagnano MW, Sierra RJ: Low risk of thromboembolic complications with tranexamic acid after primary total hip and knee arthroplasty. *Clin Orthop Relat Res* 2013;47(1):150-154.

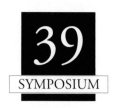

39
SYMPOSIUM

Medical and Legal Considerations in Managing Patients With Musculoskeletal Tumors

Carol D. Morris, MD, MS
B. Sonny Bal, MD, JD, MBA
Elizabeth M. D'Elia, JD, RN
Joseph Benevenia, MD

Abstract

At some point in their careers, many orthopaedic surgeons will have to navigate the legal system as it pertains to medical malpractice. An orthopaedic surgeon will find it helpful to review information on the basic legal elements of medical malpractice law along with suggestions on how he or she can assist the legal defense team if a lawsuit is filed. Surgeons who face litigation within the context of managing patients with musculoskeletal tumors should be aware of the common pitfalls in managing these patients. Knowledge of complementary strategies can provide good patient care and reduce legal risks when caring for patients with musculoskeletal neoplasms.

Instr Course Lect 2014;63:421-430.

Treating a patient with an actual or possible musculoskeletal neoplasm is challenging under the best of circumstances. When the possibility of a medical liability lawsuit is involved, the task of managing the patient becomes more difficult. Litigation affects the physician's day-to-day practice and the care of patients and is associated with substantial personal, emotional, and financial expenses. Although malpractice insurance can protect the physician from the direct costs of litigation, the indirect costs—including time away from the medical practice, stress, and damage to one's reputation—are not covered by insurance.

Civil lawsuits alleging medical malpractice filed by dissatisfied patients are a relatively common occurrence in the United States. General surgeons as well as subspecialists (including orthopaedic surgeons) have a high likelihood of facing a malpractice claim during their careers. It is estimated that approximately 14% of orthopaedic surgeons are sued annually.[1] The likelihood of an orthopaedic surgeon being sued at least once during his or her career (by age 65) is 98%. Most cases are settled or dismissed; of those cases that go to trial, the orthopaedic surgeon is successfully defended 92% of the time.[2]

The purpose of this chapter is to provide information to an orthopaedic surgeon who is facing litigation within the context of managing patients with musculoskeletal tumors. Specifically, the goals of this chapter are to help an orthopaedic surgeon understand the basic legal elements of medical malpractice law, identify common pitfalls in managing patients with musculoskeletal neoplasms, offer complementary alternative strategies that provide good patient care and reduce legal risks, and provide suggestions on how an orthopaedic surgeon can assist his or her legal defense team if a lawsuit is filed.

Dr. Morris or an immediate family member serves as a board member, owner, officer, or committee member of the American Academy of Orthopaedic Surgeons. Dr. Benevenia or an immediate family member is a member of a speakers' bureau or has made paid presentations on behalf of the Musculoskeletal Transplant Foundation; serves as an unpaid consultant to Merete NJOS; has received research or institutional support from Biomet, the Musculoskeletal Transplant Foundation, and Synthes; and serves as a board member, owner, officer, or committee member of the American Academy of Orthopaedic Surgeons, the Musculoskeletal Transplant Foundation, and the Musculoskeletal Tumor Society. Neither of the following authors nor any immediate family member has received anything of value from or has stock or stock options held in a commercial company or institution related directly or indirectly to the subject of this chapter: Dr. Bal and Ms. D'Elia.

Understanding Legal Liability in Medical Practice

Medical Malpractice Law

Medical malpractice is defined as any act or omission by a physician during patient care that falls below accepted norms of practice in the medical community and leads to an injury to the patient. Medical malpractice is a specific subset of tort law that deals with professional negligence. Tort means wrong, and tort law creates and provides remedies for civil wrongs that are distinct from contractual duties or criminal wrongs.[3] Negligence is defined as conduct that does not meet a certain standard; the most commonly used standard in tort law is that of a reasonable person. The reasonable person standard is a reference standard of reasonable conduct that a person in similar circumstances would do or not do to protect a party from a foreseeable risk of harm.

Medical malpractice law can be traced back to 19th-century English common law.[4] In the United States, medical malpractice law is under the authority of the states; the framework and rules that govern it have been established through decisions in lawsuits filed in state courts. Although state law governing medical malpractice can vary across different jurisdictions in the United States, the principles are similar.

Lawsuits alleging medical malpractice are generally filed in a state trial court. The venue (place where the case is filed) is guided by the residence of the parties involved and the location of the alleged misconduct. Trial courts have jurisdiction (the legal authority to hear and decide) medical malpractice cases. In each state, specific legal rules guide the selection of a venue and determine jurisdiction.

In the United States, the right to a jury trial is a fundamental constitutional right. A jury trial is a legal proceeding in which a group of individuals, chosen from the public, is asked to consider the evidence presented during the case and render a judgment. The choice of jurors is guided by court rules and includes the participation of attorneys representing both sides. Assuming there is no disposal of the case before trial, a physician can expect a jury trial in nearly all cases of medical malpractice.

The Adversarial System

Civil disputes, such as medical malpractice lawsuits, are resolved in an adversarial model, in which advocates for each side argue before an impartial party.[5] In contrast to the adversarial system, an inquisitorial system is usually used in continental European countries, where the civil law systems are derived from Roman law or the Napoleonic code. In such systems, magistrates and judges independently investigate the facts of the dispute and decide the outcome.

The patient who files a legal complaint and seeks remedy from the court is called the plaintiff, and the party against whom the complaint is directed is the defendant. In medical malpractice cases, the defendant is usually a physician, a medical laboratory, a hospital, or a professional organization to which the physician belongs. In litigation, cases are identified by citing the plaintiff first; thus a lawsuit is cited as plaintiff versus defendant. In the complaint, the plaintiff will set forth the specific alleged wrongs committed by the defendant physician with a demand for relief.

Legal Elements of Medical Malpractice

To gain judicial relief for the alleged harm, the plaintiff must prove four basic legal requirements, also known as elements.[6] The first element is a duty of care that is invoked whenever a professional relationship is established between the patient and the physician. The general notion of a legal duty is that, in a civilized society, each person owes a duty of reasonable care to others. Practically, this element is the easiest to prove because a duty is assumed whenever a physician undertakes the care of a patient.

The second legal requirement is to show that a breach of duty occurred; the plaintiff must invoke the concept of standard of care. The standard of care generally refers to the level of care that a reasonable, similarly situated professional would have provided to the patient. Expert witness testimony is usually needed to explain to lay jurors the standard of care that should apply to the alleged medical misconduct.

The third required element is causation. A breach of duty may be a quality concern for the doctor and/or the hospital, but a breach is legally meaningless unless it causes an injury to the patient. The plaintiff must show a causal nexus between the alleged misconduct and the injury sustained.

The fourth and final element of a medical malpractice lawsuit is that of damages that should be amenable to calculation. Because monetary damages are easy to calculate and administer, a medical malpractice claim will usually determine an amount of monetary damage suitable to compensate the injured patient. Punitive damages are rare in medical malpractice cases and typically apply only in cases of egregious conduct that society wants to deter, such as the deliberate destruction of medical records or sexual misconduct toward a patient.

Pretrial and Trial Litigation

As is the case in other civil disputes, medical malpractice lawsuits rarely reach court trial. The US legal system relies on adversarial advocacy by respective attorneys, which is intended to promote the efficient self-resolution of disputes. After a lawsuit is filed, the important phase of discovery is set in motion so that the disputing parties can exchange relevant factual information. Discovery is facilitated by requests for documents, interrogatories, and depositions. Contrary to a popular misconception, neither party can introduce surprise evidence during the court trial. Legal discovery is designed to allow the respective parties to understand the facts and the relative strengths and weaknesses of both sides of the dispute, with the hopeful goal of mutual understanding, settlement, and judicial economy.

At trial, the plaintiff (through his or her attorney) must prove (to some legally required standard of proof) each and every element required to establish medical malpractice. This generally means that the plaintiff's attorney must convince the jury that it was more likely than not that the physician was negligent. Any assertions by the physician's attorney to the contrary are called defenses. Defenses serve to negate or cast doubt on the evidence presented by the aggrieved plaintiff. The more likely than not standard of legal proof that the plaintiff must overcome is also called the preponderance of evidence standard, and it is less stringent than the beyond reasonable doubt standard required to convict criminal defendants. In medical malpractice cases, an impartial jury, after hearing and considering all of the information discovered by the respective parties, must find a greater than 50% probability that professional negligence occurred to return a verdict against the physician.

The Costs of Medical Malpractice Litigation

The trial skills of the respective attorneys can influence the outcome of medical malpractice litigation. The demeanor and presentation of the defendant physician are equally important because jurors attach great importance to the testimony of the physician. The plaintiff's attorneys are hired by the patient, usually on the basis of a contingency fee, whereby the attorneys collect a fee only if monetary damages are awarded. This system has been criticized because it can encourage medical malpractice lawsuits and unscrupulous advocacy on behalf of patients and can discourage meritorious medical malpractice lawsuits with a low chance of substantial monetary recovery.[7]

Defense attorneys are appointed on behalf of the physician by the medical malpractice insurance company; legal fees are paid by the insurance company, even though the attorney's client is the physician being represented. A physician named as a defendant in medical malpractice litigation in the United States can hire personal counsel to provide additional guidance, review, and insight at the physician's expense.

Medical malpractice lawsuits are time- and resource-consuming events and can be emotionally exhausting. Many lawsuits are settled out of court on terms agreed on by both parties, with a monetary payment made by the physician's insurance company. Medical malpractice litigation may lead to increased medical costs for patients because of increased resource consumption from defensive practices undertaken by the physician to avoid future claims.[8] Many physicians agree to settlements to avoid the nuisance, harassment, and the financial risk inherent in jury trials.[9] It is worth noting that monetary payments, even if paid through a pretrial settlement, are usually reported to a national practitioner databank, state medical licensing boards, and medical societies. Although the goal of such reporting practices may be related to quality assurance, the advantages of these mechanisms remain unproven.[10]

In addition to the substantial financial costs, there is a personal cost to medical malpractice litigation. Physicians are usually unaware of the intricate logistics, structure, and functioning of the legal system until faced with a lawsuit alleging medical malpractice. Even a jury verdict in favor of the defendant physician can take a heavy toll in terms of personal stress, discouragement, professional dissatisfaction, and time commitment to the process.

Although the losing party of a medical malpractice lawsuit can appeal the verdict, the US legal system is extremely deferential to the finality of a jury trial; successful legal appeals usually concern a specific point of law or procedure that may have been misapplied during the trial. The practical implication is that medical malpractice cases are won or lost at trial; thus, physician preparation, participation, involvement, and cooperation with the defense counsel are very important.

The Malpractice Litigation Process

Factors Influencing the Attorney's Selection of the Plaintiff's Case

Understanding how and why an attorney decides to prosecute a medical malpractice lawsuit may affect the way a physician manages his or her public persona on websites and in social media. When the patient first meets with his or her prospective attorney, an interview is generally conducted to elicit the events that transpired during treatment from the patient's perspective. Often, a patient is prompted to seek an attorney's advice because of an adverse outcome and negative feelings toward the physician. The adverse outcome may be a well-known complication of a particular procedure, such as a postoperative infection, or some completely unforeseeable event, such as a perioperative hemorrhage from a previously undiagnosed hematologic disorder. On many occasions, the physician is not aware that the patient is angry.[11,12]

After hearing the patient's story, the prospective plaintiff's attorney will perform a cost-benefit analysis to evaluate certain financial factors related to the case, including the value of the patient's injury based on similar case settlements and/or jury verdicts; the likelihood of obtaining a settlement and/or a favorable jury verdict based on an evaluation of the strength of the patient's case and the attorney's evaluation of the physician as a potential witness; the financial investment needed to cover anticipated court costs, expert witness costs, and the time and energy needed to prosecute the case; and the length of time required for the attorney to receive a return on his or her investment of time and financial resources, either through settlement or a favorable jury verdict.

The physician can influence whether the plaintiff's attorney will reject the case by leading the attorney to conclude that the patient's case is weak and/or nonexistent. Maintaining a favorable public persona and a well-documented medical record will assist the physician in deterring lawsuits.

The plaintiff's attorney will likely investigate the physician's reputation in the community, use Internet searches to locate relevant information in the public domain (such as social media sites), review published literature to determine whether the patient's care was consistent with generally accepted practices, and access website pages maintained by the physician or affiliated organizations. In addition, many jurisdictions, such as New York state, now have searchable websites that provide information on a health-

care provider's involvement in lawsuits,[13] whether there has been a settlement or adverse verdict against the provider over a set period of years,[14] or whether there are any public documents regarding professional misconduct and disciplinary actions taken against a physician.[15]

If the plaintiff's prospective attorney finds evidence that the involved physician has been named in numerous malpractice lawsuits that have resulted in either a settlement or an adverse verdict or has been subjected to professional disciplinary action, the attorney may be more likely to take the case. A history of poor outcomes for the physician in prior litigation may make it more likely that the plaintiff's attorney would obtain a settlement offer because the physician may be viewed as too high a risk for litigation. If the physician has a website or a social media presence that reflects a less-than-professional persona, either based on photographs or comments, the plaintiff's attorney may conjecture that the physician will not present himself or herself well at a deposition and/or before a jury.

Factors That Decrease the Likelihood of Being Sued

From a risk avoidance standpoint, one of the most important factors in determining whether a physician will be sued is the physician's demeanor or (more specifically) the quality of the physician's communication skills.[16,17] The well-being of patients hinges on not only the treating physician's diagnostic and technical skill level but also how well the physician communicates with the patient, the patient's family, and other healthcare providers. Disputes regarding the information communicated, when it was communicated, and who provided the communication can often result in he said/she said arguments that, in the ab-

sence of well-documented medical records, are often determined by the jury's perception of who is more credible.

Thorough medical records that adequately explain and re-create the care provided and the rationale for the medical judgments made can enhance a physician's credibility with the plaintiff's attorney and increase the likelihood of a favorable legal outcome. The physician is not expected to be correct 100% of the time, but the law requires that reasonable judgment be exercised in caring for patients and that the standard of care be met. A complete and accurate medical record can support the physician's fulfillment of these requirements.

The statute of limitations allows a period of time after an alleged malpractice incident during which a patient can file a lawsuit (for example, New York State allows 2.5 years).[18] Without thorough medical records, it is unlikely that a physician will remember the critical details of the patient's care after a lapse of months or years. A physician's lack of recall in the face of a patient's testimony that he or she clearly remembers what happened during treatment can become a focal point in the attempt to discredit the physician.

Medical records made at or near the time of the physician's care of the patient are critical in convincing a plaintiff's attorney (and a jury if the case is prosecuted) that any harm incurred by the patient was an unfortunate event but was not caused by malpractice. Good medical records are clear and concise and provide a roadmap of the physician's thoughtful assessment and reasonable investigation of the patient's complaints, subsequent appropriate treatment recommendations, and evaluation of the effectiveness of the treatment plan. The medical record should include factual and objective observations (who, what, where, when, and how) and a precise record of important comments made by the patient in quotation marks (such as "my pain is all gone") or any inappropriate behavior by the patient (yelling at the receptionist). The medical record should document key details regarding informed consent discussion with the patient, with the names of any family member or concerned parties present; the use of appropriate teaching tools, including an interpreter if needed; the patient's consent/assent to the proposed treatment course, using consent forms if appropriate; and instances of noncompliance, missed appointments, and appropriate follow-up with the patient.[19,20]

A patient who is not incapacitated can refuse to consent to a proposed diagnostic workup or treatment plan, even though the treating physician and others might deem it an unreasonable medical choice. It is critical to document the patient's refusal of any tests or treatment recommended by the physician. Depending on the potential negative effect on the patient's wellbeing, the physician should consider sending a letter to the patient that includes his or her diagnosis and recommendations, indicating why the patient should reevaluate his or her decision. A copy of the letter should be kept in the medical record.

The medical record should be devoid of pejorative or subjective comments that may create a negative impression about the physician's concern or regard for the patient. Notes should be reviewed with a critical eye. The standard of professionalism for medical record keeping applies to all written communications, including e-mails, which can be discoverable evidence.

If a critical piece of information was omitted or if some information is mistakenly included, the medical record should be amended following acceptable practices. The new entry should

be added or the incorrect information should be deleted by drawing a single line through it; the change should then be initialed with the date and time. The change of record must be obvious so that there is no allegation that the record was inappropriately altered. If medical records are altered, the case is generally indefensible because the physician has lost credibility.

Partnering With the Defense Attorney

It is critical for the physician to actively engage with his or her attorneys in preparing the defense. Litigation is a foreign and artificial environment for a physician, but the physician's medical knowledge is a valuable aspect of the defense. Although an attorney can learn much about the technical aspects involved, it is unlikely that he or she will be able to equal the physician level of knowledge, which was mastered through years of education, training, and experience.

In preparing for deposition, the physician will need to spend time with his or her attorney to become familiar with the records and anticipate the lines of questioning. The physician should answer only the questions asked and not volunteer any information. It may be difficult for a physician to refrain from trying to educate the plaintiff's attorney.

The physician's attorney may need assistance in selecting appropriately credentialed experts. Although there are many well-credentialed orthopaedic surgeons available, not all surgeons would make appropriate expert witnesses. The questions to consider are as follows: How will a jury respond to the expert? Does the expert have personality traits that might detract from his or her message? Does he or she have the expertise to be a credible witness for the case? The physician's attorney can provide advice on the credentials the

expert must have to testify because requirements vary from jurisdiction to jurisdiction.

The physician should be present at the trial to show the jury that he or she is as committed to the outcome of the trial as the patient. If scheduling will not allow the physician to attend the trial for the entire day, it is important to make an appearance for some portion of the day, especially for opening statements, the patient's testimony, the expert witness testimony, and summations.

Common Pitfalls in Managing Suspected Musculoskeletal Tumors

Pitfalls are unapparent sources of trouble or danger, hidden hazards, or unforeseen or unexpected difficulties that usually produce a negative result. Orthopaedic oncology has potential pitfalls because many neoplastic processes simulate nononcologic orthopaedic conditions. Many conditions seen in patients have similar and sometimes identical presenting signs and symptoms, imaging characteristics, and gross appearances.[21] As is the case in most medical and surgical specialty and subspecialties, an accurate diagnosis is the key to successful treatment.[22,23] In the subspecialty of musculoskeletal (orthopaedic) oncology, a correct and timely diagnosis is even more crucial.[21,24]

More than 60% of malpractice claims made in general orthopaedics are directly related to the diagnosis and performance of the correct procedure. In addition, erroneous surgical procedures result in increased morbidity for patients.[25] Local tumor recurrence and the ability to perform limb-preserving surgery are affected by misdiagnoses and performing erroneous surgical procedures.[25,26] There is some evidence that a delayed diagnosis can negatively affect a patient's chance of survival.[24]

Workup

The importance of proper musculoskeletal tumor staging cannot be overstated. Staging involves proper imaging, laboratory analyses, and biopsy.[25] Imaging always begins with plain radiography. In many instances, the differential diagnosis can be narrowed down considerably based on the radiographic findings. When a lesion is identified by radiography, the need for further imaging is based on whether the lesion is thought to be a primary bone tumor or metastatic in origin. Primary bone tumors that are believed to be malignant are further characterized with MRI of the affected bone, a whole body bone scan, and CT of the chest. For bone tumors believed to be benign, a plain radiograph alone is often sufficient, although axial imaging of the affected bone may be required for further characterization of the lesion. The workup for suspected metastatic disease typically includes a whole body bone scan and CT of the chest, the abdomen, and the pelvis to identify the primary tumor site. All processes suspicious of a malignancy should also be evaluated with a serum chemistry analysis, including alkaline phosphatase, lactate dehydrogenase, and a complete blood count. For metastatic disease, serum and urine protein analyses and electrophoresis may be included to rule out myeloma and check for the presence of some of the common cancer antigens, such as prostate-specific antigen and CA-125 protein, when indicated.

After the appropriate imaging studies are completed, a biopsy specimen must be obtained for histologic analysis to establish a diagnosis. Based on the results of the imaging studies, a differential diagnosis is formulated, and the biopsy technique can be determined.[27] Biopsy can be performed with needle, open incisional, and open excisional techniques.[27] Needle or core needle biopsies and those using an open incisional technique are the most commonly performed biopsy procedures. Open biopsies require considerable planning, including a determination of the correct approach and incision, attention to meticulous hemostasis, adequate lesion sampling, and proper wound closure.[28,29] Excisional biopsies are rarely performed by nononcologic orthopaedic surgeons and are most appropriate for small, nonmalignant tumors.[30] In many instances, small lesions treated with excisional biopsy are found to be malignant. This increases the risk of inadvertent contamination of the surrounding tissues, which leads to more complex surgery at the time of reexcision.[30] If an intraoperative frozen section is performed, the adequacy of the lesional tissue is the first priority.[31] When the definitive diagnosis is made, it must coincide with the expected differential diagnosis. If this is not the case, more tissue from another zone must be obtained or another biopsy must be performed. Inadequate tissue or negative biopsy results do not justify performing a definitive procedure.

The type of biopsy chosen usually depends on the expertise of the treating surgeon or his or her institution. The importance of following good biopsy principles cannot be overstated. The biopsy is the first step in successful limb salvage surgery. If there is high suspicion for a primary malignant bone or soft-tissue tumor, the biopsy is best performed by the surgeon who will ultimately perform the definitive procedure.

Definitive Treatment

The timing of the definitive surgical treatment is the most problematic aspect of inadvertent procedures.[25] It is unwise to proceed with any definitive treatment in the absence of a diagnosis. Many misconceptions exist that lead to untimely and inappropriate treatment of pathologic bony lesions.

(1) It is believed that the bone must be fixed regardless of the histopathologic results; however, the method used to fix the bone is dependent on the underlying pathology. For example, sarcomas always require wide excision. Even if the bone is fractured, complete excision can often be successfully performed if contamination can be controlled. Rodding a sarcoma will almost always lead to amputation.

(2) It is believed that the lesion needs to be removed; however, the method used to remove the lesion is dependent on the pathologic diagnosis. Removing tumors in a piecemeal fashion increases the area of contamination that must be addressed at the time of the definitive procedure.

(3) It is believed that reaming material can be sent for biopsy analysis; however, intramedullary reaming materials are burnt, crushed pieces of tissue that are very difficult for a pathologist to analyze. Often, reaming material is nondiagnostic and should never be sent as the true biopsy sample.

(4) It is believed that a definitive procedure is appropriate because the needle biopsy result was negative. Any biopsy, but especially a needle biopsy, can render a false negative result. If the biopsy result does not match the suspected clinical or imaging diagnosis, the biopsy should be repeated. After the definitive diagnosis is made, the definitive procedure can be performed.

Case Examples

The following case examples are helpful in demonstrating some common pitfalls and errors in the treatment of patients with musculoskeletal tumors.

Case 1

A 32-year-old woman with hip pain and a limp for 2 months presented for treatment with an avulsion fracture of

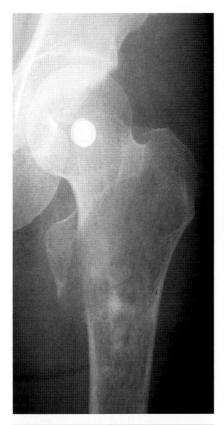

Figure 1 AP radiograph of the proximal femur and hip of a patient with an avulsion fracture of the lesser trochanter, which is a common indication for malignancy. The femur also shows increased radiodensities that are consistent with malignant bone formation.

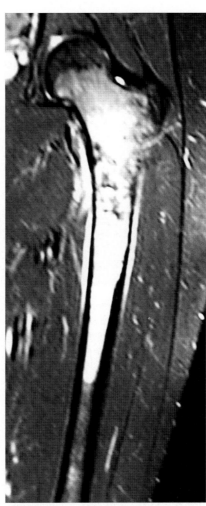

Figure 2 T2-weighted coronal MRI scan showing extensive bone marrow replacement of the femoral shaft is suspicious for malignancy.

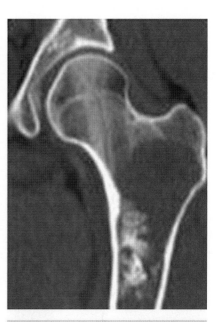

Figure 3 Coronal CT scan showing new bone formation in the endosteal space is suspicious for osteosarcoma.

the lesser trochanter of the femur (**Figure 1**). The presumptive diagnosis of an aneurysmal bone cyst was made.

MRI and CT scans were obtained (**Figures 2** and **3**). The patient was treated with osteosynthesis using a sliding hip screw and polymethyl methacrylate cement (**Figure 4**). Tissue sent for routine pathologic analysis revealed a high-grade osteosarcoma. The patient subsequently was treated with neoadjuvant chemotherapy and tumor restaging. Extensive surgery was required, including a large soft-tissue resection and subtotal femoral replacement.

The pitfalls in treating this patient were (1) assuming an incorrect diagno-

sis of an aneurysmal bone cyst, (2) performing a definitive procedure after the biopsy but before the biopsy results were available, and (3) performing a surgical procedure inadequate to treat the high-grade osteosarcoma found in the final diagnosis.

In formulating a differential diagnosis, the clinical and imaging features indicating a possible malignancy included the presence of indolent hip pain in a 32-year-old woman, radiographic evidence of an avulsion fracture of the lesser trochanter matrix, and radiodensities in the lesion seen on the CT scan.

Case 2

A 60-year-old man presented to the emergency department after a low-energy traumatic fall. Plain radiography showed a base cervical hip fracture (**Figure 5**). A presumptive diagnosis of metastatic disease was made, and the patient underwent a surgical procedure (**Figure 6**). Reamings were sent to pathology. The final pathology results showed high-grade intramedullary sarcoma. To obtain a clear margin, a high amputation was required because of massive contamination from the large soft-tissue mass.

The pitfalls in treating this patient included (1) the limited staging of the lesion with a lack of necessary imaging (CT and MRI) before surgery, (2) assuming an incorrect diagnosis (metastatic carcinoma), (3) performing a surgical procedure before the biopsy results were obtained, and (4) performing a surgical procedure that was inadequate based on the final diagnosis.

The initial imaging studies showed a suspected malignant lesion (tumor).

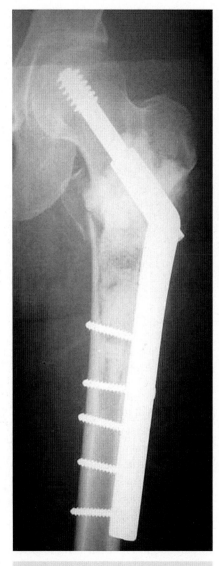

Figure 4 Postoperative AP radiograph after intralesional excision and osteosynthesis with a sliding hip screw and cement on a lesion found to be osteosarcoma.

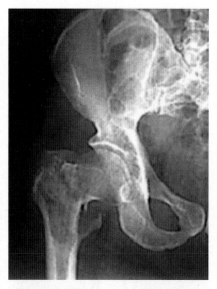

Figure 5 AP radiograph of the hip of a 60-year-old man with a pathologic peritrochanteric fracture with the appearance of metastatic carcinoma.

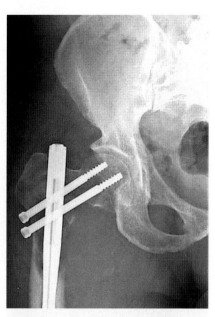

Figure 6 AP radiograph of the hip of the patient in Figure 5 after nailing of the peritrochanteric pathologic fracture. Note the absence of polymethyl methacrylate cement and the insufficient fracture fixation.

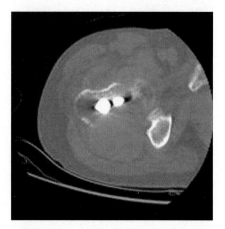

Figure 7 CT scan of the trochanter of the patient in Figure 5 showing the postoperative nail in place adjacent to a large soft-tissue mass.

The diagnosis of presumed metastatic disease cannot be definitively made without staging, which should include CT, laboratory analyses (including prostate-specific antigen and serum and urine protein electrophoresis) to evaluate for the most common primary malignancies in a male patient. The CT and MRI studies obtained after the surgical procedure showed a large soft-tissue mass, which is typical for a sarcoma and would have prompted a biopsy, not a definitive surgical procedure (**Figure 7**).

Case 3

An 11-year-old boy fell from a trampoline and sustained an injury (**Figure 8**). There also was a fallen fragment sign. MRI showed a lesion consistent with a fibrous tumor (**Figure 9**). The differential diagnosis included a bone cyst and a fibrous lesion. At the time of surgery, some of the lining of the lesion was sent for pathologic analysis, but the cystic nature of the lesion could not be confirmed. Because of the benign appearance of the lesion and the fallen fragment sign, a benign process was assumed; however, a decision was made to place the patient in skeletal traction and wait for the final pathology findings. The pathology results showed telangiectatic osteosarcoma. The patient was placed in a long-leg spica cast and started on neoadjuvant therapy. Three months later, the patient was treated with limb-preserving intercalary resection and allograft placement.

The pitfall in treating this patient was assuming an incorrect diagnosis of a benign process; however, after biopsy, the treating medical team chose the correct approach by deciding not to proceed without a definitive diagno-

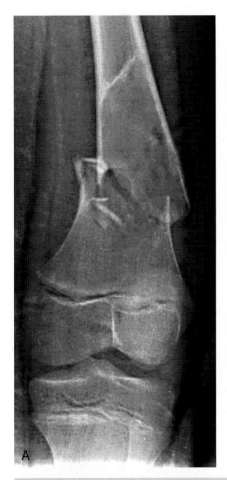

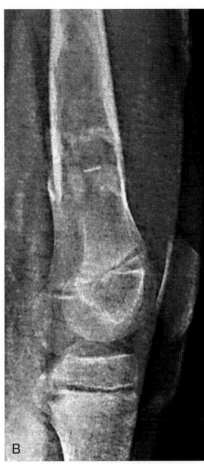

Figure 8   AP (**A**) and lateral (**B**) radiographs of the distal femur showing a benign-appearing lesion and an apparent fallen fragment sign, indicating a possible bone cyst.

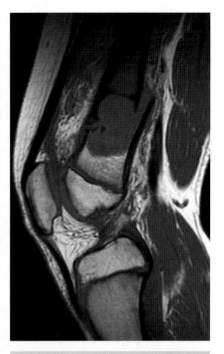

Figure 9   Sagittal T1-weighted MRI scan of a benign-appearing intramedullary lesion of the distal femur.

sis because the cystic nature of the lesion had not been confirmed by pathology.

Making the correct diagnosis is mandatory in orthopaedics, especially for suspected musculoskeletal lesions. Staging and adequate biopsy results are required. Confirming a final pathologic diagnosis that conforms to the differential diagnosis is required before surgical intervention.

Summary

Avoiding common pitfalls in managing patients with suspected musculoskeletal neoplasms is the key to good patient care. Although musculoskeletal tumors are uncommon, the associated pitfalls in managing patients with these tumors are common. The most common pitfalls leading to allegations of medical malpractice involve obtaining an incorrect diagnosis and performing the procedure for that diagnosis. When faced with a medical malpractice lawsuit, familiarity with aspects of the malpractice litigation process will be helpful to an orthopaedic surgeon.

References

1. Jena AB, Seabury S, Lakdawalla D, Chandra A: Malpractice risk according to physician specialty. *N Engl J Med* 2011;365(7):629-636.

2. Lundy DW: Trends in medical liability coverage for orthopaedic surgeons: Fellowship survey finds 92 percent of trial cases decided for defendant. *AAOS Now*. Feb 2012. http://www.aaos.org/news/aaosnow/feb12/managing5.asp. Accessed April 29, 2013.

3. White GE: *Tort Law in America: An Intellectual History.* New York, NY, Oxford University Press, 2003.

4. Speiser SM, Krause CF, Gans AW: *The American Law of Torts.* Rochester, NY, Lawyers Cooperative Publishing Company, 1987.

5. Richards EP, Rathbun KC: *Medical Care Law.* New York, NY, Aspen Publishers, 1999.

6. Gittler GJ, Goldstein EJ: The elements of medical malpractice: an overview. *Clin Infect Dis* 1996;23(5):1152-1155.

7. Fisher TL: Medical malpractice in the United States: A review. *Can Med Assoc J* 1974;110(1):102-103.

8. Roberts B, Hoch I: Malpractice litigation and medical costs in Mississippi. *Health Econ* 2007; 16(8):841-859.

9. Peeples R, Harris CT, Metzloff TB: Settlement has many faces: Physicians, attorneys and medical malpractice. *J Health Soc Behav* 2000;41(3):333-346.

10. Paterick TJ, Paterick TE, Waterhouse BE: The fundamentals of liability insurance: Physician and organization perspectives. *J Med Pract Manage* 2007;23(3): 151-156.

11. Clark A: Discovery by plaintiff of defendant, in *NYSBA CLE Coursebook: Medical Malpractice 2012.* Albany, NY, New York State Bar Association, 2012, pp 167-170.

12. Regan J, Lange F: Discovery/ deposition (by plaintiff of defendant), in *NYSBA CLE Coursebook: Medical Malpractice 2012.* Albany, NY, New York State Bar Association, 2012, pp 195-199.

13. eCourts: Web civil local. New York State Unified Court System website. https:// iapps.courts.state.ny.us/ webcivilLocal/LCMain. Accessed July 25, 2013.

14. New York State Physicians Profile website. http:// www.nydoctorprofile.com/. Accessed July 25, 2013.

15. Physician and physician assistants disciplinary and other actions. New York State Department of Health website. http:// www.health.ny.gov/professionals/ doctors/conduct/. Accessed July 25, 2013.

16. ECRI Institute: Healthcare Risk Control Supplement A: Communication. 2009. https:// www.ecri.org/Forms/Documents/ Communication.pdf. Accessed April 30, 2013.

17. Hickson GB, Jenkins AD: Identifying and addressing communication failures as a means of reducing unnecessary malpractice claims. *N C Med J* 2007;68(5): 362-364.

18. New York Code, Civil Practice Law and Rules. Article 2, Section 214-a: Action for medical, dental or podiatric malpractice to be commenced within two years and six months: Exceptions. New York, CVP Law § 214-a.

19. Rozovsky F: *Consent to Treatment: A Practical Guide*, ed 4. New York, NY, Aspen Publishers, 2007, pp 12.3-12.18

20. CRICO staff: Documentation dos and don'ts. Controlled Risk Insurance Company (CRICO) and Risk Management Foundation of the Harvard Medical Institutions. 2002. https:// www.rmf.harvard.edu/Clinician-Resources/Article/2002/ Documentation-Dos-and-Donts. Accessed April 30, 2013.

21. Gould CF, Ly JQ, Lattin GE Jr, Beall DP, Sutcliffe JB III: Bone tumor mimics: Avoiding misdiagnosis. *Curr Probl Diagn Radiol* 2007;36(3):124-141.

22. Epstein JB, Sciubba JJ, Banasek TE, Hay LJ: Failure to diagnose and delayed diagnosis of cancer: Medicolegal issues. *J Am Dent Assoc* 2009;140(12):1494-1503.

23. Kern KA: Medicolegal analysis of the delayed diagnosis of cancer in 338 cases in the United States. *Arch Surg* 1994;129(4):397-403, discussion 403-404.

24. Rougraff BT, Davis K, Lawrence J: Does length of symptoms before diagnosis of sarcoma affect patient survival? *Clin Orthop Relat Res* 2007;462:181-189.

25. Ayerza MA, Muscolo DL, Aponte-Tinao LA, Farfalli G: Effect of erroneous surgical procedures on recurrence and survival rates for patients with osteosarcoma. *Clin Orthop Relat Res* 2006; 452:231-235.

26. Gandhi TK, Kachalia A, Thomas EJ, et al: A study of closed malpractice claims. *Ann Intern Med* 2006;145(7):488-496.

27. Adams SC, Potter BK, Pitcher DJ, Temple HT: Office-based core needle biopsy of bone and soft tissue malignancies: An accurate alternative to open biopsy with infrequent complications. *Clin Orthop Relat Res* 2010;468(10): 2774-2780.

28. Bickels J, Jelinek JS, Shmookler BM, Neff RS, Malawer MM: Biopsy of musculoskeletal tumors: Current concepts. *Clin Orthop Relat Res* 1999;368:212-219.

29. Weber KL: What's new in musculoskeletal oncology. *J Bone Joint Surg Am* 2005;87(6):1400-1410.

30. Mankin HJ, Lange TA, Spanier SS: The hazards of biopsy in patients with malignant primary bone and soft-tissue tumors. *J Bone Joint Surg Am* 1982;64(8): 1121-1127.

31. Ashford RU, McCarthy SW, Scolyer RA, Bonar SF, Karim RZ, Stalley PD: Surgical biopsy with intra-operative frozen section: An accurate and cost-effective method for diagnosis of musculoskeletal sarcomas. *J Bone Joint Surg Br* 2006;88(9):1207-1211.

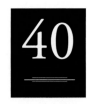

Contemporary Management of Metastatic Bone Disease: Tips and Tools of the Trade for General Practitioners

Robert H. Quinn, MD
R. Lor Randall, MD
Joseph Benevenia, MD
Sigurd H. Berven, MD
Kevin A. Raskin, MD

Abstract

Metastatic bone disease has a significant effect on a patient's mortality and health-related quality of life. An aging US population and improved survival rates of patients with cancer have led to an increase in the incidence of symptomatic bony metastatic lesions that may require orthopaedic care. Skeletal-related events in neoplastic disease include pain, pathologic fracture, hypercalcemia, and neural compression, including spinal cord compression. The clinical evaluation and diagnostic study of a patient with a skeletal lesion of unknown etiology should be approached carefully.

In patients with widespread metastatic disease, the treatment of a skeletal-related event may be limited to stabilization of the pathologic fracture or local disease control. The treatment of metastatic bone disease is guided by the nature of the skeletal-related event, the responsiveness of the lesion to adjuvant care, and the overall condition and survival expectations of the patient. Impending pathologic fractures are often more easily treated, with less morbidity and easier recovery for patients, than completed fractures. Quality of life is the most important outcome measure in these patients.

When surgery is indicated, the approach, choice of fixation, and use of adjuvant should allow for immediate and unrestricted weight bearing. Because metastatic lesions to the skeleton have a limited capacity for spontaneous healing, surgical fixation should be durable for the life expectancy of the patient. In the epiphyseal region of long bones, replacement arthroplasty is generally preferred over internal fixation. Metaphyseal and diaphyseal regions can generally be addressed with intramedullary nailing or plate fixation with adjuvant. The specific treatment of acetabular lesions is dictated by the anatomy and the degree of bone loss. Spinal stability and neural compromise are important considerations in choosing a strategy for managing spine tumors. Effective surgical approaches to metastatic disease of the spine may include vertebral augmentation or open decompression and realignment of the spinal column with internal fixation. Radiation therapy is an important adjunctive modality in the treatment of metastatic bone disease. Medical management consists of symptom control, cytotoxic chemotherapy, and targeted therapy. Emerging technologies, including radiofrequency ablation, cementoplasty, and advances in intraoperative imaging and navigation, show promise in the treatment of metastatic bone disease.

Instr Course Lect 2014;63:431-441.

Metastatic bone disease has a substantial effect on mortality and health-related quality of life. The aging of the population in the United States and the improved survival rate of patients with cancer have led to an increase in the prevalence of osseous metastatic lesions that are symptomatic and may require orthopaedic care. Skeletal-related events in neoplastic disease include pain, pathologic fracture, hypercalcemia, and neural compression,

Table 1
Tumor Characteristics

Primary Tumor	Common Type of Bone Destruction	Fracture Healing[a] (%)	5-Year Relative Survival Rates With Distant Metastases[b] (%)	Radiosensitivity[c]
Breast	Mixed	37	23.8	+++
Lung	Lytic	0	3.7	++
Thyroid	Lytic	NA	53.9	++
Kidney	Lytic	44	11.6	−
Prostate	Blastic	42	27.8	+++
Melanoma	Lytic	NA	15.1	++

[a]Data are from the study by Gainor and Buchert.[4]
[b]Data are from the American Cancer Society.[5]
[c]Radiosensitivity was rated as high (+++), intermediate (++), low (+), or none (−).
NA = not available.

including spinal cord compression. Metastatic bone disease develops annually in approximately 400,000 patient in the United States, and bone is the fourth most common metastatic site, after the lymphatic system, lung, and liver.[1-3] Bone metastases develops in 70% of patients with metastatic breast or prostate cancer compared with 20% to 30% of patients with metastatic lung or gastrointestinal cancers.[2] Patients with breast cancer experience a mean of 2.2 to 4.0 skeletal events annually, whereas patients with prostate cancer experience a mean of 1.5 skeletal events.[3] The general orthopaedic practitioner is the primary evaluator and treating physician for an increasing population of patients with skeletal events. The purpose of this chapter is to review contemporary strategies for the management of metastatic bone disease.

Prognosis in metastatic bone disease is determined by the primary tumor and cell type. **Table 1** illustrates some of these differences as well as current survival estimates.[4,5] **Figure 1** shows a pathologic fracture related to metastatic breast carcinoma that healed after internal fixation and radiation. Accurate diagnosis and staging of metastatic bone disease are fundamental to guiding an evidence-based approach to management.

Diagnosis
The clinical evaluation and diagnostic studies of a patient who presents with a skeletal lesion of unknown etiology should be approached carefully and thoughtfully. Although the approach should be individualized, a general workup might include any of the tests shown in **Table 2** in addition to a complete history and physical examination. This workup identifies 85% of primary lesions;[6] another 10% are identified by biopsy. The remaining 5% of lesions generally remain undiagnosed despite extensive workup and biopsy. It is important to recognize primary bone tumors, or solitary or oligometastatic tumors, because the goals of treatment may include complete local resection to improve survival. Even a patient with a known primary and/or known metastatic disease may warrant a biopsy of the new lesion for confirmation, especially if the patient has been disease free for a prolonged period of time, and if the lesion is not characteristic of the known primary tumor.

Indications for Treatment
Treatment of metastatic bone disease is guided by the nature of the skeletal-related event, the responsiveness of the

Dr. Quinn or an immediate family member serves as a board member, owner, officer, or committee member of the American Academy of Orthopaedic Surgeons, the Musculoskeletal Tumor Society, and the Wilderness Medical Society. Dr. Randall or an immediate family member has received research or institutional support from the Musculoskeletal Transplant Foundation and serves as a board member, owner, officer, or committee member of the American Academy of Orthopaedic Surgeons, the American Orthopaedic Association, the American Society of Clinical Oncology, the Association of Bone and Joint Surgeons, Children's Oncology Group, the Connective Tissue Oncology Society, the Musculoskeletal Transplant Foundation, the Musculoskeletal Tumor Society, the National Comprehensive Cancer Network, and the MHE Research Foundation. Dr. Benevenia or an immediate family member is a member of a speakers' bureau or has made paid presentations on behalf of the Musculoskeletal Transplant Foundation; serves as an unpaid consultant to Merete; has received research or institutional support from Biomet, the Musculoskeletal Transplant Foundation, and Synthes; and serves as a board member, owner, officer, or committee member of the Musculoskeletal Transplant Foundation and the Musculoskeletal Tumor Society. Dr. Berven or an immediate family member has received royalties from Medtronic; is a member of a speakers' bureau or has made paid presentations on behalf of Medtronic Sofamor Danek, DePuy, and Globus Medical; has stock or stock options held in Baxano, Simpirica, Providence Medical, Asix, and AccuLif; has received research or institutional support from the Orthopaedic Research and Education Foundation, the AO Foundation, and Medtronic Sofamor Danek; and serves as a board member, owner, officer, or committee member of Bone and Joint Decade USA, the North American Spine Society, and the Scoliosis Research Society. Dr. Raskin or an immediate family member serves as an unpaid consultant to Kinetic Concepts.

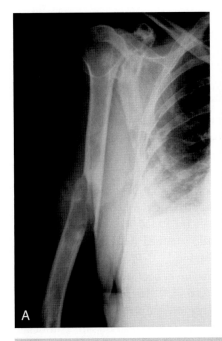

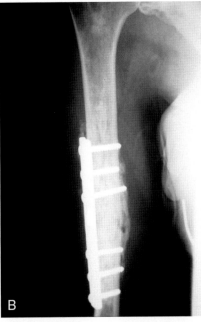

Figure 1 A pathologic fracture of the humerus developed in a patient with metastatic breast carcinoma. **A,** Preoperative AP radiograph of the humerus shows the pathologic fracture. **B,** Radiograph made after internal fixation and radiation therapy shows healing of the fracture.

Table 2

Testing Considerations for Workup of a New Skeletal Lesion

Laboratory Studies

Complete blood cell count with differential

Electrolytes, blood urea nitrogen, and/or creatinine

Erythrocyte sedimentation rate

Liver function tests

Urinalysis

Calcium

Prostate-specific antigen

Carcinoembryonic antigen

Serum protein electrophoresis and immunoelectrophoresis

Radiographic Studies

CT of chest, abdomen, and pelvis

Whole-body bone scan

Whole-body PET and/or CT scan

PET = positron emission tomography.

lesion to adjuvant care, and the overall condition and survival expectation of the patient. Pathologic fractures are an important cause of morbidity and mortality in patients with metastatic bone disease. Pathologic fractures have a diminished ability to heal spontaneously. Fracture stabilization with internal fixation or arthroplasty may substantially improve patient mobility and quality of life. In the lower extremity and spine, internal fixation should be performed in most patients expected to survive another 6 to 12 weeks. Although morbidity and even mortality (8% for a total hip replacement) can be high, intervention substantially improves the quality of remaining life.[7] In the upper extremity, conservative measures are more likely to be successful, particularly in patients with a limited life expectancy.

Impending pathologic fractures are often more easily treated, with less morbidity and easier recovery, than completed fractures. The rating system

Table 3

Mirels Rating System for the Prediction of Pathologic Fracture Risk

Score	Site	Nature	Size[a]	Pain
1	Upper extremity	Blastic	< 1/3	Mild
2	Lower extremity[b]	Mixed	1/3 to 2/3	Moderate
3	Peritrochanteric	Lytic	> 2/3	Functional

[a]Relative proportion of bone width involved by tumor.
[b]Nonperitrochanteric lower extremity.

described by Mirels[8] (**Table 3**) is the most widely used predictor of pathologic fracture, and its use has demonstrated 91% sensitivity and 35% specificity.[9] Prophylactic fixation is recommended with a score of 9 or more and should be considered with a score of 8. Those with a score of less than 8 should be considered for local irradiation. The final decision to perform surgery should also consider individual patient-related factors, such as the patient's size and activity level.

The Spine Instability Neoplastic Score (SINS) classification system was developed by an expert panel to estimate the stability of tumors affecting the spinal column[10] (**Table 4**). The SINS classification is based on tumor behavior and the radiographic and clinical presentation of the patient with a tumor affecting the spine. Patients with a score of less than 8 points have a stable spinal column and are at low risk for spontaneous vertebral fracture. Patients with a score of 8 to

Table 4
Spinal Instability Neoplastic Score (SINS; May 2008)

Description	Score (Points)[a]
I. Location (3-point maximum)[b]	
Junctional (Occ–C2, C-T, TL, LS)	3
Midcervical (C3-C6) or lumbar (L2-L4)	2
Thoracic (T3-T9)	1
Sacroiliac	1
II. Pain (4-point maximum)	
Movement-related pain[c] (VAS score of > 5)	4
Movement-related pain (VAS score of < 5)	2
III. Bone response (2-point maximum)	
Lytic	2
Mixed	1
Other	0
IV. Radiographic features (6-point maximum)	
A. Alignment	
Subluxation and/or translation (> 3 mm)	6
De novo deformity (scoliosis and/or kyphosis)	2
B. Bone involvement (lytic only)	
Bilateral PLC involvement	2
Unilateral PLC involvement	1
Vertebral body lytic region of more than 50% (no collapse)	1
C. Collapse and/or fracture (lytic only)	
Bilateral PLC involvement	4
Unilateral PLC involvement	3
Vertebral body collapse of ≥ 50%	3
Vertebral body collapse of < 50%	2

[a]The maximum score is 15 points. A score less than 8 points indicates stability; 8 to 12 points, possible instability; and more than 12 points, instability.
[b]Use the highest scoring region if lesion spans multiple regions.
[c]Structural or neural pain, localized to the level of the tumor.
Occ = occiput, C-T = cervical to thoracic, TL = thoracolumbar, LS = lumbosacral region, VAS = visual analog scale, PLC = posterolateral complex (includes occipital condyles, facets, pedicles, and costovertebral joints).
(Adapted with permission from Fisher CG, DiPaola CP, Ryken TC, et al: A novel classification system for spinal instability in neoplastic disease: An evidence-based approach and expert consensus from the Spine Oncology Study Group. *Spine (Phila Pa 1976)* 2010;35(22):E1221-1229.)

12 points are at intermediate risk of spinal column fracture or deformity, and patients with a score of more than 12 points are at high risk.

General Considerations of Surgical Treatment

Occasionally, the patient with a solitary or oligometastatic disease should have a resection of the disease. Although cure likely occurs quite rarely, evidence has suggested that aggressive management of an isolated metastasis can prolong patient survival and improve palliation.[11,12] These benefits are most likely to become manifest in patients with an isolated metastasis occurring after a prolonged disease-free interval after treatment of a localized primary tumor. Aggressive surgical management of a solitary thyroid metastasis much more often results in cure or at least substantial prolongation of survival.

Improved quality of life is the goal. When surgical intervention is indicated, the surgical approach, choice of fixation, and use of adjuvant (polymethyl methacrylate [PMMA] or bone graft alternatives) should allow immediate and unrestricted weight bearing without splint, cast, brace, or assistive device. Surgical fixation should be durable for the life expectancy of the patient. PMMA is often used to provide immediate strength to the fixation.[13-18] PMMA is most beneficial in noncontained metaphyseal or acetabular defects when combined with internal fixation, and it can improve screw fixation in pathologic bone. The exothermic polymerization reaction may kill tumor cells and minimize blood loss.[19] Biologic agents not only require time for incorporation (during which activity must often be restricted) but also may be limited by treatment and host factors. The surgical construct should be expected to last for the lifetime of the patient and, depending on the primary tumor and its susceptibility to adjuvants, may need to incorporate the possibility of local tumor progression.

All areas of weakened bone present at the time of surgery as well as all areas likely to be weakened subsequently should be addressed in any planned reconstruction. Perioperative planning should include imaging of the entire bone and whole-body bone scan. CT and three-dimensional reconstructions are recommended for metastatic lesions in the periacetabular region and the spine to estimate the extent of osteolysis and compromise of cortical boundaries. MRI is useful to assess epidural extension of the tumor and neural compromise in patients with metastatic disease affecting the spine. In the peripheral skeleton, MRI may overestimate the extent of tumor involvement to the bone and soft tissues and offers poor assessment of the integrity of bone cortices and internal architecture. Other advanced imaging may include preoperative arteriography for assessing the vascularity of metastatic lesions. Highly vascular lesions, including renal cell cancer, may benefit from preoperative embolization before resection or instrumentation to limit intraoperative bleeding.[20]

In the extremity long bones, both intramedullary and plate fixation are viable options, and current evidence, beyond biomechanical theory, does not support one intervention over the other. Intramedullary fixation provides the option of including most of the long bone in the reconstruction so that local extension of disease will have a limited effect on the stability of the fracture; however, the need to do so remains controversial. At least one study has demonstrated that prophylactic treatment of uninvolved areas of the bone has a much higher chance of causing complications related to the extended fixation than generating a benefit from the prophylaxis because substantial disease progression in uninvolved areas is a rare event.[21] In more limited areas of bone involvement, plate fixation allows better segmental defect reconstruction and realignment. Plate fixation is generally superior for addressing metaepiphyseal lesions, except in the proximal aspect of the femur. Although specific recommendations regarding the choice of implant and the extent of fixation are not well supported by evidence, the general principle is that the chosen reconstruction should allow immediate and unrestricted weight bearing, should not require osseous healing for success, and should allow for some degree of disease progression. It would follow, therefore, that intramedullary devices should be statically locked, locking plates should be considered where appropriate, and

the extent of fixation proximal and distal to the lesion should be sufficient to best ensure a solid construct and allow for some local tumor progression. Endoprosthetic reconstruction is generally the procedure of choice for tumors with extensive epiphyseal involvement and periarticular fractures not amenable to stable fixation. Specific strategies for surgical management of metastatic disease to skeletal regions are detailed in the following section.

Upper Extremity

The management of metastatic disease to the bones of the upper extremity is more elective than the treatment of metastatic disease to the lower extremity because the patient can usually be comfortable and active with nonsurgical treatment, although surgical fixation often improves function.

This chapter's authors recommend curettage and reconstruction with a plate, screws, and PMMA for lesions in the proximal part of the humerus if there is sufficient bone; otherwise, a cemented hemiarthroplasty is recommended if the tuberosities are preserved or proximal humeral endoprosthetic replacement if they are not. Diaphyseal lesions without segmental bone loss may be treated with plate fixation and PMMA or intramedullary rod with or without PMMA. When there is a large segmental loss, an intercalary replacement (endoprosthesis or allograft) is often necessary. Distal humeral lesions should be treated with column reconstruction using plate fixation and PMMA. Olecranon osteotomy should be avoided if possible because healing may be impaired by radiation. Total elbow replacement should be considered with substantial epiphyseal destruction.

Metastatic involvement distal to the elbow is rare. Lesions of the forearm are generally best treated with plate fixation and PMMA.

Lower Extremity
Pelvis and/or Acetabulum

Patients with painful metastases involving the non–weight-bearing areas of the ilium, ischium, pubis, and sacroiliac joints are treated effectively with radiation therapy.

Tumors involving the periacetabular pelvis are challenging.[22-24] **Table 5** shows a contemporary adaptation of the classic Harrington system for classifying and managing acetabular deficiencies. This chapter's authors recommend nonsurgical management initially because many patients respond favorably to radiation. Protrusion of the femoral head into the pelvis is not an emergency, is not associated with intrapelvic complications, and does not dramatically alter the reconstruction; therefore, prophylactic surgery done solely in an effort to prevent protrusio is not warranted. **Figure 2** shows an example of an acetabular metastasis with protrusio before and after reconstruction.

Femoral Head and Neck

Endoprosthetic reconstruction is the treatment of choice in this location because of the high risk of failure associated with internal fixation of existing or impending pathologic fractures.[25,26]

Intertrochanteric Femoral Involvement

In the presence of limited bone loss, curettage of the tumor, packing of the defect with PMMA, and stabilization with a hip screw side plate or an intramedullary hip screw are satisfactory options. Beyond biomechanical theory, there is a lack of evidence to support one technique over the other. PMMA strengthens the reconstruction, particularly with a noncontained defect. There is no evidence to support curettage of the tumor per se beyond what is necessary to facilitate the reconstruction. With more extensive bone loss, endoprosthetic reconstruc-

Table 5

Contemporary Adaptation of the Harrington Classification System

Acetabular Defect Type	Anatomic Description	Method of Reconstruction
I	Lateral cortices and superior and medial parts of wall are structurally intact	Conventional cemented THA
II	Medial wall is deficient	Reconstruction of defect with PMMA and protrusio cup with cemented THA
III	Superior and lateral walls are deficient	Reconstruction of defect with PMMA reinforced with screws, protrusio cup, and cemented THA
IV	Pelvic discontinuity	Reconstruction of defect with PMMA reinforced with screws, protrusio cage with ischial fixation, and cemented THA
V	Total acetabular destruction or resection for cure	Saddle prosthesis or durable reconstruction (structural allograft, custom prosthesis) if cure potential is high

PMMA = polymethyl methacrylate, THA = total hip arthroplasty.
(Reproduced from Quinn RH: Surgical management of lower extremity metastatic disease, in Schwartz HS, ed: *Orthopaedic Knowledge Update Musculoskeletal Tumors*, ed 2. Rosemont, IL, American Academy of Orthopaedic Surgeons, 2007, pp 383-391.)

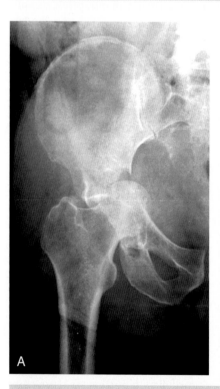 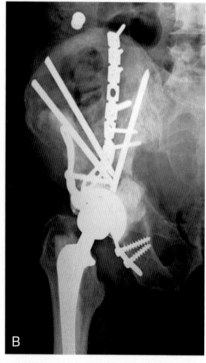

Figure 2   **A,** Preoperative AP radiograph showing a pathologic fracture of the acetabulum with protrusion in a patient with acetabular metastasis. **B,** Radiograph made after reconstruction with internal fixation, PMMA, a protrusion cage, a constrained liner, and a cemented femoral stem.

tion should be considered with reconstruction of the calcar through implant selection or PMMA. In the presence of extensive involvement of the greater trochanter, a proximal femoral replacement prosthesis is indicated.

Subtrochanteric Femoral Involvement

Forces in this region may reach six times body weight, placing extreme demands on fixation devices.[27] Second- and third-generation intramedullary re- construction nails are generally the treatment of choice in this area and allow for an array of fixation alternatives in both proximal and distal interlocking. The use of a proximal femoral replacement prosthesis should be considered when proximal bone is unlikely to provide stable fixation with nails despite the use of PMMA, if previous fixation has failed, or with extensive peritrochanteric tumor involvement. The disadvantages of the routine use of these prostheses include cost, the need for increased exposure, bleeding, neurovascular injury, and hip abductor muscle weakness.[28,29]

Femoral Shaft

Closed intramedullary nailing is appropriate for small tumors. Larger lesions with open section defects may require open curettage with PMMA in addition to internal fixation. Routine treatment of the entire bone with a reconstruction type of intramedullary nail remains controversial but should be considered in patients with prolonged life expectancy and multiple myeloma. A few large diaphyseal lesions require a modular intercalary prosthesis. Rarely, a total femoral replacement is needed for the patient with extensive involvement of the femur.

Distal Part of the Femur and Proximal Part of the Tibia

Smaller lesions in this area may be treated with osteosynthesis and PMMA. Large destructive lesions in the distal aspect of the femur and proximal part of the tibia should be treated with plate fixation when the articular surface can be maintained and the joint is otherwise normal. When the articular surface cannot be maintained, or the patient has advanced osteoarthritis, a total knee replacement is indicated. With extensive bone loss, proximal tibial replacement may be required. The extensor mechanism should be preserved when possible. When the patellar tendon attachment cannot be preserved, extensor mechanism reconstruction can be performed; however, the necessary use of muscle flaps and the complex rehabilitation required must be balanced with patient survival considerations.

Tibial Shaft and Distal End of the Leg

Lesions in the tibia and foot are rare. Small radiosensitive lesions can be treated with plate fixation and PMMA. Intramedullary nailing is a favorable option in the tibial shaft. As in the femoral and humeral shafts, segmental defects may be addressed with a modular intercalary prosthesis if necessary (**Figure 3**). Occasionally, below-knee amputation is required for advanced refractory disease that is causing substantial impairment.

Spine

The spine represents the most common site for metastatic disease to the skeleton. Tumors affecting the spinal column have a substantial and measurable effect on health-related quality of life in affected patients. Specific do-

mains affected include pain, physical function, neural function, mental health, and social function. Outcome instruments specific for patients with tumors affecting the spine may be more responsive to change than generic health outcomes measurement instruments.[30]

Spinal stability measured by the SINS classification system and neural compromise are important considerations in choosing a strategy for managing tumors affecting the spine. For patients with a stable spine and a radioresponsive tumor, radiation therapy is generally considered the treatment of choice. Confocal beam radiation may considerably improve the dose of radiation at the site of the tumor while protecting adjacent tissues. However, radiation therapy has limited use in patients with an unstable spine, a fracture of a vertebra, or neural impairment caused by a tumor or bone compressing the neural elements.

Effective surgical approaches to metastatic disease include vertebral augmentation or open decompression and realignment of the spinal column with internal fixation. Vertebral augmentation with kyphoplasty or vertebroplasty can be effective in stabilizing a pathologic vertebral fracture in most levels of the spine.[31] A percutaneous approach to vertebral augmentation permits stabilization of the spine with limited morbidity. Vertebral augmentation is especially effective for patients with myeloma of the spine and patients with vertebral lesions without extension to the epidural space and without neural compromise.[32] Vertebral augmentation may be followed within days by radiation therapy to limit local recurrence of disease.

Patients with metastatic disease affecting the spinal column and neural compromise as a result of epidural extension of tumor or fracture or spinal deformity are candidates for open de-

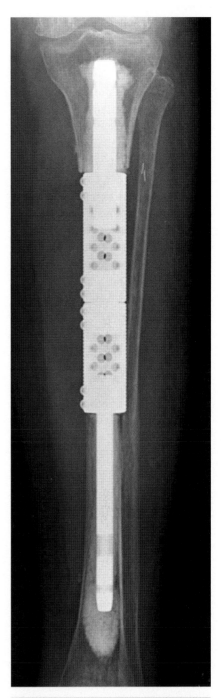

Figure 3 Radiograph showing an intercalary prosthesis used to reconstruct a segmental tibial defect.

compression of the neural elements and primary reconstruction of the spine with internal fixation with or without vertebral augmentation. Patchell et al[33] reported considerably better improvements with regard to pain and neural function in patients with metastatic tumor affecting the spine and spinal cord compression who were treated with open decompression and stabilization of the spine with instrumentation and radiation compared with those who had radiation therapy alone. Tokuhashi et al[34] developed a scoring system for tumors affecting the spine that is useful in guiding a surgical approach to patients with metastatic disease affecting the spine. This system considers the primary tumor type, the stage of disease, the overall patient condition, and the neural status of the patient in recommending options including nonsurgical and surgical care.

En bloc resection may be indicated for solitary and oligometastatic disease with treatable metastases. An effective en bloc resection requires an excision of the affected segments of the spinal column, including extraosseous extension of the tumor. Survival in selected patients treated with an en bloc resection is improved compared with intralesional approaches.[35,36] The surgical staging system of Boriani et al[37] is useful in planning margins for resection. The en bloc resection is not appropriate for patients with tumor extending to the epidural space or patients with substantial comorbidities and limited life expectancy.

Adjuvant and Alternative Modalities

Radiation Therapy

Radiation therapy is an important adjunctive modality in the treatment of metastatic bone disease. It may be used prophylactically for lesions at risk for subsequent fracture. Perioperative external beam radiation therapy is associated with a decrease in the rates of secondary procedures and the improved functional status of patients with previously unirradiated long bone, acetabular, and spinal lesions. Additionally, it

minimizes disease progression and risk of implant failure.[38] Postoperative irradiation does not appear to have a significant effect on callus formation and does not adversely affect PMMA strength.[39] Hypofractionation (single dose) compared with standard course (approximately 2-week) therapy is currently under investigation at some centers. Confocal beam radiation may be useful in targeting tumor specifically and limiting damage to surrounding radiosensitive tissues, especially for metastatic bone lesions affecting the spine and epidural space. Confocal beam radiation therapy may also permit repeat treatment of regions that have been treated previously with a maximal tolerable dose of external beam therapy.

All tumors are sensitive to radiation therapy; however, the doses required to achieve a response are widely variable by tumor type. So-called radiosensitive or radioresponsive tumors tend to respond to lower doses of irradiation and include myeloma, lymphoma, breast, and prostate carcinomas (**Table 1**). So-called radioresistant tumors, such as renal cell carcinomas and sarcomas, require much higher doses. Lung and thyroid carcinomas and melanoma generally demonstrate intermediate responsiveness.

Medical Management

Medical management consists of symptom control, cytotoxic chemotherapy, and targeted therapy. Although a detailed discussion of these modalities is beyond the scope of this chapter, a concise review of targeted therapy is relevant.

Bisphosphonates, pyrophosphate analogs that bind calcium and concentrate in bone, are ingested by osteoclasts, causing inhibition of pyrophosphate and osteoclast cell death. Bisphosphonates also inhibit growth in tumor cell lines, decrease the motil-

ity of tumor cells, demonstrate synergy with cytotoxic chemotherapy, decrease metastatic spread in mouse models, and may have immunomodulatory properties on T cell activation.

In clinical trials of breast cancer patients, intravenous bisphosphonates have decreased skeletal-related events, improved symptoms, and decreased locoregional and distant recurrence.[40] Improvement with regard to symptoms and skeletal-related events also has been shown with prostate and lung cancers and multiple myeloma. Oral forms have shown equivocal results. Risks of bisphosphonates include renal insufficiency, hypocalcemia, osteonecrosis of the jaw, and subtrochanteric stress fractures.

Angiogenesis inhibitors (thalidomide and bevacizumab) selectively target endothelial cells, thus inhibiting tumor angiogenesis.

Osteoblastic metastases are mediated by osteoblasts. Breast and prostate cancer models implicate endothelin-1, which stimulates osteoblasts, in this process. Prostate-specific antigen affects parathyroid hormone-related protein and may activate other growth factors. Calcitriol (vitamin D_3) and endothelin-A receptor inhibitors (atrasentan and ZD4054) selectively target osteoblast activity.

Osteolytic metastases are mediated by osteoclast activity. In tumor models, interleukin-6 upregulation affects tumor cells and osteoclasts; receptor activator of nuclear factor-κB ligand (RANKL) elaboration from tumor cells decreases production of osteoprotegerin; and parathyroid hormone-related protein binding to stromal parathyroid hormone receptor-1 increases RANKL, which increases osteoclast activity. These factors, along with other complex factors within the bone-tumor milieu, precipitate bone demineralization, which releases bone morphogenetic protein, insulin-like growth factor-1, and transforming growth factor-β, which in turn feed tumorigenesis, resulting in a vicious cycle. The drug denosumab directly binds RANKL, downregulating osteoclast activity, and may be beneficial.

Emerging Technologies
Radiofrequency Ablation

Radiofrequency ablation is a high-frequency alternating current used to destroy tumor cells. Radiofrequency ablation can be used to control local tumor growth, prevent recurrence, palliate symptoms, and extend survival duration for patients with certain tumors. It can be performed as an open surgical procedure, laparoscopically, or percutaneously with ultrasound or CT. Radiofrequency ablation may be combined with conventional therapies or other percutaneous treatments such as cementoplasty.

Cementoplasty

Percutaneous injection of PMMA, with or without radiofrequency ablation, has demonstrated proven utility in the treatment of metastatic bone disease in both the spine and extremities. Although long-term results for the treatment of osteoporotic compression fractures have been equivocal,[41,42] improved results have been demonstrated in the treatment of osseous spine metastases.[31,32] Palliative improvements in the extremities, acetabulum, and sacrum have also been reported.[43-48]

Although these procedures are often performed by physicians who are not orthopaedic surgeons, it is important to maintain a multidisciplinary approach with orthopaedic input in an effort to minimize complications.[49] The ability to care for spinal metastasis with comprehensive approaches, ranging from percutaneous to open approaches, empowers the orthopaedic surgeon to remain central to patient care through the spectrum of metastatic bone disease.

Summary

Metastatic bone disease remains a challenging orthopaedic problem. However, appropriate multidisciplinary interventions can decrease the prevalence of skeletal-related events and have a profound effect on the quality of life of affected patients. Interventions on the horizon show promise in improving the ability to address challenges and further improve patient care and outcomes.

References

1. Mundy GR: Metastasis to bone: Causes, consequences and therapeutic opportunities. *Nat Rev Cancer* 2002;2(8):584-593.

2. Coleman RE, Rubens RD: The clinical course of bone metastases from breast cancer. *Br J Cancer* 1987;55(1):61-66.

3. Body JJ: New developments for treatment and prevention of bone metastases. *Curr Opin Oncol* 2011;23(4):338-342.

4. Gainor BJ, Buchert P: Fracture healing in metastatic bone disease. *Clin Orthop Relat Res* 1983;178: 297-302.

5. *American Cancer Society: Cancer Facts & Figures 2012.* Atlanta, GA, American Cancer Society, 2012.

6. Rougraff BT, Kneisl JS, Simon MA: Skeletal metastases of unknown origin: A prospective study of a diagnostic strategy. *J Bone Joint Surg Am* 1993;75(9):1276-1281.

7. Quinn RH, Drenga J: Perioperative morbidity and mortality after reconstruction for metastatic tumors of the proximal femur and acetabulum. *J Arthroplasty* 2006; 21(2):227-232.

8. Mirels H: Metastatic disease in long bones: A proposed scoring system for diagnosing impending pathologic fractures. *Clin Orthop Relat Res* 1989;249:256-264.

9. Damron TA, Morgan H, Prakash D, Grant W, Aronowitz J, Heiner J: Critical evaluation of Mirels' rating system for impending pathologic fractures. *Clin Orthop Relat Res* 2003;(415):S201-S207.

10. Fisher CG, DiPaola CP, Ryken TC, et al: An evidence-based approach and expert consensus from the Spine Oncology Study Group. *Spine (Phila Pa 1976)* 2010; 35(22):E1221-E1229.

11. Jung ST, Ghert MA, Harrelson JM, Scully SP: Treatment of osseous metastases in patients with renal cell carcinoma. *Clin Orthop Relat Res* 2003;409:223-231.

12. Alt AL, Boorjian SA, Lohse CM, Costello BA, Leibovich BC, Blute ML: Survival after complete surgical resection of multiple metastases from renal cell carcinoma. *Cancer* 2011;117(13):2873-2882.

13. Harrington KD, Johnston JO, Turner RH, Green DL: The use of methylmethacrylate as an adjunct in the internal fixation of malignant neoplastic fractures. *J Bone Joint Surg Am* 1972;54(8):1665-1676.

14. Harrington KD, Sim FH, Enis JE, Johnston JO, Diok HM, Gristina AG: Methylmethacrylate as an adjunct in internal fixation of pathological fractures: Experience with three hundred and seventy-five cases. *J Bone Joint Surg Am* 1976;58(8):1047-1055.

15. Jacofsky DJ, Haidukewych GJ: Management of pathologic fractures of the proximal femur: State of the art. *J Orthop Trauma* 2004; 18(7):459-469.

16. Li Z, Butala NB, Etheridge BS, Siegel HJ, Lemons JE, Eberhardt AW: A biomechanical study of periacetabular defects and cement filling. *J Biomech Eng* 2007; 129(2):129-136.

17. Murray PJ, Damron TA, Green JK, Morgan HD, Werner FW: Contained femoral defects: Bio-

mechanical analysis of pin augmentation in cement. *Clin Orthop Relat Res* 2004;420:251-256.

18. Weiner M, Damron TA, Patterson FR, Werner FW, Mann KA: Biomechanical study of pins in cementing of contained proximal tibia defect. *Clin Orthop Relat Res* 2004;419:232-237.

19. Toy PC, France J, Randall RL, Neel MD, Shorr RI, Heck RK: Reconstruction of noncontained distal femoral defects with polymethylmethacrylate and crossed-screw augmentation: A biomechanical study. *J Bone Joint Surg Am* 2006;88(1):171-178.

20. Owen RJ: Embolization of musculoskeletal bone tumors. *Semin Intervent Radiol* 2010;27(2):111-123.

21. Alvi HM, Damron TA: Prophylactic stabilization for bone metastases, myeloma, or lymphoma: Do we need to protect the entire bone? *Clin Orthop Relat Res* 2013;471(3):706-714.

22. Harrington KD: The management of acetabular insufficiency secondary to metastatic malignant disease. *J Bone Joint Surg Am* 1981;63(4):653-664.

23. Benevenia J, Cyran FP, Biermann JS, Patterson FR, Leeson MC: Treatment of advanced metastatic lesions of the acetabulum using the saddle prosthesis. *Clin Orthop Relat Res* 2004;426:23-31.

24. Wunder JS, Ferguson PC, Griffin AM, Pressman A, Bell RS: Acetabular metastases: Planning for reconstruction and review of results. *Clin Orthop Relat Res* 2003;(415):S187-S197.

25. Keating JF, Burke T, Macauley P: Proximal femoral replacement for pathological fracture. *Injury* 1990;21(4):231-233.

26. Lane JM, Sculco TP, Zolan S: Treatment of pathological fractures of the hip by endoprosthetic replacement. *J Bone Joint Surg Am* 1980;62(6):954-959.

27. Frankel VH, Burstein AH: *Orthopaedic Biomechanics: The Application of Engineering to the Musculoskeletal System*. Philadelphia, PA, Lea & Febiger, 1970, pp 24-28.

28. Sim FH, Frassica FJ, Chao EY: Orthopaedic management using new devices and prostheses. *Clin Orthop Relat Res* 1995;312:160-172.

29. Ashford RU, Hanna SA, Park DH, et al: Financial implications for sarcoma units. *Int Orthop* 2010;34(5):709-713.

30. Street J, Lenehan B, Berven S, Fisher C: Introducing a new health-related quality of life outcome tool for metastatic disease of the spine: Content validation using the International Classification of Functioning, Disability, and Health; on behalf of the Spine Oncology Study Group. *Spine (Phila Pa 1976)* 2010;35(14):1377-1386.

31. Fourney DR, Schomer DF, Nader R, et al: Percutaneous vertebroplasty and kyphoplasty for painful vertebral body fractures in cancer patients. *J Neurosurg* 2003;98(1):21-30.

32. Hussein MA, Vrionis FD, Allison R, et al: The role of vertebral augmentation in multiple myeloma: International Myeloma Working Group Consensus Statement. *Leukemia* 2008;22(8):1479-1484.

33. Patchell RA, Tibbs PA, Regine WF, et al: Direct decompressive surgical resection in the treatment of spinal cord compression caused by metastatic cancer: A randomised trial. *Lancet* 2005;366(9486):643-648.

34. Tokuhashi Y, Matsuzaki H, Oda H, Oshima M, Ryu J: A revised scoring system for preoperative evaluation of metastatic spine tumor prognosis. *Spine (Phila Pa 1976)* 2005;30(19):2186-2191.

35. Cloyd JM, Acosta FL Jr, Ames CP: En bloc resection for primary and metastatic tumors of the spine: A systematic review of the literature. *Neurosurgery* 2010;67(2):435-444, discussion 444-445.

36. Tomita K, Kawahara N, Murakami H, Demura S: Total en bloc spondylectomy for spinal tumors: Improvement of the technique and its associated basic background. *J Orthop Sci* 2006;11(1):3-12.

37. Boriani S, Weinstein JN, Biagini R: Primary bone tumors of the spine: Terminology and surgical staging. *Spine (Phila Pa 1976)* 1997;22(9):1036-1044.

38. Townsend PW, Smalley SR, Cozad SC, Rosenthal HG, Hassanein RE: Role of postoperative radiation therapy after stabilization of fractures caused by metastatic disease. *Int J Radiat Oncol Biol Phys* 1995;31(1):43-49.

39. Murray JA, Bruels MC, Lindberg RD: Irradiation of polymethylmethacrylate: In vitro gamma radiation effect. *J Bone Joint Surg Am* 1974;56(2):311-312.

40. Theriault RL, Lipton A, Hortobagyi GN, et al: Pamidronate reduces skeletal morbidity in women with advanced breast cancer and lytic bone lesions: A randomized, placebo-controlled trial. Protocol 18 Aredia Breast Cancer Study Group. *J Clin Oncol* 1999;17(3):846-854.

41. Kallmes DF, Comstock BA, Heagerty PJ, et al: A randomized trial of vertebroplasty for osteoporotic spinal fractures. *N Engl J Med* 2009;361(6):569-579.

42. Buchbinder R, Osborne RH, Ebeling PR, et al: A randomized trial of vertebroplasty for painful osteoporotic vertebral fractures. *N Engl J Med* 2009;361(6):557-568.

43. Anselmetti GC, Manca A, Ortega C, Grignani G, Debernardi F, Regge D: Treatment of extraspinal painful bone metastases with percutaneous cementoplasty: A pro-

spective study of 50 patients. *Cardiovasc Intervent Radiol* 2008; 31(6):1165-1173.

44. Basile A, Giuliano G, Scuderi V, et al: Our experience. *Radiol Med* 2008;113(7):1018-1028.

45. Carrafiello G, Laganà D, Pellegrino C, et al: Percutaneous imaging-guided ablation therapies in the treatment of symptomatic bone metastases: Preliminary experience. *Radiol Med* 2009; 114(4):608-625.

46. Munk PL, Rashid F, Heran MK, et al: Combined cementoplasty and radiofrequency ablation in the treatment of painful neoplastic lesions of bone. *J Vasc Interv Radiol* 2009;20(7):903-911.

47. Jakanani GC, Jaiveer S, Ashford R, Rennie W: Computed tomography-guided coblation and cementoplasty of a painful acetabular metastasis: An effective palliative treatment. *J Palliat Med* 2010;13(1):83-85.

48. Basile A, Tsetis D, Cavalli M, et al: Sacroplasty for local or massive localization of multiple myeloma. *Cardiovasc Intervent Radiol* 2010;33(6):1270-1277.

49. Dayer R, Peter R: Percutaneous cementoplasty complicating the treatment of a pathologic subtrochanteric fracture: A case report. *Injury* 2008;39(7):801-804.

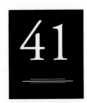

The Basic Science Behind Biologic Augmentation of Tendon-Bone Healing: A Scientific Review

Kenneth D. Weeks III, MD
Joshua S. Dines, MD
Scott A. Rodeo, MD
Asheesh Bedi, MD

Abstract

Rotator cuff tears are common musculoskeletal injuries that often require surgical repair. Despite advances in surgical techniques, including progression from a single row of anchors to double-row constructs, recurrent tearing or failure to heal still complicates 10% to 94% of repairs. The surgical treatment of rotator cuff tears is aimed at providing the best mechanical environment for tendon healing. Despite appropriate surgical management and a normal healing response, the resultant tendon healing does not regenerate the tendon-bone architecture initially formed during prenatal development. Instead, a mechanically weaker, fibrovascular scar is formed, leading to suboptimal healing rates and/or higher retear rates. Biologic augmentation strategies aim to improve healing rates by introducing higher concentrations of growth factors and cytokines, mesenchymal stem cells, and enzymatic antagonists to the repair site in the hope of directing a more sophisticated healing response. Biologic augmentation and tissue engineering to improve tendon-to-bone healing remains promising but will require more study before its clinical application is realized.

Instr Course Lect 2014;63:443-450.

Rotator cuff tears are common musculoskeletal injuries that often require surgical repair. Despite advances in ar-throscopy and minimally invasive surgical techniques, including progression from a single row of anchors to double-row constructs, recurrent tearing or failure to heal still complicates the repair of many large and massive tear patterns.[1,2] A recent systematic review by Duquin et al[3] showed that in all tears larger than 1 cm, double-row constructs, including arthroscopic transosseous equivalent repairs, led to improved healing rates. However, despite the superiority of double-row repairs, the rate of recurrent tears still approached 25%. Poorer clinical outcomes and reduced strength have been documented in patients with persistent rotator cuff defects compared with patients with structurally intact repairs. For this reason, improving structural healing rates continues to be a focus of basic science research.[4] A better understanding of the biology of tendon-to-bone healing may suggest novel therapeutic options that will lead to improved rates of healing at the enthesis after a surgical repair.

Tendon-to-Bone Healing: Overview

Before evaluating the role of biologic augmentation to improve healing of the tendon-bone interface after a rota-

Dr. Dines or an immediate family member has received royalties from Biomet; serves as a paid consultant to or is an employee of Biomimetic, CONMED Linvatec, and Tornier; and has received research or institutional support from Biomimetic. Dr. Rodeo or an immediate family member serves as a paid consultant to or is an employee of Smith & Nephew and has stock or stock options held in Cayenne Medical. Dr. Bedi or an immediate family member serves as a paid consultant to or is an employee of Smith & Nephew; has stock or stock options held in A3 Surgical; and serves as a board member, owner, officer, or committee member of the American Orthopaedic Society for Sports Medicine. Neither Dr. Weeks nor any immediate family member has received anything of value from or has stock or stock options held in a commercial company or institution related directly or indirectly to the subject of this chapter.

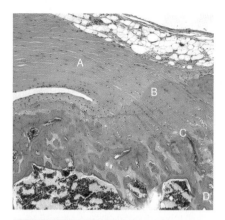

Figure 1 Histology of the rotator cuff enthesis. The native tendon-bone interface is composed of four distinct transition zones, which are defined by their collagen content. (A) The tendinous zone contains fibroblast and mainly types I and III collagen. (B) The unmineralized fibrocartilage zone contains fibrochondrocytes and types I, II, and III collagen. (C) The mineralized fibrocartilage zone contains hypertrophic fibrochondrocytes and primarily types I, II, and X collagen. (D) The bone portion of the enthesis contains osteoblasts, osteocytes, and osteoclasts and only type I collagen.

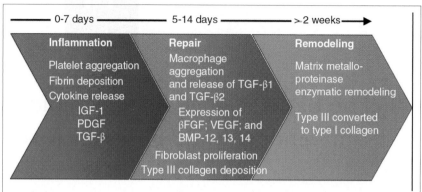

Figure 2 Illustration of the three phases of tendon-bone healing. BMP = bone morphogenetic protein, IGF-1 = insulin-like growth factor-1, PDGF = platelet-derived growth factor, VEGF = vascular endothelial growth factor.

tor cuff repair, it is helpful to review the developmental biology of the rotator cuff enthesis and the biologic process that occurs during healing. The native tendon-bone interface is composed of four distinct transition zones: the tendon proper, the unmineralized fibrocartilage, the mineralized fibrocartilage, and the bone[5] (**Figure 1**). The function of the insertion-site architecture is to minimize stress forces propagated to the bone from the muscle-tendon unit. The four transition zones are defined by their differences in collagen content. The tendinous zone is composed mainly of type I and III collagen, whereas the fibrocartilaginous zone contains types I, II, and III collagen. The mineralized fibrocartilaginous zone has primarily types I, II, and X collagen, whereas the

bone portion of the enthesis consists solely of type I collagen.

Tendon-to-bone healing occurs through a three-phase repair process of inflammation, repair, and remodeling (**Figure 2**). During the early stages of the inflammatory phase, fibrin and fibronectin are deposited by platelets within the hematoma. In addition, platelets release key cytokines, including insulin-like growth factor-1, platelet-derived growth factor (PDGF), and transforming growth factor-β (TGF-β), which signal an influx and aggregation of macrophages at the repair site.[6] The inflammatory phase is classically considered to last 7 to 8 days after injury or surgery. Macrophages then release TGF-β1, TGF-β2, and, to a lesser extent, TGF-β3, resulting in fibroblastic cell proliferation and early matrix (scar) formation. This process marks the transition from the inflammatory phase to the repair phase. The activation of fibroblasts leads to the expression of many new growth factors, including basic fibroblast growth factor (FGF), insulin-like growth factor-1, PDGF-β, vascular endothelial growth factor, and bone morphogenetic protein (BMP)-12, BMP-13, and BMP-14, as well as the deposition of type III collagen. During

the final remodeling phase, the scar, composed primarily of type III collagen, undergoes significant remodeling of type III to type I collagen over the course of weeks to months, which is largely mediated by a set of enzymes known as matrix metalloproteinases (MMPs).[7]

Surgical treatment of rotator cuff tears is aimed at providing the best mechanical environment for tendon healing; however, the resultant tendon healing does not regenerate the native tendon-bone architecture. Instead, an interposed fibrovascular scar is formed at the tendon-bone interface that remodels with time, leading to a histologically and mechanically inferior repair. Many factors are currently being investigated for use in rotator cuff repair (**Figure 3**).

Growth Factors

The first phase of tendon-bone healing is defined by inflammatory cell influx to the repair site. Within this inflammatory milieu is a large quantity of cytokines and growth factors (PDGF, TGF-β, BMP, and FGF) that play a critical role in cell proliferation, differentiation, and matrix synthesis. Significant preclinical investigation has been undertaken to gain a better understanding of the temporal expression

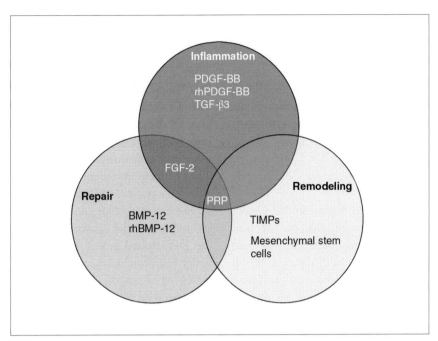

Figure 3   Illustration of the relationship between biologic augmentation therapies and healing phases. rhPDGF = recombinant human platelet-derived growth factor, rhBMP = recombinant human bone morphogenetic protein, PRP = platelet-rich plasma, TIMPs = tissue inhibitors of matrix metalloproteinases.

and importance of these growth factors, as well as opportunities to use them to improve healing at the rotator cuff enthesis. Cytokines have long been studied for their role in improving connective tissue healing. The basic rationale is that cytokines play fundamental roles in cell proliferation, chemotaxis, angiogenesis, and matrix synthesis. However, the traditional cytokines that have been studied the most (PDGF, TGF-β, and FGF) are well known to lead to fibrosis. These cytokines improve the structural properties of the tissue by inducing the formation of scar tissue, but the microstructure and the composition of the tissue remains abnormal, and the material properties are not improved. The factors that may be able to positively affect the cellular and molecular aspects of tendon biology include transcription factors and other novel signaling molecules. Several of these factors are reviewed in this chapter.

Platelet-Derived Growth Factor

PDGF comes from both platelets and smooth muscle cells. Its highest concentration occurs between 7 and 14 days after a tendon injury, which corresponds to the terminal portion of the inflammatory phase and the beginning of the repair phase.[8] PDGF is composed of two subunits (A and B) and exists in three main isoforms (AA, BB, and AB). In its role in tendon-bone healing, PDGF-BB has been found to stimulate cell chemotaxis and cell division, type I collagen synthesis, and TGF-β1 production.[8,9] Early studies identified the ability of PDGF to enhance and accelerate healing of ligamentous and tendon injuries by increasing cell proliferation and matrix remodeling.[7,10,11] The structural improvements found at the microscopic level did not correspond to improvements in tensile biomechanical strength, but given the positive histo-

logic findings, several investigators have further studied the potential benefits of PDGF augmentation.[9,12,13]

Using a rat rotator cuff model, Uggen et al[12] demonstrated that the application of a polyglycolic acid scaffold containing cells expressing PDGF-BB restored normal collagen architecture and crimp pattern. As a corollary, Uggen et al[9] examined the effects of recombinant human (rh)PDGF-BB impregnated sutures on rotator cuff healing in a sheep model. They found enhanced histologic scores within the treatment group at 6 weeks but no difference between groups in load-to-failure testing. In a more recent study, the dose-dependent nature of rhPDGF-BB in an ovine rotator cuff model was investigated.[13] An interposition graft of type I collagen matrix and low, medium, or high doses (75, 150, or 500 mg) of rhPDGF-BB was used to repair the rotator cuff. At 12 weeks after the repair, the low- and medium-dose groups had statistically significant improvements in tendon-to-bone interdigitation and attachment strength compared with the control- and high-dose group. Interestingly, the group that received the highest dose did not produce similar improvements, highlighting that the dose-response curve is not linear. Negative feedback loops may play a role in limiting the effectiveness of these exogenous factors at higher doses. Additional studies have shown similar improvements in Achilles tendon healing using PDGF-BB, garnering further support for its potential use as an augment to improve tendon healing.[14,15]

Transforming Growth Factor-β

TGF-β is a family of cytokines that is believed to play an important role in tendon healing by improving cellular proliferation, differentiation, and matrix synthesis.[8] There are three isoforms within this family: TGF-β1,

TGF-β2, and TGF-β3. Much attention has been focused on the latter (TGF-β3) because this isoform is expressed at a higher level during prenatal development. The inferred potential for this growth factor as an augment stems from the fact that healing of a wound in the prenatal period results in no scar formation. In a study examining these benefits, Manning et al[16] applied TGF-β3 to the healing of supraspinatus tendon in a rat model using a heparin-based delivery system. The authors reported improved cellularity, vascularity, and cell proliferation at early time points. Significant differences in the structural and material properties of the tendon were also seen in the treated group at both 28 and 56 days after repair. Using a different delivery method, Kovacevic et al[17] delivered TGF-β3 to repaired rat supraspinatus tendon using injectable calcium-phosphate. The authors reported a significant increase in strength of the rotator cuff at 1 month postoperatively and an improvement in the ratio of type I/III collagen. Given these findings using various delivery mechanisms, TGF-β3 has demonstrated considerable potential for improving tendon-bone healing.

Bone Morphogenetic Proteins

BMPs are a group of factors within the TGF-β superfamily that have been shown to mediate bone, tendon, and cartilage formation. Specific to rotator cuff healing, BMP-12, BMP-13, and BMP-14 have been specifically shown to improve the formation of new tendon.[18,19] Seeherman et al[20] investigated the application of recombinant human BMP-12 delivered via several carriers in a sheep rotator cuff repair model and found it to have beneficial effects on healing. The investigators reported an increase in glycosaminoglycan content and improved collagen fiber continuity at the bone-tendon interface compared with a control group. In addition, repairs treated with BMP on collagen or hyaluronan paste sponges were 2.7 and 2.1 times stronger than repairs in the control group and the group with hyaluronan paste sponges, respectively. The findings of this study highlight not only the potential efficacy of BMP but also the need to identify the most effective delivery vehicle.

In a more recent study, Gulotta et al[21] evaluated the use of bone marrow-derived mesenchymal stem cells transduced with the gene for human BMP-13 in rotator cuff healing in a rat model. In contrast to previous work showing the utility of BMP, they found no differences in collagen formation, matrix organization, or mechanical properties compared with a control group. The results of this study highlight the poor understanding of the intricate signaling pathways necessary to regenerate the native insertion-site architecture.

Fibroblastic Growth Factors

FGFs are a family of 23 related polypeptides that show an affinity for heparin-binding sites. Their primary role in tendon repair is promoting angiogenesis by stimulating cell division of capillary endothelial cells as well as mesenchymal cells. Of the 23 isoforms, FGF-1 and FGF-2 have been found to be the most highly concentrated FGFs in adult tissue.[8,22,23] Their involvement in the early phase of tendon healing has been implicated as peak levels have been found to occur at 7 to 9 days after repair.[24]

Examining the effects of FGF-2 on rotator cuff tendons, Ide et al[23] applied growth factor and a fibrin sealant to repaired rat supraspinatus tendons. The authors reported that the treatment group had statistically improved mechanical and histologic scores at the early time point of 2 weeks postoperatively. These improvements, however, were not maintained at postoperative weeks 4 and 6. In another study, the same group evaluated the use of FGF-2 applied to an acellular dermal matrix to enhance rat rotator cuff repairs.[22] Although the growth factor improved healing, the results differed from their previous work. At the early 2-week time point, there was no difference between control and treatment supraspinatus tendon morphology or strength. At 6 and 12 weeks, however, the FGF-treated group demonstrated better histologic scores and tendon attachment strength. Most recently, Buchmann et al[25] evaluated the use of continuous infusion of FGF and granulocyte colony stimulating factor in a chronic rotator cuff rat model. The authors found an improvement in tendon remodeling after repair with continuous infusion of these growth factors over 20 days compared with the control group. These preclinical studies provide evidence that FGF-2 is capable of accelerating and enhancing tissue remodeling. The temporal expression of FGF-2 and its optimal time of application during the repair process require further investigation.

Other Signaling Molecules

There are several other signaling molecules that may hold more promise for improving tendon healing. Some of these, such as type I MMP, have been identified based on their role in tendon insertion-site formation during embryonic development.[26] In addition to proteins and cytokines, transcription factors may be exploited to improve tendon healing. Transcription factors are proteins that bind to specific DNA sequences and regulate transcription of DNA into RNA. Candidate transcription factors that appear promising include scleraxis (tenocyte differentiation) and SOX-9 (chondrocyte differentiation).[27]

Platelet-Rich Plasma

Given the previously described benefits of isolated growth factors, platelet-rich plasma (PRP) has been evaluated in tendon and ligament healing. The rationale for using PRP is the presence of numerous cytokines, all derived from an autologous source. PRP contains several cytokines (such as PDGF, vascular endothelial growth factor, TGF-β, FGF-2, and insulin-like growth factor-1), as well as other plasma proteins that may play a role in the reparative process. The current evidence, however, has not shown conclusive efficacy in improved healing after tendon-to-bone repair.

Recent clinical studies evaluating the effects of PRP on rotator cuff healing have not conclusively demonstrated a beneficial effect on healing rates, range of motion, strength, or functional scores compared with control groups.[28-30] A recent level I study by Randelli et al[31] reported significantly decreased pain scores at 1 month and improved clinical outcomes at 3 months postoperatively. These improvements, however, were not maintained at the 6-, 12-, or 24-month follow-ups, suggesting a positive influence of PRP on early tendon healing. Three additional level I studies did not find that PRP improved the outcome of rotator cuff repair.[32-34] The first study, by Castricini et al,[32] reported no differences in structural or functional outcomes (determined by MRI and Constant scores, respectively) at any time point while using PRP augmentation. Rodeo et al[33] examined the vascularity and clinical outcomes after rotator cuff repair using platelet-rich fibrin matrix and found no significant difference between augmented repairs and repairs in control subjects. In addition, the authors found a lower percentage of intact repairs at follow-up in the pa-tients treated with platelet-rich fibrin matrix (67% in the platelet-rich fibrin matrix group compared with 81% in the control group), suggesting a potential detrimental effect of platelet-rich fibrin matrix on tendon healing. In the most recent randomized controlled trial by Weber et al,[34] platelet-rich fibrin matrix was not shown to significantly improve perioperative morbidity, clinical outcomes, or structural integrity at any time point during the first year after single row rotator cuff repair. At this time, it appears that PRP alone does not improve healing rates after rotator cuff repair. Future studies are necessary to identify the potential benefit of PRP combined with cell-based approaches to augment healing.

Mesenchymal Stem Cells

The augmentation strategies that have been discussed thus far are based on the assumption that exogenous cytokines and growth factors placed within a healing tendon injury will stimulate local tenocytes and fibroblasts to heal in a more efficient manner. However, many of the studies previously described reported improved histologic scores but no improvement in structural properties. It is hypothesized that the lack of efficacy may be the result of an insufficient number of target cells to respond to these signaling molecules. This chapter's authors believe that approaches that combine cytokines and growth factors in conjunction with undifferentiated mesenchymal cells may improve healing.

Mesenchymal stem cells have the ability to self-renew and differentiate into several different cell lines, including adipocytes, osteocytes, tenocytes, and chondrocytes. It is hypothesized that cell-based approaches may improve healing via three potential mechanisms: direct participation in the repair process, the paracrine effect by stimulating local or distant cells, and an anti-inflammatory/immunomodulatory role. Currently, available autologous mesenchymal stem cells are isolated from bone marrow, although techniques are being developed to isolate these cells from adipose tissue. In one study, mesenchymal stem cells were harvested from suture anchor holes in the proximal humerus at the time of rotator cuff repair, illustrating a potential graft harvest site with low morbidity.[35]

Several studies have been performed using animal models to investigate enhanced tendon regeneration with mesenchymal stem cells. Using a rat rotator cuff model, Gulotta et al[36] found no improvement in histologic or biomechanical properties with the use of isolated bone marrow–derived mesenchymal stem cells. However, further work found positive effects when the mesenchymal stem cells were used in conjunction with specific factors.[37] For example, bone marrow–derived mesenchymal stem cells were transduced with the gene for the transcription factor scleraxis (adenoviral-mediated scleraxis) and then applied to the repaired rat rotator cuff in a similar manner. Scleraxis is a transcription factor that has been found to play a key role in cell differentiation within the developing tendon-bone insertion site.[36,37] The authors reported improved tendon attachment strength, stiffness, and ultimate stress at failure at 4 weeks after repair in the group with adenoviral-mediated scleraxis mesenchymal stem cell augmentation compared with control subjects. More studies are needed to further define the appropriate signals for directing mesenchymal stem cells to their target cell line within the healing enthesis.

Matrix Metalloproteinases

Recent studies have demonstrated that MMPs and their inhibitors may play a critical role in the pathophysiology of rotator cuff tears.[38,39] The MMPs are a group of at least 24 zinc-dependent endopeptidases that are responsible for enzymatic degradation of extracellular matrix, which includes fibrillar collagens. The MMPs that have been identified as playing a specific role in rotator cuff pathophysiology are MMP-1, MMP-8, and MMP-13. In contrast, tissue inhibitors of MMPs (TIMPs) play an antagonistic role to MMPs and their degradative potential. The dynamic process of tissue breakdown and remodeling is directed by an intricate homeostatic balance of expression and timing between these enzymes and their antagonists. Although the process is not yet fully understood, it provides a potential site for biologic manipulation during healing.

Lo et al[40] found elevated mRNA levels of MMP-13 and decreased levels of TIMP-2, TIMP-3, and TIMP-4 in patients with full-thickness rotator cuff tears. McDowell et al[41] reported that MMP-mediated tissue degradation led to weakening of the tendon around the suture construct after surgical repair. Given these findings, more recent research has explored the positive effects of selectively inhibiting MMPs.[38]

Doxycycline is a potent broad-spectrum MMP inhibitor, albeit nonselective. The antibiotic works by binding to the zinc-binding site of the MMP and inhibiting MMP gene expression. It is most efficacious at inhibiting MMP-1, MMP-2, MMP-7, MMP-8, MMP-9, MMP-12, and MMP-13. Using a rat Achilles tendon model, Pasternak and Aspenberg[38] were able to show that sutures coated with doxycycline improved the holding capacity during early tendon healing. In a similar study using a rat rotator cuff repair model, Bedi et al[39] noted histologic and biomechanical improvements with inhibition of MMP-13 using doxycycline and a local MMP inhibitor at the healing en-

thesis. Because of the nonselective nature of the inhibition from doxycycline, more research is needed to evaluate the specific mechanism of improved healing demonstrated in these studies. In addition, broad-spectrum inhibition of MMPs may impede appropriate and desired tendon remodeling during the late phase of healing.

Summary

The native rotator cuff insertion architecture is not recapitulated after surgical repair. Instead, a reactive fibrovascular scar, which is weaker and therefore prone to recurrent tearing with mechanical load, is formed at the enthesis. The biologic augmentation strategies discussed in this chapter aim to improve healing rates by introducing higher concentrations of growth factors, cytokines, mesenchymal stem cells, and antagonists to degradative enzymes at the repair site in the hope of directing a more organized healing response. Clinical and preclinical research has reported some positive results using these techniques. However, the ultimate goal of regenerating native tissue rather than enhanced scar tissue is still elusive. Future directions for research will need to focus on the optimal combination of stem cells and growth factors and identify the optimal dosing, timing, and delivery methods to achieve this goal. Biologic augmentation and tissue engineering to improve tendon-to-bone healing remains promising but will require further study before its clinical application is realized.

References

1. Galatz LM, Ball CM, Teefey SA, Middleton WD, Yamaguchi K: The outcome and repair integrity of completely arthroscopically repaired large and massive rotator cuff tears. *J Bone Joint Surg Am* 2004;86(2):219-224.

2. Dines JS, Bedi A, ElAttrache NS, Dines DM: Single-row versus double-row rotator cuff repair: Techniques and outcomes. *J Am Acad Orthop Surg* 2010;18(2):83-93.

3. Duquin TR, Buyea C, Bisson LJ: Which method of rotator cuff repair leads to the highest rate of structural healing? A systematic review. *Am J Sports Med* 2010;38(4):835-841.

4. Jost B, Pfirrmann CW, Gerber C, Switzerland Z: Clinical outcome after structural failure of rotator cuff repairs. *J Bone Joint Surg Am* 2000;82(3):304-314.

5. Bland YS, Ashhurst DE: Fetal and postnatal development of the patella, patellar tendon and suprapatella in the rabbit: Changes in the distribution of the fibrillar collagens. *J Anat* 1997;190(pt 3):327-342.

6. Gulotta LV, Rodeo SA: Growth factors for rotator cuff repair. *Clin Sports Med* 2009;28(1):13-23.

7. Letson AK, Dahners LE: The effect of combinations of growth factors on ligament healing. *Clin Orthop Relat Res* 1994;308:207-212.

8. Oliva F, Via AG, Maffulli N: Role of growth factors in rotator cuff healing. *Sports Med Arthrosc* 2011;19(3):218-226.

9. Uggen C, Dines J, McGarry M, Grande D, Lee T, Limpisvasti O: The effect of recombinant human platelet-derived growth factor BB-coated sutures on rotator cuff healing in a sheep model. *Arthroscopy* 2010;26(11):1456-1462.

10. Hildebrand KA, Woo SL, Smith DW, et al: The effects of platelet-derived growth factor-BB on healing of the rabbit medial collateral ligament: An in vivo study. *Am J Sports Med* 1998;26(4):549-554.

11. Thomopoulos S, Zaegel M, Das R, et al: PDGF-BB released in tendon repair using a novel delivery system promotes cell prolifera-

tion and collagen remodeling. *J Orthop Res* 2007;25(10):1358-1368.

12. Uggen JC, Dines J, Uggen CW, et al: Tendon gene therapy modulates the local repair environment in the shoulder. *J Am Osteopath Assoc* 2005;105(1):20-21.

13. Hee CK, Dines JS, Dines DM, et al: Augmentation of a rotator cuff suture repair using rhPDGF-BB and a type I bovine collagen matrix in an ovine model. *Am J Sports Med* 2011;39(8):1630-1639.

14. Shah V, Bendele A, Dines JS, et al: Dose-response effect of an intra-tendon application of recombinant human platelet-derived growth factor-BB (rhPDGF-BB) in a rat Achilles tendinopathy model. *J Orthop Res* 2013;31(3):413-420.

15. Cummings SH, Grande DA, Hee CK, et al: Effect of recombinant human platelet-derived growth factor-BB-coated sutures on Achilles tendon healing in a rat model: A histological and biomechanical study. *J Tissue Eng* 2012;3(1):2041731412453577.

16. Manning CN, Kim HM, Sakiyama-Elbert S, Galatz LM, Havlioglu N, Thomopoulos S: Sustained delivery of transforming growth factor beta three enhances tendon-to-bone healing in a rat model. *J Orthop Res* 2011;29(7):1099-1105.

17. Kovacevic D, Fox AJ, Bedi A, et al: Calcium-phosphate matrix with or without TGF-β3 improves tendon-bone healing after rotator cuff repair. *Am J Sports Med* 2011;39(4):811-819.

18. Aspenberg P, Forslund C: Enhanced tendon healing with GDF 5 and 6. *Acta Orthop Scand* 1999;70(1):51-54.

19. Cheng H, Jiang W, Phillips FM, et al: Osteogenic activity of the fourteen types of human bone morphogenetic proteins (BMPs). *J Bone Joint Surg Am* 2003;85(8):1544-1552.

20. Seeherman HJ, Archambault JM, Rodeo SA, et al: rhBMP-12 accelerates healing of rotator cuff repairs in a sheep model. *J Bone Joint Surg Am* 2008;90(10):2206-2219.

21. Gulotta LV, Kovacevic D, Packer JD, Ehteshami JR, Rodeo SA: Adenoviral-mediated gene transfer of human bone morphogenetic protein-13 does not improve rotator cuff healing in a rat model. *Am J Sports Med* 2011;39(1):180-187.

22. Ide J, Kikukawa K, Hirose J, Iyama K, Sakamoto H, Mizuta H: The effects of fibroblast growth factor-2 on rotator cuff reconstruction with acellular dermal matrix grafts. *Arthroscopy* 2009;25(6):608-616.

23. Ide J, Kikukawa K, Hirose J, et al: The effect of a local application of fibroblast growth factor-2 on tendon-to-bone remodeling in rats with acute injury and repair of the supraspinatus tendon. *J Shoulder Elbow Surg* 2009;18(3):391-398.

24. Kobayashi M, Itoi E, Minagawa H, et al: Expression of growth factors in the early phase of supraspinatus tendon healing in rabbits. *J Shoulder Elbow Surg* 2006;15(3):371-377.

25. Buchmann S, Sandmann GH, Walz L, et al: Influence of continuous growth factor application on tendon structure. *J Orthop Res* 2013;31(2):300-305.

26. Holmbeck K, Bianco P, Chrysovergis K, Yamada S, Birkedal-Hansen H: MT1-MMP-dependent, apoptotic remodeling of unmineralized cartilage: A critical process in skeletal growth. *J Cell Biol* 2003;163(3):661-671.

27. Yang Z, Huang CY, Candiotti KA, et al: Sox-9 facilitates differentiation of adipose tissue-derived stem cells into a chondrocyte-like phenotype in vitro. *J Orthop Res* 2011;29(8):1291-1297.

28. Jo CH, Kim JE, Yoon KS, et al: Does platelet-rich plasma accelerate recovery after rotator cuff repair? A prospective cohort study. *Am J Sports Med* 2011;39(10):2082-2090.

29. Bergeson AG, Tashjian RZ, Greis PE, Crim J, Stoddard GJ, Burks RT: Effects of platelet-rich fibrin matrix on repair integrity of at-risk rotator cuff tears. *Am J Sports Med* 2012;40(2):286-293.

30. Barber FA, Hrnack SA, Snyder SJ, Hapa O: Rotator cuff repair healing influenced by platelet-rich plasma construct augmentation. *Arthroscopy* 2011;27(8):1029-1035.

31. Randelli P, Arrigoni P, Ragone V, Aliprandi A, Cabitza P: Platelet rich plasma in arthroscopic rotator cuff repair: A prospective RCT study, 2-year follow-up. *J Shoulder Elbow Surg* 2011;20(4):518-528.

32. Castricini R, Longo UG, De Benedetto M, et al: A randomized controlled trial. *Am J Sports Med* 2011;39(2):258-265.

33. Rodeo SA, Delos D, Williams RJ, Adler RS, Pearle A, Warren RF: The effect of platelet-rich fibrin matrix on rotator cuff tendon healing: A prospective, randomized clinical study. *Am J Sports Med* 2012;40(6):1234-1241.

34. Weber SC, Kauffman JI, Parise C, Weber SJ, Katz SD: Platelet-rich fibrin matrix in the management of arthroscopic repair of the rotator cuff: A prospective, randomized, double-blinded study. *Am J Sports Med* 2013;41(2):263-270.

35. Mazzocca AD, McCarthy MB, Chowaniec DM, Cote MP, Arciero RA, Drissi H: Rapid isolation of human stem cells (connective tissue progenitor cells) from the proximal humerus during arthroscopic rotator cuff surgery. *Am J Sports Med* 2010;38(7):1438-1447.

36. Guotta LV, Kovacevic D, Ehteshami JR, Dagher E, Packer JD, Rodeo SA: Application of bone marrow-derived mesenchymal stem cells in a rotator cuff repair model. *Am J Sports Med* 2009;37(11):2126-2133.

37. Gulotta LV, Kovacevic D, Packer JD, Deng XH, Rodeo SA: Bone marrow-derived mesenchymal stem cells transduced with scleraxis improve rotator cuff healing in a rat model. *Am J Sports Med* 2011;39(6):1282-1289.

38. Pasternak B, Aspenberg P: Metalloproteinases and their inhibitors: Diagnostic and therapeutic opportunities in orthopedics. *Acta Orthop* 2009;80(6):693-703.

39. Bedi A, Fox AJ, Kovacevic D, Deng XH, Warren RF, Rodeo SA: Doxycycline-mediated inhibition of matrix metalloproteinases improves healing after rotator cuff repair. *Am J Sports Med* 2010; 38(2):308-317.

40. Lo IK, Marchuk LL, Hollinshead R, Hart DA, Frank CB: Matrix metalloproteinase and tissue inhibitor of matrix metalloproteinase mRNA levels are specifically altered in torn rotator cuff tendons. *Am J Sports Med* 2004; 32(5):1223-1229.

41. McDowell CL, Marqueen TJ, Yager D, Owen J, Wayne JS: Characterization of the tensile properties and histologic/biochemical changes in normal chicken tendon at the site of suture insertion. *J Hand Surg Am* 2002;27(4):605-614.

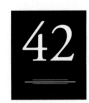

42

Biologic Augmentation of Tendon-to-Bone Healing: Scaffolds, Mechanical Load, Vitamin D, and Diabetes

Sarah Nossov, MD
Joshua S. Dines, MD
George A.C. Murrell, MD, PhD
Scott A. Rodeo, MD
Asheesh Bedi, MD

Abstract

Biologic and synthetic scaffolds, mechanical loads, vitamin D, and diabetes can affect tendon and tendon-to-bone healing, muscle recovery, and growth in the perioperative period. Despite important advances in technical approaches to achieve surgical repair of soft tissues in a minimally invasive fashion, structural healing after tendon-to-bone repair remains a formidable challenge that is complicated by our incomplete knowledge of complex natural biologic processes and a diverse patient population with various comorbidities and deficiencies. Scientific research has led to promising strategies for promoting a structural repair that recapitulates the native anatomy of the tendon or enthesis. Augmentation with scaffolds may reinforce the initial repair biomechanically and can be coupled with growth factors to promote a favorable biologic environment for healing. Careful consideration of the implications of postoperative rehabilitation and endocrine and nutritional deficiencies on structural healing and muscle recovery are also critical to optimize patient outcomes.

Instr Course Lect 2014;63:451-462.

Tissue engineering emerged at the turn of the 21st century from early research started in the late 1980s. The aim of tissue engineering is to resolve problems related to impaired healing and the loss of load-bearing tissue by providing substrates and scaffolds for regrowth. Three-dimensional scaffolds can be made of xenografts, allografts, or various synthetic or nonbiologic materials that are electrically spun using nanotechnology. Continued interest in the use of scaffolds is fueled by the substantial rate of recurrent tears and structural failures after primary tendon repair.[1] Scaffolds serve as architectural guides, with or without the addition of cytokines or seeding with mesenchymal or differentiated cells, to encourage host tissue growth and augment healing after injury. Scaffolds can further stimulate cells by virtue of their surface receptors and chemistry.[2]

Biologic Scaffolds

Scaffolds composed of biologic materials, or mammalian extracellular matrix (ECM), are believed to offer more benefits than synthetic scaffolds because of the potential for remodeling afforded by their natural structure and favorable protein composition. The substantial variations in products from animal origins and among various tissue types make it difficult to generalize

Dr. Dines or an immediate family member has received royalties from Biomet; serves as a paid consultant to or is an employee of Biomimetic, CONMED Linvatec, and Tornier; and has received research or institutional support from Biomimetic. Dr. Murrell or an immediate family member has received royalties from Novan and has received research or institutional support from Arthrocare and Arthrex. Dr. Rodeo or an immediate family member serves as a paid consultant to or is an employee of Smith & Nephew and has stock or stock options held in CAYENNE. Dr. Bedi or an immediate family member serves as a paid consultant to or is an employee of Smith & Nephew; has stock or stock options held in A3 Surgical; and serves as a board member, owner, officer, or committee member of the American Orthopaedic Society for Sports Medicine. Neither Dr. Nossov nor any immediate family member has received anything of value from or has stock or stock options held in a commercial company or institution related directly or indirectly to the subject of this chapter.

performance and form complex comparisons. Scaffolds are available from several major orthopaedic manufacturers and are procured from human, porcine, bovine, and equine sources, which are derived from dermis, small intestine submucosa, and the pericardium. Overall, scaffolds are predominantly composed of type 1 collagen. Important considerations for evaluating and comparing ECMs include the rate of degradation and the immune response. These factors appear to relate to biomechanical strength, healing, and, ultimately, patient satisfaction and perception of the clinical success facilitated by the ECM.

Cellular Responses

All ECMs induce a significant initial cellular response. Over time, this response results in various morphologies, which are related to properties of cross-linking and degradation.[3] ECMs are processed by decellularization and/or chemical cross-linking intended to remove or obscure graft antigenicity. Although a limited initial response to an implanted material is expected, a prolonged or severe immune response to ECM scaffolds is concerning and has been attributed to a mammalian Gal epitope, remnant DNA, and other residual cellular materials.[4,5] In mouse studies of small intestinal submucosa ECM, a type 2 versus a type 1 cell-mediated immune response was believed to predominate and has been associated with a non-macrophage response and transplant acceptance.[4] A randomized controlled trial was aborted after 4 of 19 patients (21%) had a severe local inflammatory reaction requiring surgical intervention after rotator cuff repair augmentation with the Restore (DePuy) non–cross-linked, porcine small intestine submucosa implant.[6]

Remodeling

ECM scaffolds are intended to provide temporary structural support. Host integration is intended to commence and eventually replace the foreign implant; ideally, the rate of remodeling and the loss of scaffold material would be matched to maintain mechanical strength throughout healing. Degradation is unique to each implant product and is related to cross-linking and other variables; the variable ECM deposition is associated with changes in material properties. It is not clear if matrix deposition is sufficiently strong to mimic native tendon strength. The seeding of ECM with factors or cells was designed to accelerate repair to maintain homeostasis and balance the rate of degradation. Bovine collagen ECM that was seeded with human tenocytes demonstrated reduced degradation, increased ECM deposition, and increased Young modulus and failure stress at 26 days in media.[7]

Host Response

Histologic studies help identify the host response to the spectrum of ECM products. A broad comparison of several commercially available ECMs (GraftJacket, Wright Medical Technology; Restore; CuffPatch, Arthrotek; TissueMend, TEI Biosciences; and Permacol, Covidien) along with an autologous implant control was studied in an abdominal tissue defect in a rat model that examined the host histologic responses.[8] Cellular infiltration was found to be greatest in the ECMs that degraded quickly (the Restore autologous patch). Evidence of chronic inflammation with giant cells and more dense disorganized tissue was found in the more slowly degrading ECMs (CuffPatch, TissueMend, and Permacol) and appeared to correlate with clinical outcomes. Connective tissue organization was most similar to native tissue at 112 days with the Re-store patch. Although an immunologic response occurred with all of the ECMs, the structural morphology and the type of host cell replacement for the ECM was variable.

Mechanical Properties

Mechanical properties are used to compare surgical repairs with uninjured tendon and in head-to-head comparisons of different ECMs. Stiffness and load-to-failure are quantified to gauge the strength of the construct under physiologic force. As degradation and the loss of the scaffold over time can weaken an initially strengthened repair, chemical cross-linking of the tissue is used to hasten the rate of scaffold integration,[9] possibly at the cost of extended foreign body exposure. Data suggest that cross-linking is correlated with poor incorporation.[10,11] Soler et al[10] reported on the use of Permacol, a porcine dermal biologic, that is cross-linked with noncalcifying hexamethylene diisocyanate. In a study of four patients in which the biologic implant was used to bridge irreparable rotator cuff defects, failure of the repairs was reported, with no detectable graft and a severe inflammatory response determined by MRI and histologic evaluation. Microscopic evaluation revealed necroinflammatory exudate with fibrinous material and chronic synovitis. Nirmalanandhan et al,[11] reported that mechanical properties were increased in vitro but decreased in vivo at 12 weeks in specimens cross-linked with ultraviolet irradiation. The authors suggested that increased stiffness and alterations in the scaffold pore size may shield cells from the mechanical stimulation necessary to meet the preinjury level of strength. A study by Deeken et al[12] used a porcine model of incisional hernia repair to compare the long-term outcomes of cross-linked (Peri-Guard, Synovis; Permacol) and non–cross-linked (Alloderm, LifeCell Products; Veritas, Synovis) repairs. Augmented repairs were very similar in strength at 1, 6, and 12 months after repair, and the stiffness of any of the implants was not significantly greater than native tissue. The authors noted that the stiffness measurement relies on strain at the time of measurement. Histologic evaluation showed that cross-linking may hinder infiltration in the short-term, but, in the long-term, both the cross-linked and the non–cross-linked meshes showed equivalent infiltration.

Outcomes

Animal and human cadaver models of biologic scaffolds for tendon repair have yielded equivocal results. Infraspinatus repairs augmented with acellular dermal matrix in a canine model reported no differences in strength at time zero and 12 weeks; weaker strength was found at 6 weeks.[13] A similar study using a hybrid poly-L-lactic acid (PLLA) reinforced human fascial patch found early improvement only in mechanical properties.[14] Bovine ECM demonstrated less gap formation with high cyclic physiologic loading in augmented repairs of cadaver Achilles tendon compared with controls. The authors noted that because of cross-linking, particular attention was given to orienting the stiffest axis of the graft so that it was aligned in the direction of the long axis of the tendon. A trial test found greater gapping with perpendicular orientation without an effect on ultimate failure; further isotropic study was recommended.[15]

In the few available randomized trials in humans, outcome measures are based on imaging comparisons and clinical surveys. Acellular human dermal matrix (GraftJacket) was evaluated as an augmentation patch in a randomized controlled trial of two-tendon rotator cuff repairs for 3- to 5-cm defects. Improved clinical outcomes were reported in the scaffold group; MRI at a follow-up of 12 months or longer found intact rotator cuffs in 85% of the patients treated with an augmented repair versus 40% in the group treated with a nonaugmented repair.[16] An earlier randomized control trial, however, found no significant difference in outcomes using porcine small intestine mucosa for augmentation in human chronic two-tendon large to massive rotator cuff tears.[17] Satisfaction scores were correlated with healing, but no difference in outcomes was seen. The augmentation group also did not have an improved rate of healing. Another small series that evaluated massive rotator cuff repairs augmented with interpositional porcine small intestine mucosa did not show evidence of improved healing on MRI at 6 months, and there was no improvement in patient satisfaction scores.[18] Similar data have been reported at 2-year follow-up in a small group of patients with large rotator cuff defects whose repairs were supplemented with xenograft augmentation.[6] The disappointing clinical outcomes in human studies in contrast to the promising results in animal studies may be attributed to incongruent rates of degradation and cell proliferation, along with host reaction to remnant porcine DNA in small intestine mucosa augments.[19,20] It also has been shown that skin grafts have a higher load to failure compared with small intestine mucosa grafts,[21] which supports the findings in a randomized controlled trial by Barber et al[16] using acellular human dermal matrix (GraftJacket).

Few scientific data are available to provide clear guidelines for clinical decision making regarding the use of biologic ECM to augment tendon or tendon-to-bone repairs. Six clinical grades of pathology in rotator cuff tears have been described by Derwin et al[22] (**Table 1**). The authors recommend augmentation in small to medium grade III tears, large to massive repairable grade IV tears, and in selected cases for interposition in massive grade V tears that are otherwise irreparable.

Synthetic Scaffolds

Synthetic scaffolds are composed of chemical compounds and are designed to provide a temporary three-dimensional surface area for cells to attach, grow, and differentiate. Using nanotechnology, biodegradable polymers are structured to imitate native ECMs to encourage gap healing in tendons and unload significant tensile forces on the primary suture repair.[2] Immunogenicity, manufacturing irregularities, and the risk of infection are presumably minimized with synthetic devices compared with biologic scaffolds. The promise of greater supply availability also makes synthetic scaffolds an attractive alternative to biologic allografts.

Composition

The engineering of synthetic scaffolds relies on a chemical base, a healthy population of cells, and inductive signals such as growth factors. The rate of degradation, which will optimally coincide with infiltration of adequate host tissue, can be orchestrated in synthetic scaffolds and depends on the chemistry of the composed material, the scaffold design, and processing techniques.[3] Synthetic scaffolds are composed of synthetic polymers, such as PLLA, polylactide-co-glycolide (PLGA), or polyurethane, and are generally stronger than biologic ECMs.[23] Both PLLA and PLGA are aliphatic polyesters. PLLA is a homopolymer composed of renewable sources (such as corn starch), and PLGA is a copolymer whose degradation is affected by

Table 1
Clinical Grades of Rotator Cuff Pathology

Grade	Rotator Cuff Indication	Current Treatment	Outcomes	Graft Indication
6	Massive, retracted, irreparable tear with intra-articular pathology	Open reverse total shoulder replacement (aggressive)	Adequate but limited function	Not indicated
5	Large, massive tear (3 to 5 cm, 2 to 3 tendons); irreparable (unable to reappose to tuberosity with low tension)	Open or arthroscopic attempts at repair, muscle transfer, débridement, and/or partial repair	High failure rate (≥ 50% retear rate and/or low outcome scores)	Interpositional in selected instances
4	Large, massive tear (3 to 5 cm, 2 to 3 tendons); reparable	Open or arthroscopic repair	Moderate failure rate (≥ 30% retear rate; 85% pain free but reduced function)	Augmentation
3	Small to medium tear (< 3 cm, 1 tendon)	Arthroscopic repair	Moderate failure rate (5% to 10% retear rate; 85% pain free but > 50% reduced function)	Augmentation
2	Partial-thickness tear (> 50% of articular or bursal surface	Arthroscopic decompression/ débridement or repair with acromioplasty	40% failure rate with 5 years with débridement only; 95% heal when repaired	Not indicated
1	Partial-thickness tear (< 50% of articular or bursal surface	Arthroscopic decompression/ débridement or repair with acromioplasty	95% heal when repaired	Not indicated

(Adapted with permission from Derwin KA, Badylak SF, Steinmann SP, Iannotti JP: Extracellular matrix scaffold devices for rotator cuff repair. *J Shoulder Elbow Surg* 2010;19(3):467-476.)

the content of glycolide units. Other biologic materials, such as silk and collagen, can be used as a base for synthetic scaffolds. Over a period of months, aliphatic polyesters degrade into easily metabolized components, whereas nondegradable materials (such as Teflon [DuPont] would be expected to remain.

Host Response

Residual synthetic scaffold structures can support growth but may also exacerbate an unfavorable host response. In vitro studies of PLGA nanofiber scaffolds with rotator cuff fibroblasts demonstrated that scaffold alignment and structure influenced the mechanical properties of new cell growth even after degradation.[24] Host reactions to synthetic scaffolds include a foreign body response, which sometimes progresses to chronic inflammation and fibrous tissue formation.[25] Issues with long-term biocompatibility and chronic inflammation from synthetic

tendon and ligament prostheses resulted in regulatory intervention in the 1980s.[23] Bioincompatibility can result in various complications, such as higher incidences of postoperative infection, osteolysis, chronic inflammation, and potentially toxic by-products such as lactic acid and glycolic acid.

Mechanical Properties

Although growth induction is not improved compared with biologic scaffolds, synthetic scaffolds have excellent mechanical strength. Recent studies have evaluated PLGA, PLLA, and polyurethane patches for rotator cuff repair. PLGA has a relatively fast rate of degradation; is composed of a strong absorbable monofilament; and enhances cell-to-cell interaction, which may stimulate ECM production.[26] In a rabbit model of a rotator cuff tear repair, PLGA served as an interpositional graft to bridge a 1 cm defect of the infraspinatus tendon.[27] At 4 and 16 weeks, the PLGA graft had

more favorable mechanical properties compared with a more slowly degrading polymer graft. At 24 weeks, the PLGA graft was completely resorbed, had been replaced with fibrous tissue, and produced minimal foreign body reactions.

Biomechanical testing in human cadavers of a simulated infraspinatus rotator cuff repair using a PLLA scaffold reported that augmentation should result in a 25% higher yield load and 16% greater stiffness than nonaugmented repairs at time zero. Both augmented and nonaugmented repairs were most affected by the material properties of the tendon-to-bone repair and the increased demand on the scaffold to sustain 45% of the load in the immediate postoperative period.[28] These results are comparable with other animal rotator cuff repair models using PLLA augmentation. A sheep model showed 25% increased strength with PLLA augmentation, and a canine model showed greater strength and increased stiffness with PLLA augmentation compared with repairs made without scaffold augmentation.[29-31]

In a study of 10 female patients without comparative controls, a nonresorbable reticulated polycarbonate polyurethane patch was hypothesized to be capable of maintaining more permanent structural support to resist retearing in small- to medium-sized rotator cuff tears.[32] No adverse events occurred. The evaluation (using MRI and ultrasound) at 12 months postoperatively showed a 10% retear rate. A study of chronic rotator cuff tears in an ovine model demonstrated a significantly greater load to failure with a polyurethane scaffold mesh augment versus suture anchor repair at 12 weeks and recovery of approximately 40% of native stiffness.[33] In a rat model of rotator cuff repair, Cole et al[34] reported no evidence of inflammatory reaction to polycarbonate polyurethane augmentation and an 80% rate of tissue ingrowth by 6 weeks after surgery.

Although bioengineered augmentation may enhance the strength of a surgical repair and potentially influence cell integration, the ultimate outcome of monophasic scaffolds relies on the presumed inherent ability of the body to re-create the complex multilayered cell transitions of the tendon-to-bone junction. Multiphasic scaffolds have been designed in an attempt to recapitulate the native anatomy of the enthesis. These scaffolds are modeled after the uninjured zonal distribution of cell types at tendon-to-bone and ligament-to-bone junctions, with an intermediate fibrocartilage zone. This organized architecture is not achieved after tendon-to-bone repair alone, in which an interposed fibrovascular scar tissue layer organizes and matures over time. Interactions between the various cell types at the boundaries of these scaffold zones are believed to establish the native architecture and strength of the

enthesis and avoid simple fibrocartilage replacement. An in vitro evaluation of a graft seeded with synthetic triphasic bovine culture yielded promising early results, including the identification of distinct cellular regions.[35] Gradients in mineral composition using calcium phosphate on a PLGA scaffold result in a gradual transition of mechanical properties, which can influence the activity of cells, such as the adherence of preosteoblasts.[36]

Cell-sheet engineering may be the future of "scaffoldless" tissue bridging. Scaffold failures are related to low cellular proliferation rates, degradation-proliferation mismatches, bioincompatibility, and low rates of cellular induction. Using tendon-derived stem cells treated with connective tissue growth factor and vitamin C, a scaffold-free tendon tissue was found to induce neotendon formation in preliminary results in a mouse model.[37]

The Effect of Mechanical Loads on Tendon-to-Bone Healing

Mechanical loading affects the mechanical properties of native and engineered tendon tissues via influences on direct cellular differentiation and ECM production.[38,39] In vitro, cyclic tension was shown to enhance fibroblast appearance and healing in the flexor tendons of chickens, whereas stress deprivation resulted in decreased tensile modulus in canine flexor digitorum profundus tendon.[40,41] Decreased loading alters the homeostasis of ECM production and degradation by matrix metalloproteinase enzymes such that degradation occurs more rapidly. The extent of changes in the tendon resulting from a decreased load is related to the type of insertion; indirect insertions are seen to lose much osseous integration. This is illustrated by increased weakening at the medial collateral ligament (indirect insertion)

with immobilization compared with a knee cruciate ligament (direct insertion). Conversely, repetitive loading in a physiologic range can increase the matrix deposition and organization of tendons and the strength of the enthesis.[42] Uninjured, immobilized rabbits showed increased osteoclastic activity and decreased stiffness in ligaments, which were partially reversed with restoration of activity.[43]

Muscle forces are necessary for the normal development and function of the enthesis.[44] The favorable influence of loading on mechanical properties is maintained even for mature tendon and ligament tissues. The influence of mechanical loading with physiologic muscle forces on tendon-to-bone healing was studied in flexor digitorum profundus tendons in canine paws. Improved function and biomechanical properties were reported. The authors theorized that mechanical loading resulted in increased matrix production and improved collagen organization in comparison with an immobilized group.[45] Tensile loading of healing tendon encourages fibers to align parallel to the direction of tensile loading, induces gene expression, and can accelerate healing.[42,46]

Although mechanical loading is important to develop and maintain the ECM of soft tissues, rest in the acute inflammatory period after initial tissue repair and before mechanical loading begins may be beneficial. In a recent study of rotator cuff repair in a rat model, improved mechanical properties were observed in the healing enthesis when the shoulder was immobilized postoperatively.[47] Mechanical properties were evaluated at 2, 8, and 12 weeks. More significant differences were found at the longest follow-up period, with a higher level of tissue organization and a closer resemblance to normal tissue. The authors hypothesized that early loading at the insertion may impede collagen organization and integration into bone and promote disorganized scar formation. Similar results have been reported using chemical immobilization techniques in the postoperative period. In a rat model of acute rotator cuff repair, a group of rats treated with chemical immobilization of the supraspinatus using botulinum toxin showed improved histologic organization at 4 weeks compared with a control group treated with the repair alone; however, thereafter, no benefit in mechanical properties was observed, suggesting that early immobilization may be beneficial.[48] An Achilles tendon repair model in rats used botulinum toxin perioperatively to decrease motion in treated tendons. The authors reported a threefold decrease in spontaneous rerupture and increased tendon rupture force only in the first 3 weeks after repair.[49]

Vitamin D and Tendon-to-Bone Healing

Hypovitaminosis D has been known for nearly 100 years to be associated with skeletal pathology. Low levels of vitamin D are associated with numerous health problems, including rickets, cardiovascular disease, cancer, diabetes, bone fragility, and stress fractures.[50]

Vitamin D is a group of fat-soluble secosteroids, also known as cholecalciferol or vitamin D_3. More accurate serum measurements evaluate inactive 25-hydroxyvitamin D (calcifediol) because it has a greater half-life of 3 weeks compared with the 24-hour half-life of cholecalciferol. Vitamin D levels reflect endogenous synthesis from sun exposure as well as dietary intake. Fortified foods are the major source of dietary intake in the United States and Canada, but ultraviolet B radiation–mediated conversion of 7-dehydrocholesterol to vitamin D_3 in the skin is the primary source in most

persons.[50] This inactive form, which is also available in the diet, is absorbed through the intestine and must undergo hydroxylation in the liver followed by enzymatic conversion in the kidney to its active hormonal form, 1,25-dihydroxyvitamin D or calcitriol.

Active vitamin D circulates bound to a protein receptor and acts by regulating the concentration of calcium and phosphate in the bloodstream and promoting the growth and remodeling of bone. Vitamin D also affects neuromuscular functions; affects inflammatory and immune responses, and influences the expression of genes that regulate the proliferation, differentiation, and apoptosis of cells.[51]

Calcitriol behaves agonistically at the vitamin D receptor located on the nuclei of target cells.[52] A functional polymorphism of the vitamin D receptor has been described and implicated in a phenotype that suggests vitamin D resistance; homozygous expression results in growth retardation, osteomalacia, secondary hypoparathyroidism, and alopecia.[53]

Release of parathyroid hormone secondary to low serum calcium and phosphate levels stimulates the production of calcitriol. This process is inhibited by high serum levels of calcitriol and fibroblast growth factor secreted by osteocytes. Optimal serum vitamin D levels are disputed; however, the Institute of Medicine defines adequate levels as 20 ng/mL (≥ 50 nmol) and deficiency as less than 12 ng/mL (< 30 nmol), whereas more than 50 ng/mL (125 nmol) may be toxic.[54]

A lack of exposure to sunlight; obesity; malabsorption syndromes; antiseizure, antiretroviral, and cholesterol-lowering medications; and acquired and genetic disorders can contribute to hypovitaminosis D.[55] In an effort to preserve adequate serum calcium levels in the presence of hypovitaminosis D,

the parathyroid gland induces 1,25-dihydroxyvitamin D production and thus increases serum calcium via bone resorption.[56] In a Cochrane review, Avenell et al[57] concluded that the administration of vitamin D alone did not reduce the risks of hip fractures in elderly patients, whereas vitamin D and calcium supplementation may result in fewer hip fractures. Because of the action of 1,25-dihydroxyvitamin D, it has been suggested that dietary supplementation with vitamin D alone may aggravate osteomalacia.[56]

Although clinical studies have examined the relationship between vitamin D levels and fragility fractures, there is a paucity of data on the effect of vitamin D on tendon-to-bone healing after injury or surgical repair. However, increased tendinopathy and the spontaneous rupture of patellar, quadriceps, Achilles, supraspinatus, subscapularis, distal biceps, and oblique internal abdominal tendons have been reported in patients with hyperparathyroidism and calcium-associated metabolic disorders (such as patients with chronic kidney disease undergoing dialysis).[58-62] Tendon ruptures are associated with potential osteolysis at the tendon insertion and repetitive microtrauma, as evidenced in histologic samples.

Serum vitamin D levels can affect muscle health and function. Muscle metabolism and growth is stimulated by 1,25-dihydroxyvitamin D. Mice who are deficient in vitamin D receptors have smaller muscle fibers. Hypovitaminosis D is associated with proximal muscle weakness, which is characterized by type II muscle fiber atrophy and necrosis and fatty muscle infiltration.[63,64] These may be a sequelae of calcium and phosphate imbalance that impairs glycolysis.[65] Low vitamin D and high parathyroid hormone levels were associated with low muscle bulk in elderly patients.[66] A recent study reported a significant negative correlation between low serum vitamin D levels and fatty degeneration of the rotator cuff muscle and a positive correlation with isokinetic muscle torque.[67] The study evaluated 366 patients with shoulder disorders; 228 patients had a full-thickness rotator cuff tear, and 138 patients had no tear. All of the patients were evaluated with magnetic resonance arthrography and an isokinetic muscle performance test. Multivariate linear regression analysis revealed that a low serum level of vitamin D was an independent predictor for fatty degeneration of the supraspinatus and infraspinatus muscles.

Studies directly correlating clinical outcomes of tendon repairs with vitamin D levels do not exist despite the evidence suggesting that hypovitaminosis D may contribute to tendon and muscle pathology.[67-69] A recent animal model of rotator cuff repair correlated vitamin D deficiency with decreased mechanical strength at 2 weeks, decreased fibrocartilage formation, and inferior collagen organization.[70] Consideration for evaluating serum vitamin D levels in patients with risk factors may prove to optimize successful healing and recovery from difficult tendon repairs. Identification and supplementation of vitamin D deficiency may reduce the incidence or extent of tendon damage if an injury occurs.

Diabetes and Tendon-to-Bone Healing

Metabolic changes present in patients with diabetes mellitus include glycosylation of proteins, microvascular abnormalities, and collagen accumulation. Although these metabolic changes are known to contribute to vascular and neuropathic disease, they can also affect the health of the musculoskeletal system.[71] Diabetes mellitus is associated with numerous orthopaedic manifestations, which appear to more significantly involve the upper extremity. Common diabetic orthopaedic issues include trigger finger, Dupuytren contracture, adhesive capsulitis, calcific tendinosis, osteomyelitis related to foot infections, and neuropathic Charcot joints. An increased incidence of diffuse idiopathic skeletal hyperostosis of the spine as well as an increased rate of calcaneal avulsion fractures also occur in patients with diabetes. In a cross-sectional population study of 6,237 Finnish patients, both types 1 and 2 diabetes mellitus were associated with increased shoulder pain and rotator cuff tendinitis in men.[72] High fasting glucose levels may be a risk factor for rotator cuff tears, and diabetes mellitus has been identified as an independent risk factor for failure of healing and restricted range of motion after rotator cuff repair.[73-75]

Tendon abnormalities related to metabolic changes have been documented in patients with diabetes. Spontaneous tendon failure is uncommon in patients with diabetes mellitus but has been described in patients with long-standing disease involving the flexor digitorum profundus, flexor digitorum superficialis, tibialis anterior, and Achilles tendons.[76-78] These ruptures have been attributed to chronic changes related to nonenzymatic glycosylation, vascular abnormalities, and repetitive trauma. The ruptured tendons have increased size and material property attrition, which may predispose them to failure during lower-energy traumatic events. Ultrasound measurements of supraspinatus and proximal biceps tendons in 150 diabetic patients identified a significant increase in tendon thickness in patients with diabetes compared with a group of control patients without diabetes. Patients with diabetes are 22 times more likely to have increased tendon thickness in the right supraspinatus tendon than are nondiabetic patients, 24 times more likely for the left supraspinatus tendon, 16 times more likely for the right biceps tendon, and 60 times more likely for the left biceps.[79] This apparent increase in tendon volume does not correlate with improved material properties. Despite the gross size microscopically, the collagen fibers are smaller, denser, and stiffer.[80] A reduced Young modulus and higher likelihood of midsubstance tears have been shown in patellar tendons of diabetic rats compared with controls.[81,82] Advanced glycosylation by-products contribute to collagen cross-linking, resulting in the disorganized structure of tendons that can lead to failure via loss of viscoelasticity and fiber-fiber sliding.[83] This process occurs in normal aging but is advanced and more pronounced in patients with diabetes mellitus.

Diabetes and insulin resistance can affect healing and outcomes after rotator cuff repair. A study by Clement et al[84] reported improvement in pain and function in patient after arthroscopic rotator cuff repair but found less improvement than in euglycemic control patients matched for age, sex, size of tear, and other medical comorbidities. A survey of 309 patients treated with arthroscopic rotator cuff repair showed that diabetes mellitus, older age, female sex, and participation in low-level sport activities were associated with low postoperative ($\geq$ 12 months) physical health-related quality-of-life scores measured by the Medical Outcomes Study 36-Item Short Form.[85] The multivariate analysis did not find that failure of the rotator cuff repair, the preoperative pain level, or the level of fatty infiltration of the supraspinatus had a significant effect on the quality-of-life score.

Type 1 diabetes mellitus is associated with shoulder stiffness and a propensity toward postoperative wound complications and infection. Chen et al[86] compared the results of open repair for full-thickness rotator cuff tears in 30 patients with diabetes and a matched, nondiabetic population. No differences were observed in preoperative range of motion; however, at a mean of 34 months, substantial differences in active and passive shoulder range of motion were found postoperatively. Five of 30 patients (17%) with diabetes had complications, with 2 failures (7%) and 3 infections (10%). In nondiabetic patients, there was one failed repair (3%) and no infections.

Sustained hyperglycemia can impair tendon-to-bone healing after rotator cuff repair and may have important implications for the preoperative workup and counseling of patients with poor glycemic control regarding expected outcomes of soft-tissue repair or reconstructive procedures. In a rat model of acute rotator cuff repair, diabetic animals had substantially less fibrocartilage and organized collagen at the healing enthesis, as well as the deposition of diffusely increased advanced glycation end products at the tendon-bone interface.[87] The healing enthesis in diabetic animals demonstrated a significantly reduced ultimate load to failure and stiffness compared with control animals with euglycemia.

The biochemical environment of the subacromial bursa may be altered in patients with diabetes, and this may further contribute to inferior outcomes after shoulder injury or rotator cuff repair surgery. A substantial increase in the expression of vascular endothelial growth factor and an abnormal angiogenesis process were identified in patients with type 2 diabetes with shoulder contracture and rotator cuff disease compared with nondiabetic patients.[88] This finding suggests that synovial proliferation is increased in patients with diabetes and

may contribute to increased pain and reduced range of motion in the postoperative period. A study by Chbinou and Frenette[89] reported an impaired inflammatory response to tendon injury in patients with diabetes.

In managing an orthopaedic patient with diabetes, it is important to conduct a multidisciplinary perioperative evaluation and maintain diligent glycemic control to reduce morbidity and improve outcomes.[90] Strict glycemic management may minimize complications, including infection, in this at-risk population.

The Use of Augmentation in Muscle Recovery and Growth

Optimizing surgical outcomes in the future will require approaches that not only achieve successful structural healing of tendon-to-bone and tendon-to-tendon interfaces but also expedite and facilitate full recovery of function and limit or prevent muscular atrophy. An improved understanding of the relationship of cell development and growth factors, reactive oxygen species regulators, and the balance of catabolic enzymes and anabolic supplements will likely guide further attempts to enhance muscle recovery.

It has been well established that disuse and immobilization results in muscle atrophy. Reducing activity decreases myofibril volumes and the muscular oxidative capacity in just weeks, but immobilization causes much more rapid muscle degradation.[91] After 1 week of immobilization in rats, gastrocnemius muscle atrophy was 30%.[92] In contrast, low tension, high repetition muscle loading increases endurance, and high tension, low repetition loading increases strength.[42] Myofibers respond to persistent changes in activity by passive stretching and active contraction, which alters the cell structure, volume, and function.[93]

Using a model of chronic rotator

cuff disease in sheep, Gerber et al[94] found that partial muscle recovery was induced with traction. Rotator cuff tears were allowed to retract for 4 months after they were created via infraspinatus tendon release and an osteotomy of the greater tuberosity. The tears were subsequently repaired. An implanted traction device then retensioned the muscle 1 mm per day to correct retraction. This process resulted in an arrest of fatty infiltration and improvement in atrophy to a muscle square area of 78% of the contralateral side. After recovery and rehabilitation, there was an increase in both muscle quality and architecture. The increase in mass resulted from increased muscle length; no increase in the diameter of fibers was observed.

Serum levels of circulating growth factors and inhibitors can affect muscle recovery after surgical repair. Myostatin, also known as growth differentiation factor 8, is a protein that originates in skeletal muscle cells and is a member of the transforming growth factor beta family.[95] Myostatin negatively regulates muscle growth, with animal knockout models demonstrating significant hypertrophy and force production of many muscle groups. In a recent study focusing on quadriceps atrophy and recovery after anterior cruciate ligament reconstruction, elevated serum levels of myostatin were present in the immediate postoperative period.[96] The authors suggested that inhibition of myostatin may prevent muscle atrophy and aid in maintaining preoperative muscle mass, which would potentially enhance recovery and indirectly decrease osteoarthritis. In a level I clinical trial, a therapeutic decoy myostatin receptor developed to treat diseases such as muscular dystrophy resulted in a small increase in lean muscle mass when administered to healthy postmenopausal women. This finding may suggest promise for this agent in patients undergoing elective orthopaedic procedures.[97]

Summary

Despite the important advances in technical approaches to achieve the surgical repair of soft tissues in a minimally invasive fashion, structural healing after tendon-to-bone repair remains challenging. Scientific research has led to promising strategies for promoting a structural repair that recapitulates the native anatomy of the tendon or the enthesis. Augmentation with scaffolds may reinforce the initial repair biomechanically and can be coupled with growth factors to promote a favorable biologic environment for healing. Careful consideration of the implications of postoperative rehabilitation and endocrine and nutritional deficiencies on structural healing and muscle recovery are also critical to optimize results.

References

1. Nho SJ, Brown BS, Lyman S, Adler RS, Altchek DW, MacGillivray JD: Prospective analysis of arthroscopic rotator cuff repair: Prognostic factors affecting clinical and ultrasound outcome. *J Shoulder Elbow Surg* 2009;18(1): 13-20.

2. Deng M, James R, Laurencin CT, Kumbar SG: Nanostructured polymeric scaffolds for orthopaedic regenerative engineering. *IEEE Trans Nanobioscience* 2012;11(1): 3-14.

3. Ricchetti ET, Aurora A, Iannotti JP, Derwin KA: Scaffold devices for rotator cuff repair. *J Shoulder Elbow Surg* 2012;21(2):251-265.

4. Badylak SF, Gilbert TW: Immune response to biologic scaffold materials. *Semin Immunol* 2008;20(2): 109-116.

5. Xu H, Sandor M, Qi S, et al: Implantation of a porcine acellular dermal graft in a primate model of rotator cuff repair. *J Shoulder Elbow Surg* 2012;21(5):580-588.

6. Walton JR, Bowman NK, Khatib Y, Linklater J, Murrell GA: Restore orthobiologic implant: Not recommended for augmentation of rotator cuff repairs. *J Bone Joint Surg Am* 2007;89(4): 786-791.

7. Tilley JM, Chaudhury S, Hakimi O, Carr AJ, Czernuszka JT: Tenocyte proliferation on collagen scaffolds protects against degradation and improves scaffold properties. *J Mater Sci Mater Med* 2012; 23(3):823-833.

8. Valentin JE, Badylak JS, McCabe GP, Badylak SF: Extracellular matrix bioscaffolds for orthopaedic applications: A comparative histologic study. *J Bone Joint Surg Am* 2006;88(12):2673-2686.

9. Liang HC, Chang Y, Hsu CK, Lee MH, Sung HW: Effects of crosslinking degree of an acellular biological tissue on its tissue regeneration pattern. *Biomaterials* 2004;25(17):3541-3552.

10. Soler JA, Gidwani S, Curtis MJ: Early complications from the use of porcine dermal collagen implants (Permacol) as bridging constructs in the repair of massive rotator cuff tears: A report of 4 cases. *Acta Orthop Belg* 2007; 73(4):432-436.

11. Nirmalanandhan VS, Juncosa-Melvin N, Shearn JT, et al: Combined effects of scaffold stiffening and mechanical preconditioning cycles on construct biomechanics, gene expression, and tendon repair biomechanics. *Tissue Eng Part A* 2009;15(8):2103-2111.

12. Deeken CR, Melman L, Jenkins ED, Greco SC, Frisella MM, Matthews BD: Histologic and biomechanical evaluation of crosslinked and non-crosslinked biologic meshes in a porcine model of ventral incisional hernia repair. *J Am Coll Surg* 2011;212(5):880-888.

13. Adams JE, Zobitz ME, Reach JS Jr, An KN, Steinmann SP: Rotator cuff repair using an acellular dermal matrix graft: An in vivo study in a canine model. *Arthroscopy* 2006;22(7):700-709.

14. Baker AR, McCarron JA, Tan CD, Iannotti JP, Derwin KA: Does augmentation with a reinforced fascia patch improve rotator cuff repair outcomes? *Clin Orthop Relat Res* 2012;470(9): 2513-2521.

15. Magnussen RA, Glisson RR, Moorman CT III: Augmentation of Achilles tendon repair with extracellular matrix xenograft: A biomechanical analysis. *Am J Sports Med* 2011;39(7):1522-1527.

16. Barber FA, Burns JP, Deutsch A, Labbé MR, Litchfield RB: A prospective, randomized evaluation of acellular human dermal matrix augmentation for arthroscopic rotator cuff repair. *Arthroscopy* 2012;28(1):8-15.

17. Iannotti JP, Codsi MJ, Kwon YW, Derwin K, Ciccone J, Brems JJ: Porcine small intestine submucosa augmentation of surgical repair of chronic two-tendon rotator cuff tears: A randomized, controlled trial. *J Bone Joint Surg Am* 2006;88(6):1238-1244.

18. Sclamberg SG, Tibone JE, Itamura JM, Kasraeian S: Six-month magnetic resonance imaging follow-up of large and massive rotator cuff repairs reinforced with porcine small intestinal submucosa. *J Shoulder Elbow Surg* 2004; 13(5):538-541.

19. Zhang X, Bogdanowicz D, Erisken C, Lee NM, Lu HH: Biomimetic scaffold design for functional and integrative tendon repair. *J Shoulder Elbow Surg* 2012; 21(2):266-277.

20. Zheng MH, Chen J, Kirilak Y, Willers C, Xu J, Wood D: Porcine small intestine submucosa (SIS) is not an acellular collagenous matrix and contains porcine DNA:

Possible implications in human implantation. *J Biomed Mater Res B Appl Biomater* 2005;73(1): 61-67.

21. Barber FA, Herbert MA, Coons DA: Tendon augmentation grafts: Biomechanical failure loads and failure patterns. *Arthroscopy* 2006; 22(5):534-538.

22. Derwin KA, Badylak SF, Steinmann SP, Iannotti JP: Extracellular matrix scaffold devices for rotator cuff repair. *J Shoulder Elbow Surg* 2010;19(3):467-476.

23. Chen J, Xu J, Wang A, Zheng M: Scaffolds for tendon and ligament repair: Review of the efficacy of commercial products. *Expert Rev Med Devices* 2009;6(1):61-73.

24. Moffat KL, Kwei AS, Spalazzi JP, Doty SB, Levine WN, Lu HH: Novel nanofiber-based scaffold for rotator cuff repair and augmentation. *Tissue Eng Part A* 2009; 15(1):115-126.

25. Mikos AG, McIntire LV, Anderson JM, Babensee JE: Host response to tissue engineered devices. *Adv Drug Deliv Rev* 1998; 33(1-2):111-139.

26. Lu L, Zhu X, Valenzuela RG, Currier BL, Yaszemski MJ: Biodegradable polymer scaffolds for cartilage tissue engineering. *Clin Orthop Relat Res* 2001;(391): S251-S270.

27. Yokoya S, Mochizuki Y, Nagata Y, Deie M, Ochi M: Tendon-bone insertion repair and regeneration using polyglycolic acid sheet in the rabbit rotator cuff injury model. *Am J Sports Med* 2008; 36(7):1298-1309.

28. Aurora A, McCarron JA, van den Bogert AJ, Gatica JE, Iannotti JP, Derwin KA: The biomechanical role of scaffolds in augmented rotator cuff tendon repairs. *J Shoulder Elbow Surg* 2012;21(8): 1064-1071.

29. Koh JL, Szomor Z, Murrell GA, Warren RF: Supplementation of rotator cuff repair with a bioresorbable scaffold. *Am J Sports Med* 2002;30(3):410-413.

30. Derwin KA, Codsi MJ, Milks RA, Baker AR, McCarron JA, Iannotti JP: Rotator cuff repair augmentation in a canine model with use of a woven poly-L-lactide device. *J Bone Joint Surg Am* 2009;91(5): 1159-1171.

31. MacGillivray JD, Fealy S, Terry MA, Koh JL, Nixon AJ, Warren RF: Biomechanical evaluation of a rotator cuff defect model augmented with a bioresorbable scaffold in goats. *J Shoulder Elbow Surg* 2006;15(5):639-644.

32. Encalada-Diaz I, Cole BJ, Macgillivray JD, et al: Preliminary results at 12 months' follow-up. *J Shoulder Elbow Surg* 2011;20(5): 788-794.

33. Santoni BG, McGilvray KC, Lyons AS, et al: Biomechanical analysis of an ovine rotator cuff repair via porous patch augmentation in a chronic rupture model. *Am J Sports Med* 2010;38(4):679-686.

34. Cole BJ, Gomoll AH, Yanke A, et al: Biocompatibility of a polymer patch for rotator cuff repair. *Knee Surg Sports Traumatol Arthrosc* 2007;15(5):632-637.

35. Spalazzi JP, Doty SB, Moffat KL, Levine WN, Lu HH: Development of controlled matrix heterogeneity on a triphasic scaffold for orthopedic interface tissue engineering. *Tissue Eng* 2006;12(12): 3497-3508.

36. Li X, Xie J, Lipner J, Yuan X, Thomopoulos S, Xia Y: Nanofiber scaffolds with gradations in mineral content for mimicking the tendon-to-bone insertion site. *Nano Lett* 2009;9(7):2763-2768.

37. Ni M, Rui YF, Tan Q, et al: Engineered scaffold-free tendon tissue produced by tendon-derived stem cells. *Biomaterials* 2013;34(8): 2024-2037.

38. Altman GH, Horan RL, Martin I, et al: Cell differentiation by mechanical stress. *FASEB J* 2002; 16(2):270-272.

39. Garvin J, Qi J, Maloney M, Banes AJ: Novel system for engineering bioartificial tendons and application of mechanical load. *Tissue Eng* 2003;9(5):967-979.

40. Tanaka H, Manske PR, Pruitt DL, Larson BJ: Effect of cyclic tension on lacerated flexor tendons in vitro. *J Hand Surg Am* 1995;20(3):467-473.

41. Hannafin JA, Arnoczky SP, Hoonjan A, Torzilli PA: Effect of stress deprivation and cyclic tensile loading on the material and morphologic properties of canine flexor digitorum profundus tendon: An in vitro study. *J Orthop Res* 1995;13(6):907-914.

42. Buckwalter JA, Grodzinsky AJ: Loading of healing bone, fibrous tissue, and muscle: Implications for orthopaedic practice. *J Am Acad Orthop Surg* 1999;7(5): 291-299.

43. Woo SL, Gomez MA, Sites TJ, Newton PO, Orlando CA, Akeson WH: The biomechanical and morphological changes in the medial collateral ligament of the rabbit after immobilization and remobilization. *J Bone Joint Surg Am* 1987;69(8):1200-1211.

44. Schwartz AG, Lipner JH, Pasteris JD, Genin GM, Thomopoulos S: Muscle loading is necessary for the formation of a functional tendon enthesis. *Bone* 2013;55(1): 44-51.

45. Thomopoulos S, Zampiakis E, Das R, Silva MJ, Gelberman RH: The effect of muscle loading on flexor tendon-to-bone healing in a canine model. *J Orthop Res* 2008; 26(12):1611-1617.

46. Bedi A, Kovacevic D, Fox AJ, et al: Effect of early and delayed mechanical loading on tendon-to-bone healing after anterior cruciate ligament reconstruction. *J Bone Joint Surg Am* 2010; 92(14):2387-2401.

47. Thomopoulos S, Williams GR, Soslowsky LJ: Tendon to bone healing: Differences in biomechanical, structural, and compositional properties due to a range of activity levels. *J Biomech Eng* 2003;125(1):106-113.

48. Hettrich CM, Rodeo SA, Hannafin JA, Ehteshami J, Shubin Stein BE: The effect of muscle paralysis using Botox on the healing of tendon to bone in a rat model. *J Shoulder Elbow Surg* 2011;20(5):688-697.

49. Ma J, Shen J, Smith BP, Ritting A, Smith TL, Koman LA: Bioprotection of tendon repair: Adjunctive use of botulinum toxin A in Achilles tendon repair in the rat. *J Bone Joint Surg Am* 2007; 89(10):2241-2249.

50. Patton CM, Powell AP, Patel AA: Vitamin D in orthopaedics. *J Am Acad Orthop Surg* 2012;20(3): 123-129.

51. Puthucheary Z, Skipworth JR, Rawal J, Loosemore M, Van Someren K, Montgomery HE: Genetic influences in sport and physical performance. *Sports Med* 2011;41(10):845-859.

52. Uitterlinden AG, Fang Y, Van Meurs JB, Pols HA, Van Leèuwen JP: Genetics and biology of vitamin D receptor polymorphisms. *Gene* 2004;338(2):143-156.

53. Erben RG, Soegiarto DW, Weber K, et al: Deletion of deoxyribonucleic acid binding domain of the vitamin D receptor abrogates genomic and nongenomic functions of vitamin D. *Mol Endocrinol* 2002;16(7):1524-1537.

54. Chung M, Balk EM, Brendel M, et al: A systematic review of health outcomes. *Evid Rep Technol Assess (Full Rep)* 2009;183:1-420.

55. Binkley N, Ramamurthy R, Krueger D: Low vitamin D status: Definition, prevalence, consequences, and correction. *Rheum Dis Clin North Am* 2012;38(1):45-59.

56. Lieben L, Carmeliet G: Vitamin D signaling in osteocytes: Effects on bone and mineral homeostasis. *Bone* 2013;54(2):237-243.

57. Avenell A, Gillespie WJ, Gillespie LD, O'Connell D: Vitamin D and vitamin D analogues for preventing fractures associated with involutional and post-menopausal osteoporosis. *Cochrane Database Syst Rev* 2009;2:CD000227.

58. Chen CM, Chu P, Huang GS, Wang SJ, Wu SS: Spontaneous rupture of the patellar and contralateral quadriceps tendons associated with secondary hyperparathyroidism in a patient receiving long-term dialysis. *J Formos Med Assoc* 2006;105(11):941-945.

59. Park JH, Kim SB, Shin HS, Jung GH, Jung YS, Rim H: Spontaneous and serial rupture of both Achilles tendons associated with secondary hyperparathyroidism in a patient receiving long-term hemodialysis. *Int Urol Nephrol* 2013;45(2):587-590.

60. De Franco P, Varghese J, Brown WW, Bastani B: Secondary hyperparathyroidism, and not beta 2-microglobulin amyloid, as a cause of spontaneous tendon rupture in patients on chronic hemodialysis. *Am J Kidney Dis* 1994; 24(6):951-955.

61. Basic-Jukic N, Juric I, Racki S, Kes P: Spontaneous tendon ruptures in patients with end-stage renal disease. *Kidney Blood Press Res* 2009;32(1):32-36.

62. Ryuzaki M, Konishi K, Kasuga A, et al: Spontaneous rupture of the quadriceps tendon in patients on maintenance hemodialysis: Report of three cases with clinicopathological observations. *Clin Nephrol* 1989;32(3):144-148.

63. Endo I, Inoue D, Mitsui T, et al: Deletion of vitamin D receptor gene in mice results in abnormal skeletal muscle development with deregulated expression of myoregulatory transcription factors. *Endocrinology* 2003;144(12): 5138-5144.

64. Schott GD, Wills MR: Muscle weakness in osteomalacia. *Lancet* 1976;1(7960):626-629.

65. Birge SJ, Haddad JG: 25-hydroxycholecalciferol stimulation of muscle metabolism. *J Clin Invest* 1975;56(5):1100-1107.

66. Visser M, Deeg DJ, Lips P; Longitudinal Aging Study Amsterdam: Low vitamin D and high parathyroid hormone levels as determinants of loss of muscle strength and muscle mass (sarcopenia): The Longitudinal Aging Study Amsterdam. *J Clin Endocrinol Metab* 2003;88(12):5766-5772.

67. Oh JH, Kim SH, Kim JH, Shin YH, Yoon JP, Oh CH: The level of vitamin D in the serum correlates with fatty degeneration of the muscles of the rotator cuff. *J Bone Joint Surg Br* 2009;91(12): 1587-1593.

68. Hamilton B: Vitamin D and human skeletal muscle. *Scand J Med Sci Sports* 2010;20(2):182-190.

69. Girgis CM, Clifton-Bligh RJ, Hamrick MW, Holick MF, Gunton JE: The roles of vitamin D in skeletal muscle: Form, function, and metabolism. *Endocr Rev* 2013;34(1):33-83.

70. Angeline ME, Ma R, Pascual-Garrido C, et al: Effect of diet-induced vitamin D deficiency on rotator cuff healing in a rat model. *Am J Sports Med* [published online ahead of print October 16, 2013.] PMID: 24131579.

71. Kim RP: The musculoskeletal complications of diabetes. *Curr Diab Rep* 2002;2(1):49-52.

72. Rechardt M, Shiri R, Karppinen J, Jula A, Heliövaara M, Viikari-Juntura E: Lifestyle and metabolic factors in relation to shoulder pain and rotator cuff tendinitis: A population-based

study. *BMC Musculoskelet Disord* 2010;11:165.

73. Longo UG, Franceschi F, Ruzzini L, Spiezia F, Maffulli N, Denaro V: Higher fasting plasma glucose levels within the normoglycaemic range and rotator cuff tears. *Br J Sports Med* 2009; 43(4):284-287.

74. Chung SW, Oh JH, Gong HS, Kim JY, Kim SH: Factors affecting rotator cuff healing after arthroscopic repair: Osteoporosis as one of the independent risk factors. *Am J Sports Med* 2011; 39(10):2099-2107.

75. Namdari S, Green A: Range of motion limitation after rotator cuff repair. *J Shoulder Elbow Surg* 2010;19(2):290-296.

76. El Zahran T, Collins K, Terk MR: Bilateral spontaneous rupture of the flexor digitorum superficialis and the flexor digitorum profundus in a diabetic patient. *Skeletal Radiol* 2013;42(2):297-301.

77. Rajagopalan S, Sangar A, Upadhyay V, Lloyd J, Taylor H: Bilateral atraumatic sequential rupture of tibialis anterior tendons. *Foot Ankle Spec* 2010;3(6):352-355.

78. Maffulli N, Longo UG, Maffulli GD, Khanna A, Denaro V: Achilles tendon ruptures in diabetic patients. *Arch Orthop Trauma Surg* 2011;131(1):33-38.

79. Akturk M, Karaahmetoglu S, Kacar M, Muftuoglu O: Thickness of the supraspinatus and biceps tendons in diabetic patients. *Diabetes Care* 2002;25(2):408.

80. Grant WP, Sullivan R, Sonenshine DE, et al: Electron microscopic investigation of the effects of diabetes mellitus on the Achilles tendon. *J Foot Ankle Surg* 1997;36(4):272-278.

81. de Oliveira RR, de Lira KD, Silveira PV, et al: Mechanical properties of Achilles tendon in rats induced to experimental diabetes. *Ann Biomed Eng* 2011;39(5): 1528-1534.

82. Fox AJ, Bedi A, Deng XH, et al: Diabetes mellitus alters the mechanical properties of the native tendon in an experimental rat model. *J Orthop Res* 2011;29(6): 880-885.

83. Li Y, Fessel G, Georgiadis M, Snedeker JG: Advanced glycation end-products diminish tendon collagen fiber sliding. *Matrix Biol* 2013;32(3-4):169-177.

84. Clement ND, Hallett A, MacDonald D, Howie C, McBirnie J: Does diabetes affect outcome after arthroscopic repair of the rotator cuff? *J Bone Joint Surg Br* 2010; 92(8):1112-1117.

85. Chung SW, Park JS, Kim SH, Shin SH, Oh JH: Quality of life after arthroscopic rotator cuff repair: Evaluation using SF-36 and an analysis of affecting clinical factors. *Am J Sports Med* 2012; 40(3):631-639.

86. Chen AL, Shapiro JA, Ahn AK, Zuckerman JD, Cuomo F: Rotator cuff repair in patients with type I diabetes mellitus. *J Shoulder Elbow Surg* 2003;12(5):416-421.

87. Bedi A, Fox AJ, Harris PE, et al: Diabetes mellitus impairs tendon-bone healing after rotator cuff repair. *J Shoulder Elbow Surg* 2010;19(7):978-988.

88. Handa A, Gotoh M, Hamada K, et al: Vascular endothelial growth factor 121 and 165 in the subacromial bursa are involved in shoulder joint contracture in type II diabetics with rotator cuff disease. *J Orthop Res* 2003;21(6): 1138-1144.

89. Chbinou N, Frenette J: Insulin-dependent diabetes impairs the inflammatory response and delays angiogenesis following Achilles tendon injury. *Am J Physiol Regul Integr Comp Physiol* 2004;286(5): R952-R957.

90. Rizvi AA, Chillag SA, Chillag KJ: Perioperative management of diabetes and hyperglycemia in pa-

tients undergoing orthopaedic surgery. *J Am Acad Orthop Surg* 2010;18(7):426-435.

91. Józsa L, Kannus P, Thöring J, Reffy A, Järvinen M, Kvist M: The effect of tenotomy and immobilisation on intramuscular connective tissue: A morphometric and microscopic study in rat calf muscles. *J Bone Joint Surg Br* 1990;72(2):293-297.

92. Järvinen MJ, Lehto MU: The effects of early mobilisation and immobilisation on the healing process following muscle injuries. *Sports Med* 1993;15(2):78-89.

93. Caplan A, Carlson B, Faulkner J: Skeletal muscle, in Woo SLY, ed: *Injury and Repair of the Musculoskeletal Soft Tissues*. Park Ridge, IL, American Academy of Orthopaedic Surgeons, 1988, pp 213-291.

94. Gerber C, Meyer DC, Frey E, et al: Reversion of structural muscle changes caused by chronic rotator cuff tears using continuous musculotendinous traction: An experimental study in sheep. *J Shoulder Elbow Surg* 2009;18(2): 163-171.

95. Mendias CL, Bakhurin KI, Faulkner JA: Tendons of myostatin-deficient mice are small, brittle, and hypocellular. *Proc Natl Acad Sci USA* 2008; 105(1):388-393.

96. Mendias CL, Lynch EB, Davis ME, et al: Changes in circulating biomarkers of muscle atrophy, inflammation, and cartilage turnover in patients undergoing anterior cruciate ligament reconstruction and rehabilitation. *Am J Sports Med* 2013;41(8):1819-1826.

97. Attie KM, Borgstein NG, Yang Y, et al: A single ascending-dose study of muscle regulator ACE-031 in healthy volunteers. *Muscle Nerve* 2013;47(3):416-423.

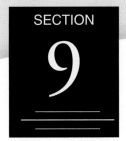

The Practice of Orthopaedics

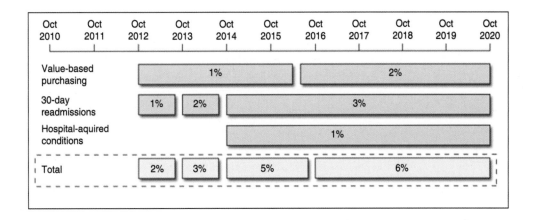

The Practice of Orthopaedics

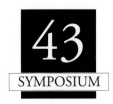

Applying Quality Principles to Orthopaedic Surgery

Gregory Katz, MD
Crispin Ong, MD
Lorraine Hutzler, BA
Joseph D. Zuckerman, MD
Joseph A. Bosco III, MD

Abstract

The unsustainable rising cost of medical care is creating financial pressures that will critically alter the way that health care is paid for and delivered. Limited resources dictate that physicians must become more efficient at providing high quality care. In an effort to provide financial incentive for delivering quality care, the federal government instituted value-based purchasing to transform Medicare from a passive payer of claims to an active purchaser of medical care. Healthcare providers must follow the basic tenants of certain quality principles to maximize reimbursement under the value-based purchasing system.

Instr Course Lect 2014;63:465-472.

The unsustainable rising cost of medical care is creating financial pressures that will critically alter the way that health care is paid for and delivered. The newly enacted Patient Protection and Affordable Care Act (PPACA) creates important changes in the economics of health care. The passage of this landmark legislation will affect all those involved in healthcare delivery, from physicians and ancillary staff to administrators and hospitals. Although the benefits and drawbacks of the legislation can be debated, the reality is that fundamental change is necessary. The United States spends $2.3 trillion annually on health care, which is one sixth of the US gross national product.[1] Population demographics indicate that this number will continue to rise in the future.

Yearly healthcare costs for individuals older than 65 years are approximately $15,000 per person (three times higher than costs of younger Americans), and the number of older Americans is projected to grow by more than 30 million over the next two decades.[2,3] Avoiding changes to the healthcare systems would keep the United States on a path to financial ruin; simply shifting who pays for medical care is an inadequate solution. There must be an evolution in what services are paid for and how the amount of payment is determined. Physicians and hospitals must make changes in the way healthcare services are delivered. The limited resources of time and money mean that a stark choice must be made—healthcare providers can either become more efficient at providing high quality care for everyone, or decisions will be required regarding who will go without care.

Because the government is the single largest purchaser of health care, new Medicare payment guidelines can dictate that hospitals must change the way that medical services are delivered. Beginning in October 2012, 2% of Medicare payments will be withheld and reallocated based on how well hospitals comply with new guidelines. Between 2012 and 2020, this percentage will

Dr. Zuckerman or an immediate family member has received royalties from Exactech; has stock or stock options held in Hip Innovation Technology and Neostem; and serves as a board member, owner, officer, or committee member of the American Orthopaedic Association. Dr. Bosco or an immediate family member has received research or institutional support from 3M and MAKO, and serves as a board member, owner, officer, or committee member of the American Orthopaedic Society for Sports Medicine and the New York State Society of Orthopaedic Surgeons. None of the following authors or any immediate family member has received anything of value from or owns stock in a commercial company or institution related directly or indirectly to the subject of this chapter: Dr. Katz, Dr. Ong, and Ms. Hutzler.

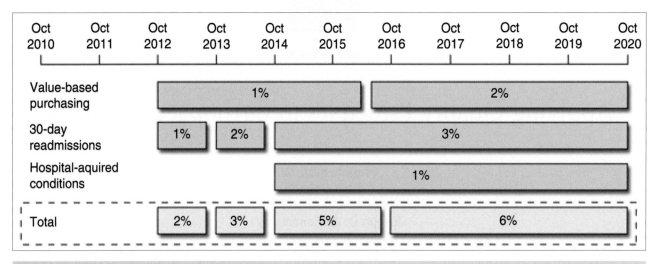

Figure 1   Timeline used by CMS to determine the payments at risk.

increase to 6%. This means that the best-performing hospitals will receive a 6% bonus, whereas the worst-performing hospitals will see their reimbursements cut by 6%. Given that the average hospital had an operating margin of 3% to 4% in 2010, these changes in reimbursement rates will have a substantial effect.[4] Making adjustments in care delivery ceases to be a choice and becomes a requirement if a hospital is to remain financially solvent.

Three provisions in the Affordable Care Act will put Medicare-associated operating margins at risk: value-based purchasing, 30-day readmissions, and hospital-acquired conditions. **Figure 1** details the timeline used by the Centers for Medicare and Medicaid Services (CMS) to determine the payments at risk. This chapter will assess these provisions by examining how the application of quality principles from the business world can help hospitals change their systems to improve both outcomes and efficiency.

Value-Based Purchasing

The goal of value-based purchasing is to transform Medicare from a passive payer of claims to an active purchaser of care.[5] For decades, healthcare systems have responded to incentives that rewarded volume regardless of quality. Value-based purchasing is an effort to change the focus of how care is paid for; in essence, the government wants value, not just quantity, for the money that it spends. Kathleen Sebelius, Secretary of Health and Human Services, says, "Under this initiative, Medicare will reward hospitals that provide high-quality care and keep their patients healthy. As hospitals work to improve their performance on these measures, all patients, not just Medicare patients, will benefit."[6] Value-based purchasing creates a model for rewarding hospitals that perform well and penalizing hospitals that perform poorly. Beginning in fiscal year 2013, incentive payments for value-based purchasing are funded by a 1% decrease in reimbursements for diagnosis-related group payments; a 2% decrease will begin in fiscal year 2017. These incentive payments will be allocated based on performance on 13 measures divided between two domains of care measures: clinical process and patient experience.

Domains of Care

The clinical process of care domain encompasses 12 performance targets in the care of acute myocardial infarction, heart failure, pneumonia, healthcare-associated infections, and surgical care. The patient experience of care domain is measured by the Hospital Consumer Assessment of Healthcare Providers and Systems (HCAHPS) score, which is a subjective measure of patients' opinions regarding care they received. Beginning in 2014, measures of mortality outcomes and iatrogenic complications will be added as a third domain. The CMS will determine a hospital's total performance score for achievement and improvement levels and will subsequently calculate appropriate incentive payments based on these measures.

Discussion of the full breadth of the CMS calculations is beyond the scope of this chapter, but the following description provides an abridged explanation. Using performance data from July 1, 2009, through March 31, 2010, CMS has established minimum achievement and benchmark thresholds for each measure of clinical care. These thresholds are calculated using the 50th and 90th percentiles of compliance in each domain. The scores for each measure will be determined based on where a hospital falls within the achievement range. Individual hospitals will be scored on both achievement and improvement during the performance period of evaluation, which runs from July 1, 2011, to March 31, 2012, with the higher score used in the assessment of each measure. The clinical process of care domain score will give equal weight to each performance measure being assessed. The total performance score will then be calculated, with clinical process of care measures accounting for 70% and patient experience measures determining the remaining 30%. Incentive payments will then be made using a linear scale, with budget neutrality determining the allocation of funds.[5]

Achieving better results in the clinical process and the patient experience domains are complementary goals, but each poses its own set of challenges and requires its own unique quality improvements. The goals of both represent an effort to improve the overall quality of medical care; however, quality means different things in different contexts. Quality can be measured via internal metrics evaluating the elimination of errors (clinical process domain) and/or via external metrics evaluating patient satisfaction (patient experience domain). As previously discussed, the principles of value-based purchasing ensure that both sets of metrics will play a role in determining the quality of care that a hospital provides. Improving clinical process domains must be guided by eliminating errors from the process of care delivery. This method of quality improvement can be approached using techniques to improve operating efficiency, reduce variation, avoid defects, and reduce waste. This complements the patient experience domain, which is focused on achieving patient satisfaction. Improvements in this latter area should be approached with the goal of enhancing long-term success through customer satisfaction.

Internal Metrics for Measuring and Improving the Quality of Care

Improving internal metrics involves detecting and correcting errors. Before this can occur, it is vital to properly identify where improvements should be made in the process of care delivery. The clinical process domains from the value-based purchasing provision in the PPACA are objective (for example, there is no ambiguity about whether a patient receives prophylactic antibiotics or appropriate anticoagulation therapy). The objective nature of internal metrics simplifies their measurement and allows straightforward calculations regarding improvement. Improving internal metrics places importance on conformance to well-designed standards and consistency in their execution. The application of quality management principles is vital in reducing defects, the standard by which clinical process domain improvement is measured.

Professionalizing Quality Management

Professionalizing quality management is a necessary part of improving internal metrics. Adjusting the role of clinical coordinators may be a useful step for hospitals to improve care delivery. A professional quality manager must be proactive and not simply reactive, working to redesign the system in anticipation of potential problems instead of formulating ad hoc solutions as difficulties arise.

Professionalizing quality management is a requirement for large organizations seeking to reduce defects and improve efficiency. If no one has the responsibility to identify and fix system problems, each member of the patient-care team will develop his or her own work-around to circumvent a breakdown or a problem in the system. This situation reduces quality and in-

creases costs by continuing systemic procedures that may be causing errors or slowing down care delivery. Six Sigma, a widely used business management strategy developed by Motorola and most famously applied by General Electric, has shown the effectiveness of creating a command chain of quality management and the need for commitment from executive leadership and project managers to achieve success.[7] Applying these principles to a hospital means that both administrative and clinical personnel need to be enlisted to properly execute quality management. Adjusting the system through the employment of quality managers means empowering staff to bring their concerns to the attention of those responsible for making changes to address problems.

Quality improvement professionals in the Toyota Production System approach improvement incrementally, using simulations to break large problems into smaller pieces and generate solutions for each step in the process. When a problem is identified, instead of asking employees what changes should be made to improve the process, quality improvement professionals inquire about specific systemic impediments that prevent people from doing their job. This approach pinpoints systemic flaws and avoids the insinuation that employees are failing to perform their duties. When problems are identified, rapid experimentation with novel solutions is used and successful interventions are incorporated into standard protocols. The result is a decrease in defects and improvements in efficiency as workarounds are gradually eliminated from daily operations.[8]

Pilot programs across the country have demonstrated the efficacy of implementing aspects of the Toyota Production System approach. The Pittsburgh Regional Health Initiative decreased central line infections by more than 50% within 3 years of implementing techniques adapted from the Toyota approach.[9] The Virginia Mason Medical Center of Seattle reduced the number of annual cases of ventilator-acquired pneumonia by approximately 90% in 2 years after adopting Toyota Production System methods. When Western Pennsylvania Hospital (Pittsburg) professionalized quality management in the surgical unit by changing the role of a clinical coordinator from an improviser of last minute solutions to a devisor of systemic improvements, 54 problems were solved over the course of 1 year.[8] Positive effects included reducing idle operating room time, eliminating the problem of incomplete laboratory results, and improving the timely availability of surgical supplies.

Critically evaluating and continually reassessing the efficacy and efficiency of established systems is a necessary part of quality improvement. This cannot be adequately achieved without the specific delegation of quality improvement monitoring and systemic adjustment to employees tasked with improving care delivery.

30-Day Readmission Rates

Readmission rates are viewed as an important barometer of quality of care. Under the current CMS program, readmission rate guidelines do not apply to most orthopaedic surgeons because hospitals will be penalized only for an excessive number of readmissions following discharges for heart failure, myocardial infarctions, and pneumonia. These penalties began at 1% of reimbursements in 2012 and increased to 2% in 2013 and 3% in 2014. It is anticipated that readmissions after total joint replacement procedures will soon be added to the guidelines, creating pressure to reduce readmission rates in these patients. Hospitals and or-

thopaedic surgeons should plan accordingly. It also should be noted that in 2012, the PPACA required CMS to conduct research on the potential expansion of penalties to postacute settings such as inpatient rehabilitation facilities, long-term care hospitals, and outpatient facilities. A fully coordinated system of clinical alignment and resource effectiveness became necessary so hospitals and health systems could ensure they were prepared to comply with guidelines encompassing acute and postacute care.

Hospital-Acquired Conditions

Hospital-acquired conditions (HACs) are familiar to orthopaedic surgeons and include retained foreign bodies after surgery, urinary tract infections after Foley catheterization, sepsis after placement of a central line, air embolisms, blood incompatibility, pressure ulcers, falls and traumatic injuries, and manifestations of poor glycemic control. At the current time, the quantitative guidelines are being determined; CMS will be publicly reporting HAC data starting in 2015. At that time, the bottom quartile of hospitals with the highest rates of HACs will be financially penalized, with an overall payment reduction of 1% for those facilities with the highest HAC rates. In their calculations of the worst-performing 25% of organizations, CMS will stratify hospitals based on patient risk, a distinction pertinent to those physicians and hospitals that treat high-risk populations. The statistics behind HACs are not trivial. According to studies reviewed by the Institute of Medicine, approximately 100,000 people die unnecessarily each year from hospital-acquired infections.[10-12] HACs have been shown to increase inpatient cost by $25,903 per patient, leading to additional overall health costs of $45 billion nationally.[13]

Of all the members of the patient care team, nurses usually have the most

powerful influence on HACs. The direct patient contact provided by nurses is the first line of defense against many of these complications. In many instances, a nurse is the first care provider to notice the earliest signs of infection and skin breakdown. This fact speaks to the importance of organizational fluidity and interdisciplinary communication. For quality measures to be truly successful, all operational disciplines and every member of the hospital staff must have the same quality goals. These domains include awareness of quality processes, compliance with protocols, appropriate skill-level achievement, system design, effective use of data, decision making that supports systemic structure, and accurate measurement of performance metrics. The level of execution across all domains determines the maturity level of operations and the success that will be achieved in reaching organizational goals.

External Metrics for Measuring and Improving the Quality of Care

Although assessing quality improvement of clinical process domains involves measuring objective internal metrics, the subjective nature of the external metrics in the patient care domain presents a different set of challenges. In the patient care domain, outcomes are governed by patient preferences, attributes, expectations, and perceptions. These factors are difficult to measure and vary from person to person and population to population. Because satisfaction cannot be assessed until each episode of care delivery is complete, the instant feedback that can be obtained with clinical process improvement is not possible, and an additional layer of complexity is added to an already daunting process. For organizations confronting this challenge, the HCAHPS score provides a method of standardization of patients' desired delivery models.

Measuring Patient Satisfaction

To improve patient satisfaction, it is imperative to be aware of the standards that comprise its evaluation. The HCAHPS survey asks a random sampling of discharged patients to answer 27 questions about their hospital stay. Eighteen core questions pertain to important aspects of the hospital experience, including communication with nurses and doctors, responsiveness of the hospital staff, cleanliness and quietness of the hospital environment, effectiveness of pain management, communication about medications, receipt of discharge information, overall rating of the hospital, and whether they would recommend the hospital to others. Four items on the survey direct patients to relevant questions, three items are included to adjust for the mix of patients across hospitals, and two items support congressionally mandated reporting. The surveys will be distributed to a broad demographic and medical cross section of patients between 2 days and 6 weeks after discharge.[14]

Expected and Received Care

There may be a divide between patients' preconceived notions of the care they expect and their perception of the care they receive. To make the necessary adjustments to improve external metrics, it is vital to understand the areas in which patient expectations may not be met. These discrepancies generally fall into one of the following five areas. (1) The design gap—Will the product as designed satisfy the intended customer? This is the gap between patient expectations and the physician understanding of what patients expect. (2) The capability gap—Is the process capable of producing the product as designed? When the patient's expecta-

tions are understood, the hospital must have the capability to provide care that meets those expectations. (3) The delivery gap—Is the product delivered to the customer as intended? If the hospital is capable of providing the expected care, it must be appropriately performed without error. (4) The experience gap—Is the product being used as intended? If care is delivered appropriately and executed properly, the patient must also experience the result he or she was anticipating. (5) The perception gap—Do customers perceive the value of the delivered product? The patient must subjectively believe that he or she received the level of care that was anticipated.

Improved physician communication can bridge these gaps. The addition of HCAHPS metrics to the CMS total performance score mandates that physicians approach interactions with patients from the perspective of satisfying a customer and not only fixing a medical disorder.

Amending Poor Outcomes

High levels of patient satisfaction are relatively easy to obtain when outcomes are favorable and there are no setbacks in treatment or recovery. It is not surprising that market researchers have found that the most satisfied customers are those who have never experienced a serious problem or product defect.[15] Patient dissatisfaction is likely when patients experience adverse side effects from treatment or are harmed by medical errors. Two concepts that must be kept in mind for these patients are service recovery and the grapevine effect.

Service recovery is the process of restoring a patient's trust and confidence in the ability of the hospital or doctor to provide high-quality care. Experts in this area provide a six-step outline for intervening in cases of patient dissatisfaction: apologize for and ac-

knowledge the error; listen, empathize, and ask open-ended questions; fix the problem quickly and fairly; offer atonement; follow-up; and remember promises made to the patient.[16]

It is recommended that a healthcare system have five components in place to handle patient complaints.[16] (1) Effective systems should be in place for inviting and encouraging customers to complain. (2) Staff should have guidelines and latitude to act on complaints and atone for mistakes. (3) A documentation and a feedback loop should be created to channel problems through service recovery into an improvement or problem elimination process. (4) Clear protocols should be established to effectively handle complaints. (5) Staff should be skilled in service recovery.

Using feedback loops to channel patient complaints into organizational problem-solving ideas is necessary to proactively evaluate and improve the external metrics of care delivery. Because most complaints are directed towards frontline staff members who do not have the authority to make systemic changes, creating a feedback loop allows a negative patient experience to become an impetus for positive change.

The grapevine effect stems from the observation that only 50% of unhappy customers complain to the offending organization, but 96% will tell 9 or 10 friends about a bad experience.[16] With the Internet democratizing reviews of physicians and hospitals, a handful of dissatisfied patients can quickly lead to a change in a physician's or hospital's reputation in the community.

Elements and Effects of Patient Satisfaction

It is important to realize that many elements of patient satisfaction are dependent on factors outside of patient-physician interactions. These factors include communication with nurses, perceptions of hospital cleanliness, and the level of noise in the hospital. Given that the time lag of HCAHPS can extend as long as 6 weeks after discharge, orthopaedic surgeons should recognize that postoperative office visits also may play a role in a patient's perceptions of the care received. Subjective beliefs about all elements of the outpatient experience, including interactions with office staff, time spent in the waiting room, and even the perceived cleanliness of the office, may have an influence on hospital HCAHPS scores. Awareness of the scope of HCAHPS satisfaction evaluations and possible quality gaps in care delivery will ensure that physicians are appropriately prepared to score well on these subjective assessments of medical care.

Excellent achievement relating to external metrics will be an important aspect of an orthopaedic surgeon's career even outside an acute hospital setting. It is likely that the results of patient satisfaction surveys will become part of the maintenance of certification process of the American Board of Orthopaedic Surgery. The coupling of external metrics to reimbursement is likely to be a permanent feature in medical finances. This coupling is already being experimented with in the private health insurance market by WellPoint (Indianapolis, IN), a large healthcare management company, and other insurers will almost certainly follow in tying reimbursement levels to patient satisfaction.[17]

Quality Leverages

Understanding at-risk payments and basic quality principles is the first step in improving the quality of care and patient outcomes. Orthopaedic surgeons should focus on useful quality leverages. The process of quality improvement should be viewed using the Pareto Principle (also known as the 80/20 rule), named after the early 20th

century Italian economist Vilfredo Pareto. He observed that 80% of the land in Italy was owned by 20% of the population. This principle, which highlights the unequal distribution between inputs and outputs, can be thought of more simply as the idea that some factors have a much larger effect on results than others. A prime example of this principle is the total distribution of healthcare costs in the United States, with 50% of total costs incurred by 5% of the population.[18]

Applying this concept to quality improvement requires distinguishing between the vital few and the trivial many. Because each hospital has its own set of metrics requiring improvement, proper stratification of an organization's flaws is essential to efficiently apply improvement efforts. The Pareto Principle says that cost-control efforts should not be equally allocated, and not all cost-control mechanisms have the same effect. The allocation of resources for improvement should be dictated by two factors: where they are most needed and where they can have the greatest effect. The former is based on an individual hospital's performance, whereas the latter can be better understood through the investigation of additional quality leverages.

Improvement efforts should focus on the concept of early detection and resolution at the source of a problem. For example, General Electric found that fixing a defect at the level of the supplier costs approximately $0.003 per unit. This cost rises by a factor of 10 at each step of the production process, culminating at a cost of $300 per unit for servicing a product that has already been purchased. In essence, the costs of poor quality exceed the costs required to provide high quality.

Drug preparation and dispensation errors are implicated in as many as 21% of medication errors.[19] Correcting a problem at the pharmacy that

prevents the timely administration of prophylactic antibiotics is much more cost effective than treating a surgical site infection. In medicine, savings from early detection are not just monetary. In the example of a surgical site infection (monetary cost as much as $30,000) the resulting morbidity may involve the long-term use of intravenous antibiotics and their associated adverse side effects, a longer hospital stay for the patient, a higher rate of readmission, and the possibility of additional surgeries.[20]

Although early detection of errors can reduce costs and improve outcomes, prevention is an even more effective measure. Methods to prevent errors can be designed into a system by establishing protocols. For example, when a right hip replacement is being performed, the operating room should be stocked with only right-sided parts and the parts should be clearly labeled to eliminate any possibility of confusion. A DePuy femoral unicondylar cemented component for the right hip is labelled LM/RL to inform the user that left is medial and right is lateral. This description is complicated and requires an unnecessary level of cognition and awareness that can lead to errors. Reducing operating room errors could be as simple as placing a large label that says "RIGHT" on the device in question. Preventive measures in organization systems can improve outcomes by eliminating the possibility of certain errors.

Discussion

In many ways, the healthcare industry has been immune to the normal monetary forces that dictate business operations. Operating under the fee-for-service model has, to a certain extent, allowed the medical profession to avoid cost control and has retarded the implementation of quality principles commonly used in other industries.

The increasing pressure to provide value presents a new set of challenges to the current healthcare practices. Although the goal of obtaining the best clinical outcome has always guided and will continue to guide medical decision making, physicians have never been forced to document quality because the primary focus has been on maximizing clinical volumes. Monetary pressure to cut costs while improving outcomes represents a new force in the marketplace. The translation of concepts from the business world to orthopaedics and to all of medicine is an invaluable method of improving both the quality and efficiency of the delivery of medical care. Applying principles of quality management is vital to comply with the changing structure of healthcare reimbursements, and, more importantly, to provide the best care for an aging population.

Summary

PPACA was enacted to deflect the cost curve associated with the unsustainable rising cost of medical care in this country. This legislation creates substantial changes in the economics of health care and affects the way that health care is paid for and delivered. The principles of quality leveraging are well tested and easily applicable to healthcare delivery. The value-based purchasing program will decrease payments to institutions that do not provide quality care. It is essential for the financial survival of healthcare institutions that they internalize these principles. The involvement of healthcare providers is necessary for the successful application of these quality strategies, so it will be increasingly imperative that orthopaedic surgeons become well versed in the quality principles needed to improve healthcare delivery while lowering costs.

References

1. US health care costs. Kaiser Edu.org website. http://www.kaiseredu.org/Issue-Modules/US-Health-Care-Costs/Background-Brief.aspx. Accessed January 14, 2013.

2. Total personal health care spending, by age group, calendar years, 1987, 1996, 1999, 2002, 2004. Centers for Medicare and Medicaid Services website. https://www.cms.gov/NationalHealthExpendData/downloads/2004-age-tables.pdf. Accessed January 14, 2013.

3. Population projections. United States Census Bureau website. http://www.census.gov/population/projections/. Accessed January 14, 2012.

4. Hospital financial performance. State of California Office of Statewide Health Planning and Development website. http://www.oshpd.ca.gov/HID/Products/Hospitals/AnnFinanData/HospFinanPerform/HospitalFinancialPerformance.pdf. Accessed January 14, 2013.

5. Medicare FFS Physician Feedback Program: Value-Based Payment Modifier: Background. Centers for Medicare and Medicaid Services. http://cms.gov/medicare/medicare-fee-for-service-Payment/PhysicianFeedbackProgram/background.html. Accessed May 20, 2013.

6. Administration implements affordable care act provision to improve care, lower costs. April 29, 2011. Department of Health and Human Services. http://www.hhs.gov/news/press/2011pres/04/20110429a.html. Accessed January 14, 2013.

7. Stamatis DH: *Six Sigma Fundamentals: A Complete Guide to the System, Methods, and Tools.* New York, NY, Productivity Press, 2004.

8. Spear SJ: Fixing health care from the inside, today. *Harv Bus Rev* 2005;83(9):78-91, 158.

9. Reduction in central-line associated bloodstream infections among patients in intensive care units: Pennsylvania, April 2001-March 2005. Morbidity and Mortality Weekly Report. Centers for Disease Control and Prevention. http://www.cdc.gov/mmwr/preview/mmwrhtml/mm5440a2.htm. Accessed May 20, 2013.

10. Burke JP: Infection control: A problem for patient safety. *N Engl J Med* 2003;348(7):651-656.

11. Jarvis WR: Infection control and changing health-care delivery systems. *Emerg Infect Dis* 2001;7(2):170-173.

12. Weinstein RA: Nosocomial infection update. *Emerg Infect Dis* 1998;4(3):416-420.

13. Scott RD II: The direct medical costs of healthcare-associated infections in US hospitals and the benefits of prevention. http://www.cdc.gov/HAI/pdfs/hai/scott_costpaper.pdf. Accessed May 20, 2013.

14. Hospital quality initiative. Centers for Medicare and Medicaid Services website. https://www.cms.gov/hospitalqualityinits/30_hospitalhcahps.asp. Accessed January 14, 2013.

15. Berry L: *Discovering the Soul of Service: The Nine Drivers of Sustainable Business Success.* New York, NY, Free Press, 1999.

16. Surveys and tools to advance patient-centered care. US Department of Health and Human Services website. Agency for Healthcare Research and Quality. Consumer Assessment of Healthcare Providers and Systems. https://www.cahps.ahrq.gov/qiguide/content/interventions/ServiceRecoverySystems.aspx. Accessed January 14, 2013.

17. Adamy J: WellPoint shakes up hospital payments. *Wall Street Journal*. May 16, 2011. http://online.wsj.com/article/SB10001424052748704281504576325163218629124.html. Accessed January 14, 2013.

18. The high concentration of US health care expenditures. US Department of Health and Human Services website. Agency for Healthcare Research and Quality. http://www.ahrq.gov/research/ria19/expendria.htm. Accessed January 14, 2013.

19. Bond CA, Raehl CL, Franke T: Medication errors in United States hospitals. *Pharmacotherapy* 2001;21(9):1023-1036.

20. Urban JA: Cost analysis of surgical site infections. *Surg Infect (Larchmt)* 2006;7(suppl 1):S19-S22.

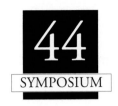

44

SYMPOSIUM

Measuring Quality in Orthopaedic Surgery: The Use of Metrics in Quality Management

Joseph A. Bosco III, MD
Ranjan Sachdev, MD, MBA, CHC
Louis A. Shapiro
Spencer M. Stein, BA
Joseph D. Zuckerman, MD

Abstract

There has been a substantial shift in the assessment of outcomes in medicine, including orthopaedic surgery. The quality movement is redefining the delivery of health care. The effect of these changes on orthopaedic surgery and orthopaedic surgeons has been significant and will become increasingly important. Orthopaedic surgeons must become active participants in the quality movement by understanding the basic principles of the movement and how they apply to patient care. A clear understanding of the different agencies (governmental and private) that are leading these initiatives is also essential. Ultimately, active participation in the quality movement will enhance the care provided to patients with musculoskeletal disorders.

Instr Course Lect 2014;63:473-485.

The quality movement in medicine is redefining the delivery of health care. The effect on orthopaedic surgery already has been substantial and will continue to increase in importance. Orthopaedic surgeons are very familiar with the terminology involved in the open reduction and internal fixation of specific fractures, the techniques of anterior cruciate ligament reconstruc-

tion, and the various approaches for total hip arthroplasty; however, they must now add many new terms to the orthopaedic lexicon, including value-based purchasing, quality, clinical practice guidelines, appropriate-use criteria, accountable care organizations, bundled payment systems, and episodes of care. This chapter will provide orthopaedic surgeons with insights into the effects of the quality movement on the daily practice of orthopaedic surgery and, more importantly, strategies for participation in the quality movement.

Many definitions of quality have been proposed. The definition proposed by the Institute of Medicine and modified from the ideas of W. Edwards Deming is particularly helpful.[1] Quality consists of the degree to which health services for individuals in populations increase the likelihood of desired health outcomes (quality principles), are consistent with current professional knowledge (professional practitioner skills), and meet the expectations of healthcare users (the marketplace). The understanding of value is

Dr. Bosco or an immediate family member has received research or institutional support from 3M and MAKO and serves as a board member, owner, officer, or committee member of the American Orthopaedic Society for Sports Medicine and the New York State Society of Orthopedic Surgeons. Dr. Sachdev or an immediate family member has stock or stock options held in Bristol-Myers Squibb, Eli Lilly, General Electric, Johnson & Johnson, Pfizer, Procter & Gamble, Sanofi-Aventis, Stryker, Zimmer Founder, and Exscribe. Dr. Zuckerman or an immediate family member has received royalties from Exactech; has stock or stock options held in Hip Innovation Technology and Neostem; has received nonincome support (such as equipment or services), commercially derived honoraria, or other non–research-related funding (such as paid travel) from Orthonet; and serves as a board member, owner, officer, or committee member of the American Orthopaedic Association. Neither of the following authors nor any immediate family member has received anything of value from or has stock or stock options held in a commercial company or institution related directly or indirectly to the subject of this chapter: Mr. Shapiro and Mr. Stein.

intrinsic to the understanding of quality. Value has been defined as patient health outcomes per dollar expensed (value is equal to the health outcome divided by the cost of delivering the outcome). Understanding value requires that outcomes are measured and costs are understood. Both of these areas are now of utmost importance in the practice of orthopaedic surgery.

The Centers for Medicare and Medicaid Services (CMS) has taken the lead in defining value and quality. In 2005, the Deficit Reduction Act identified the concept of hospital-acquired conditions.[2] In 2007, the US Department of Health and Human Services further defined eight hospital-acquired conditions that would be considered "never events."[3] These occurrences are discussed in greater detail later in this chapter. In 2009, value-based purchasing was introduced as a demonstration project. However, in 2012, value-based purchasing took effect for all hospitals providing services to Medicare and Medicaid patients.[4] Physicians are currently in the initial phases of value-based purchasing, but in 2015, the value-based modifier will be phased in for physicians. At that time, it will no longer be only the healthcare institutions that are required to respond to value-based purchasing; rather, this concept will apply to individual physicians also. In 2017, the value-based modifier will no longer be a demonstration project and will be applied to all physicians.[5] Although these changes have been directed by the CMS, their importance is expected to extend to all patients. Past experience has shown that policies instituted by the CMS with respect to hospital and physician reimbursement are likely to be adopted by commercial payors. With respect to value and quality, this trend has already been noted.

Measuring Quality

Quality is a metaphysical concept that is difficult to define and quantitate. However, defining quality is essential to any organization aiming to understand and improve the level of care it provides to patients. Many management strategies use metrics to define and measure items of interest. Quality can and must be measured using metrics. To quantitatively measure a variable, it is necessary to first define and then discern what will be measured. In general, items that are measured are items that are valued; therefore, items such as infection rates, the length of the hospital stay, hospital readmissions, and the frequency of never events are all currently considered quality indicators that are amenable to measurement.

Measuring items that are important to an institution is a simple yet challenging concept. Too many metrics, too many numbers, and too many charts tend to dilute the importance of any of the individual metrics. This concept is termed metric fatigue. Metric fatigue entails overanalyzing and overproducing meaningless data that drown out meaningful data. However, defining and reporting metrics is crucial and must be linked to the strategy of an organization. Metrics must be presented on a scorecard, maintaining a balance between what is easy to measure and what is most important to the institution. Any complex organization, such as a hospital, an orthopaedic department, or a medical practice, must be managed with data. Data provide objective criteria for both performance and change management. The data must be transparent, and the definitions and rules governing the collection of data must be understood by all involved parties. The data must be presented in an impartial, impassionate manner so that "the numbers speak for

themselves." In this way, performance can be evaluated, and change strategies can be defined.

Increasing healthcare costs are forcing a basic philosophic change regarding payments for healthcare services; this change involves factors ranging from reimbursement for provided services to paying for quality, efficiency, and cost-effective care as opposed to clinical volume. The Institute of Medicine's defined goals for improvements in the quality of care include the features of safe, effective, patient-centered, timely, and equitable care.[6]

Public Sector Initiatives to Improve Quality

Physician Quality Reporting System

In 2015, the physician quality reporting system (PQRS) mandated by the Affordable Care Act will use a combination of incentives (1.5%) and adjustments (0.5%) based on 2013 data to encourage medical practices to submit PQRS measures. Medical practices need to submit one measure to avoid a penalty and three measures to receive a bonus. They can submit data using claims, electronic health record (EHR)–based reporting, reporting through a registry, or the group practice reporting option. For the claims-based reporting option, medical practices must meet the threshold of more than 50% of eligible claims for the time period from January 1, 2013 through December 31, 2013. For the EHR or the registry option, medical practices must meet the threshold of reporting for more than 80% of eligible patients from January 1, 2013 through December 31, 2013.[7]

A number of PQRS measures that are relevant to orthopaedic practices make it relatively easy to report three quality measures to achieve the 1.5% incentive. Orthopaedic relevant measures are listed in **Table 1**.

Table 1
Orthopaedic-Relevant Measures of the Physician Quality Reporting System

Measure No.	Description
20	Perioperative care: Timing of parenteral prophylactic antibiotic
21	Perioperative care: Selection of parenteral antibiotic
22	Perioperative care: Discontinuation of antibiotics
23	Perioperative care: Venous thromboembolism prophylaxis
24	Osteoporosis: Communication with the physician managing care after fractures of the hip, the spine, or the distal radius in men and women older than 50 years
39	Screening or therapy for osteoporosis for women at least 65 years of age
40	Osteoporosis management after fracture of the hip, the spine, or the distal radius for men and women at least 50 years of age
41	Osteoporosis: Pharmacologic therapy for men and women at least 50 years of age
46	Medication reconciliation
127	Diabetes mellitus: Evaluation of footwear
128	Preventive care and screening: Body mass index screening and follow-up
130	Documentation of current medications in medical record
131	Pain assessment and follow-up
142	Osteoarthritis: Assessment for use of anti-inflammatory or analgesic over-the-counter medications
154	Falls: Risk assessment
155	Falls: Plan of care
162	Diabetes mellitus: Foot examination
217	Functional deficit: Change in risk-adjusted functional status for patients with knee impairments
218	Functional deficit: Change in risk-adjusted functional status for patients with hip impairments
219	Functional deficit: Change in risk-adjusted functional status for patients with lower leg, ankle, and foot impairments
220	Functional deficit: Change in risk-adjusted functional status for patients with lumbar spine impairments
221	Functional deficit: Change in risk-adjusted functional status for patients with shoulder impairments
222	Functional deficit: Change in risk-adjusted functional status for patients with elbow, wrist, and hand impairments
223	Functional deficit: Change in risk-adjusted functional status for patients with neck, cranium, mandible, thoracic spine, ribs, or other general orthopaedic impairments

EHR Meaningful Use Program Clinical Quality Measures

In 2013, based on EHR meaningful use stage 1 regulations, eligible professionals will continue to report three core/alternate core and three additional measures. The eligible professional can report zero if the measures do not apply to the type of patients seen by that provider.

In 2014, when EHR meaningful use stage 2 regulations take effect, there will be a significant revamping of measures that need to be reported. Eligible professionals must then report on 9 of 64 measures. The nine measures must cover at least three of the six National Quality Strategy domains. The six domains are (1) patient and family engagement, (2) patient safety, (3) care coordination, (4) population/public health, (5) the efficient use of healthcare resources, and (6) clinical process/effectiveness. Clinical quality measures relevant to orthopaedic surgery are summarized in **Table 2**.

Bundled Payment Incentive Program

In January 2013, CMS officially launched the bundled payments for care improvement (BPCI) program, which is one of the largest financial innovation programs mandated by healthcare reform.[8] More than 500 hospitals, health systems, and other providers have enrolled in the program. The BPCI program is based on a CMS experiment with bundled payments (the concept that healthcare providers receive a lump sum payment from the payor). By participating in the BPCI program, it is believed that hospitals, physicians, and other parties will collaborate to better coordinate care, improve health outcomes, reduce readmissions, diminish duplicative care, and lower Medicare costs. CMS will provide a discounted payment for an episode of care and, in return, all involved caregivers share in the savings if the care is well delivered and efficient. Participating hospitals and providers can choose from four models for the

Table 2

Clinical Quality Measures Relevant to Orthopaedics

CMS Measure ID	NQF No.	Measure
CMS138v1	0028	Preventive care and screening: Tobacco use: Screening and cessation intervention
CMS166v2	0052	Use of imaging studies for low back pain
CMS123v1	0056	Diabetes: Foot examination
CMS68v2	0419	Documentation of current medications in the medical record
CMS69v1	0421	Preventive care and screening: Body mass index screening and follow-up
CMS139v1	0101	Falls: Screening for future fall risks
CMS50v1		Closing the referral loop: Receipt of specialist report
CMS66v1		Functional status assessment for knee replacement for patients with patient-reported functional status assessment results not more than 180 days before the primary total knee arthroplasty procedure and at least 60 days and not more than 180 days after the total knee arthroplasty procedure
CMS56v1		Functional status assessment for hip replacement for patients with patient-reported functional status assessment results not more than 180 days before the primary total hip arthroplasty procedure and at least 60 days and not more than 180 days after the total hip arthroplasty procedure

NQF = National Quality Forum.

Table 3

Four Models for Bundled Payments for Care Improvement Program

Model	Covers	DRG Codes Included	Payment
Model 1	Inpatient stay in acute care facility	All DRG codes are included	Retrospective adjustment to the usual fee for service payments
Model 2	Both inpatient stay and postacute care	Facility can choose DRG codes	Retrospective adjustment to the usual fee for service payments
Model 3	Postacute care only	Providers can choose DRG codes	Retrospective adjustment to the usual fee for service payments
Model 4	Inpatient stay in acute care facility and related readmissions	Facility can choose DRG codes	Prospective payments: hospitals agree to a price upfront on a particular DRG, and CMS pays that specific bundled price to the hospital

DRG = Diagnosis-related group, CMS = Centers for Medicare and Medicaid Services.

BPCI program (**Table 3**).

The five most common clinical bundles are major joint arthroplasty of the lower extremity (hip and knee replacements), congestive heart failure, coronary artery bypass grafting, chronic obstructive pulmonary disease (bronchitis, asthma), and percutaneous coronary intervention. Any one of the four models can be applied to a specific clinical bundle, and a proposal can be submitted to CMS for consideration. It is anticipated that each participating institution will combine the model and clinical bundle that will provide the greatest probability of success.

The Surgical Care Improvement Project

The Surgical Care Improvement Project (SCIP) is a national quality partnership of organizations interested in improving surgical care by substantially reducing surgical complications. SCIP partners include the steering committees of 10 national organizations (the Agency for Healthcare Research and Quality, the American College of Surgeons, the American Hospital Association, the American Society of Anesthesiologists, the Association of Perioperative Nurses, CMS, the Centers for Disease Control and Prevention, the Department of Veterans Affairs, the Institute for Healthcare Improvement, and the Joint Commission) who have pledged their commitment and full support for SCIP. Each SCIP target area is advised by a technical panel of experts. These groups have provided hours of technical expertise and resources to ensure that the SCIP measures are fully supported by evidence-based research.[9]

Other Initiatives

The Joint Commission continues to align with CMS with respect to performance measures for patients undergoing surgery. These measures include patient safety indicators developed by the Agency for Healthcare Research and Quality. These indicators provide information on potential in-hospital complications and adverse events after surgeries, procedures, and childbirth.[10] The Centers for Disease Control and Prevention maintains the National Healthcare Safety Network, an Internet-based surveillance system.[11] The data collected are used to estimate the magnitude of adverse events, determine trends, assist with surveillance, and evaluate and design prevention strategies. The National Institutes of Health maintains the Patient Reported Outcome Measurement System (PROMIS), which is used for chronic disease management.[12] Using a PROMIS questionnaire, patient responses are calculated into scores and used to improve communication, manage health conditions, and design treatment plans.

Private Sector Initiatives

National Quality Forum

The National Quality Forum (NQF) is a nonprofit organization that operates under a three-part mission to improve the quality of US healthcare by (1) building consensus on national priorities and goals for performance improvement and working in partnership to achieve them; (2) endorsing national consensus standards for measuring and publicly reporting on performance; and (3) promoting the attainment of national goals through education and outreach programs.

The membership of the NQF includes a wide variety of healthcare stakeholders, including consumer organizations, public and private purchasers, physicians, physician organizations (including the American Academy of Orthopaedic Surgeons), nurses, hospitals, accrediting and certifying bodies, supporting industries, and healthcare research and quality improvement organizations.[13] The breadth and diversity of its membership and NQF's unique structure enables private- and public-sector stakeholder to work together to craft and implement cross-cutting solutions to drive continuous quality improvement in the US healthcare system.

In January 2009, the NQF entered into a contract with the Department of Health and Human Services to help establish a portfolio of quality and efficiency measures for reporting on and improving healthcare quality. These measures will allow the federal government to more clearly determine how and whether healthcare spending is achieving the best results for patients and taxpayers. The contract is part of a provision in the Medicare Improvements for Patients and Providers Act of 2008.[14]

The NQF also will supervise a systematic review and synthesis of evidence relating to 20 high-priority conditions identified by the CMS and accounting for more than 95% of Medicare costs. The NQF will synthesize evidence related to these 20 high-impact conditions and prioritize them along multiple dimensions to guide the future development of performance measures. Measures 11 (hip and pelvic fractures) and 14 (rheumatoid arthritis and osteoarthritis) are of particular interest to orthopaedic practices.[15]

National Committee for Quality Assurance

The National Committee for Quality Assurance is a private, 501(c)(3) nonprofit organization dedicated to improving the quality of health care. This organization develops quality standards and performance measures for a broad range of healthcare entities. These standards and measures are tools that organizations and individuals can use to identify opportunities for improvement. The annual reporting of performance against such measures has become a focal point for the media, consumers, and health plans, which use the results to set improvement agendas for the following year.

The Healthcare Effectiveness Data and Information Set (HEDIS) is a tool used by more than 90% of US health plans to measure performance on important dimensions of care and service. Altogether, HEDIS consists of 75 measures across 8 domains of care. Because so many health plans collect HEDIS data and because the measures are so specifically defined, HEDIS makes it possible to compare the performance of health plans on an "apples-to-apples" basis. HEDIS measures address a broad range of important health issues. Among them are asthma medication use, the persistence of beta-blocker treatment after a heart attack, the control of high blood pressure, comprehensive diabetes care, breast cancer screening, antidepressant medication management, childhood and adolescent immunization status, and childhood and adult weight and body mass index assessments. Included in HEDIS is the Consumer Assessment of Healthcare Providers and Systems (CAHPS) 5.0 survey, which measures members' satisfaction with their care in areas such as claims processing, customer service, and receiving needed care quickly.[16]

Patient-Centered Specialty Recognition Program

The National Committee for Quality Assurance is reinforcing the importance of the strong connections between primary, specialty, and supporting care coordination by developing a recognition program for specialty practices engaged in the patient-centered care model.[17] This program will recognize specialty practices that successfully coordinated care with other specialty practices and their primary care colleagues and meet the goals of providing timely access to care and continuous quality improvement. In addition, the program addresses reducing the duplication of tests, measuring performance, and improving communication with patients.

Pacific Business Group on Health

Founded in 1989, the Pacific Business Group on Health is one of the nation's leading nonprofit business coalitions focused on health care. The organization helps leverage the power of 60 large purchaser–members who spend $12 billion annually to provide healthcare coverage to more than 3 million employees, retirees, and dependents in California.[18]

The Pacific Business Group on Health works to improve the quality and affordability of health care, often in close partnership with health insurance plans, physician groups, consumer organizations, and others concerned about the US healthcare system. The organization has four key strategies with specific goals and metrics to achieve its vision: (1) It attempts to engage consumers with information and incentives to choose the right care at the right price. (2) It promotes paying for value by ensuring that providers are rewarded for quality and efficiency. (3) It is redesigning care delivery by supporting the healthcare system in achieving improved outcomes at a better price. (4) It advances value-based policy by helping policymakers create public policies that improve care and reduce costs.

California Chartered Value Exchange

The California Chartered Value Exchange is a collaborative of many organizations formed to advance high-quality, patient-centered, cost-effective health care for Californians.[19] Through increased coordination of the activities of the participating organizations, the California Chartered Value Exchange provides value to Pacific Business Group on Health members and all Californians by improving the availability and accessibility of publicly reported information for plan and provider accountability and consumer engagement. The alignment of reporting initiatives and payment incentives aids in translating quality measurement results into actionable steps for quality improvement. The current foci of this organization are making measurements at the individual physician, practice site, group, and hospital level using best available data and exploring opportunities for obtaining clinical data from providers.

The Leapfrog Group

The Leapfrog Group is a voluntary program aimed at mobilizing employer purchasing power to alert the US health industry that big advances in healthcare safety, quality, and customer value will be recognized and rewarded.[20] Among other initiatives, the Leapfrog Group works with its employer members to encourage transparency and easy access to healthcare information, and it rewards hospitals that have a proven record of high-quality care. Many of the nation's largest corporations and public agencies that purchase health benefits on behalf of their enrollees are members of this group. Together, these private- and public-sector purchasers represent more than 34 million Americans and more than $62 billion in healthcare expenditures.

The Leapfrog hospital survey is the gold standard for comparing the performances of hospitals on the national standards of safety, quality, and efficiency that are most relevant to consumers and purchasers of care. Four key quality measures are computer-based physician order entry, evidence-based hospital referral for consumers, staffing of intensive care units by intensivists, and adherence to NQF safe practices. The Leapfrog group generates hospital safety scores using 26 publicly available measures. Measures that apply to orthopaedic surgeons are the timing of preoperative antibiotic administration, selection, and discontinuation; urinary catheter removal; venous thromboembolism (VTE) prophylaxis; falls and injuries; deaths; postoperative deep vein thrombosis; and postoperative wound dehiscence.

UnitedHealthcare Premium Physician Designation Program

The UnitedHealthcare Premium Physician Designation Program for providers awards one star for quality and one star for cost-effectiveness. To receive a quality star, the provider must be in the 75th percentile based on NQF-endorsed standards. To earn a star for cost-effectiveness, the provider must meet or exceed cost-effectiveness measures compared with peers in the same geographic area. Direct and ancillary fees and facility costs are considered in judging cost-effectiveness. A quality star must be earned before a cost-effectiveness star can be awarded.[21]

Healthcare Incentives Improvement Institute

The Healthcare Incentives Improvement Institute is an initiative representing the combined efforts of Aetna, Blue Cross Blue Shield, CIGNA, The 3M Company, International Business

Table 4

Quality Improvement Initiatives

Initiative	Organization	Website Address
Physician Quality Reporting System	Center for Medicare and Medicaid Services	http://www.cms.gov/Medicare/Quality-Initiatives-Patient-Assessment-Instruments/PQRS/index.html?redirect=/PQRS/
Electronic health record meaningful use clinical quality measures	Center for Medicare and Medicaid Services	http://www.cms.gov/Regulations-and-Guidance/Legislation/EHRIncentivePrograms/Meaningful_Use.html
Bundled Payments for Care Improvement program	Center for Medicare and Medicaid Services	http://innovation.cms.gov/initiatives/bundled-payments/
The Surgical Care Improvement Project	The Joint Commission	http://www.jointcommission.org/surgical_care_improvement_project/
Patient Safety Indicators	Agency for Healthcare Research and Quality	http://www.qualityindicators.ahrq.gov/modules/psi_overview.aspx
National Healthcare Safety Network	Centers for Disease Control and Prevention	http://www.cdc.gov/nhsn/
Patient Reported Outcome Measurement System	The National Institutes of Health	http://www.nihpromis.org/
Measurement endorsement and use projects	National Quality Forum	http://www.qualityforum.org/Home.aspx
The Healthcare Effectiveness Data and Information Set	National Committee for Quality Assurance	http://www.ncqa.org/HEDISQualityMeasurement.aspx
Patient-centered specialty recognition program	National Committee for Quality Assurance	http://www.ncqa.org/Programs/Recognition/PatientCenteredSpecialtyPracticeRecognition.aspx
Improve the quality of health care and moderate cost increases	Pacific Business Group on Health and California Chartered Value Exchange	http://www.pbgh.org/
Hospital safety score	The Leapfrog Group	http://www.leapfroggroup.org/
United Healthcare Premium Physician Designation Program	United HealthCare	http://www.uhc.com/physicians/care_programs/unitedhealth_premium_designation.htm
PROMETHEUS (Provider Payment Reform for Outcomes, Margins, Evidence, Transparency, Hassle-reduction, Excellence, Understanding, and Sustainability	Healthcare Incentive Improvement Institute	http://www.hci3.org/

Machines, Intel, Wellpoint, and the states of Colorado and Georgia. There is an opportunity for recognition in 1 or more of 12 clinical programs. Although most are cardiac programs, spine programs are included. For spine programs, included measures are appropriate physical therapy, avoiding unnecessary imaging, the appropriate use of epidural injections and surgery, patient education, and shared decision making.[22]

The PROMETHEUS (Provider Payment Reform for Outcomes, Margins, Evidence, Transparency, Hassle-reduction, Excellence, Understanding, and Sustainability) model packages payment around a comprehensive episode of medical care that covers all patient services related to a single illness or condition. Covered services are based on commonly accepted clinical guidelines or expert opinions that define the best methods for treating a given condition from beginning to end. The prices of all treatments are tallied to generate an evidence-informed case rate. This creates a budget for the entire care episode. Evidence-informed case rates include all covered services bundled across all providers (including the hospital, the physicians, the laboratory, the pharmacy, and the rehabilitation facility) that would typically treat a patient for the given condition. The evidence-informed case rate is adjusted for the severity and complexity of each patient's condition.[23]

It is becoming evident that future reimbursements will be linked to quality, which will be measured using validated measures. Many organizations are participating in initiatives to improve the quality of health care (**Table 4**). There is considerable overlap in the measures advocated by both public and private initiatives. A distinct effort has been made to include patient perception of care and the coordination of care as quality indicators. Many initiatives, such as the Leapfrog Group, are making certified EHR technology a prerequisite for participation in quality programs. Proper data collection and the use of technology will enable orthopaedic surgeons to successfully participate in quality-based reimbursement programs.

Implementing a Quality Program in an Academic Center

The vision of an orthopaedic group should be to transform itself from an ad hoc distributed management and decision-making organization to a centralized, data-focused enterprise and a first-class patient-care center. This vision is linked with several goals: (1) The organization should create a culture of accountability for all its workers. Metrics provide the basis for the culture of accountability. (2) The organization should achieve and demonstrate quality improvements. Metrics are essential for demonstrating numeric and objective improvements in quality. (3) The organization must achieve sustainability, which embodies an institutional ethos that is independent from the people leading the organization. (4) The organization must practice excellence as a core value of which these metrics are a part.

To achieve these transformational results, data must be objective. Institutional or practice decision making must become increasingly data driven. Subjective notions and concepts are less important than objective data. Everything must be transparent, including the exposure of data and metrics, to improve results with accuracy, timeliness, consistency, and reliability.

Never Events

Metrics are especially amenable to measuring never events. In 2002, the NQF defined 27 reportable events that met the criteria of serious, measurable, and wholly preventable.[24] The risk of occurrence of these never events is substantially influenced by the policies and practices of an organization. The original 27 never events were divided into six categories: products of service, surgical categories, patient protection, case management, environmental, and criminal. The never events that pertain to orthopaedic surgery include a retained foreign body after surgery, wrong-site surgery, wrong-patient surgery, improper procedure, and perioperative death in an American Society of Anesthesiologists class 1 patient.

Measuring never events may seem like a simple task; however, these events must be precisely defined so that each member of an institution understands which events are included and excluded from the set of surgical never events.

Retained Foreign Body

Although a retained foreign body seems to be a straightforward concept, certain foreign bodies left in a patient after surgery are not considered to be retained foreign bodies. In general, a foreign body is not considered retained if removing it would cause more harm to the patient than leaving it in place.

In 2011, NQF published a widely accepted definition of a retained foreign object event, which is defined as an event with an unintended retention of a foreign object in a patient after surgery or another invasive procedure. The definition includes medical or surgical items intentionally placed by a provider that are unintentionally left in place.[25] The definition excludes objects present before surgery or other invasive procedures that are intentionally left in place, objects intentionally implanted as part of a planned intervention, and objects not present before surgery or a procedure that are intentionally left in place when the risk of removal is deemed to exceed the risk of retention (such as microneedles and broken screws).

According to this definition, a microneedle (commonly considered as needles that are 13 mm or smaller) can be safely left in a patient. It is not observable on a routine radiograph and does not cause injury or harm. Neither a surgical screw that is broken during active insertion nor a retained screw from hardware removal is considered a retained foreign body. If a screw or drill bit is broken at the time of insertion, the bone need not be violated to remove the tip of the drill bit or the end of the screw if the surgeon judges that extraction would be harmful to the patient.

It is also important to precisely define when an object is considered retained and at what point surgery is completed. An object is considered to be retained when additional surgery is required to remove it or if the object is discovered after skin closure.[25] Therefore, the fascial layers, subcutaneous layers, and partial skin closure can be performed before an object is considered retained. If the counts of surgical instruments are incorrect or a retained foreign body is suspected, the wound need not remain open, increasing the risk of infection. The fascial subcutaneous layers of skin can be closed before obtaining a radiograph; however, the sterile operating field must remain in place, and the patient must remain under anesthesia while the radiograph is obtained if the needle or instrument count is incorrect. The definition of a retained foreign body and when an object is considered retained are essential concepts in defining the metric.

Wrong-Site Surgery

Other surgical events, including wrong-site surgery, are simpler to define. The correct patient and the correct body part must undergo the surgical procedure. This includes the concepts of laterality, left versus right, the proper digit of the hand, and the proper level in spinal surgery. For example, some institutions have written documentation requiring that all parties adhere to established guidelines to determine the levels of spinal fusion and decompression; these include marking the spinous processes with a towel clamp and obtaining radiographs. In another example, a never event occurs in a patient undergoing hand surgery if the patient had consented to surgery to treat a trigger finger and a carpal tunnel procedure was performed.

Because wrong-site surgery never events are extremely rare, any policies or procedures designed to decrease the likelihood of these events from occurring are difficult to assess using the actual incidence of the events themselves. The use of near-miss analysis is well-suited for analyzing surgical never events. Near-miss analysis began in the aviation industry. Midair airplane collisions are similar to surgical never events in that both are extremely rare. Near misses are not as rare and can be studied to decrease the likelihood of the occurrence of an actual midair plane collision.[26]

It is important to analyze near misses because they can be used to model how small failures can develop into adverse outcomes. This modeling can expose weaknesses in recovery systems and a poor culture of safety. Studying near misses also allows a more robust quantitative analysis of strategies to decrease the likelihood of near misses. The analysis of near misses also encourages institutional awareness of safety. For example, each time an incorrectly scheduled case as a result of a misidentified laterality is reported back to the surgeon, it increases the awareness of the surgeon and staff of the importance of vigilance for wrong-site surgery and reinforces an awareness of the culture of safety.

Value-Based Purchasing

Value-based purchasing has highlighted the importance of measuring and understanding quality and its relationship to the use of metrics.[27,28] As previously discussed, the value-based purchasing program allows the federal government to reward high-quality outcomes and penalizes poor-quality outcomes by augmenting payments to higher preforming hospitals and withholding Medicare payments to poorly performing hospitals. Value-based purchasing is graded on 25 dimensions, 70% of which are process of care measurements. For orthopaedic surgery, the processes of care measurements include prophylactic antibiotics administered before incision, proper antibiotic selection, antibiotic discontinuation 24 hours after surgery, adherence to recommended VTE prophylactic guidelines, and beginning VTE prophylaxis within 24 hours of surgery.

Thirty percent of the value-based purchasing metric is based on patient experience, including communication with doctors and nurses. Measurement of 30-day readmissions are also included as part of value-based purchasing. Effective in 2015, the 30-day readmission measure will include readmission after total hip and total knee arthroplasties.[29]

Quality Indicators

Length of Hospital Stay

The length of the hospital stay is a measure of quality and efficiency; however, there is a certain complexity to this metric. The observed length of stay is the number of days a patient stays in the hospital. There is also an expected length of stay, which is calculated by the type of procedure performed and the medical comorbidities associated with the particular patient. These data are compared so that the length of stay can be reported as an observed/expected length of stay ratio (< 1 is desirable). In this way, the expected length of stay takes into account patient and procedural characteristics, which affect the length of stay. The measure also accounts for interhospital and interphysician comparisons because data are stratified by patient risk factors and the type of procedure performed.

Surgical Site Infection

The number of surgical site infections (SSIs) is a metric that is publicly reported by several states, including the state of New York.[30] For the past 3 years, New York has publicly reported the rate of SSIs after hip replacement. The New York guidelines combine total hip arthroplasties and revision hip arthroplasties in the same metric; however, the actual SSI rate is adjusted for complexity, which takes into account the number of revision surgeries performed.

SSIs must be precisely defined, with most reports including only deep infections. The National Healthcare Safety Network and the Centers for Disease Control and Prevention define deep infections as those that involve deep soft tissues (for example, fascial and muscle layers).[31] A patient with a deep infection also has one of the following factors: purulent drainage from the deep incision; a deep incision that spontaneously dehisces or is deliberately opened by a surgeon and is culture positive or is not cultured and the patient has fever or localized pain and tenderness; an abscess or other evidence of infection found on direct examination during an invasive procedure, histopathologic examination, or imaging test; or a diagnosis of deep incision SSI infection by a surgeon or an attending physician.

The reporting of SSIs may be poorly performed by surgeons. All SSIs should be reported by an epidemiologist in the hospital's infection control department. Epidemiologists can screen all positive cultures within their hospital, search for readmissions, and determine which patients are receiving parenteral antibiotics. Using this process, patients with infected prostheses can be detected. It is important that epidemiologists work with the operating surgeons to accurately define which patients are infected; however, the hospital epidemiologist should make the final determination regarding patients with a deep SSI.

Venous Thromboembolism

VTE is another quality indicator that must be measured and quantified. The actual rate of VTE is easily measurable when all positive Doppler studies and spiral CTs are readily available for analysis. However, the actual rate of VTE is a function of the aggressiveness of screening and diagnosis because there are a certain number of false-positive results or positive CT scans that have little clinical importance.

Most payors and government bodies are not as focused on the actual rate of VTE as they are on certain metrics associated with VTE, such as prophylaxis started within 24 hours of surgery based on the American College of Chest Physicians guidelines and proper patient selection for prophylaxis.[32] It has been theorized that proper patient selection for prophylaxis, adherence to the American College of Chest Physicians guidelines, and timely administration will result in the lowest possible rate of VTE.

Readmissions

Readmissions are considered a barometer of quality in hospital systems and the physician care of patients. The CMS is interested in measuring readmissions within 30 days of hospital discharge. The overall rate of Medicare readmissions 30 days after discharge

was 19.6% but recently fell to 17.8% in the final quarter of 2012.[33] The cooperation of clinicians is needed to obtain and analyze administrative data defining readmissions. In an examination of the administrative data of a single orthopaedic hospital regarding 30-day readmissions from 2007 to 2009, McCormick et al[34] detailed concerns regarding the accurate reporting of hospital readmissions. The authors found that 27% of all 30-day readmissions were actually planned readmissions, including staged procedures. Some readmissions were actually cancelations, rescheduled procedures, or the transfer of a patient from one part of a hospital to another.

Each readmission should be evaluated by a hospital's documentation service and the involved clinicians to ascertain whether it represents an unplanned readmission for a complication or a planned readmission. A close collaboration and working relationship with the clinical documentation specialist or coders is important to accurately portray the rate of readmissions.

In 2015, readmissions after total knee and total hip arthroplasties will become part of value-based purchasing. Hospitals with a higher than average readmission rate may lose a percentage of their Medicare payments. Metrics can be used to compare institutions with other institutions and physicians with other physicians. The interphysician analyses and comparisons included in the physician-specific metrics are a vital part of any high-quality practice or institution. Physician-specific metrics increase performance awareness in comparison with their peers and between institutions. They also differentiate high performers from low performers, allowing analysis and understanding of the differences between these groups.

Best Practice

It is important that physician-specific metrics are transparent and available between peers. To be effective, these metrics must be displayed in a nonpejorative manner and discussed in terms of improving patient care. Physician-specific metrics can be used to improve the performance of an individual physician and decrease the differences between high- and low-performing physicians, allowing for more uniform and high-quality patient care across physicians.

An example of a physician-specific metric is the operating time for a specific type of procedure. The operating room time for a total hip replacement is included in this metric (**Figure 1**). It is imperative that physicians understand that the time to perform a procedure is not just the period from the time the incision is made until the incision is closed; it is the entire amount of time the patient is in the operating room. Different healthcare providers often "own" different parts of the operating room time. For example, the anesthesiologist and nurses own the first part of the surgical period from the patient's entry into the operating room until the incision is made. The surgeon takes ownership of the time from the incision until incision closure, and anesthesiologists and nurses own the third portion of the operating room period from closure of the incision until the patient leaves the room. The surgeon is in charge and should be available to help position the patient and perform an adequate preprocedural briefing and debriefing to decrease the total time in the operating room.[35-37] This metric is particularly useful in increasing physician awareness of exactly how much time is required to perform a procedure and how to properly schedule procedures to fit into the allotted time block.

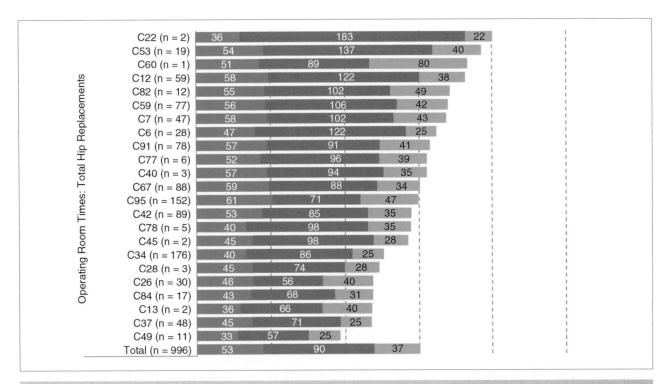

Figure 1   Bar graph showing surgeon-specific operating room times for total hip replacement from data gathered at the New York Hospital for Joint Diseases. The blue portion of each bar represents the time (in minutes) from the patient's arrival in the operating room until the time that the first incision is made. The red portion of the bar is the time from the first incision until the time the incision is closed. The green portion of each bar is the time from incision closure until the patient leaves the operating room. The specific surgeon is identified by a letter and number (C22, C23, etc), and "n" represents the number of cases analyzed to obtain the data in the bar graph.

The Role of the Hospital Administration

Although physicians view quality initiatives in one context, the view of the hospital administration (chief executive officer [CEO]) may be different. A CEO must review the quality movement as a business imperative. This mind-set is essential for healthcare institutions to survive and thrive in the current environment. A CEO of a healthcare institution should partner with physicians to achieve the quality goals established for the institution. In doing so, it is important to identify aspirational goals and gain the support of physicians and all hospital personnel. To be successful, the established goals must cascade through the entire organization, beginning at the board level and extending through administrative management and the medical

staff. Quality data, before and after interventions, must be available for review by people at all levels of the organization who are involved in achieving the desired outcome. For example, when addressing the issue of SSIs, the CEO should work with the medical staff leadership to establish goals and with each relevant department within the organization to achieve those goals. It is essential to have longitudinal data that show the effect of the measures taken. These data should be reviewed by the leadership, including the board of directors, to ensure that the goals are being achieved.

To achieve quality-related goals, it is often helpful to establish a hospital quality council to oversee the initiative. The hospital quality council can be supported by a variety of quality coordinating committees, each with subcommit-

tees to address specific areas within the institution, such as ambulatory care, inpatient care, perioperative services, medical staff, and housekeeping staff.

Identifying a value stream also can be helpful. A value stream consists of people, processes, technologies, information, and material flows that come together to deliver a valuable product or service to the patient. The value stream can be applied to each portion of the organization that is required to achieve quality goals. Specific areas, including patient satisfaction, preventing in-hospital falls, achieving SCIP measures, SSI prevention, and reducing the rate of readmissions and postoperative thrombophlebitis will benefit from a value-stream approach. An institutional commitment at every level is needed to measure, communicate, and improve results.

Administrators should recognize that creating, improving, and demonstrating value is the key to achieving success within an rganization. Although strong physician leadership is necessary to drive the initiative, the institution's CEO will also play a key role by forging the important partnership between the medical staff and the administrative staff. Value in health care will be achieved by leveraging physician leadership within the organization's structure and designing processes to deliver consistently high results.

Summary

Measuring quality in medicine has gained increasing attention from those involved in the healthcare system. Physicians, patients, policy makers, and payors all have a stake in ensuring continuation on the path toward a high-quality and high-value healthcare system. The quality metrics and payment initiatives reviewed in this chapter represent an evolving approach to ensuring that the US healthcare system is patient centered, sustainable, and delivers high-quality care. As orthopaedic surgeons, staying involved and aware of the changing policy landscape will be increasingly important as more quality metrics are added to specifically measure the quality of orthopaedic care. Within the past decade, the healthcare delivery system has witnessed enormous changes, and quality improvement will remain a part of future changes through the next decade.

References

1. Porter ME, Teisberg EO: *Redefining Health Care: Creating Value-Based Competition on Results*. Boston, MA, Harvard Business School Press, 2006.

2. Deficit Reduction Act of 2005, 1932-27, 109th Cong, 2nd Sess (2006). http://www.gpo.gov/fdsys/pkg/BILLS-109s1932enr/pdf/BILLS-109s1932enr.pdf. Accessed June 5, 2013.

3. Centers for Medicare and Medicaid Services: Fact Sheet: Incorporating Selected National Quality Forum and Never Events Into Medicare's List of Hospital-Acquired Conditions. http://www.cms.gov/apps/media/press/factsheet.asp?Counter=3043&intNumPerPage=10&checkDate=&checkKey=2&srchType=2&numDays=0&srchOpt=0&srchData=never+events&keywordType=All&chkNewsType=6&intPage=&showAll=1&pYear=&year=0&desc=&cboOrder=date. Accessed November 5, 2013.

4. Centers for Medicare and Medicaid Services: Hospital Value-Based Purchasing. http://www.cms.gov/Medicare/Quality-Initiatives-Patient-Assessment-Instruments/hospital-value-based-purchasing/index.html?redirect=/hospital-value-based-purchasing. Accessed May 16, 2013.

5. Centers for Medicare and Medicaid Services: Summary of 2015 Physician Value-based Payment Modifier Policies. http://www.cms.gov/Medicare/Medicare-Fee-for-Service-Payment/PhysicianFeedbackProgram/Downloads/CY2015ValueModifierPolicies.pdf. Accessed June 5, 2013.

6. Centers for Medicare and Medicaid Services: CMS Quality Improvement Roadmap: Executive Summary. http://www.cms.gov/Medicare/Coverage/CouncilonTechInnov/downloads/qualityroadmap.pdf. Accessed June 5, 2013.

7. Centers for Medicare and Medicaid Services: Physician Quality Reporting System. http://www.cms.gov/Medicare/Quality-Initiatives-Patient-Assessment-Instruments/PQRS/index.html?redirect=/PQRS/. Accessed June 5, 2013.

8. Centers for Medicare and Medicaid Services: Bundled Payments for Care Improvement (BPCI) Initiative: General Information. http://innovation.cms.gov/initiatives/bundled-payments/. Accessed June 5, 2013.

9. The Joint Commission: Surgical Care Improvement Project. http://www.jointcommission.org/surgical_care_improvement_project/. Accessed June 5, 2013.

10. Agency for Healthcare Research and Quality: Patient Safety Indicators Overview. http://www.qualityindicators.ahrq.gov/modules/psi_overview.aspx. Accessed June 5, 2013.

11. Centers for Disease Control and Prevention: National Healthcare Safety Network. http://www.cdc.gov/nhsn/. Accessed June 5, 2013.

12. National Institutes of Health: PROMIS: Dynamic Tools to Measure Health Outcome From the Patient Perspective. http://www.nihpromis.org/. Accessed June 5, 2013.

13. National Quality Forum website. http://www.qualityforum.org/. Accessed June 5, 2013.

14. Medicare Improvements for Patients and Providers Act of 2008, Pub L No. 110-275, 122 Stat 2494. http://www.gpo.gov/fdsys/pkg/PLAW-110publ275/pdf/PLAW-110publ275.pdf. Accessed June 5, 2013.

15. National Quality Forum: Committee Report: Prioritization of High-Impact Medicare Conditions and Measure Gaps. http://www.qualityforum.org/Publications/2010/05/Committee_Report,_Prioritization_of_High-Impact_Medicare_Conditions_and_Measure_Gaps.aspx. Accessed June 5, 2013.

16. National Committee for Quality Assurance: HEDIS & Performance Measurement. http://www.ncqa.org/HEDISQualityMeasurement.aspx. Accessed June 5, 2013.

17. National Committee for Quality Assurance: Patient-Centered Speciality Practice Frequently Asked Questions. http://www.ncqa.org/Programs/Recognition/PatientCenteredSpecialtyPractice Recognition/PatientCenteredSpecialtyPractice-FAQs.aspx. Accessed June 5, 2013.

18. Pacific Business Group on Health website. http://www.pbgh.org. Accessed June 5, 2013.

19. Pacific Business Group on Health: California Chartered Value Exchange. http://www.pbgh.org/key-strategies/engaging-consumers/166-ccve. Accessed June 5, 2013.

20. The Leapfrog Group website. http://www.leapfroggroup.org. Accessed June 5, 2013.

21. UnitedHealthcare website. UnitedHealth Premium Physician Designation Program: Detailed Methodology. https://www.unitedhealthcareonline.com/ccmcontent/ProviderII/UHC/en-US/Assets/ProviderStaticFiles/ProviderStaticFilesPdf/Unitedhealth%20Premium/UnitedHealth_Premium_Detailed_Methodology_2012.pdf. Accessed June 5, 2013.

22. Health Care Incentives Improvement Institute website. http://www.hci3.org. Accessed June 5, 2013.

23. Health Care Incentives Improvement Institute: What is the PROMETHEUS Payment? http://www.hci3.org/what_is_prometheus. Accessed June 5, 2013.

24. National Quality Forum: List of SREs. http://www.qualityforum.org/Topics/SREs/List_of_SREs.aspx. Accessed June 5, 2013.

25. National Quality Forum. Serious Reportable Events in Healthcare 2011. http://www.qualityforum.org/Publications/2011/12/Serious_Reportable_Events_in_Healthcare_2011.aspx. Accessed June 5, 2013.

26. Aspden P, Corrigan J, Wolcott J, Erickson S: *Patient Safety: Achieving a New Standard for Care.* Washington, DC, National Academies Press, 2004.

27. Shoemaker P: What value-based purchasing means to your hospital. *Healthc Financ Manage* 2011;65(8):60-68.

28. VanLare JM, Conway PH: Value-based purchasing: National programs to move from volume to value. *N Engl J Med* 2012;367(4):292-295.

29. Premier Healthcare Alliance: CMS FY 2014-2016 Measures for CMS Payment Determination. https://www.premierinc.com/quality-safety/tools-services/safety/topics/guidelines/downloads/CMS_measures_for_payment FY14FY16_b.pdf. Accessed June 5, 2013.

30. New York State Department of Health: Hospital-Acquired Infections (HAI) Rates in New York State Hospitals. http://www.health.ny.gov/statistics/facilities/hospital/hospital_acquired_infections/. Accessed June 5, 2013.

31. Centers for Disease Control: National Healthcare Safety Network: Surgical Site Infection (SSI) Event, Procedure-Associated Events, 2013. http://www.cdc.gov/nhsn/pdfs/pscmanual/9pscssicurrent.pdf. Accessed June 5, 2013.

32. Geerts WH, Bergqvist D, Pineo GF, et al: American College of Chest Physicians Evidence-Based Clinical Practice Guidelines (8th Edition). *Chest* 2008:133:381S-453S.

33. Statement of Jonathan Blum, Acting Principal Deputy Administrator and Director, Centers for Medicare and Medicaid Services, on Delivery System Reform: Progress Report from CMS Before the US Senate Finance Committee, February 28, 2013. http://www.finance.senate.gov/imo/media/doc/CMS%20Delivery%20System%20Reform%20Testimony%202.28.13%20(J.%20Blum).pdf. Accessed June 5, 2013.

34. McCormack R, Michels R, Ramos N, Hutzler L, Slover JD, Bosco JA: Thirty-day readmission rates as a measure of quality: Causes of readmission after orthopedic surgeries and accuracy of administrative data. *J Healthc Manag* 2013;58(1):64-76.

35. DeFontes J, Surbida S: Preoperative safety briefing project. *Permanente J* 2004;8:21-27.

36. Bandari J, Schumacher K, Simon M, et al: Surfacing safety hazards using standardized operating room briefings and debriefings at a large regional medical center. *Jt Comm J Qual Patient Saf* 2012;38(4):154-160.

37. Berenholtz SM, Schumacher K, Hayanga AJ, et al: Implementing standardized operating room briefings and debriefings at a large regional medical center. *Jt Comm J Qual Patient Saf* 2009;35(8):391-397.

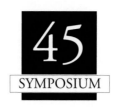

How Do You Educate Someone to Have the Skills of an Orthopaedic Surgeon?

Gregory Lopez, MD

Paul Tornetta III, MD

Augustus D. Mazzocca, MD, MS

Peter J. Stern, MD

Nathanael Heckmann, MD

Ranjan Gupta, MD

Abstract

The landscape of orthopaedic surgical education is changing because of many factors, including advances in surgical procedures and musculoskeletal basic science along with an increased focus on ethics and patient education. Over the course of 5 years, a training program must navigate resident physicians through many rotations and effectively teach trainees to become competent orthopaedic surgeons. Each rotation must best balance service requirements and educational experiences to optimize resident education and patient outcomes. Factors such as the 80-hour work week and the current medicolegal climate limit the ability of residents to learn basic surgical skills in the operating room. The benefits of performing simulator-based surgical procedures in cadavers and using simulation for other procedures are becoming increasingly important to teach basic psychomotor skills to residents.

Allowing a technically incompetent resident to graduate is a disservice to the medical profession, society, patients, and (ultimately) to the resident. Dealing with such a resident is challenging but necessary to ensure that residency programs continue to graduate competent medical professionals.

Instr Course Lect 2014;63:487-494.

Dr. Tornetta or an immediate family member has received royalties from Smith & Nephew. Dr. Mazzocca or an immediate family member serves as a paid consultant to or is an employee of Arthrex and has received research or institutional support from Arthrex and Arthrosurface. Dr. Gupta or an immediate family member is a member of a speakers' bureau or has made paid presentations on behalf of Arthrex and Integra; has received research or institutional support from Arthrex, Smith & Nephew, Synthes, Medartis, and SpineArt; and serves as a board member, owner, officer, or committee member of the American Academy of Orthopaedic Surgeons, the American Society for Surgery of the Hand, and the Orthopaedic Research Society. None of the following authors nor any immediate family member has received anything of value from or has stock or stock options held in a commercial company or institution related directly or indirectly to the subject of this chapter: Dr. Lopez, Dr. Stern, and Dr. Heckmann.

After completing medical school, a young physician who wishes to pursue a career in orthopaedics must match into an orthopaedic training program where he or she will begin the task of acquiring the skills to become a competent orthopaedic surgeon. With the many advances in surgical procedures, the continual increase in general orthopaedic knowledge, and an increased focus on ethics and patient satisfaction, it is necessary to judiciously use the available time in the new, hour-restricted, 5-year residency programs to ensure that the young physician acquires the necessary skills to become a successful orthopaedic surgeon. This chapter reviews the current status of orthopaedic residency education, discusses potential new avenues for teaching surgical principles and techniques, and addresses the issue of a resident who is not functioning at the expected competency level.

Service Versus Education

After the first year of residency, the Accreditation Council for Graduate

Medical Education (ACGME) requires an orthopaedic surgery resident to learn from the multitude of orthopaedic subspecialties within a four-year period. Because these subspecialties often have their own dedicated rotation, training programs must recognize that each rotation has its own service-related and educational components. The balance between those components varies with each rotation, and, importantly, the perception of the balance between service and education may be viewed differently by residents and faculty.

Resident and Faculty Perceptions

Sanfey et al[1] reported that program directors tend to rank tasks as being more educational than the residents who perform the tasks. In this study, 105 program directors and 407 residents were asked to rank 24 activities on a five-point Likert scale. Based on the survey results, 87.5% of the program directors rated the activities as more educational than the residents did. The reasons for the differing opinions varied depending on the postgraduate year (PGY) of the resident. PGY-1 and PGY-2 respondents reported that the tasks lacked educational value because the skill set had already been acquired; the faculty provided inadequate teaching; and the tasks were needlessly stressful, offered limited autonomy, and had time constraints. In contrast, PGY-3 through PGY-5 respondents attributed the lack of educational value to the lack of continuity, the resident's need to perform administrative duties, and the belief that the tasks should be performed by junior residents.

A survey by Reines et al[2] found similar results. Attending physicians ranked rounds to be more educational than the residents did, whereas residents believed performing surgical procedures with limited supervision was more educational compared with the attending physician's perception of that training aspect. Forty percent of the residents surveyed believed that more than 50% of their training experience was strictly service oriented. This belief was experience dependent, with 60% of the PGY-1 residents and 34% of the PGY-5 residents indicating that more than 50% of their residency experience was strictly service oriented and not educational. In contrast, only 10% of the attending physicians believed that more than 50% of the residency experience was strictly service oriented.

Factors in Improving Patient Outcomes

Service duties performed by residents include taking patients' histories and performing physical examinations, detailing medications, writing daily notes, performing discharge summaries, participating in patient meetings, writing clinic notes, and completing clinic forms. Interestingly, the service portion of a resident's responsibilities is the area where most medical errors occur. In a survey of factors that negatively affect clinical care, residents included incomplete handoffs, inexperience or lack of knowledge, insufficient ancillary personnel, and excessive workloads.[3] Most residents did not believe that a further reduction in work hours would improve patient outcomes and suggested that system changes to address factors such as inexperience and lack of knowledge would more likely affect patient outcomes.

Because of the 80-hour work week restriction, interresident communication is crucial to avoid medical errors. Studies have shown that handoff training improves patient outcomes.[4] In conjunction with handoff communication, an appropriate workload for the skill level of the resident is also beneficial. A study by Coit et al[5] reported that internal medicine residents who had a more manageable workload wrote substantially better discharge summaries containing more of the required elements of the patient's history, the inpatient course, and the discharge plan and provided better continuity of care than those with a heavier workload. The authors concluded that establishing an appropriate workload for a resident's level of knowledge and ability and providing tools for successful handoff practices would help minimize medical errors.

Improvements in the quality of patient care have not been readily apparent since the onset of work-hour restrictions. In a study of patient care before and after the implementation of resident work-hour restrictions in a level I trauma center, Helling et al[6] concluded that the restriction did not have an obvious beneficial effect on patient care. In a study of 107,006 neurotrauma admissions at teaching hospitals and 115,604 neurotrauma admissions at nonteaching hospitals, Hoh et al[7] reported that resident work-hour restrictions led to a 23% increase in complications at teaching hospitals but no change in the complication rate at nonteaching hospitals.

Balance

These studies illustrate the importance of maintaining a balance between education and service so that residents have the opportunity to learn the important skills needed to provide comprehensive patient care after graduation; however, they also indicated the need for further improvements in the residency education system. The primary goal of the program director, department chair, and faculty is to prepare residents for practice, regardless of the subspecialty. It is important to teach and expose orthopaedic residents to the fundamentals of orthopaedic surgery: performing physical examinations, ordering tests, consulting ancillary services, performing surgery, and determining appropriate postoperative care. This broad curriculum is often at odds with a resident's desire to concentrate primarily on performing surgical procedures.

Training a Competent Surgeon

Skill Sets

To train competent surgeons, residency programs must teach residents a real skill set, including the ability to thoroughly and accurately assess a patient's condition, apply sound clinical and surgical judgment, demonstrate communication and surgical skills, and obtain an appropriate understanding of perioperative management. This skill set must be taught using an apprenticeship model, not a classroom model or independent teaching. Although it remains challenging to teach these multiple skills in the environment of work-hour restrictions for residents, Baskies et al[8] reported that the number of surgical hours for PGY-2 through PGY-4 orthopaedic residents was unchanged after the implementation of work-hour restrictions, and, surprisingly, there was an increase in the number of surgical hours for PGY-5 residents after the change. Although the amount of surgical time does not appear to have been changed by work-hour restrictions, it is highly plausible that other important aspects of a resident's education (such as clinical time and patient management) have been compromised.

Effect of Midlevel Practitioners and Team Care

Assistance provided by midlevel practitioners has played a crucial role in freeing residents from many service-related patient issues. In a survey of residents' attitudes toward midlevel practitioners, most of the respondents reported that midlevel practitioners were an asset because they decreased the workload of residents and provided a better environment for teaching and patient care.[9] However, when implementing the use of midlevel practitioners, it is important to ensure that routine service tasks are still learned and performed by residents. Activities such as taking a patient's history, making daily notes, writing discharge summaries, meeting with patients, taking clinic notes, and completing clinic forms are important tasks for an orthopaedic resident to learn because they must be performed proficiently by the conclusion of training and as independent orthopaedic surgeons. These skills should be taught, reviewed, and documented.

A team environment (faculty, ancillary personnel, nursing staff, operating room personnel, and clinic staff) is necessary to provide optimal patient care while maximizing the time available for resident education. A well-functioning team will provide better treatment for patients. With the successful integration of midlevel practitioners into an orthopaedic service, residents can benefit from increased conference time, operating room participation, improved clinic experience, better patient management, and increased time in learning skills. The attending physician is a mentor, a teacher, and a team leader and is responsible for clearly explaining the need for activities, showing appreciation for the resident's work, and providing assistance when needed.

Surgical Skills Laboratory

The American Academy of Orthopaedic Surgeons (AAOS) along with its specialty organizations have recognized the need for creating educational opportunities for members to learn and master surgical skills in settings outside the operating room. The AAOS Orthopaedic Learning Center offers surgical skills courses to provide such opportunities.

Many factors influencing residency education have prompted the consideration of including surgical skills laboratories in resident training programs. These factors include the likely decrease in clinical experience because of the 80-hour work week and an increased focus on decreasing medical errors and complications. Surgical skills laboratories are tools in developing a proficiency-based curriculum. These laboratories allow residents to learn arthroscopic and open surgical techniques in a controlled environment. Surgical simulator training allows both experienced and novice surgeons to optimize their technical skills at an individual pace using a structured curriculum without the associated risk of patient morbidity.

Achieving Proficiency

O'Neill et al[10] reported on a survey, which included 164 orthopaedic department chairs and fellowship program directors, asking for an estimate of the number of procedures required to attain proficiency in various types of arthroscopic procedures. The respondents noted that a substantial number of repetitions is required to attain proficiency in various arthroscopic procedures, and the number of repetitions varies considerably depending on the procedure. In August 2011, the Residency Review Committee for Orthopaedic Surgery determined that at least 30 knee and 30 shoulder arthroscopic procedures be performed during a 5-year residency program. Vitale et al[11] reported on 1,074 responses from surgeons listed on the AAOS website who performed shoulder surgery, arthroscopic surgery, and/or sports medicine surgery. The orthopaedic surgeons were asked to rank the relative importance of a resource in training for rotator cuff repair. The respondents ranked the top three resources as a sports medicine fellowship, hands-on courses, and arthroscopic practice on cadaver specimens. Multiple studies have validated the survey data and demonstrated that practicing arthroscopic procedures improves performance. A strong correlation was found between the performance of basic arthroscopic tasks in a simulator model and performance of the same tasks in a cadaver model.[12] A study by Gomoll et al[13] reported that the performance of residents trained on a simulator had improved on retesting compared with their initial performance 3 years earlier. This improvement in performance with additional experience was similar to improvements seen in surgeons trained with traditional methods.

Laboratory Design and Development

At several academic institutions around the country, surgical skills laboratories provide residents and fellows with the opportunity for hands-on learning. Most laboratories resemble a mock-up of outpatient and inpatient suites. The development of a successful skills laboratory can be an intensive undertaking involving many steps, including negotiations with the university administration for space and funds, partnerships with industry for equipment and instruments, and obtaining grants and extramural funds to maintain the facility. One example of a successful laboratory is the biologic skills laboratory of the Department of Orthopaedic Surgery at the University of Connecticut. It has 691 square feet of dedicated space, with six arthroscopy stations, one dry laboratory station, and an adjacent 299 square foot preparation room with 10 freezers and an area where specimens are stored and prepped.

When planning a skills laboratory, it is important to recognize that equipment cost will be substantial. For example, the approximate cost for an arthroscopy center will include the costs for the articulating arm for an arthroscopy monitor tower ($4,600), the power system ($6,200), the monitor ($400), the water pump ($8,215), the light source ($10,000), the camera box ($17,500), and the ablation generator ($18,200). Typically, many of these items can be purchased used or refurbished for approximately 50% of the list price. Each arthroscopy station also requires a vacuum source and, often, an air source, which cost approximately $400 to $500 per vacuum or air line installation. Surgical instrument sets are also expensive, with a single set costing between $5,000 and $40,000. A skills laboratory also benefits from having a variety of instrument sets, such as a knee (anterior cruciate ligament) set ($5,000), a shoulder retractor set ($10,000), a shoulder set ($25,000), an ankle fracture set ($25,000), and a hip scope master set ($40,000). Other equipment costs can include C-arms, radiolucent tables, and lights. In addition to fixed costs, variable costs include cadaver specimens and shipping, storage, and disposal of the specimens. Administrative costs include laboratory and maintenance supplies and the salary of a dedicated laboratory manager who is responsible for all aspects of the laboratory administration and maintaining compliance with all university regulations.

Although surgical skills laboratories require a substantial financial commitment from residency programs and hospitals, they are a very valuable educational asset to residents, faculty, and community physicians and can improve patient care. These laboratories are also increasingly expected to be part of orthopaedic residency and fellowship training programs.

Surgical Simulation
Background
n 1889, Sir William Halsted introduced a residency training system at Johns Hopkins Hospital.[14] The system, which emphasized graded responsibility and hands-on learning, remained the cornerstone of surgical training in North America for more than a century. Over the past few decades, the concept of learning by doing has become less acceptable, particularly when invasive procedures and high-risk care are involved. In 2000, a report by the Institute of Medicine drew attention to preventable medical errors, brought the issue of patient safety to prominence, and raised ethical concerns about trainees learning basic skills by practicing on patients.[15] These issues have led to calls for a separation of practice and performance in healthcare delivery. Financial constraints, work-hour restrictions, and expanded skill requirements also pose new challenges in residency education. Educating residents requires efficient methods for learning, accountability for patient safety, and the incorporation of new technology into teaching modalities.

The past decade has seen a substantial increase in the available tools to enhance medical education, including web-based resources, virtual reality, and high-fidelity patient simulations. In 2006, several general surgery associations, including the American Board of Surgery, the American College of Surgeons, and the American Surgical Association, created a Surgical Council on Resident Education to develop a standardized national curriculum and a website, the General Surgery Resident Curriculum Portal.[16]

Despite the fact that other professions require many hours of simulator training, surgical simulation training in orthopaedic surgery remains in its infancy. For example, more than 200 hours of flight simulation training are required before a pilot can fly an F18 aircraft and an average of 6 to 8 hours of logged simulation time is required before each flight. If a pilot does not fly an aircraft for more than 15 days, he or she must complete the full curriculum, including simulated flying, to meet proficiency requirements.

Reducing the Number of Medical Errors

Approximately 98,000 deaths each year are attributed to medical errors.[15] Simulation training has been proposed as a means of reducing errors. A study by Barsuk et al[17] reported that simulation-based training can be used to reduce catheter-related bloodstream infections in patients in the intensive care unit. Traditional central venous catheter insertion training, which consisted of 4 hours of didactics, was replaced with simulation training, which included 1 hour of didactics and 3 hours of simulated ultrasound-guided practice to proficiency in inserting a central venous catheter. The newer training methods resulted in fewer catheter-related bloodstream infections (0.50 infections per 1,000 catheter-days) compared with the baseline results before the intervention of 3.20 infections per 1,000 catheter-days ($P = 0.001$) and with 5.03 infection per 1,000 catheter-days ($P = 0.001$) in another intensive care unit in the same hospital that did not have the simulation training.

Key Elements

Simulation is defined as the imitation of some real thing, state of affairs, or process for the purpose of learning or practice. The key elements of simulation surgery and medical procedures are (1) the repetitive practice of skills to a prescribed proficiency, without patient involvement; (2) immediate feedback about errors or complications encountered during training and the opportunity for repractice; (3) learner-centered rather than patient-centered learning; and (4) objective, measurable proficiency. Simulation allows for repetition of a task, thereby building important physiologic connections without the risk of patient morbidity.

Acquiring Skills

The acquisition of motor skills is often divided into two phases.[18] During phase I (fast learning) gamma-aminobutyric acid (GABA)–related neural processes select optimal neural pathways for the performance of a task.[19] During phase II (slow learning) a process occurs involving the long-term structural modifications of basic motor modules and time-dependent strengthening of links between motor neurons in different areas of the brain. Hands-on learning in a simulated environment may help develop the neural links necessary to acquire surgical skills. Learning at spaced intervals provides better long-term retention of knowledge and surgical skills than a single learning experience.[20,21] Because of the sporadic nature and periodicity of surgery, ideally spaced surgical learning experiences are not readily available. Simulation training in surgical procedures may help bridge this gap by providing training at regular intervals.

Practice using surgical simulation in the immediate preoperative time period may also improve surgeon performance. Unlike athletes and musicians, most surgeons perform without any preoperative warm-up. Multiple prospective randomized trials across surgical specialties have shown simulation used as a preoperative warm up improves surgeon performance.[22,23] Pre-operative warm-up results in better attention and focus, smoother hand and instrument motion, less distraction, and improved technical performance.

Implementation in Other Surgical Fields

A curriculum based on simulation training has been validated in the field of general surgery. The fundamentals of laparoscopic surgery (FLS) program is a proficiency-based curriculum that simulates basic laparoscopic skills applicable to many surgical procedures and offers an online curriculum that coincides with those skills.[24] In a randomized controlled trial, Sroka et al[25] reported that training to proficiency using the FLS training program resulted in substantial improvements in surgical performance. Junior-level residents who participated in the training program performed better than the control group.

The FLS program is the only simulation training curriculum that has been fully integrated into a nationwide residency curriculum. The FLS program meets certain necessary criteria for a surgical simulation exercise. These criteria include face validity (how well the simulation reproduces a real-world situation), content validity (how much of the real-world situation is reproduced in the simulator model), construct validity (the ability of an assessment to distinguish between advanced and novice practitioners), and predictive validity (the ability of the assessment to predict future intraoperative performance). The face and content validity of FLS were assessed by 44 experienced laparoscopic surgeons who detailed the motor skills fundamental to laparoscopic surgery. These skills were broken down into 11 skills, which were then incorporated into one or more exercises. Construct validity was assessed in multiple studies that showed the performance of experienced surgeons was better than that of junior-level residents.[26-28] Fried et al[26] demonstrated predictive validity in a study showing that the total FLS score had a high correlation with intraoperative measurements of technical skills in the operating room.

Because the costs of implementing an FLS program are manageable, FLS has been embraced by both large academic centers and community programs. As of 2009, the American Board of Surgery requires FLS certification, and this surgical simulation training is a requirement in all general surgery residency curriculums as outlined by the American College of Surgeons. Interestingly, insurance carriers have started to sponsor FLS training sessions for practicing surgeons and may require FLS training as a criteria for plan participation.[29] Over time, it is likely that the American Board of Surgery will require FLS certification for surgeons performing laparoscopic surgery and maintaining certification.

The field of urology is also incorporating simulation training into the residency training curriculum.[30] In several programs, surgical simulation has become an integral part of residency training in laparoscopic and robotic surgery and has provided a platform for new technologic advances. Simulator training gives urologists an opportunity to practice and maintain complex surgical skills, prepare for difficult cases, and provide methods to improve team communication. Currently, the American Urological Association is in the process of validating the simulation training curriculum.[31]

Simulation Training in Orthopaedics

In 2011, the AAOS hosted an orthopaedic surgery simulation summit to discuss the current status and direction of simulation training in orthopaedic education. Currently, three main proj-

ects are available or being developed. The ArthroSim (Touch of Life Technologies) is a virtual reality knee arthroscopy simulator that has been purchased by 14 residency programs; a shoulder simulator is being developed. The AAOS and the Orthopaedic Trauma Association are working on a simulation project and educational curriculum for PGY-1 and PGY-2 residents that focuses on hip fractures. The third project is TraumaVision (Swemac), a simulation system providing an interactive training environment for learning new surgical techniques and practicing tasks in both two-dimensional (radiographic view) and three-dimensional (computer-generated three-dimensional view) environments. The system provides haptic feedback, allowing the practicing surgeon to "feel" the simulated procedure.

Substantial costs are associated with the use and the acquisition of each current program or project that has been or is being developed. Unlike the general surgery simulation curriculum, orthopaedic simulation programs are not readily available to all residency programs and may not be accessible to all training programs because of the costs. The goal of future simulation training in orthopaedics will be to develop a program that simulates the fundamentals of orthopaedic surgery in a cost-effective manner.

The Technically Incompetent Resident

Ideally, all orthopaedic residents will complete their residency programs with a solid foundation in the principles of orthopaedic surgery, have the ability to make sound clinical and intraoperative decisions, and acquire superb technical skills. In reality this is not the case. The talent levels of residents are spread across a spectrum of ability levels. Dealing with an incom-

petent resident is difficult and allowing such a resident to graduate does a disservice to the profession, society, patients, and (ultimately) the resident.

Survey Results

A telephone survey regarding resident trainability was conducted by one of this chapter's authors (PS). Eleven current or past orthopaedic department chairs who had served in that position for at least 10 years (mean, 20.2 years; range, 10 to 32 years) and two orthopaedic surgeons were surveyed. The respondents reported that, on average, approximately 2% (range, 0% to 6%) of orthopaedics residents are untrainable. The consensus was that almost any resident is trainable, but there remains substantial variability in the rate at which residents can acquire skills.

The respondents were also asked to define technical incompetence. Replies included "I know it when I see it" and more detailed responses, including "an effective surgeon divides operations into predefined, sequential steps, but a technically incompetent resident cannot"; and the "inability to perform routine procedures in an efficient, timely, and safe fashion." The respondents also unanimously agreed that it was not possible to accurately measure technical competence, which revealed both a deficiency in resident education assessment and a need to develop an accurate and standardized mode of assessment. For general surgery, a validated system known as the Objective Structured Assessment of Technical Skills (OSATS) has been developed and includes a checklist and a global rating scale to assess surgical skills. This type of system is needed for orthopaedic-specific surgical procedures.

Survey respondents were also questioned about screening medical students for technical competence during interviews. Most of the respondents said that they did not screen students. One respondent had students complete sawbones exercises but believed the results were difficult to standardize, expensive, and of negligible value. The survey also found that most technical deficiencies are identified during a resident's second year of training.

Providing Support

Helping residents who require additional support can be difficult for social and psychological reasons. A resident's ego may limit his or her ability to address learning problems. Some residents are aware of problems and recognize the need to change fields. When poorly performing residents will not acknowledge deficits, effective remediation is precluded.

If a resident acknowledges a learning deficit, an accurate assessment of his or her problem is paramount to successful remediation. The problem may be multifactorial, including the cognitive, affective, and organizational domains. Consulting an educational psychologist may help to accurately identify learning difficulties. After a thorough assessment of a resident's needs, a dedicated mentor can be selected to serve as an advisor and coach and can guide the resident through supervised cadaver dissections and arthroscopy laboratories to improve psychomotor skills. Other considerations should include vision testing and the possibility of repeating a year of training.

Many respondents reported stories of trainees who had lacked adequate technical skills at some point in their training but had gone on to lead successful careers. Many of these individuals avoided subspecialization in technically demanding domains, such as microsurgery. Based on information provided in the survey, it also appears that most residents who cannot successfully complete the remediation

process choose a different specialty; therefore, it is rarely necessary to terminate a resident from an orthopaedic residency program because of inadequate surgical skills.

The field of orthopaedic residency education is evolving. A competency-based curriculum may need to be considered instead of allowing a resident to move on to the next program year because certain case log numbers have been met and baseline evaluations have been passed. Such a competency-based system would allow a resident to work at his or her own pace. Those capable of faster learning could complete the residency program earlier, and slower learners could be given more time to attain necessary skills.

Summary

Resident training is a complex undertaking that involves resident, faculty, and staff commitments as well as a continual willingness to adapt to the educational changes needed to maintain an efficient and effective training curriculum. Sufficient ancillary staff support is important to free residents from performing unnecessary or redundant service-based activities. Specific needs vary depending on the institution. Maintaining open lines of communication between residents and faculty allows for appropriate assessments of the residents' needs. Teaching basic surgical skills outside of the operating room is imperative in the current medicolegal climate. This need can be addressed by implementing a surgical skills laboratory. Although these laboratories are expensive and time consuming to develop and maintain, they provide educational benefits for residents, faculty, and community physicians. Creating a low-cost surgical simulator is less costly than using cadaver specimens. An orthopaedic-specific simulator can provide an objective measure of a resident's psychomotor

competence and is a tool for teaching and learning orthopaedic skills. Simulator training may also help educators better identify areas for improvement for individual residents and reduce the number of technically incompetent residents. Significant strides have been made over the past decade in improving orthopaedic residency education, but further change is still needed.

References

1. Sanfey H, Cofer J, Hiatt JR, et al: In the eye of the beholder. *Arch Surg* 2011;146(12):1389-1395.

2. Reines HD, Robinson L, Nitzchke S, Rizzo A: Defining service and education: The first step to developing the correct balance. *Surgery* 2007;142(2): 303-310.

3. Borman KR, Jones AT, Shea JA: Duty hours, quality of care, and patient safety: General surgery resident perceptions. *J Am Coll Surg* 2012;215(1):70-77, discussion 77-79.

4. Mueller SK, Call SA, McDonald FS, Halvorsen AJ, Schnipper JL, Hicks LS: Impact of resident workload and handoff training on patient outcomes. *Am J Med* 2012;125(1):104-110.

5. Coit MH, Katz JT, McMahon GT: The effect of workload reduction on the quality of residents' discharge summaries. *J Gen Intern Med* 2011;26(1):28-32.

6. Helling TS, Kaswan S, Boccardo J, Bost JE: The effect of resident duty hour restriction on trauma center outcomes in teaching hospitals in the state of Pennsylvania. *J Trauma* 2010;69(3):607-612, discussion 612-613.

7. Hoh BL, Neal DW, Kleinhenz DT, Hoh DJ, Mocco J, Barker FG II: Higher complications and no improvement in mortality in the ACGME resident duty-hour restriction era: An analysis of

more than 107,000 neurosurgical trauma patients in the Nationwide Inpatient Sample database. *Neurosurgery* 2012;70(6):1369-1381, discussion 1381-1382.

8. Baskies MA, Ruchelsman DE, Capeci CM, Zuckerman JD, Egol KA: Operative experience in an orthopaedic surgery residency program: The effect of work-hour restrictions. *J Bone Joint Surg Am* 2008;90(4):924-927.

9. Reines HD, Robinson L, Duggan M, O'Brien BM, Aulenbach K: Integrating midlevel practitioners into a teaching service. *Am J Surg* 2006;192(1):119-124.

10. O'Neill PJ, Cosgarea AJ, Freedman JA, Queale WS, McFarland EG: Arthroscopic proficiency: A survey of orthopaedic sports medicine fellowship directors and orthopaedic surgery department chairs. *Arthroscopy* 2002;18(7):795-800.

11. Vitale MA, Kleweno CP, Jacir AM, Levine WN, Bigliani LU, Ahmad CS: Training resources in arthroscopic rotator cuff repair. *J Bone Joint Surg Am* 2007;89(6):1393-1398.

12. Martin KD, Belmont PJ, Schoenfeld AJ, Todd M, Cameron KL, Owens BD: Arthroscopic basic task performance in shoulder simulator model correlates with similar task performance in cadavers. *J Bone Joint Surg Am* 2011;93(21):e1271-e1275.

13. Gomoll AH, Pappas G, Forsythe B, Warner JJ: Individual skill progression on a virtual reality simulator for shoulder arthroscopy: A 3-year follow-up study. *Am J Sports Med* 2008;36(6):1139-1142.

14. Cameron JL: William Stewart Halsted: Our surgical heritage. *Ann Surg* 1997;225(5):445-458.

15. Kohn LT, Corrigan J, Donaldson MS, eds: *To Err is Human: Building a Safer Health System.* Washington, DC, National Academy Press, 2000.

16. SCORE: Surgical Council on Resident Education website. http://www.surgicalcore.org/. Accessed August 9, 2013.

17. Barsuk JH, Cohen ER, Feinglass J, McGaghie WC, Wayne DB: Use of simulation-based education to reduce catheter-related bloodstream infections. *Arch Intern Med* 2009;169(15):1420-1423.

18. Karni A, Meyer G, Rey-Hipolito C, et al: Fast and slow experience-driven changes in primary motor cortex. *Proc Natl Acad Sci USA* 1998;95(3):861-868.

19. Ziemann U, Muellbacher W, Hallett M, Cohen LG: Modulation of practice-dependent plasticity in human motor cortex. *Brain* 2001;124(pt 6):1171-1181.

20. Stransky D, Wilcox LM, Dubrowski A: Mental rotation: Cross-task training and generalization. *J Exp Psychol Appl* 2010;16(4):349-360.

21. Kerfoot BP, Fu Y, Baker H, Connelly D, Ritchey ML, Genega EM: Online spaced education generates transfer and improves long-term retention of diagnostic skills: A randomized controlled trial. *J Am Coll Surg* 2010;211(3):331-337, e1.

22. Lee JY, Mucksavage P, Kerbl DC, et al: Laparoscopic warm-up exercises improve performance of senior-level trainees during laparoscopic renal surgery. *J Endourol* 2012;26(5):545-550.

23. Calatayud D, Arora S, Aggarwal R, et al: Warm-up in a virtual reality environment improves performance in the operating room. *Ann Surg* 2010;251(6):1181-1185.

24. Fundamental of Laparoscopic Surgery: The Definitive Laparoscopic Skills Enhancement and Assessment Module. http://www.flsprogram.org/. Accessed August 9, 2013.

25. Sroka G, Feldman LS, Vassiliou MC, Kaneva PA, Fayez R, Fried GM: Fundamentals of laparoscopic surgery simulator training to proficiency improves laparoscopic performance in the operating room: A randomized controlled trial. *Am J Surg* 2010;199(1):115-120.

26. Fried GM, Feldman LS, Vassiliou MC, et al: Proving the value of simulation in laparoscopic surgery. *Ann Surg* 2004;240(3):518-525, discussion 525-528.

27. Swanstrom LL, Fried GM, Hoffman KI, Soper NJ: Beta test results of a new system assessing competence in laparoscopic surgery. *J Am Coll Surg* 2006;202(1):62-69.

28. Okrainec A, Soper NJ, Swanstrom LL, Fried GM: Trends and results of the first 5 years of Fundamentals of Laparoscopic Surgery (FLS) certification testing. *Surg Endosc* 2011;25(4):1192-1198.

29. Derevianko AY, Schwaitzberg SD, Tsuda S, et al: Malpractice carrier underwrites Fundamentals of Laparoscopic Surgery training and testing: A benchmark for patient safety. *Surg Endosc* 2010;24(3):616-623.

30. Ehdaie B, Tracy C, Reynolds C, et al: Evaluation of laparoscopic curricula in American urology residency training. *J Endourol* 2011;25(11):1805-1810.

31. Sweet RM, Beach R, Sainfort F, et al: Introduction and validation of the American Urological Association Basic Laparoscopic Urologic Surgery skills curriculum. *J Endourol* 2012;26(2):190-196.

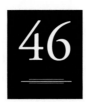

Volunteer Opportunities for Orthopaedic Surgeons in the Developing World

Iain S. Elliott, BS
David Spiegel, MD
Richard A. Gosselin, MD, MPH, MSC, FRCS
Peter G. Trafton, MD
R. Richard Coughlin, MD, MSc

Abstract

Orthopaedic surgeons have consistently shown interest in volunteering to aid needy populations throughout the world. Service missions, building surgical capacity, and disaster relief have benefited from the volunteer efforts of orthopaedic surgeons. The burden of musculoskeletal disease is high and will continue to increase as motorization and development reach more people. The increasing burden of musculoskeletal disease requires thoughtful, well-planned, and effectively executed interventions. A framework for action will help orthopaedic surgeons use the many avenues available for involvement in international volunteer work.

Instr Course Lect 2014;63:495-503.

Orthopaedic surgeons have a long history of volunteering their services in a variety of capacities in low- and middle-income countries. Volunteer work includes service missions, teaching and training, disaster relief, and involvement in activities aimed at building surgical capacity. Overseas volunteerism offers opportunities to care for patients in need and share knowledge and skills with health professionals in developing countries. It also provides valuable insights into the diagnosis and treatment of musculoskeletal disorders that are rarely seen in developed countries. Although most medical conditions will be familiar, an unfamiliar presentation of a familiar condition may be encountered (such as neglected or late presenting cases of trauma or infection, congenital or angular deformities, or tumors), or the surgeon may encounter a typical presentation of an unfamiliar condition (such as polio, tuberculosis, or rickets).

It is not necessary to travel overseas to find opportunities to care for patients without access to medical care or the ability to pay for services; however, many low- and middle-income countries have a large number of patients with severe conditions that strongly appeal to humanitarian interests and attract an increasing number of potential volunteers. Providing care for patients in need offers great fulfillment for interested surgeons, and its effect is immediately and readily perceived. However, it is impossible for volunteers to treat all needy patients; therefore, helping poorer countries develop their own resources for health care is an alluring challenge. For volunteer surgeons, improving health care involves creating sustainable, long-term partnerships focused on training and education that will increase the volume

Dr. Spiegel or an immediate family member serves as a board member, owner, officer, or committee member of the Pediatric Orthopaedic Society of North America and the American Academy of Orthopaedic Surgeons. Dr. Trafton or an immediate family member serves as a paid consultant to Illuminoss Medical; has stock or stock options held in Johnson & Johnson; and serves as a board member, owner, officer, or committee member of Orthopaedics Overseas, the American Academy of Orthopaedic Surgeons, the US Bone & Joint Initiative, and AO North America. Dr. Coughlin or an immediate family member serves as a board member, owner, officer, or committee member of the American Academy of Orthopaedic Surgeons. Neither of the following authors nor any immediate family member has received anything of value from or has stock or stock options held in a commercial company or institution related directly or indirectly to the subject of this chapter: Mr. Elliott and Dr. Gosselin.

and quality of locally available health care. Building human, technical, material, and financial capacity may be the volunteer's most effective contribution.[1-5] Although a volunteer's personal contribution to building capacity may not be immediately obvious, progress can be seen over time through return visits, personal relationships with local surgeons, and participation in communities of involved volunteers.

This chapter describes the magnitude and effect of musculoskeletal conditions in low-and middle-income countries, characterizes barriers to the delivery of orthopaedic services at the population level, outlines avenues for volunteer involvement in orthopaedic care in poorer countries, and discusses the pearls and pitfalls of these engagements. The section on disaster relief addresses the healthcare needs of a region that has been overwhelmed by a natural catastrophe or human conflict. Volunteers responding to a disaster must contend with a broad variety of challenges that extend beyond providing health care.

Magnitude of the Problem

The worldwide trend for increased economic development has led to increases in life expectancy, urban living, and motorization.[6] These changes have been associated with an epidemiologic transition in which the burden of communicable diseases has been reduced while the burden of noncommunicable diseases and injuries has increased.[7,8] Although the burden of diseases requiring surgery has not been accurately quantified using existing metrics, it is estimated to represent approximately 11% of the world's disability adjusted life years (DALYs).[6,9] DALYs incorporate both fatal and nonfatal outcomes, addressing years lived with a disability in addition to mortality secondary to a particular condition. Injuries have been implicated as the cause of 9.8% of all deaths and 12.3% of the world's burden of disease in 2004.[6] Ninety-five percent of all deaths caused by injury occur in low- and middle-income countries.[6] By the year 2030, based on the number of DALYs lost, injuries are projected to become the third largest contributor to disease burden after cardiovascular disease and mental health issues.[10,11]

With the aim of addressing the growing burden of traumatic injuries worldwide, the United Nations has designated the decade from 2011 through 2020 as a Decade of Action for Traffic Safety.[12] The World Health Organization also has several initiatives aimed at addressing the burden of surgical disease.[13,14] Although injury prevention is an essential part of addressing this epidemic, strategies to improve the treatment of injured patients also must be appropriately funded and developed.[1,2,15]

Quantifying the burden of musculoskeletal disease is challenging because only limited information is available. Epidemiologic studies are needed; data can then be further analyzed using health metrics such as DALYs. A 2008 study found that the prevalence of musculoskeletal disease in Rwanda was 5.2%, with substantial variations in etiology based on age groups.[7] The authors estimated that 180,000 surgical procedures would be required to treat the musculoskeletal conditions of Rwanda's 2005 population of 8.4 million people. These data can likely be extrapolated to other countries with a similar socioeconomic status.[8]

Barriers to Orthopaedic Surgical Care

It is recognized that there is an enormous burden from surgical conditions worldwide, including orthopaedics, but data on the unmet need for surgical care have been sparse.[7,8,15] Low- and middle-income countries share a disproportionate amount of unmet surgical need, with the poorest third of the world's population receiving only 3.5% of the total worldwide surgical care provided.[16] To address the unmet need for orthopaedic surgical care, the various barriers to the delivery of services must be considered. Barriers, which can vary within and among countries, may be encountered in accessing services (system level) and using existing health services (individual level).[17] A lack of access to health services may be caused by deficiencies in infrastructure and resources, human resources (number, distribution, and training of health providers), referral networks, and other system issues (such as the distribution of health facilities).[18,19] Patients may not use existing services because of social, cultural, financial (direct or indirect costs), physical (geographic), and/or religious reasons or perhaps because of the perception that the quality and the effectiveness of the services are low.[19] Out-of-pocket expenditures are a major concern, and several million families are pushed below the poverty line each year because of catastrophic health expenditures.[17,19] To truly improve the delivery of orthopaedic services, all barriers to access and use must be addressed.

Opportunities for Involvement

The goals of volunteering abroad are numerous; are unique to each individual; and may include a desire to give back, personal development, or the challenge of working in a situation that is very different from the physician's home institution. When working abroad, orthopaedic surgeons are challenged to be creative, learn from their hosts, and expand their treatment ar-

Table 1

Trip Length Considerations

Trip Length	Opportunities and Realities	Pros	Cons
Less than 2 weeks	Some relief work can be accomplished, mostly service oriented; teaching is a bonus, not the goal.	Not away from home or practice for too long; less expensive	Cannot travel too far; no substantial follow-up is possible; limited contact with local people; relies on good infrastructure for screening, follow-up; all work and no play
2 to 6 weeks	Relief work and service-oriented trips are viable. Teaching and training are usually the main goals for residents, faculty, students, and other healthcare workers.	Longer lasting, multiplier effect; allow opportunity for better follow-up; can impact all aspects of disease and treatment; more contact with local people; no geographic limitations; more margin of error permissible in relation to local infrastructure; easier to plan for family rest and relaxation	More time away from practice; more expensive; some lack of follow-up
More than 6 weeks	Long-term relief work, teaching, training, research, surveillance programs, and administration are all possible.	Depends on personal goals; cultural immersion; only way to meet long-term teaching goals	Substantial decrease in income; personal health and safety issues

mamentarium.[5,20,21] These opportunities are often classified as service missions, teaching and training programs, and disaster relief missions, although there can be a degree of overlap.

Overseas volunteerism may reinvigorate and stimulate an orthopaedic surgeon, and the interaction with medical students, residents, local hosts, and patients will undoubtedly alter his or her perception of orthopaedics.[22] Many surgeons believe that they derive more benefits from the experience than they are able to contribute. Opportunities exist for surgeons at various stages of training. The key is to find an activity that resonates with an individual's skill set and level of experience. The length of time available for volunteer service is also an important consideration (**Table 1**).

Service Missions

Service missions involve direct patient care and may or may not be associated with surgical capacity–building activities. Orthopaedic surgeons trained in trauma and pediatrics are typically in high demand around the world.[7] Short trips (less than 2 weeks) are usually service oriented, although teaching activities may be included. Consultation for facility assessment, program evaluations, or systems analysis can be accomplished during this time frame. These trips limit the time away from a surgeon's practice, are less expensive, and, if well organized, can maximize the number of patients treated. Service missions also can be counterproductive, such as in instances when the organizers and participants are insensitive to the presence of local physicians and/or other groups working in the area.[23-25] Contextual variables are important and will always influence the treatment plan.[26] The visiting surgeon should be aware of the local culture, the resources available, the healthcare delivery system, whether adequate rehabilitation services are available, and how his or her surgical patients will receive follow-up evaluation and treatment. Organizations such as Orthopedics Overseas, Operation Rainbow, Operation Walk, Medical Missions International, and many other secular and faith-based organizations offer opportunities for overseas service missions.

Teaching and Training Programs

Programs that focus on teaching and training have the potential for the greatest long-term effect on the delivery of orthopaedic services to a community. Local health professionals are ultimately the people who will care for the population, so any improvement in their education, knowledge, capacity, or systems will affect care at the population level. Educational activities include didactic lectures, hands-on skills workshops, teaching during direct patient care, or simply providing educational resources that are not accessible to local providers. Teaching is typically geared toward orthopaedic residents and faculty but can include medical students and other healthcare providers. Sustainable initiatives require a long-term commitment to a particular country or site that sends volunteers to well-established sites, with a strong focus on teaching and training to empower local providers.[27] Sustainable educational programs are sometimes developed through long-term relationships between academic institutions.[28] Mid-length trips ranging from 2 to 6 weeks are usually required.

As an example from outside the field of surgery, Partners in Health has demonstrated that building capacity at

Table 2

Selected Organizations That Respond to Disasters or Provide Medical Needs in Conflict Zones

Type	Website Uniform Resource Locator (URL)
Relief	
International Committee of the Red Cross	http://www.icrc.org
Doctors Without Borders: Médecins Sans Frontiéres	http://www.msf.org
International Medical Corps	http://www.internationalmedicalcorps.org
The International Rescue Committee	http://www.theirc.org
Médecins du Monde	http://www.medecinsdumonde.org
Merlin	http://www.merlin.org.uk
Emergency USA	http://www.emergencyusa.org
SIGN	http://www.sign-post.org
Service	
Heath Volunteers Overseas (Orthopaedics Overseas)	http://www.hvousa.org
Operation Rainbow	http://www.operationrainbow.org
Operation Walk	http://www.operationwalk.org
Mercy Ships	http://www.mercyships.org
Medical Missions International	http://www.medicalmission.ca
Educational	
Global HELP	http://www.global-help.org
Health Volunteers Overseas (Orthopaedics Overseas)	http://hvousa.org/volunteerToolkit/knownet.shtml

the local level can drive improvements in the health of a particular community.[1,2] Partners in Health has set up partnerships with organizations operating hospitals around the world in which local physicians practice. Visitors from high-income countries work alongside local physicians for long-term assignments, support these institutions through education and service, and have mechanisms in place for long-term follow-up and structural support.[2]

Educational exchange can be accomplished at the resident level, and several programs have developed international electives. For example, residents at the University of California at San Francisco are offered the opportunity to spend 4 to 7 weeks abroad working at a partner institution under the direct supervision of local faculty. Recently, residents from the University of Pennsylvania have been offered exposure to overseas work through a partnership with Health Volunteers Overseas. These experiences expose trainees to a different spectrum of pathology, emphasize the importance of clinical skills over modern imaging modalities (which are rarely available), require adaptation of surgical approaches when standard implants are not available, and expose residents to the social and cultural context of working abroad.[29-31] Participation during medical training has been shown to correlate with continued interest in volunteerism and caring for indigent patients throughout orthopaedic surgeons' careers.[32]

Diaster Relief Missions

Disaster relief has become a specialized field. The International Committee of the Red Cross, Doctors Without Borders (Médecins Sans Frontiéres), Médecins du Monde, the International Medical Corps, the International Rescue Committee, Merlin, and Emergency USA are organizations that respond to disasters or provide medical needs in conflict zones (**Table 2**). The volunteer should be aware that there are several phases after a disaster, and specific training and experience are required to function effectively in the setting of disasters (or conflicts). The initial response involves stabilization and requires the most specific preparation. The treatment of serious injuries with limited resources in an austere environment is done differently compared with typical North American trauma centers. Surgeons must be trained to stabilize traumatic injuries quickly. After this initial phase, there is a sustained phase in which more definitive treatment will be provided.[20,33]

An evaluation of the response to the 2010 Haitian earthquake suggests that the willingness to help does not mean that adequate results will always be achieved, and there are numerous lessons to be learned.[33-38] In the absence of a coordinated effort, which is an essential component of disaster response, well-meaning individuals may cause more problems than they solve.[32,34,35,39,40] Ample anecdotal evidence after the Haitian earthquake of 2010 indicates that many individuals not affiliated with a coordinated effort put strain on already tenuous food and water supplies, had difficulty coordinating patient care with established programs, and were not prepared to treat the types of injuries encountered.[34,40] Important issues to consider include the organization and logistics of diaster response, personal immuni-

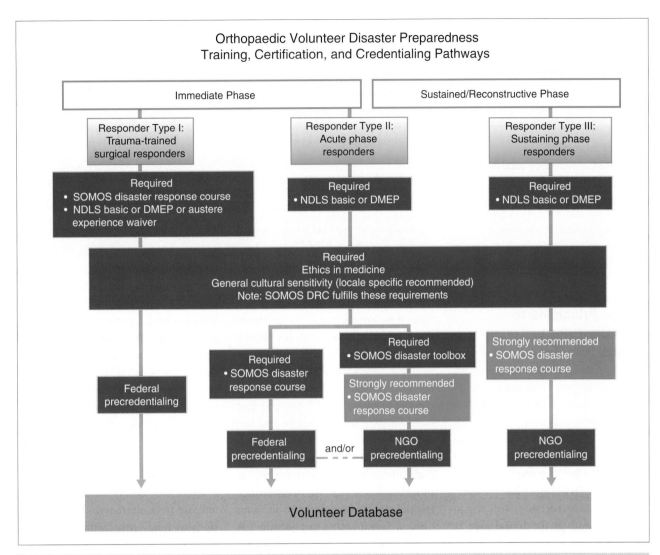

Figure 1   This flow diagram illustrates the AAOS orthopaedic volunteer disaster preparedness training, certification, and credentialing pathways. SOMOS = Society of Military Orthopaedic Surgeons; NDLS = national disaster life support; DMEP = disaster management and emergency preparedness; DRC = disaster response course; NGO = nongovernmental agencies. (Reproduced from Born CT, Teuscher D, Dowling L: AAOS approves disaster preparedness plan. *AAOS Now.* 2011;5(8). Available at http://www.aaos.org/news/aaosnow/aug11/clinical2.asp.)

zations and safety plans, liability insurance, cultural sensitivity, and patient follow-up procedures.[35]

In an effort to improve orthopaedic response to future disasters, the Society of Military Surgeons, the Orthopedic Trauma Association, the American Academy of Orthopedic Surgeons (AAOS), and the Pediatric Orthopedic Society of North America have developed a course designed to teach appropriate disaster response procedures to prospective volunteers.[41] This training

program is designed for civilian orthopaedic surgeons wishing to serve in disaster situations abroad. The course prepares surgeons for functioning in an austere environment with limited equipment and details the complex social situations that are present during disasters. Goals include preparing for deployment as a member of a disaster response team, familiarity with commonly encountered injuries in the disaster environment, awareness of challenges unique to the austere envi-

ronment of disaster situations, and knowledge of cultural and ethical considerations in caring for disaster victims.[42] The AAOS has developed a database for disaster response volunteers.[43] The process for inclusion in the database emphasizes the importance of training as well as affiliation with and precredentialing by appropriate governmental or nongovernmental organizations (**Figure 1**).

Table 3

Questions to Evaluate a Volunteer Opportunity

Pretrip communication with the hosts is essential to understanding their expectations. The following questions will help in preparation:

Who will be trained?

What pathologies will be encountered?

What resources are available?

What educational materials are available?

Is patient rehabilitation available?

Who will provide patient follow-up after the volunteer physician leaves?

Table 4

Technical Pearls for Practicing Orthopaedic Medicine Overseas

The guiding principle is to do no harm.

Most patient care is likely to involve trauma and infection, not reconstruction.

All treatment will be contextually based (such as resources, follow-up, and rehabilitation).

Use the simplest and most cost-effective strategy to reduce complications.

The absence of fluoroscopy will negate the use of many minimally invasive strategies.

Strive for nonsurgical care. Recognize that orthopaedic surgery is an industry-driven, technologically dependent specialty in the Western world.

The physician must have access to information concerning unusual conditions not seen with frequency at home and management principles for conditions seen with frequency at home but which present in an unfamiliar way (such as neglected traumatic injuries and infections).

Ethical Principles to Consider Prior to Travel

The same ethical principles that guide treatment and patient care in economically developed countries should guide treatment in economically underdeveloped countries.[2,26,44-47] The principles for volunteering internationally mirror those of conducting international clinical research,[48] including those of DeCamp.[44] Establishing a collaborative partnership with the local community is the foundation on which the rest of the project can be built. Site selection should be fair. (For example, if the volunteer activity will benefit a particular individual politically or financially there is an inherent conflict of interest, and the relationship must be critically evaluated.) The individual volunteer and the organization that he or she is affiliated with should commit to tangible goals that will benefit the community. Capacity-building activities, which might include educating the local community and enhancing local infrastructure, are essential if any long-term effect on the community's health care is to be realized.[44] Continuing ethical review of actions and interventions is necessary to ensure the appropriateness of the projects.[44,45]

Ethical evaluation also applies to the donation of services and goods. The donation of goods (instruments, implants, medicine, and educational materials) is considered by many overseas volunteers, but such donations can pose ethical issues with respect to conflict of interest and long-term benefit. Donating medical equipment may appear to be an ideal choice because of its complex nature and limited local availability; however, without an appropriate action plan for maintenance, training, and use prior to the donation, such equipment can become a financial and safety liability for the recipients.[49] Donations of free goods can negatively affect developing local economies; such an effect has been described for goods such as t-shirts and food.[50,51] The World Health Organization has established guidelines on appropriate and ethical methods for donating medical equipment.[49,52]

Trip Preparation: Pearls and Pitfalls

Preparing for international work in orthopaedic care requires consideration of logistics, clinical care, and personal expectations. Some questions for evaluating a volunteer opportunity prior to travel are listed in **Table 3**, and technical limitations to assist planning are shown in **Table 4**. Common misconceptions can hinder positive or productive interaction with local colleagues and patients (**Table 5**). Keeping these key points in mind will allow for a positive volunteer experience. The Global-Help and Health Volunteer Overseas websites offer publications and resources to assist the volunteer in service delivery, teaching, and training.

Discussion

There are a variety of opportunities, ranging from short-term medical missions to long-term commitments, for orthopaedic surgeons to work internationally. Adequate preparation is needed prior to travel, including logistics and physical, emotional, and technical considerations. Surgeons should familiarize themselves with the pathologies likely to be encountered, such as late-presenting musculoskeletal trauma, adult presentations of congenital orthopaedic disorders, and chronic osteoarticular infections.

It is essential to be aware of the benefits of collaboration with a local host group. Prior to travel, the volunteer should communicate with the host group concerning expectations, local needs, and the work environment. Predeparture communication with previous volunteers can be valuable. The volunteer should have a plan for safety,

Table 5

Common Misconceptions That Can Have an Adverse Effect on the Volunteer Experience

Misconception	Explanation
The volunteer physician knows more than local physicians and is a better surgeon.	This might be true at home for the volunteer's particular field of expertise, but local physicians know more and are likely better than volunteer physicians in diagnosing and treating locally prevalent disorders, such as musculoskeletal tuberculosis, chronic osteomyelitis, or a neglected shoulder dislocation.
Resources will be available to do proper medical investigations and perform treatment.	This is actually rarely the case, but with a minimum of investigative capacity and clinical judgment, the proper course of action (given the context) can usually be reached.
Everybody will be happy about the presence of the volunteer physician and will feel gratitude.	This is not always the case. The volunteer's presence may foster resentment or political tensions between colleagues and administrators or between colleagues and academia. It also can be difficult for an outsider to appropriately assess the political determinants and repercussions of his or her presence.
The volunteer can be useful just by being there.	On the contrary, in the early phases of disaster relief, the volunteer's presence can be a greater burden than help if the volunteer is not properly prepared.
The volunteer can change the way things are done.	This is partially true. The volunteer may change the way a colleague performs a particular part of a procedure but will be unlikely to change the anesthesia schedule or convince the operating room staff to start earlier than usual.

treatment, follow-up, and future involvement.

Orthopaedic surgeons interested in training as disaster responders should take advantage of the program being developed by the AAOS, in collaboration with the Society of Military Surgeons, the Orthopedic Trauma Association, and the Pediatric Orthopedic Society of North America. The appropriate way to provide surgical assistance in a disaster is to work with a well-prepared group that has expertise in this special type of volunteer activity. The AAOS offers essential resources for interested volunteers.[43]

Beneficial long-term effects can become a reality when working in developing countries through thoughtful preparation and collaboration with a group that is based in the target area. Ultimately, the goal is to provide the community with lasting benefits, which are best achieved through long-term partnerships and a focus on education and building surgical capacity.

Summary

The burden of musculoskeletal disease in low- and middle-income countries is great, and the systems currently in place are not robust enough to deal with the enormity of the need. Orthopaedic surgeons from the developed world can help alleviate part of this burden through various actions, including volunteering their surgical skills and building local surgical capacity through education and direct work efforts. Having a positive effect in any volunteer setting is challenging and requires thoughtful preparation, analysis of the situation, and collaboration with local partners. Volunteer service in the developing world has the potential to be one of the most meaningful experiences in the life of an orthopaedic surgeon.

References

1. Ivers LC, Garfein ES, Augustin J, et al: Surgery as a public good for public health. *World J Surg* 2008; 32(4):537-542.

2. Farmer PE, Kim JY: Surgery and global health: A view from beyond the OR. *World J Surg* 2008;32(4): 533-536.

3. Gosselin RA, Gyamfi YA, Contini S: Challenges of meeting surgical needs in the developing world. *World J Surg* 2011;35(2): 258-261.

4. Dobson M: Training the trainers. *Anaesthesia* 2007;62(suppl 1): 96-102.

5. Dormans JP: Orthopaedic surgery in the developing world: Can orthopaedic residents help? *J Bone Joint Surg Am* 2002;84(6):1086-1094.

6. Mathers CD, Ma Fat D, Boerma JT; World Health Organization: *The Global Burden of Disease: 2004 Update.* Geneva, Switzerland, World Health Organization, 2008.

7. Atijosan O, Rischewski D, Simms V, et al: Prevalence, causes and service implications. *PLoS One* 2008;3(7):e2851.

8. Groen RS, Samai M, Stewart KA, et al: A cluster randomised, cross-sectional, countrywide survey. *Lancet* 2012;380(9847):1082-1087.

9. Debas HT, Gosselin R, McCord C, Thind A: Surgery, in Jamison DT, ed: *Disease Control Priorities in Developing Countries*, ed 2. Washington, DC, The International Bank for Reconstruction and Development/The World Bank Group, 2006.

10. Hughes BB, Kuhn R, Peterson CM, et al: Projections of global health outcomes from 2005 to 2060 using the International Futures integrated forecasting model. *Bull World Health Organ* 2011; 89(7):478-486.

11. Mathers CD, Loncar D: Projections of global mortality and burden of disease from 2002 to 2030. *PLoS Med* 2006;3(11):e442.

12. World Health Organization: Violence and Injury Prevention. Global status report on road safety 2009. http://www.who.int/violence_injury_prevention/road_safety_status/2009/en/. Accessed January 4, 2013.

13. Bickler SW, Spiegel D: Improving surgical care in low- and middle-income countries: A pivotal role for the World Health Organization. *World J Surg* 2010;34(3): 386-390.

14. Mock C, Cherian M, Juillard C, et al: Furthering the link between surgery and public health policy. *World J Surg* 2010;34(3):381-385.

15. Bae JY, Groen RS, Kushner AL: Surgery as a public health intervention: Common misconceptions versus the truth. *Bull World Health Organ* 2011;89(6):394.

16. Weiser TG, Regenbogen SE, Thompson KD, et al: A modelling strategy based on available data. *Lancet* 2008;372(9633): 139-144.

17. Irfan FB, Irfan BB, Spiegel DA: Barriers to accessing surgical care in Pakistan: Healthcare barrier model and quantitative systematic review. *J Surg Res* 2012;176(1): 84-94.

18. Kushner AL, Cherian MN, Noel L, Spiegel DA, Groth S, Etienne C: Addressing the Millennium Development Goals from a surgical perspective: Essential surgery and anesthesia in 8 low- and middle-income countries. *Arch Surg* 2010;145(2):154-159.

19. Grimes CE, Bowman KG, Dodgion CM, Lavy CB: Systematic review of barriers to surgical care in low-income and middle-income countries. *World J Surg* 2011;35(5):941-950.

20. Gosselin RA: War injuries, trauma, and disaster relief. *Tech Orthop* 2005;20(2):97-108.

21. Pezzella AT: Volunteerism and humanitarian efforts in surgery. *Curr Probl Surg* 2006;43(12): 848-929.

22. Coughlin RR: Overseas volunteering: The antidote to managed care. Hospital Physician. June, 2000. http://www.hospitalphysician.com/pdf/hp_jun00_overseas1.pdf. Accessed January 4, 2012.

23. Bermúdez LE: Humanitarian missions in the third world. *Plast Reconstr Surg* 2004;114(6):1687-1689, author reply 1689.

24. Dupuis CC: Humanitarian missions in the third world: A polite dissent. *Plast Reconstr Surg* 2004; 113(1):433-435.

25. Robinson OG Jr: Humanitarian missions in the third world. *Plast Reconstr Surg* 2006;117(3):1040-1041, author reply 1041.

26. Wall A: The context of ethical problems in medical volunteer work. *HEC Forum* 2011;23(2): 79-90.

27. Health Volunteers Overseas website. http://www.hvousa.org. Accessed May 6, 2013.

28. Kelly NA, Moroz LA, Dormans JP: Short-term volunteers: Channeling the energy and maximizing the impact. *Tech Orthop* 2005; 20(2):76-80.

29. Ozgediz D, Roayaie K, Debas H, Schecter W, Farmer D: Surgery in developing countries: Essential training in residency. *Arch Surg* 2005;140(8):795-800.

30. Ozgediz D, Wang J, Jayaraman S, et al: Initial results of a 5-year partnership with a surgical training program in a low-income country. *Arch Surg* 2008;143(9): 860-865, discussion 865.

31. Debas HT: Surgery: A noble profession in a changing world. *Ann Surg* 2002;236(3):263-269.

32. Disston AR, Martinez-Diaz GJ, Raju S, Rosales M, Berry WC, Coughlin RR: The international orthopaedic health elective at the University of California at San Francisco: The eight-year experience. *J Bone Joint Surg Am* 2009; 91(12):2999-3004.

33. Born CT, Cullison TR, Dean JA, et al: Lessons learned from international events. *J Am Acad Orthop Surg* 2011;19(suppl 1):S44-S48.

34. Steinman M, Lottenberg C, Pavao OF, et al: As bad as it gets. *Injury* 2012;43(3):386-387.

35. Sonshine DB, Caldwell A, Gosselin RA, Born CT, Coughlin RR: Critically assessing the Haiti earthquake response and the barriers to quality orthopaedic care. *Clin Orthop Relat Res* 2012; 470(10):2895-2904.

36. Chu K, Stokes C, Trelles M, Ford N: Improving effective surgical delivery in humanitarian disasters: Lessons from Haiti. *PLoS Med* 2011;8(4):e1001025.

37. McIntyre T, Hughes CD, Pauyo T, et al: Partners in Health and Zanmi Lasante experience. *World J Surg* 2011;35(4):745-750.

38. Chackungal S, Nickerson JW, Knowlton LM, et al: Best practice guidelines on surgical response in disasters and humanitarian emergencies: Report of the 2011 Humanitarian Action Summit Working Group on Surgical Issues within the Humanitarian Space. *Prehosp Disaster Med* 2011;26(6): 429-437.

39. Knowlton LM, Gosney JE, Chackungal S, et al: Consensus statements regarding the multidisciplinary care of limb amputation patients in disasters or humanitarian emergencies: Report of the

2011 Humanitarian Action Summit Surgical Working Group on amputations following disasters or conflict. *Prehosp Disaster Med* 2011;26(6):438-448.

40. Benjamin E, Bassily-Marcus AM, Babu E, Silver L, Martin ML: Principles and practice of disaster relief: Lessons from Haiti. *Mt Sinai J Med* 2011;78(3):306-318.

41. Leahy M: Course prepares members for disaster service. *AAOS Now*, October 2011. American Academy of Orthopaedic Surgeons website. http://www.aaos.org/news/aaosnow/oct11/clinical9.asp. Accessed May 15, 2013.

42. Berry BH: Diaster relief course: How to get involved. Lesson learned from Haiti. *AAOS 2012 Annual Meeting Proceedings*. CD-ROM. Rosemont, IL, American Academy of Orthopaedic Surgeons, 2012, pp 257-260.

43. Born CT, Teuscher D, Dowling L: AAOS approves disaster preparedness plan. *AAOS Now*. August 2011. http://www.aaos.org/news/aaosnow/aug11/clinical2.asp. Accessed January 7, 2012.

44. DeCamp M: Ethical review of global short-term medical volunteerism. *HEC Forum* 2011;23(2):91-103.

45. Wall LL: Ethical concerns regarding operations by volunteer surgeons on vulnerable patient groups: The case of women with obstetric fistulas. *HEC Forum* 2011;23(2):115-127.

46. Ott BB, Olson RM: Ethical issues of medical missions: The clinicians' view. *HEC Forum* 2011;23(2):105-113.

47. Langowski MK, Iltis AS: Global health needs and the short-term medical volunteer: Ethical considerations. *HEC Forum* 2011;23(2):71-78.

48. Council for Organizations of Medical Sciences: International Ethical Guidelines for Biomedical Research Involving Human Subjects. 2002. http://www.fhi360.org/training/fr/retc/pdf_files/cioms.pdf. Accessed January 4, 2013.

49. Gatrad AR, Gatrad S, Gatrad A: Equipment donation to developing countries. *Anaesthesia* 2007;62(suppl 1):90-95.

50. Frazer G: Used-clothing donations and apparel production in Africa. *Econ J* 2008;118(532):1764-1784.

51. Isenman PJ, Singer HW: Food aid: Disincentive effects and their policy implications. *Econ Dev Cult Change* 1977;25(2):205-237.

52. World Health Organization: Guidelines for Health Care Equipment Donations. March 2000. http://www.who.int/hac/techguidance/pht/1_equipment%20donationbuletin82WHO.pdf. Accessed May 15, 2013.

Planning for Life After Orthopaedics

Joseph S. Barr Jr, MD
Michael J. McCaslin, BA, CPA
Cynthia K. Hinds, CLU, ChFC, MSFS

Abstract

The word retirement is going out of fashion. Many orthopaedic surgeons want to work in some capacity when they stop performing surgery. Making a smooth transition from a busy orthopaedic practice to alternative work demands advanced planning. The surgeon must consider personal issues that involve how to use human capital (his or her accumulated knowledge and experience). New ventures, hobbies, travel, and spending time with family and friends are some possibilities. Plans for slowing down or leaving the practice should be discussed and agreed on well ahead of time. Agreements for buyouts may be difficult to work out and will require creative thinking. The solo practitioner can close the practice or hire a successor. Financial planning is perhaps the most important consideration and should be started by approximately age 40. It is recommended that the surgeon develop a portfolio of secure investments and annuities to provide adequate income for as long as is needed and then to turn the residual income to one's family, favorite charities, or other desired cause. A team of competent advisors is needed to help develop and achieve one's goals, create financial security, and provide the discipline to carry out the needed planning for life after orthopaedics.

Instr Course Lect 2014;63:505-509.

The word retirement is not used in the title of this chapter for good reasons. The tradition of receiving a gold watch and a handshake at age 65 is a thing of the past. Most orthopaedic surgeons will want a smooth transition from a busy practice to the next stage of life. Suggestions for achieving a successful transition in the areas of personal issues, practice management, and financial planning are discussed in this chapter.

Is There Life After Surgery?

Many years are given to education, training, and practice to become competent in the field of orthopaedic surgery. How can an orthopaedic surgeon best move away from a busy surgical practice toward partial or full retirement or perhaps into an entirely different endeavor? There are many possible pathways, nothing is cast in stone, and no two pathways will be exactly alike. In a 2010 article by Ranawat and Rothman,[1] the question was raised concerning whether a surgeon could judge his or her own competence. However, the true objectivity of peer review also can be questioned. Intellectual ability, emotional toughness, physical fitness, and professional competence all need to be taken into account when judging competence. For physicians older than 65 years, the authors suggested a mandatory evaluation every 2 years involving an internist, a neurologist, an ophthalmologist, and a fellow specialist. Many hospitals and medical organizations now have bylaws and guidelines that address these issues.

Slowing down can present a difficult psychological hurdle. The surgeon's self image must change, and there may be a period of denial. Discussions with family, friends, and colleagues are needed. It is helpful to develop new activities and interests and to do the financial planning in advance. To decrease work stressors and

Mr. McCaslin or an immediate family member has stock or stock options held in Pfizer. Neither of the following authors nor any immediate family member has received anything of value from or has stock or stock options held in a commercial company or institution related directly or indirectly to the subject of this chapter: Dr. Barr and Ms. Hinds.

improve lifestyle, various steps can be taken, such as stopping on-call service, changing the surgical workload, and passing complex medical cases to colleagues. Working as a locum tenens will produce income and provide travel, living expenses, and malpractice insurance; however, a surgeon must eventually stop performing surgery. Hopefully, this can be a reasoned decision and not one mandated by physical or mental health. There is no set age to cease performing surgery, although other professions have such requirements. For example, the mandatory retirement age is 65 years for airline pilots.

Do surgical skills decline with increasing age? Waljee et al[2] reviewed surgical mortality rates and found a slight increase for surgeons older than 60 years performing pancreatectomies, coronary bypass procedures, and carotid endarterectomies. Other procedures did not show differences, although no orthopaedic procedures were evaluated. Age alone does not seem to be an important factor in surgical skills.

Career satisfaction and physician burnout, which is characterized by depression, decreased job satisfaction, difficulty in dealing with increasing stressors, and a decreased quality of life, are other important factors. The medical world is changing rapidly, and physicians are less in control of their practices. More than 50% of orthopaedic surgeons are now employed by hospitals, accountable care organizations, health maintenance organizations, and other large groups.[3,4] Shanafelt et al[5] reported on a 2008 survey of members of the American College of Surgeons regarding surgeon burnout. Approximately 7,900 surveys were returned. The respondents had been in practice for a median of 18 years, worked 60 hours per week, and provided on-call service two nights per week. Results

showed that 40% of surgeons were burned out, 30% had symptoms of depression, and 28% had a quality-of-life score more than one half SD below the population norm. Only 36% of the respondents believed that they had enough time for family life, and only 50% would recommend that their children pursue a medical career. Are orthopaedic surgeons more satisfied and happier than physicians in other specialties? Perhaps, because orthopaedics has led the surgical specialties in innovating new procedures and treatments and the future appears promising for those trends to continue. Because physical and mental health also play an important role in job satisfaction, it is vital to take care of one's own needs and exercise, sleep, recreate, and plan and enjoy family activities.

After orthopaedic surgery, there are many activities and choices to use one's accumulated human capital (knowledge and experience). It may be necessary for financial reasons to continue to generate an income or a surgeon may just want to continue working in some capacity. Nonsurgical orthopaedics, which involves consultations, independent medical examinations, and teaching, is growing as a specialty. Forensic orthopaedics, which includes the evaluation of personal injury or workers' compensation cases and malpractice issues, may appeal to some orthopaedic surgeons. The American Academy of Orthopaedic Surgeons (AAOS) offers an annual course dealing with workers' compensation issues.[6] The legal profession needs accurate and unbiased opinions, reports, and testimony from orthopaedic surgeons who want to work as expert witnesses. The AAOS has established standards of professionalism to govern expert witness testimony.[7] Any surgeon providing expert witness testimony should read and understand these standards.

A retiring orthopaedic surgeon should develop leisure activities such as reading, cooking, exercise, and spending quality time with family and friends. Adult education courses are available to keep up with the electronic revolution. Individual travel or group travel with alumni and faculty are attractive options. Overseas volunteer opportunities are available with such groups as Health Volunteers Overseas[8] and Medecins Sans Frontieres.[9] The physician may want to lecture on medicine and orthopaedics to local groups or write books. There are many options to occupy the time of a nonoperating orthopaedist. The important concept is to learn to enjoy change.

Practice Management Considerations

The complexity of medical practice management is constantly increasing. The transition to electronic health records is expensive and time-consuming. In October of 2014, the International Classification of Diseases-Tenth Revision (ICD-10) will be introduced and will increase the number of diagnostic codes from 13,000 to 68,000. The potential costs for adopting the ICD-10 changes is estimated to range from approximately $80,000 to $2.7 million depending on the size of the practice.[10] Keeping up with these changes is becoming more difficult, requires constant effort and competent advisors, and is an important consideration in retirement planning.

In a group practice, many individual and group decisions are needed as a physician nears retirement. It must be determined how many years of compensation are needed by the retiring surgeon, whether work efforts will slowly or quickly be changed, whether on-call coverage will decrease or cease, and if the retiring surgeon will decrease the complexity of the surgical procedures performed or stop performing surgery entirely. Will the retiring surgeon continue to practice office orthopaedics, do independent medical evaluations, provide expert witness testimony, or work in the administration of the group practice?

The retiring surgeon will need to negotiate a lower overhead rate as his or her income decreases. The group will need to reach decisions based on an assessment of the market, patient demands on the practice, and merger possibilities (whether to join an accountable care organization or sell the practice to a hospital). The group must develop policies dealing with the length of time a physician will continue as a member of the practice. These decisions will also affect how ancillary facilities will be treated during the retirement period in terms of a buy-out or cash-out of assets. It will be necessary to make decisions regarding assets such as MRI and CT scanners and real estate, physical therapy, and surgical centers. These policies require good advice and should be in place before a physician decides to retire from a group practice In addition, the practice members and the retiring physician will have to agree on valuation and payout of accounts receivable assets. The group must determine the value to be paid to the departing physician for each of these assets.

The group will also need to consider the concept of the sale value to a third party (such as a hospital, ambulatory surgical center, management company, or a larger group practice) versus the internal value agreed on among the physicians in the group. The valuation among the group's physicians must consider the ongoing needs of the practice to avoid creating a scenario that bankrupts the practice. The internal valuation of these assets for transactions among the physicians should

be agreed on in advance and legally documented by such means as a buy-sell agreement, an employment agreement, and a deferred compensation agreement.

How can a physician put a value on his or her employees? Good will has little worth in these negotiations. It is also important to anticipate how the group will deal with partial or total disability of a physician or premature death. If there is a tail on the liability insurance policy (a tail payment insures against a loss regardless of when it is reported), it should be established in advance how that will be paid off and who will be responsible for the payments.

Large practice groups may be able to negotiate favorable contracts with insurance companies or provide value based on the number of patients they care for. Small groups may have to consider merging to become large enough to access a bigger population or may need to consider hospital employment or similar arrangements if they are unable to successfully recruit orthopaedic surgeons to perpetuate the practice. Ongoing evaluation of the local practice environment is critical to allow the group to make favorable deals rather than to be forced into less advantageous arrangements. The increasing number of rules and regulations may convince more small group practices to seek employment with larger organizations.

The solo practitioner is usually solo as a personal choice made for reasons of freedom and control. A solo practitioner has basically two succession planning choices: close the practice and liquidate the assets or transfer ownership of the practice to a successor. The practice location and environment may dictate the best choice. Young physicians have often been advised not to "buy in" to a practice. An alternative method is the cashless

buyin, whereby the new associate agrees to forego some income for 1 to 3 years, with the retiring physician receiving more income to effectively pay him or her for the practice. Outright sales of a practice are rare. The retiring physician and the successor should enlist the help of certified public accountants, attorneys, and practice management specialists to transfer ownership of the practice.

Financial Considerations
Generating Income and Preserving Assets

When planning for retirement from orthopaedics, a thorough financial review is needed. Investment strategies, designated beneficiaries, retirement plan documents, insurance policies (including life and disability), and the estate plan should be reviewed. All assets and liabilities should be listed. Healthcare proxy and power of attorney designations should be made or reviewed.

A team of financial experts, including a primary advisor, a certified public accountant, an attorney, an insurance agent, and a financial consultant and/or a broker, is recommended. These advisors should be carefully chosen based on recommendations from trusted associates and friends. The surgeon should work with his or her advisors to analyze and determine objectives, create a plan, and review it regularly. Methods of paying these team members vary: an hourly retainer or rate, a project fee, or an asset-based fee. A broker or financial consultant who trades stocks and bonds should be paid by basis points depending on the size of the account; this arrangement discourages an excessive number of trades to "churn" the account.

Because people are living longer, retirement funds will have to last longer. Original Social Security Administration calculations were made based on an average life expectancy of 72 years; this meant that the average recipient would collect retirement benefits for approximately 7 years. With longer life expectancies, this assumption is no longer valid. Investment returns may be less than calculated, as occurred in 2008 when many 401(K) pension plans lost value. Higher living expenses and taxes are likely. Inflation averaged 3.24% a year from 1913 through 1999 and has increased to 4.5% yearly since 2000. At this rate of inflation, the amount of retirement income needed will increase 50% every 8 to 10 years. Because health care is a major expense for many older Americans, long-term healthcare insurance may be advisable. When all these issues are considered, it may be necessary to delay retirement to avoid running out of funds. Formulas are available to calculate how much savings can be spent each year without spending the corpus of one's retirement fund (approximately 4% to 5%).

The 2013 tax law changes should be considered in retirement planning. The highest income tax rate increases from 35% to 39.6%. There is a 3.8% surtax on unearned income to help fund the Affordable Care Act. The tax rate on capital gains and dividends increases from 15% to 20%. Pretax contributions for flexible spending accounts decrease from $5,000 to $2,500. Estate taxes increase from 35% to 40%, but there was a $5.12 million exemption in 2012 for funds going to the surviving spouse. This exemption has been indexed to inflation and will be $5.25 million in 2013. The annual gift tax exemption increased to $14,000. Slight increases have been adopted for yearly contributions to individual retirement accounts and 401(K) pension plans. The 2013 tax law increased payroll taxes from 4.2% to 6.2% of salary, up to $113,700 annually.

A retiree will need approximately 70% of his or her preretirement income to maintain a comfortable lifestyle. A budget is necessary for retirement. A retiree should consider whether he or she will need to cut down on some expenses, pay off the mortgage and other debts, or move to smaller living quarters to lower the costs of home heating, maintenance, and taxes. Lifestyle expenses also may need to be decreased. Options and decisions need to be considered regarding Social Security retirement benefits.[11] A detailed analysis of expected benefits should be done to review the benefits available at varying ages. The age selected for retirement can make a substantial difference in the amount of the monthly Social Security benefits received.[12]

It is important to balance fixed expenses against fixed and variable income. Types of income include guaranteed income (such as annuity payments, pension payments, and Social Security retirement benefits), fixed income (such as bond dividends), and variable income (salary, capital gains, and some annuity payments). A retirement investment portfolio should be structured into short-term (such as savings, certificates of deposit, short-term bonds) and longer-term (such as longer-term bonds, variable annuities, and stocks) investments. Income needs and risk tolerance must be factored into investment decisions. Various types of annuities are available, such as those with a guaranteed step-up provision or income base, a death benefit, surrender or market value, and even a nursing home rider. Municipal bonds provide steady, tax-free income. A structured portfolio should be designed at least 2 years before retirement and reviewed annually. The key to financial security in retirement is good planning and having reserves, a diversified portfolio with a blended tax rate, and the discipline to take the ac-

tions necessary to achieve these objectives.

Internal Revenue Service Rules and Distribution Planning

There are penalties if money is withdrawn from a qualified retirement plan before age 59.5 years, and harsher penalties if the required amount of money is not withdrawn after age 70.5 years. The required minimum distribution must be calculated per Internal Revenue Service (IRS) tables and taken annually. The distribution rate is approximately 5% initially and slowly increases with age. The system is designed to allow retirement funds to last throughout the retiree's life, but also to allow the IRS to take a portion of this qualified money that has grown tax free. These distributions are taxed at the recipient's tax rate in the year received. Currently, there is a provision allowing up to $100,000 per year in charitable donations without taxation.

Qualified pension funds can be distributed in several ways. Before age 59.5 years, equal periodic payments can avoid the 10% penalty tax. A lump sum rollover can be done and the money annuitized. At death, there are other options for money remaining in the pension plan. A designated beneficiary must be named or the entire fund will be paid out to the estate in 1 to 5 years, with income taxes due at the time of payout. The single most important step is to designate beneficiaries; they may be primary, contingent, successor, or restricted. This allows payout of the money during the period of the beneficiaries' life expectancy. A stretch-out individual retirement account can be used for the surviving spouse and children.

Assets can be transferred at death through joint accounts, beneficiary designation of individual retirement account funds, annuities, life insurance, wills, and trusts. Gift and estate taxes occur at the time of transfer; however, transfers between spouses are not taxed. There is an annual gift tax exclusion of $14,000 per donor per donee. Each spouse can give $14,000 to a child in 1 year. The lifetime gift limit is $1,000,000, and at death it is currently $5,000,000.

Trusts are a useful method of protecting and distributing wealth. Assets are granted to a trust, and the trustee makes payments to the beneficiaries. The advantages of a trust are greater control, protection from creditors, the ability to meet special needs, proper distribution in the event of a second marriage, and avoidance of a spendthrift frittering away his or her share of the money. Disadvantages of a trust are that they must remain open during the life expectancy of all the beneficiaries, there are administrative costs, the trust must meet the requirements of a see-through trust, and the stretch-out option is not available. Trusts enable the grantor to plan ahead to avoid possible taxes, costs, and fees.

There are several different types of trusts: marital (A trust), family (B trust), irrevocable life insurance trust, charitable trust, qualified personal residence trust, and offshore trust. Asset titles must be coordinated with the estate plan. Joint tenancy could result in a loss of unified credit. Assets should be equalized between spouses to optimize estate taxes.

Insurance is basically a risk management tool. Insurance policies provide money to replace the loss of income or assets. Many types of insurance policies are available: homeowner's, automobile, disability (premiums should be paid by the policyholder to avoid tax on a payout, not available after age 65 years), long-term care, life, and umbrella policies for better protection.

Planning for retirement is a complex process that should be taken seriously and done with the help of financial professionals. The objectives are to make sure the money lasts throughout the retiree's lifetime and to ensure that any residual funds pass to loved ones or chosen causes in a timely and tax-efficient manner.

Summary

There is no perfect pathway in making the transition from a busy orthopaedic surgical practice to a more relaxed lifestyle, but principles of structured planning in the areas of practice management and financial issues are common to all plans. Planning should start years before the transition. A team of consultants should be carefully chosen, and their recommendations should be discussed, followed, and regularly updated. Personal consideration will be quite variable, but thought and planning are still needed.

References

1. Ranawat CS, Rothman RH: A surgeon's transition: When to retire from surgical practice. *J Bone Joint Surg Am* 2010;92(8):e7.

2. Waljee JF, Greenfield LJ, Dimick JB, Birkmeyer JD: Surgeon age and operative mortality in the United States. *Ann Surg* 2006; 244(3):353-362.

3. Rosenstein AH: Physician Stress and Burnout: Prevalence, Cause, and Effect. *AAOS Now*. Rosemont, IL, American Academy of Orthopaedic Surgeons, August, 2012, p 31.

4. Rosenstein AH: Physician Stress and Burnout: Taking Care of Yourself. *AAOS Now*. Rosemont, IL, American Academy of Ortho-

paedic Surgeons, September, 2012, p 33.

5. Shanafelt TD, Balch CM, Bechamps GJ, et al: Burnout and career satisfaction among American surgeons. *Ann Surg* 2009; 250(3):463-471.

6. 15th Annual AAOS Occupational Orthopaedics and Workers' Compensation Course: A Multidisciplinary Perspective. AAOS website: CME courses. http://www7.aaos.org/education/courses/course_detail.aspx?ProductId=25135. Accessed June 25, 2013.

7. Standards of Professionalism: Orthopaedic Expert Opinion and Testimony. Amended May 12, 2010. http://www3.aaos.org/member/profcomp/ewtestimony_May_2010.pdf. Accessed June 25, 2013.

8. Health Volunteers Overseas website. http://www.hvousa.org/. Accessed June 25, 2013.

9. Medecins Sans Frontieres website. http://www.msf.org/. Accessed June 25, 2013.

10. Bresnick J: Estimating the costs of ICD-10 implementation. November 1, 2012. EHR intelligence website. http://ehrintelligence.com/2012/11/01/estimating-the-costs-of-icd-10-implementation/. Accessed September 20, 2013.

11. Social Security: The Official Website of the Social Security Administration. http://www.socialsecurity.gov/. Accessed June 25, 2013.

12. Social Security Timing website. https://www.socialsecuritytiming.com/. Accessed June 25, 2013.

Index